Pathology for Medical Professionals

Pathology for Medical Professionals

Edited by Hans Affleck

hayle medical
New York

Hayle Medical,
750 Third Avenue, 9th Floor,
New York, NY 10017, USA

Visit us on the World Wide Web at:
www.haylemedical.com

ISBN: 978-1-63241-512-7

Printed in China.

Cataloging-in-Publication Data

Pathology for medical professionals / edited by Hans Affleck.
p. cm.
Includes bibliographical references and index.
ISBN 978-1-63241-512-7
1. Pathology. 2. Pathology--Practice. I. Affleck, Hans.
RB37.6 .P38 2018
616.07--dc23

Table of Contents

Preface

As a sub-field of medicine, pathology is concerned with four major areas of disease study namely its cause, its mechanism of development, the alterations it causes in a cell and lastly, the consequences of these changes. It is a vast field of study, encompassing different techniques like forensic pathology, anatomical pathology, histopathology, dermatopathology, etc. This book provides significant information about this discipline to help develop a good understanding of pathology and its related fields. The various studies that are constantly contributing towards advancing technologies and evolution of this area are examined in detail. Students, researchers, experts and all associated with pathology will benefit alike from the book.

Various studies have approached the subject by analyzing it with a single perspective, but the present book provides diverse methodologies and techniques to address this field. This book contains theories and applications needed for understanding the subject from different perspectives. The aim is to keep the readers informed about the progresses in the field; therefore, the contributions were carefully examined to compile novel researches by specialists from across the globe.

Indeed, the job of the editor is the most crucial and challenging in compiling all chapters into a single book. In the end, I would extend my sincere thanks to the chapter authors for their profound work. I am also thankful for the support provided by my family and colleagues during the compilation of this book.

Editor

1

Bone Marrow Mesenchymal Stem Cells Ameliorates Seawater-Exposure-Induced Acute Lung Injury by Inhibiting Autophagy in Lung Tissue

Qiu-ping Liu,[1] Dang-xia Zhou,[2] Li Sun,[3] Luo Ling,[4] Chang-gui Wu,[5] Pu Lin,[6] and Shui-ping Han[2]

[1] *Third Ward of VIP, 323 Hospital of PLA, Xi'an 710054, China*
[2] *Pathology Department, Medical School, Xi'an Jiaotong University, Xi'an 710061, China*
[3] *Ward of VIP, Shaanxi People's Hospital, Xi'an 710068, China*
[4] *Department of Endocrinology, The First Hospital of PLA, Lanzhou 730000, China*
[5] *Department of Respiratory Medicine, Xijing Hospital, Fourth Military Medical University, Xi'an 710038, China*
[6] *Electric Power Science Research Institute of Shaanxi Province, Xi'an 710054, China*

Correspondence should be addressed to Dang-xia Zhou; dangxia75@163.com

Academic Editor: Piero Tosi

Seawater drowning can lead to acute lung injury (ALI). Several studies have shown that bone marrow mesenchymal stem cells (BMSC) treatment could attenuate ALI. However, the mechanisms underlying this phenomenon still remain elusive. Therefore, this study aimed to investigate whether BMSC treatment can ameliorate seawater-induced ALI and its underlying mechanisms in a rat model. In this study, arterial blood gas, lung weight coefficient, and TNF-α, and IL-8 in bronchoalveolar lavage fluid (BALF), as well as histopathology examination, were used to detect the lung injury of seawater exposure. Moreover, western blot and RT-PCR were used to explore autophagy in lung tissues. The results demonstrated that seawater exposure induced ALI including impaired arterial blood gas, pulmonary edema, histopathologic changes, and inflammatory response in lung tissues. What is more, these changes were partly ameliorated by BMSC treatment through inhibition of autophagy in lung tissues. The application of BMSC may be a potential effective treatment for seawater-induced ALI.

1. Introduction

Drowning is one of important causes of accidental deaths. It has been shown that drowning accounts for approximately half a million deaths each year in the world [1]. Acute pulmonary injury (ALI)/and its more severe form, acute respiratory distress syndrome (ARDS), are common symptoms of drowning [2]. As seawater has high osmolarity and its NaCl concentration is about 3-fold of that in physiologic saline, ALI, including lung edema, hypoxemia, and inflammatory reaction, is more serious in seawater drowning compared to those in freshwater drowning [3]. However, currently there are no effective strategies to treat it.

Bone marrow mesenchymal cells (BMSCs) are multiple differentiation progenitor cells derived from bone marrow, which have the ability to differentiate into endothelial cells, vascular smooth muscle cells, bone, cartilage, muscle, and other connective tissues [4]. BMSCs are being studied with increasing intensity because of their potential use as a therapeutic tool [5]. Several studies have demonstrated that the BMSC transplantation might attenuate ALI/ARDS in lung tissue by decreasing mortality rate and maintaining the normal pulmonary endothelial and epithelial function as well as participating in modulating the inflammatory responses that are involved in ALI [6–9]. BMSC-based therapy seems to be a promising treatment for ALI/ARDS. However, little is known about the therapeutic effects of BMSC transplantation on ALI induced by seawater exposure.

Although BMSCs are being studied as potential therapeutic tool for ALI, the discrete mechanisms underlying this phenomenon still remain unclear. Autophagy is an evolutionarily conserved physiological process which provides a membrane-dependent mechanism for the sequestration, transport, and lysosomal turnover of subcellular components, including proteins and organelles [10]. Autophagy occurs at low basal levels in cells to execute homeostatic function. However, it could be rapidly upregulated under various stress conditions such as hypoxia, ischemia, oxidative stress, and endoplasmic reticulum stress [11]. Recently, it is increasingly clear that autophagy is relevant to many pulmonary diseases including ALI, and autophagy-blocking agents might rescue cell death and ameliorate ALI [12–14]. Our earlier studies also demonstrated that seawater exposure triggered autophagy, and autophagy might be a damaging factor responsible for ALI induced by seawater [15]. However, as far as is known, there is little evidence of whether BMSC transplantation has therapeutic effects on seawater-induced ALI by inhibiting autophagy in lung tissues.

Therefore, the current study was aimed to investigate whether BMSC treatment can ameliorate seawater-induced ALI and its underlying mechanisms, focusing on the changes of autophagy in particular. Understanding the role of BMSC in the seawater exposure will contribute to further disclosing the therapy effects of BMSC in ALI/ARDS.

2. Materials and Methods

2.1. Animals Preparation. Healthy adult male Sprague-Dawley rats weighing 180–200 g from Experimental Animal Center of Xi'an Jiaotong University were obtained and housed in solid-bottomed polycarbonate cages in SPF animal laboratory with a temperature 21–25°C and a relative humidity of 40–60%. Rats were acclimatized at a 12 h light/12 h dark cycle and fed a standard diet and tap water *ad libitum* before the experiments. Experiments were performed in accordance with the Animal Experimentation Committee Regulation of Xi'an Jiaotong University.

2.2. Seawater and Bone Marrow Stem Cells (BMSCs) Preparation. According to the methods of previous study [16], seawater (osmolality 1300 mmol/l, SW 1.05, pH 8.2, NaCl 26.518 g/l, $MgSO_4$ 3.305 g/l, $MgCl_2$ 2.447 g/l, $CaCl_2$ 1.141 g/l, KCl 0.725 g/l, $NaHCO_3$ 0.202 g/l, and NaBr 0.083 g/l) was prepared.

BMSCs (RASMX-01001) of SD rats were purchased from Cyagen Biotechnology Ltd. in Guangzhou, China. The cells were further cultured in Iscove's modified Dulbecco's medium (IMDM, Hyclone) with 20% fetal bovine serum at 37°C. After subculturing 3–5 times, the BMSCs were used for the following experiments.

2.3. Establishment of Seawater-Induced Acute Lung Injury Model. Seawater group (SG): According to the methods of Han et al. study [16]. The rats in the experimental groups were anesthetized with 20% urethane (5 mL/kg) intraperitoneally and maintained in the supine position during experiments. A tube was inserted into trachea through a tracheostomy and then 3 mL/kg of seawater was aspirated into trachea within 5 min.

In BMSC group (BG), the rats were given an intravenous (through caudal vein) injection of BMSC (2×10^6 cells) at 10 min after seawater instillation as in SG, and the other treatment conditions were the same as those in SG.

In naive group (NG), neither seawater nor BMSC was given in this group. And the other treatment conditions were same as those in SG.

2.4. Arterial Blood Gas Analysis. The rats were sacrificed by aortic puncture at the indicated time points. The blood samples were immediately taken for arterial blood gas analysis. Hydrogen ion concentration (pH), arterial oxygen tension (PaO_2), and arterial carbon dioxide tension ($PaCO_2$) were measured with a blood gas analyzer.

2.5. Lung Weight Coefficient. The lung weight coefficient was determined as an index of pulmonary edema. The lung tissue were immediately removed and weighed after the surface blood was aspirated. The lung weight coefficient was calculated by dividing the lung weight by body weight in each rat.

2.6. Measurement of TNF-α and IL-8 in Bronchoalveolar Lavage Fluid (BALF). The bronchoalveolar lavage fluid was taken by a method as described by Han et al. [16]. Briefly, the left lungs were excised integrally from rats in each group, the bronchoalveolar lavage (BAL) was made with intratracheal injections of 2 mL of physiological saline at 37°C three times. The BALF was retrieved and centrifuged, and TNF-α and IL-8 were then determined by the ELISA method (R&D Systems Inc., Minneapolis, MN, USA).

2.7. Histopathological Examination. Lung tissue for histological study was fixed in fresh 4% formaldehyde solution for 24 h and then dehydrated and embedded in paraffin, finally 4 μm sections were cut and stained with hematoxylin-eosin (H&E). The tissue sections were observed under a light microscope for the lung histopathology. Lung injury was evaluated according to the degree of alveolar edema, interstitial edema, neutrophil infiltration, and hemorrhage.

2.8. RT-PCR. Total RNA was extracted from lung tissue using the Trizol reagent and reverse-transcribed into cDNA using commercial kits (Fermentas, Lithuania). PCR was carried out in 20 ul reaction volumes, containing 7 μL of PCR Mix (10x Taq Buffer with $(NH_4)_2SO_4$, 0.2 mmol/L dNTP, 1.5 mmol/L $MgCl_2$), 1 μL of each primer, 9 μL ddH_2O, and 2 μL of genomic DNA. PCR cycling was performed using the MyCycler Thermal Cycler (Bio-Rad) with following conditions: at 95°C, 5 min, followed by 35 cycles of 30 sec at 95°C, 30 sec at 60°C, and 45 sec at 72°C, after cycles at 72°C, 10 min. The primer sequences and the expected sizes of PCR products were as follows. LC3 (sense): 5′-CCATGCCGTCCGAGA-AGACCTTC-3′ and (antisense) 5′-GACCAGCTTCCG-CTGGTAACGTC-3′ (452 bp). GAPDH: (sense) 5′-GCA-AGTTCAACGGCACAG-3′ and (antisense) 5′-GCCAGT-AGACTCCACGACAT-3′ (140 bp).

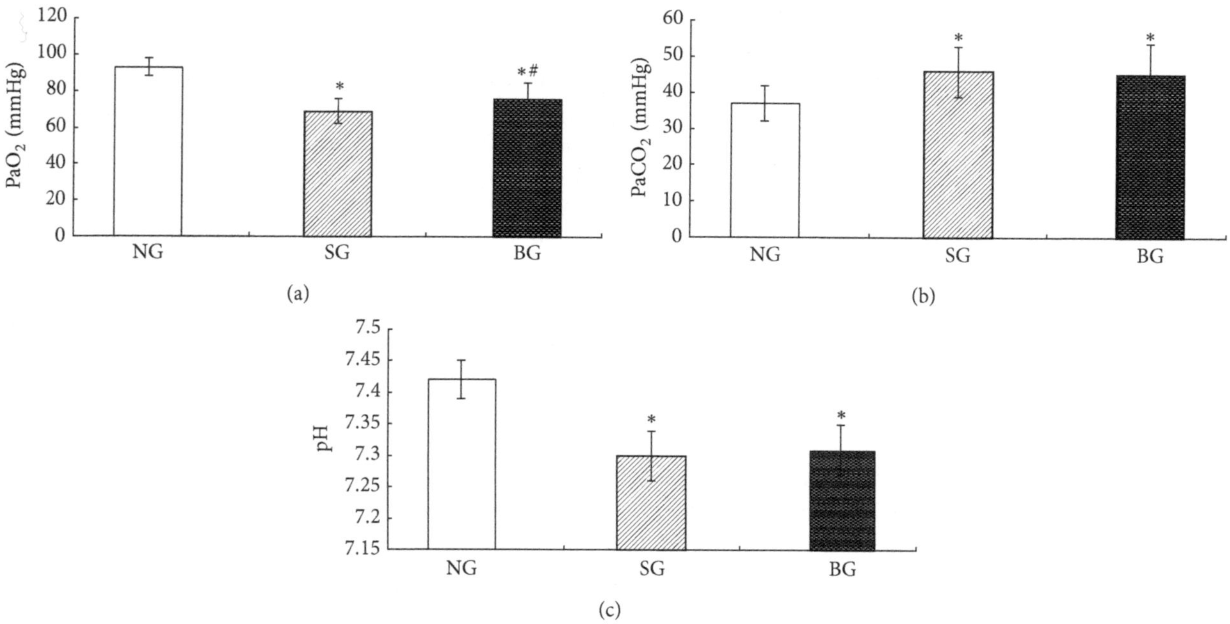

FIGURE 1: Effects of BMSC treatment on changes in arterial blood gas parameters at 2 h after seawater exposure. (a) PaO_2; (b) $PaCO_2$; (c) pH. Data are expressed as mean ± S.D. $^*P < 0.05$ compared to NG group. $^\#P < 0.05$ compared to SG group.

2.9. Western Blotting. In brief, lung tissue in each group was homogenized in ice-cold RIPA lysate buffer (Sigma) and centrifuged at 15000 ×g for 15 min at 4°C. The total protein concentration was determined with a UV 3000 ultraviolet spectrophotometer (Nano Drop, Wilmington, DE). The samples (100 ug protein per lane) were separated with 15% gradient SDS-PAGE gel and then transferred onto a PVDF membrane. Nonspecific binding to the membrane was blocked with 5% nonfat milk in Tris buffered saline-Tween 20 (TBST, pH 7.4) for 2 h at room temperature. After that the membranes were incubated overnight with rabbit polyclonal antibody against LC3 (1 : 1000 dilution, Cell signaling technology) and β-actin (1 : 1000 dilution, Sigma). After washed repeatedly with TBST, the membrane were incubated in goat anti-rabbit IgG (1 : 5000 dilution, Beijing Zhongshan Biotechnology Co., Ltd., Beijing, China) for 2 h, and bands were visualized by using the ECL kit (Proteintech, USA). The ratio of LC3 level II/LC3I level was used as an indicator of autophagic level.

2.10. Statistical Analysis. All statistical analyses were carried out using SPSS statistical software version 13.0 (SPSS, Chicago, USA). Data were summarized as mean ± SD; one-way ANOVA and post hoc comparisons were used to determine the difference among multiple groups. $P < 0.05$ was regarded as statistically significant.

3. Results

3.1. Effects of BMSC Treatment on Arterial Blood Gas. The previous study and our earlier experiments all found that the most obvious inflammatory response and autophagy of lung tissues occurred at about 2 h after seawater exposure [16]. Therefore the 2 h time point was considered suitable for the following studies.

TABLE 1: Effects of BMSC treatment on changes in TNF-α and IL-8 in bronchoalveolar lavage fluid after seawater exposure in rats.

Group	TNF-α (pg/mL)	IL-8 (pg/mL)
NG	21.67 ± 6.86	30.61 ± 5.28
SG	52.83 ± 16.74*	55.50 ± 8.96*
BG	52.17 ± 10.36*	52.01 ± 11.31*

$^*P < 0.05$, compared with NG.

Compared with the control group, seawater exposure caused significant changes in the arterial blood gas parameters, which was manifested by an obvious decrease in PaO_2 and pH value, as well as a significant increase in $PaCO_2$ (Figure 1).

As shown in Figure 1(a), the decrease of PaO_2 induced by seawater instillation were significantly reversed by treatment of BMSC; however, the changes of $PaCO_2$ and pH value were not significantly reversed (Figures 1(b) and 1(c)).

3.2. Effects of BMSC Treatment on Lung Weight Coefficient. Lung weight coefficient was significantly increased in the seawater group when compared with that in the control group. Moreover, lung weight coefficient was partly ameliorated by treatment of BMSC (Figure 2).

3.3. Effects of BMSC Treatment on TNF-α and IL-8 in Bronchoalveolar Lavage Fluid (BALF). As shown in Table 1, TNF-α and IL-8 levels in bronchoalveolar lavage fluid (BALF) significantly increased in the SG when compared with those in the NG. In contrast, IL-8 level in bronchoalveolar lavage fluid (BALF) was slightly attenuated by treatment of BMSC when compared with SG (Table 1). However, TNF-α level in bronchoalveolar lavage fluid (BALF) was not obviously ameliorated by treatment of BMSC (Table 1).

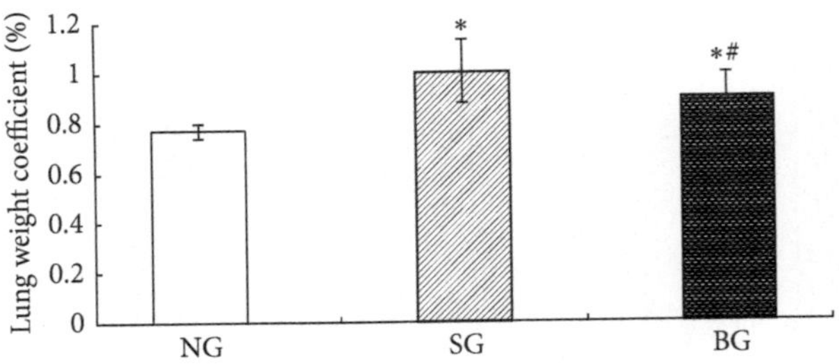

FIGURE 2: Effects of BMSC treatment on changes in lung weight coefficient at 2 h after seawater exposure. Data are expressed as mean ± S.D. $^{*}P < 0.05$ compared to NG group. $^{\#}P < 0.05$ compared to SG group.

3.4. Effects of BMSC Treatment on Lung Histopathological Changes. As H&E (haematoxylin and eosin) stained sections showed, normal lung tissue structures and clear alveoli existed in rats of NG group (Figure 3(a)). Seawater exposure induced prominent lesions, such as edema and hemorrhage, collapse, and inflammatory exudation in alveolar (Figure 3(b)). In contrast, these changes were partly ameliorated by BMSC treatment.

3.5. Effects of BMSC Treatment on LC3 mRNA Level by RT-PCR. Autophagy-related (Atg) proteins are eukaryotic factors participating in various stages of the autophagic process. Thus far 34 autophagy-related genes (Atg) have been identified in yeast [17]. Recently, the orthologs of Atg genes have been isolated and functionally characterized in mammals [18]. LC3 is a mammalian homologues protein of yeast Atg8 protein; LC3 gene is one of critical genes involved in autophagy [19]. Therefore, we focused on the changes of LC3 gene in this study. RT-PCR results showed that there was a notable upregulation of LC3 mRNA level in rat lung tissue of SG group when compared with NG group (Figure 4). Furthermore, the activation of LC3 after seawater exposure was slightly reversed by BMSC treatment.

3.6. Effects of BMSC Treatment on LC3 Conversion by Western Blotting. The conversion of LC3-I to LC3-II is a necessary step during the process of autophagy. The level of LC3-II is known to correlate well with the number of autophagosomes. Our studies showed that the LC3-II protein was hardly detectable in normal lung tissue by using western blotting analysis. However, there was a marked upregulation of the ratio of LC3-II/LC3-I in rats of SG group (Figure 5). What is more, these changes were partly reversed by BMSC treatment.

4. Discussion

In the present study, we investigated the role of BMSC transplantation for early seawater-induced ALI in a rat model. The results demonstrated that seawater exposure induced ALI including impaired arterial blood gas, pulmonary edema, histopathologic changes, and inflammatory response in lung tissues. What is more, these changes were partly ameliorated by BMSC treatment through inhibiting autophagy in lung tissues.

Drowning is one of the most common causes of accidental deaths in the world [16]. Actually, there are mostly two kinds of outcomes after drowning. Some victims might die of apnoea soon after drowning; other patients might survive initial apnoea and then suffer acute lung injury [20]. The aim of this study was to explore the therapeutic effect of BMSC transplantation in early seawater-induced ALI, so we only chose the rats that survived the early stage after seawater intratracheal instillation for further experiments. Furthermore, previous studies and our earlier experiments showed that the most obvious inflammatory response and autophagy of lung tissues occurred at about 2 h after seawater exposure [15, 16]. Therefore the 2 h time point was selected for the following studies.

In this study, we found that seawater exposure could cause lung injury, which was characterized by decreased PaO_2 and increased $PaCO_2$, lung weight coefficient, and TNF-α and IL-8 in bronchoalveolar lavage fluid (BALF) in a rat model. The results were consistent with histopathologic findings. All these data suggested that the intratracheal exposure of seawater in the rat model induced topical acute lung injuries (ALI), which was also in accordance with the findings of other authors and our previous study [2, 15, 16, 21].

In addition, we explored whether or not the BMSC treatment played a role in early seawater-induced ALI in a rat model. We found that PaO_2, lung weight coefficient, histopathologic changes, and inflammatory responses induced by seawater exposure were partly attenuated by treatment of BMSC. It indicated that BMSC might play a protective effect on the ALI induced by seawater exposure. Bone mesenchymal stem cells (BMSC) were originally identified more than 120 years ago as a component population among the predominant hematopoietic cells of the bone marrow [22]. Furthermore, BMSC express no major histocompatibility complex class II; they are the viable therapeutic methods across tissue typing [23]. It also has been shown to differentiate into a variety of mesenchymal cell types, including fibroblasts, myofibroblasts, osteoblasts, chondroblasts, adipocytes, and myoblasts, as well as epithelial cells [5]. In addition, BMSC might provide a number of potent cytokines and growth factors to protect lung injury [5]. Our current finding is in agreement with other studies which have shown an ameliorating effect of BMSC treatment in other models of ALI [6–9]. Xu et al. found that intravenous transplantation of BMSCs could maintain the integrity of the pulmonary alveolar-capillary barrier and modulate the inflammatory response to attenuate oleic-acid-inducing the experimental ALI, and transplantation of BMSCs could be a novel cell-based therapeutic strategy for prevention and treatment of ALI [6]. Huang et al. reported that BMSCs had a protective effect on paraquat-induced ALI in rats, and the effect was closely related to the transplantation time and number of transplanted BMSCs [7]. The study of Curley et al. showed that BMSC therapy enhanced lung repair following ventilator-induced ALI via a paracrine mechanism that might be dependent on keratinocyte growth factor [8]. Islam et al. argued that BMSC protected against ALI by restituting alveolar bioenergetics through Cx43-dependent alveolar attachment and mitochondrial transfer [9].

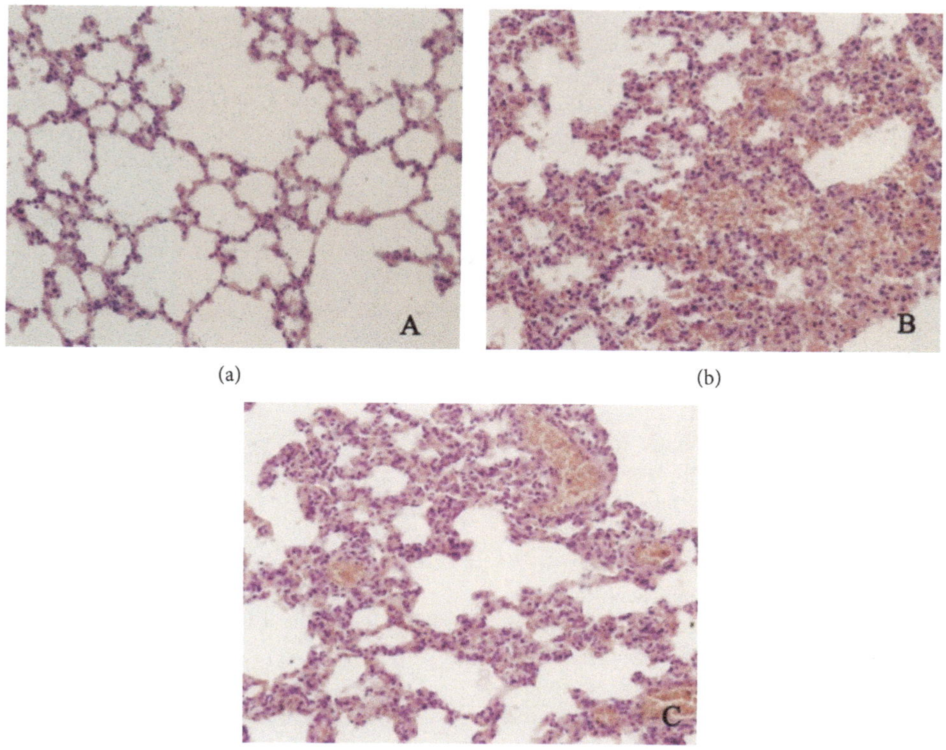

(a) (b) (c)

FIGURE 3: Light micrographs of lung tissues stained with haematoxylin-eosin (H&E) (×400). (a) Lung tissue in a rat of NG group. (b) Lung tissue in a rat of SG group. Hemorrhage, edematous changes, collapse, and inflammatory exudation in alveolar were observed. (c) Lung tissue in a rat of BG group. Lung injury was alleviated and less damage was observed compared with the SG group.

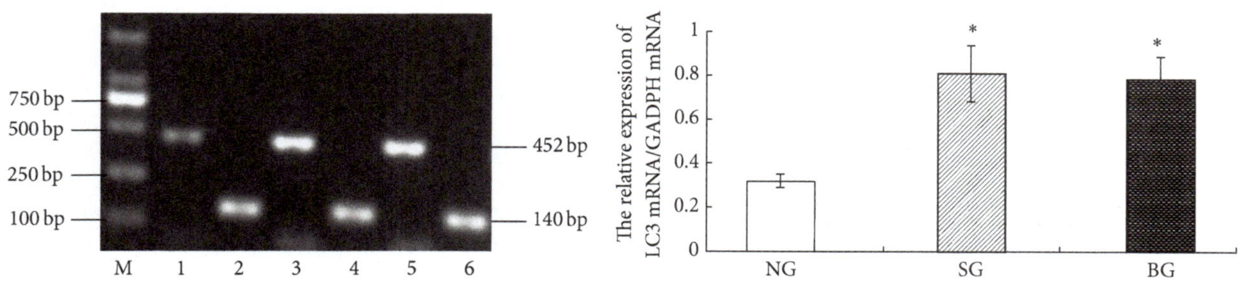

(a) (b)

FIGURE 4: Effects of BMSC treatment on LC3 mRNA level in rat lung tissue. (a) Electrophorogram picture for LC3 mRNA in lung tissues in different groups. (b) The ratio of LC3 mRNA/GADPH mRNA was presented in bar chart. $^{*}P < 0.05$, compared with NG group. M: marker; lanes 1, 3, and 5 represent the LC3 mRNA expression (452 bp) in NG, SG, and BG groups, respectively; lanes 2, 4, and 6 represent the GADPH mRNA expression (140 bp) in NG, SG, and BG groups, respectively.

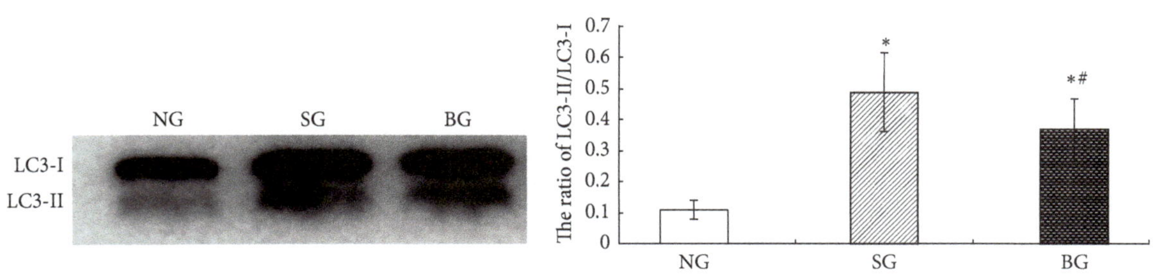

(a) (b)

FIGURE 5: Effects of BMSC treatment on LC3 conversion in rat lung tissue. (a) Western blot picture for LC3 in lung tissues in different groups. (b) The ratio of LC3-II/LC3-I was presented in bar chart. $^{*}P < 0.05$, compared with NG group. $^{\#}P < 0.05$ compared to SG group.

Furthermore, our present study, reported that ALI induced by seawater exposure was ameliorated by BMSC through inhibiting autophagy of lung tissues in a rat model. Autophagy, a process in which de novo formed membrane-enclosed vesicles engulf and consume cellular components, has been shown to induce type II programmed cell death when it is inappropriately activated [24]. Evidence of autophagy in the pathogenesis of ALI has gradually accumulated in recent years [14]. For example, Sun et al. concluded that the autophagic cell death of alveolar epithelial cells likely plays a crucial role in the high mortality rate of H5N1 infection and autophagy-blocking agents might be useful as prophylactics and therapeutics against infection of humans by the H5N1 virus [13]. Li et al. reported that nanoparticles triggers autophagic cell death and the autophagy inhibitor 3-methyladenine might rescue cell death and ameliorate ALI caused by nanoparticles in mice [12]. Our data showed that LC3 II, an indicator of autophagosome formation, was attenuated by BMSC treatment. The alterations of autophagy were basically consistent with the changes in arterial blood gas, lung weight coefficient, TNF-α and IL-8 in bronchoalveolar lavage fluid (BALF), and histopathologic changes. These results demonstrated that autophagy was involved in the ALI pathophysiological process. Moreover, this is the first evidence, to our knowledge, that BMSC treatment protects against seawater-induced ALI by inhibition of autophagy in lung tissue. Taken together, our study provides evidence to further support the view that autophagy-blocking might be useful therapy for ALI.

In summary, data in this study demonstrated that BMSC treatment may exert some protective effects on ALI induced by seawater exposure, partly through inhibiting autophagy in lung tissue. The application of BMSC may be a potential effective treatment for ALI. However, further investigations on the effect of BMSC in long time are still needed in the future.

Conflict of Interests

The authors declare that there is no conflict of interests regarding the publication of this paper.

Acknowledgments

This research was financially supported by the National Natural Science Funding of China (no. 81273018), Science Technical Development Project Funding of Lanzhou Military District (nos. CLZ11JA17 and CLZ12JB26), and Science Funding of Health Department, Shaanxi Province (2012D58).

References

[1] J. Soar, C. D. Deakin, J. P. Nolan et al., "European Resuscitation Council . European Resuscitation Council guidelines for resuscitation 2005. Section 7. Cardiac arrest in special circumstances," *Resuscitation*, vol. 67, supplement 1, pp. S135–S170, 2005.

[2] J. Li, M. Xu, Q. Fan et al., "Tanshinone IIA ameliorates seawater exposure-induced lung injury by inhibiting aquaporins (AQP) 1 and AQP5 expression in lung," *Respiratory Physiology and Neurobiology*, vol. 176, no. 1-2, pp. 39–49, 2011.

[3] F. Salomez and J. Vincent, "Drowning: a review of epidemiology, pathophysiology, treatment and prevention," *Resuscitation*, vol. 63, no. 3, pp. 261–268, 2004.

[4] Z. Zhang, Y. Lu, Y. Luan, and J. Zhao, "Effect of bone marrow mesenchymal stem cells on experimental pulmonary arterial hypertension," *Experimental and Therapeutic Medicine*, vol. 4, no. 5, pp. 839–843, 2012.

[5] A. R. Brody, K. D. Salazar, and S. M. Lankford, "Mesenchymal stem cells modulate lung injury," *Proceedings of the American Thoracic Society*, vol. 7, no. 2, pp. 130–133, 2010.

[6] Y. Xu, Y. Liu, Q. Wang, G. Li, X. Lü, and B. Kong, "Intravenous transplantation of mesenchymal stem cells attenuates oleic acid induced acute lung injury in rats," *Chinese Medical Journal*, vol. 125, no. 11, pp. 2012–2018, 2012.

[7] Y. Huang, W. Yin, X. M. Zhang et al., "Optimal conditions of bone marrow mesenchymal stem cells on paraquat -induced acute lung injury in rats," *Zhonghua Lao Dong Wei Sheng Zhi Ye Bing Za Zhi*, vol. 30, no. 9, pp. 645–649, 2012.

[8] G. F. Curley, M. Hayes, B. Ansari et al., "Mesenchymal stem cells enhance recovery and repair following ventilator-induced lung injury in the rat," *Thorax*, vol. 67, no. 6, pp. 496–501, 2012.

[9] M. N. Islam, S. R. Das, M. T. Emin et al., "Mitochondrial transfer from bone-marrow-derived stromal cells to pulmonary alveoli protects against acute lung injury," *Nature Medicine*, vol. 18, no. 5, pp. 759–765, 2012.

[10] S. W. Ryter, K. Nakahira, J. A. Haspel, and A. M. K. Choi, "Autophagy in pulmonary diseases," *Annual Review of Physiology*, vol. 74, pp. 377–401, 2012.

[11] J. Zhang, J. S. Wang, Z. K. Zheng et al., "Participation of autophagy in lung ischemia-reperfusion injury in vivo," *Journal of Surgical Research*, vol. 182, no. 2, pp. e79–e87, 2013.

[12] C. Li, H. Liu, Y. Sun et al., "PAMAM nanoparticles promote acute lung injury by inducing autophagic cell death through the Akt-TSC2-mTOR signaling pathway," *Journal of Molecular Cell Biology*, vol. 1, no. 1, pp. 37–45, 2009.

[13] Y. Sun, C. Li, Y. Shu et al., "Inhibition of autophagy ameliorates acute lung injury caused by avian influenza A H5N1 infection," *Science Signaling*, vol. 5, no. 212, article ra16, 2012.

[14] P. S. Tang, M. Mura, R. Seth, and M. Liu, "Acute lung injury and cell death: how many ways can cells die?" *American Journal of Physiology—Lung Cellular and Molecular Physiology*, vol. 294, no. 4, pp. L632–L641, 2008.

[15] Q. P. Liu, D. X. Zhou, X. L. Gao, L. Pan, and F. G. Jin, "Participation of autophagy in acute lung induced by seawater," *Experimental Lung Research*, vol. 39, no. 10, pp. 441–452, 2013.

[16] F. Han, Y. Luo, Y. Li et al., "Seawater induces apoptosis in alveolar epithelial cells via the Fas/FasL-mediated pathway," *Respiratory Physiology & Neurobiology*, vol. 182, no. 2-3, pp. 71–80, 2012.

[17] T. Shpilka, H. Weidberg, S. Pietrokovski, and Z. Elazar, "Atg8: an autophagy-related ubiquitin-like protein family," *Genome Biology*, vol. 12, no. 7, article 226, 2011.

[18] E. Ferraro and F. Cecconi, "Autophagic and apoptotic response to stress signals in mammalian cells," *Archives of Biochemistry and Biophysics*, vol. 462, no. 2, pp. 210–219, 2007.

[19] C. Otomo, Z. Metlagel, G. Takaesu, and T. Otomo, "Structure of the human ATG12~ATG5 conjugate required for LC3 lipidation in autophagy," *Nature Structural and Molecular Biology*, vol. 20, no. 1, pp. 59–66, 2013.

[20] L. M. Ibsen and T. Koch, "Submersion and asphyxial injury," *Critical Care Medicine*, vol. 30, no. 11, pp. S402–S408, 2002.

[21] Q. Fan, P. Zhao, J. Li et al., "17β-Estradiol administration attenuates seawater aspiration-induced acute lung injury in rats," *Pulmonary Pharmacology and Therapeutics*, vol. 24, no. 6, pp. 673–681, 2011.

[22] D. J. Prockop, "Marrow stromal cells as stem cells for nonhematopoietic tissues," *Science*, vol. 276, no. 5309, pp. 71–74, 1997.

[23] A. S. de la Garza-Rodea, M. C. Verweij, H. Boersma et al., "Exploitation of herpesvirus immune evasion strategies to modify the immunogenicity of human mesenchymal stem cell transplants," *PLoS ONE*, vol. 6, no. 1, Article ID e14493, 2011.

[24] A. Eisenberg-Lerner, S. Bialik, H. U. Simon, and A. Kimchi, "Life and death partners: apoptosis, autophagy and the cross-talk between them," *Cell Death and Differentiation*, vol. 16, no. 7, pp. 966–975, 2009.

2

Endoscopic-Ultrasound-Guided Fine-Needle Aspiration and the Role of the Cytopathologist in Solid Pancreatic Lesion Diagnosis

Shahzad Iqbal,[1] David Friedel,[1] Mala Gupta,[2] Lorna Ogden,[2] and Stavros N. Stavropoulos[1]

[1] *Division of Gastroenterology, Department of Medicine, Winthrop-University Hospital, Mineola, NY 1150, USA*
[2] *Department of Pathology, Winthrop-University Hospital, Mineola, NY 1150, USA*

Correspondence should be addressed to Shahzad Iqbal, siqbal@winthrop.org

Academic Editor: Hanlin L. Wang

Endoscopic ultrasound (EUS) is the most sensitive imaging modality for solid pancreatic lesions. The specificity, however, is low (about 75%). It can be increased to 100% with an accuracy of 95% by the addition of fine-needle aspiration (FNA). Cytopathology plays an important role. The final diagnosis is based upon the correlation of clinical, EUS, and cytologic features. A close interaction with the cytopathologist is required in improving the diagnostic yield. In this paper, we present an overview of the role of EUS-guided FNA and importance of close interaction with the cytopathologist. Day to day examples of different solid pancreatic lesions have been presented at the end.

1. Introduction

Endoscopic ultrasound (EUS) is an emerging imaging modality. EUS-guided fine-needle aspiration (FNA) plays an important role in solid pancreatic lesions. A close interaction with cytopathology is vital in improving the diagnostic yield. The final diagnosis is based upon correlation of clinical, EUS, and cytologic features. In this paper, we will discuss the role of EUS-FNA, and the importance of cytopathology in the diagnosis of solid pancreatic lesions. We will describe the history and safety of EUS, indications for an EUS-FNA, and a short description of the technique of EUS-FNA. We will also discuss the importance of arranging an onsite cytopathologist and alternatives if that is not feasible. Finally, we will present the clinical, EUS, and key cytologic features of a few representative solid pancreatic lesions.

2. Endoscopic Ultrasound (EUS): Background

Endoscopic ultrasound (EUS) was first introduced by Dr. Eugene DiMagno in the 1980s by combining a high-frequency ultrasound transducer to an endoscope [1]. Initial echoendoscopes were radial, which scan perpendicular to scope's axis and provide 360-degree images similar to computerized tomography (CT) (Figure 1). In 1991, convex linear-array echoendoscope was introduced by Pentax (FG-32). These linear scopes scan parallel to the longitudinal axis of the scope and enable fine needle aspiration (FNA) and different therapeutic applications (Figure 2).

Different imaging modalities are available to help diagnose solid pancreatic lesions including transabdominal ultrasound, computerized tomography (CT), magnetic resonance imaging (MRI), endoscopic retrograde cholangiopancreatography (ERCP), EUS, and positron emission tomography (PET). EUS is considered one of the most sensitive imaging modalities to detect pancreatic masses, with an accuracy of 78–94% for T (local tumor) stage and 64–82% for N (lymph node) stage [2–4]. EUS is an outpatient procedure and can be done under conscious sedation, like a standard upper endoscopy. The pancreas is imaged from the stomach and duodenum.

Overall, EUS is a safe procedure with most of the complications related only to FNA. The complications include bleeding (0–1.3%) [5–7], perforation 0–0.4% [5, 6], infection (0.3%) [5, 6], and pancreatitis (1-2%) [5]. The risk of bacteremia is low, and prophylactic antibiotics are not recommended except for EUS-FNA of pancreatic cystic lesions [8]. The risk of tumor seeding is significantly lower as compared to percutaneous approach [9] with only four case reports so far. The risk of tumor seeding is further

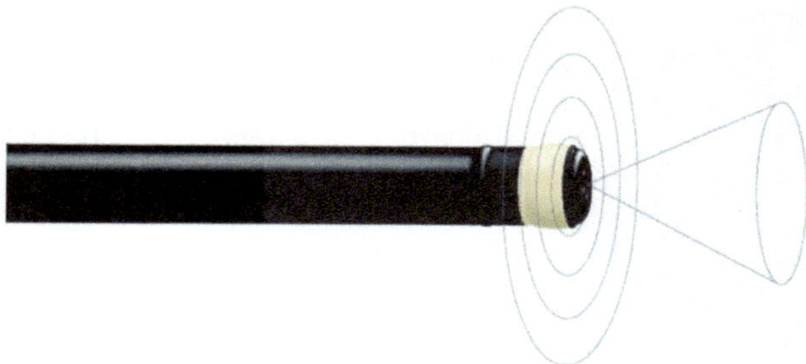

Figure 1: Radial echoendoscope. The tip of the scope scans perpendicular to its axis, providing 360-degree view.

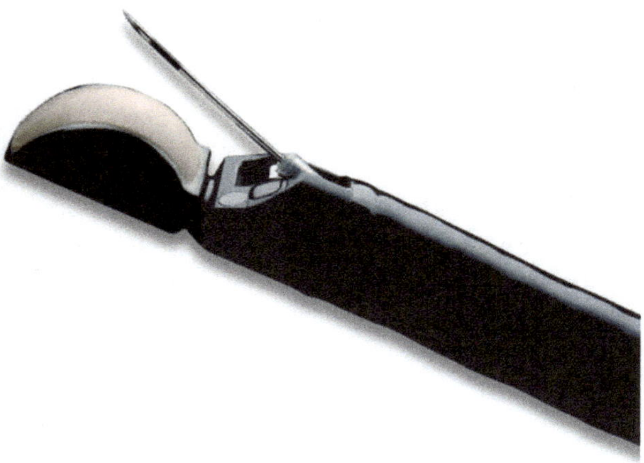

Figure 2: Linear echoendoscope. The tip scans parallel to its longitudinal axis. An FNA needle is seen coming out of the scope channel.

diminished due to the inclusion of needle tract in the resection field of pancreatic head lesions.

3. EUS-Guided Fine Needle Aspiration (EUS-FNA): Indications, Accuracy, and Technique

Although EUS is a very sensitive imaging modality, its ability to differentiate benign inflammatory and malignant pancreatic masses is low. The specificity is only about 75% [10]. The specificity can be increased to 100% with FNA with an accuracy of 95% [11]. However, the negative predictive value of EUS-FNA is low (56%) [12], and a negative result does not completely exclude malignancy. Hence, the need for routine EUS-FNA of potentially resectable pancreatic mass lesions noted on other imaging modalities is controversial [13]. In a review article by Varadarajulu and Eloubeidi [14], EUS-FNA was indicated in the following cases.

(1) Unresectable mass as a prerequisite for adjuvant chemotherapy or radiation.

(2) Suspected other tumor types like lymphoma, small cell metastasis, or neuroendocrine tumors that require different therapy.

(3) When the pretest probability of malignancy is low.

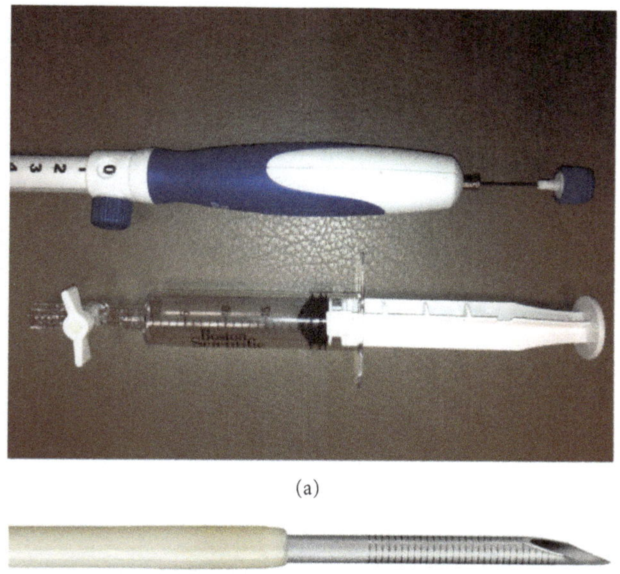

(a)

(b)

Figure 3: EUS-FNA needle. (a) The handle of the FNA needle is shown with a stylet inside and a suction syringe. (b) The tip of the FNA needle used for puncturing the tissue is shown.

(4) Patient refuses major surgery without a definitive diagnosis.

EUS-FNA is done under real-time EUS imaging [15]. The needle device is inserted into the biopsy channel of the linear echoendoscope. The stylet is withdrawn a few millimeters to expose the sharp tip of the needle, followed by advancement of the tip into the target lesion (Figure 3). Doppler is used to avoid any vessels. Once the needle is inside the target tissue, the stylet is first pushed in to expel any needle tract tissue and then removed out of the needle. Suction is applied by attaching a 10–20 mL syringe. The needle is moved to and fro about 10–20 times in a fanlike pattern inside the lesion. The suction syringe is released, the needle is withdrawn into the catheter, and the whole device is removed from the echoendoscope. The material is sprayed onto glass slides by using either air-filled syringe or the stylet, with half of the material fixed in ethanol (for Papanicolaou staining) and the remainder air-dried for onsite cytologic evaluation using Diff-Quik staining (Figure 4). Material for cell block is then obtained by recovering tissue fragments or clot from slides and also rinsing the EUS needle with sterile saline. Pancreatic adenocarcinoma and lymph node metastases of known origin can be usually diagnosed with smears alone. However with suspected neuroendocrine tumor, metastasis of unknown primary, mesenchymal neoplasms, lymphoproliferative disorders, or any other unusual case, sufficient material is needed in cell block for immunocytochemistry [16]. With suspected lymphoma, a separate sample in Roswell Park Memorial Institute (RPMI) solution is preferred for flow cytometry [17].

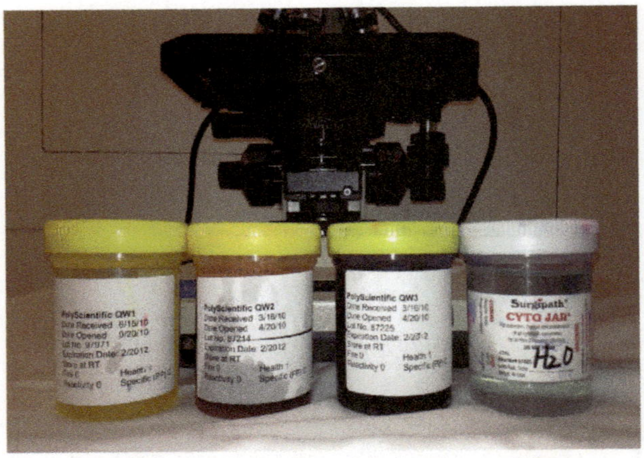

FIGURE 4: Diff-Quik staining method. Air-dried smears are stained in three steps and takes about 10–20 seconds each. The smear is first fixed in methyl alcohol solution, followed by staining with solution I containing L-xanthene (an eosin variant), and then solution II containing methylene blue and azure A. The slide is then rinsed with water and the wet slide is viewed under the microscope.

4. Diagnostic Yield of EUS-FNA and the Importance of an Onsite Cytopathologist

The diagnostic yield of EUS-FNA for solid pancreatic lesion is 86.8–98.5% for cytologic and 68.9–89% for histologic examinations, while 65–100% for lymph nodes [18]. However, there are certain variables that can affect the accuracy and diagnostic yield of EUS-FNA. These can be categorized as either endoscopist or cytopathologist related.

The success rate of EUS-FNA increases with endoscopist experience. The American Society of Gastrointestinal Endoscopy (ASGE) has recommended at least 150 supervised EUS procedures, including 50 EUS-FNAs (of which half are pancreatic and another half nonpancreatic) to achieve comprehensive competency [19]. Getting the target lesion in good view, selecting proper needle size, and proper FNA technique are associated with increased diagnostic yield [20]. The available needles are 25, 22, and 19 gauges. For solid pancreatic lesions, the 25-gauge needle is at least equivalent [21–24] or even superior for cytological diagnosis [25, 26] due to less blood contamination as compared to the standard 22-gauge needle. However, certain tumors such as malignant lymphomas, rare pancreatic neoplasms, well-differentiated adenocarcinoma, mesenchymal tumors, as well as benign conditions, such as autoimmune pancreatitis may be difficult to diagnose based on cytology alone. In such cases, core biopsies can be obtained using 22- or 19-gauge aspiration needles [27]. A spring-loaded 19-gauge Tru-Cut needle is also available for histologic diagnosis. However, it is difficult to deploy especially for pancreatic head lesions [28].

The diagnostic success of EUS-FNA also depends on the cytopathologist's experience. Unlike percutaneous biopsies, EUS-FNA material is contaminated by gastrointestinal epithelium [29, 30] leading to errors in diagnosis. It is important for the cytopathologist to be aware of the route traversed by the needle for proper evaluation of the smears. Training courses are required for cytopathologist with no previous experience with EUS-FNA [31, 32]. Proper handling and triaging of EUS-FNA material following immediate onsite cytologic evaluation are very helpful [33]. Immediate cytologic evaluation not only improves the diagnostic yield, but can potentially reduce the number of needle passes, procedure time, and patient risk [34]. However, it is expensive and many of the centers may not have an onsite cytopathologist. In a study by Savoy et al. [35], even experienced endosonographers were less reliable than cytotechnologists in evaluating onsite adequacy macroscopically. When either an onsite cytopathologist or cytotechnologist is not available, options are to use multiple needle passes or telecytopathology.

The optimal number of EUS FNA needle passes range from two to six [36]. In study by Erickson et al. [34] where onsite cytopathologist was not available, 5-6 passes were needed for diagnosis of pancreatic masses and 2-3 for liver metastases and lymph nodes. However in another study [36], at least 7 passes were needed for pancreatic and miscellaneous masses (including mediastinal, perirectal, and subepithelial) and 5 passes into lymph nodes for correct diagnosis. In a retrospective multicenter study [37], gross or macroscopic assessment of the specimen for adequacy by the endosonographer ("one or more small-core biopsy cylinders") resulted in limitation of the number of needle passes to only 1-2 in 92% of the patients with solid pancreatic lesions. However, the macroscopic assessment was wrong in 13.5% of the cases due to presence of fibrous tissue, gastrointestinal contamination, or occasionally clot. However in another study [38], neither endosonographers nor cytotechnologists were able to provide a reliable assessment of FNA adequacy for solid pancreatic lesions by using gross visual inspection of the specimen on a slide. Another emerging concept is telecytopathology which may be a valid substitute to onsite cytopathologic evaluation. The slides are initially prepared and prescreened by a cytotechnologist or pathology resident and then analyzed by an offsite cytopathologist using real-time remotely operated system (MedMicro System; Trestle Corporation of Irvine, CA). In a retrospective study [39], telecytopathology was statistically equivalent in accuracy to onsite cytopathologist for pancreatic carcinoma.

5. EUS and Cytologic Features of Different Pancreatic Solid Lesions

The clinical and radiological findings should correlate with the FNA results on whether the pancreatic lesion is benign or malignant [40]. It is the composite picture of cell type, microarchitecture, and nuclear and cytoplasmic features that determine the cytologic diagnosis. The smear is first examined under low magnification for cellularity, cell types, and cohesiveness, followed by high-magnification examination of nuclear and cytoplasmic features. Specific nuclear features determine malignancy, whereas cytoplasmic features and microarchitecture determine differentiation. Malignant cells exhibit disorganization and discohesion (loosely aggregated

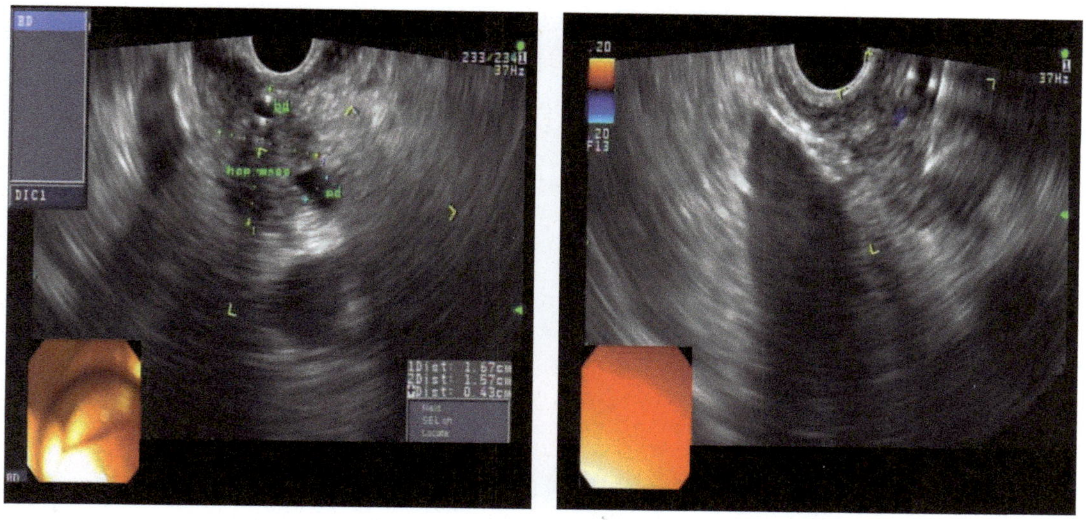

(a) (b)

Figure 5: Pancreatic ductal adenocarcinoma. (a) EUS showed a 17 mm by 15 mm hypoechoic and homogenous solid mass in the pancreatic head area obstructing the distal common bile duct (CBD) and main pancreatic duct (PD) near ampulla. (b) A single FNA was done using 25-gauge needle via transduodenal approach.

or single cells). Nuclear features of malignant cells include enlarged nuclei (higher nuclear to cytoplasmic ratio), variation in nuclear size and shape from cell to cell (anisonucleosis), hyperchromasia (increase amount of chromatin), multiple or irregular nucleoli, and abnormal mitotic figures. Cytoplasmic features (mucin in adenocarcinoma and fine red granules in neuroendocrine tumors) and microarchitecture (glands or papillae) help classify the tumor. In poorly differentiated or metastatic lesions, immunohistochemical staining of the cell blocks may be needed to determine the origin.

6. Examples of Different Solid Pancreatic Lesions

Next, we will discuss the clinical, EUS, and cytologic features of different solid pancreatic lesions.

(1) Pancreatic ductal adenocarcinoma: a 67-year-old gentleman presented with painless jaundice. MRI abdomen showed dilated bile and pancreatic ducts, but no obvious pancreatic mass was noted. EUS showed a 17 mm by 15 mm hypoechoic and homogenous mass in the pancreatic head area obstructing the distal common bile duct (CBD) and main pancreatic duct (PD) near ampulla (Figure 5). One FNA was done using 25-gauge needle via transduodenal approach. The specimen was analyzed by an onsite cytopathologist for adequate cellularity.

Onsite evaluation for a poorly differentiated adenocarcinoma is relatively easy because of increased cellularity and markedly atypical clusters with a 3-dimensional appearance (Figure 6). Necrosis may be evident in the background. On the other hand, a well-differentiated adenocarcinoma can be challenging even on alcohol fixed and Papanicolaou-stained smears. The key is to establish at least one completely normal ductal epithelium which would have uniformly sized, bland nuclei, equidistant from each other, giving it a honeycombed appearance (Figure 7). All other cell groups are compared to this normal standard. In a well-differentiated adenocarcinoma, the four most outstanding differences from normal epithelium are overall larger nuclei as compared to normal; nuclear size variation such that the largest nucleus in the group may be three times the smallest nucleus; unequal spacing of nuclei resulting in a loss of polarity, also referred to as "drunken honeycombs"; nuclear grooves and nuclear membrane irregularities [41]. If these features are not specifically sought, a false negative diagnosis may be rendered.

(2) Intraductal papillary mucinous neoplasm (IPMN): a 68-year-old female with history of acute pancreatitis of unclear etiology and associated large pancreatic tail pseudocyst was referred for EUS evaluation and possible endoscopic drainage of the pseudocyst. EUS showed a 13 mm by 10 mm irregular anechoic cystic lesion with hypoechoic solid component within the tail of pancreas (suspicious for cystic neoplasm). It was communicating with the main PD. The PD was itself dilated upstream of this lesion and was leading into a large anechoic pseudocyst (Figure 8). One FNA pass was done of the cystic-solid lesion using 22-gauge needle via transgastric approach. The specimen was analyzed by onsite cytopathologist for adequate cellularity.

This case was a classic example with thick viscid mucin that did not spread easily nor air-dry readily. Microscopy revealed classic papillary fronds and numerous macrophages in a mucinous background (Figure 9). The diagnosis of IPMN is made based on the characteristic EUS findings and cytological features of viscid mucin, macrophages, and epithelium arranged in finger like papillae [42]. However, in addition, the diagnosis of in situ or invasive malignancy within the IPMN has to be evaluated separately, applying the usual criteria for malignancy. A note of caution should be added to the report that, even if no features of malignancy

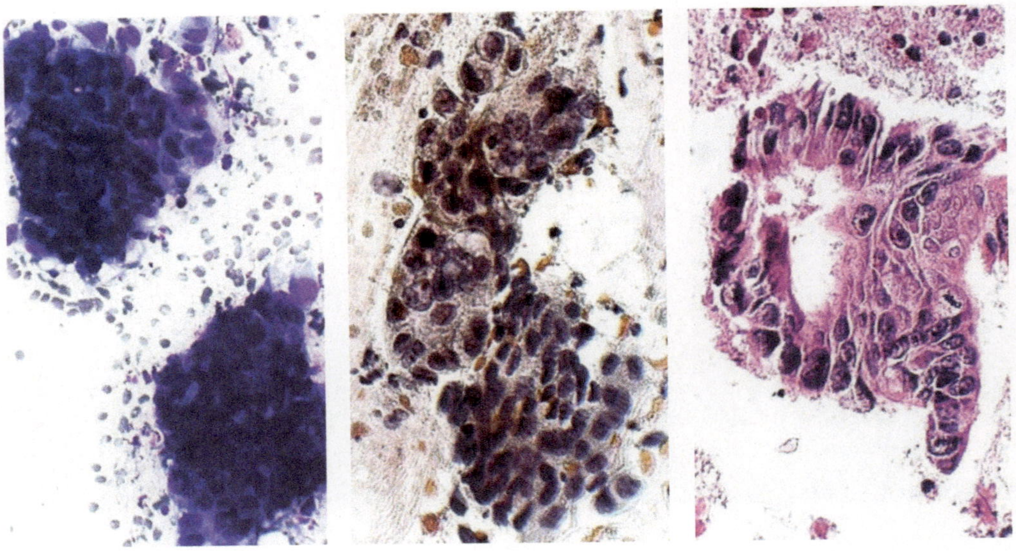

(a) (b) (c)

Figure 6: Pancreatic ductal adenocarcinoma, poorly differentiated: three-dimensional clusters in (a) Diff-Quik stain at 200x; (b) Papanicolaou's stain at 200x; (c) mitosis and hyperchromatic nuclei in cell block, H&E at 200x.

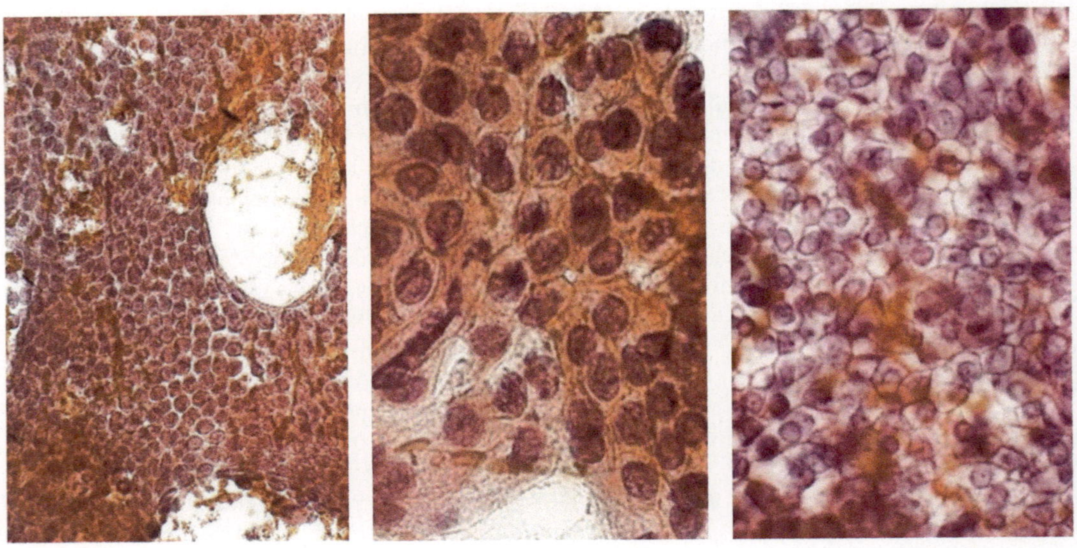

(a) (b) (c)

Figure 7: Pancreatic ductal adenocarcinoma, well-differentiated: (a) normal pancreatic ductal epithelium, Papanicolaou stain at 400x; (b) nuclear membrane irregularities, Papanicolaou stain at 600x; (c) well-differentiated adenocarcinoma with "drunken honeycombs," Papanicolaou stain at 400x.

are present in the current aspirate smears, the lesion may still harbor malignancy in unsampled areas and, therefore, should be treated surgically.

(3) Pancreatic neuroendocrine tumor: a 48-year-old gentleman was admitted with recent onset headaches and hypertensive urgency. MRI abdomen with and without contrast showed a hypervascular 19 mm by 9 mm pancreatic body/tail solid lesion. EUS showed an 18.9 mm by 9.6 mm hypoechoic mass with anechoic microcystic (most likely necrotic) components in body/tail of the pancreas (Figure 10). Three FNA passes were obtained via transgastric approach. The specimen was analyzed by onsite cytopathologist for adequate cellularity.

Pancreatic neuroendocrine tumors (NETs) have a variety of appearances. They can mimic normal pancreatic acinar parenchyma (Figure 11(a)), a gland forming adenocarcinoma, an acinar cell carcinoma, or even a plasmacytoma [43]. Only a small percentage show the classic "salt and pepper" nuclear detail on alcohol fixed smears and H&E of cell block. In fact, a single prominent nucleolus is not

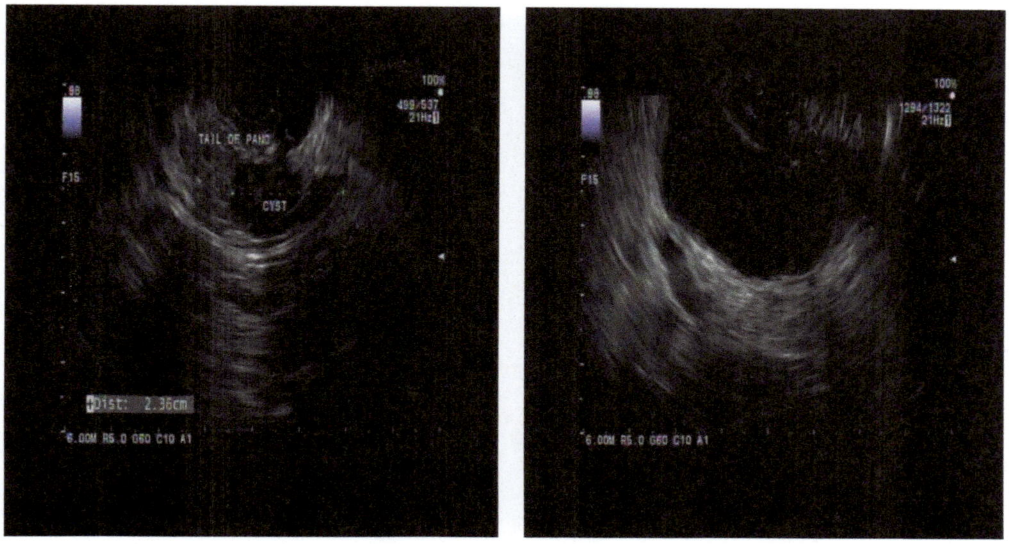

(a) (b)

Figure 8: Intraductal papillary mucinous neoplasm (IPMN). (a) An irregular anechoic cystic lesion with hypoechoic solid component was noted within the tail of pancreas (suspicious for cystic neoplasm). It was communicating with the main PD. (b) The PD was itself dilated upstream of this lesion and was leading into a large anechoic pseudocyst.

an uncommon finding. On air-dried Romanowsky-stained smears, the nuclear details are not as helpful as in alcohol fixed preparations. The key to a successful diagnosis is to keep this possibility in the differential diagnosis and obtain adequate material in cell block to do the relevant immunoperoxidase stains for neuroendocrine markers, such as chromogranin and synaptophysin (Figures 11(e) and 11(g)). Synaptophysin is more sensitive than chromogranin, but less specific. A quirky detail to be aware of is that gastrointestinal neuroendocrine tumors, including pancreatic NET, may occasionally be cytokeratin AE1 : AE3 negative. It is therefore important to include Cam 5.2, which is more reliably positive. As of now, it is not a requirement to do a Ki67 on the cell block for World Health Organization (WHO) grading based on proliferative index, but a mitotic count should be attempted if there is adequate material in the cell block [44]. As per the WHO classification of neuroendocrine tumors <2 mitosis/10 hpf is classified as a neuroendocrine tumor, 2–20 mitosis/10 hpf is classified as a well-differentiated neuroendocrine carcinoma, and >20 mitosis/10 hpf is a high-grade neuroendocrine carcinoma [45]. A note of caution: sometimes the aspiration needle may pick up incidental pancreatic endocrine microadenoma (<5 mm) or islet cell proliferations in pancreatic atrophy. Under these circumstances it is best to correlate with EUS for their relevance.

(4) High-grade neuroendocrine carcinoma: a 87-year-old gentleman status after Billroth II surgery and history of choledocholithiasis with multiple ERCP procedures in the past presented with a new onset of biliary obstruction. CT abdomen showed multiple liver lesions and retroperitoneal/portal lymphadenopathy suspicious for malignancy. EUS showed a 29 mm by 27 mm pancreatic body hypoechoic and homogenous solid lesion (Figure 12). Two FNAs passed were done via transgastric approach. The specimen was analyzed by onsite cytopathologist for adequate cellularity. Celiac lymphadenopathy and multiple liver lesions were also noted, consistent with metastases.

Immediate onsite evaluation with Diff-Quik revealed abundant cellularity and necrosis with closely packed tumor cells that could be described generically as a "small, blue, round cell tumor" (Figure 13). The combination of nuclear molding, nuclear streaking artifact, mitosis, single-cell necrosis, polar cytokeratin staining, and positive neuroendocrine markers is diagnostic of a high-grade neuroendocrine carcinoma. The differential diagnosis during an onsite evaluation of these lesions includes a high-grade lymphoma. Immunoperoxidase stains, preferably on a cell block, help to sort out these two entities by a binary algorithm. Lymphoma is LCA+/CK− while high-grade neuroendocrine carcinoma is LCA−/CK+. Since high-grade neuroendocrine carcinoma occurs rarely in the pancreas, a metastasis from a lung primary should be ruled out. Clinical and chest CT findings are more important in establishing a metastasis than immunohistochemistry, because TTF1 does not reliably differentiate the two primaries as TTF1 may be positive in extrapulmonary small cell carcinoma [46]. As mentioned earlier, per WHO guidelines, a high-grade neuroendocrine carcinoma of pancreas would require a mitotic count >20/10 high power field (hpf) or a Ki-67 index >20%.

(5) Acinar cell carcinoma: a 47-year-old female with prior history of cholecystectomy presented with epigastric pain. CT abdomen showed a 21 mm distal pancreatic body cystic lesion. EUS showed a 25 mm by 23 mm hypoechoic solid lesion with few anechoic cystic areas (most likely necrosis) in distal pancreatic body (Figure 14). Five passes were done

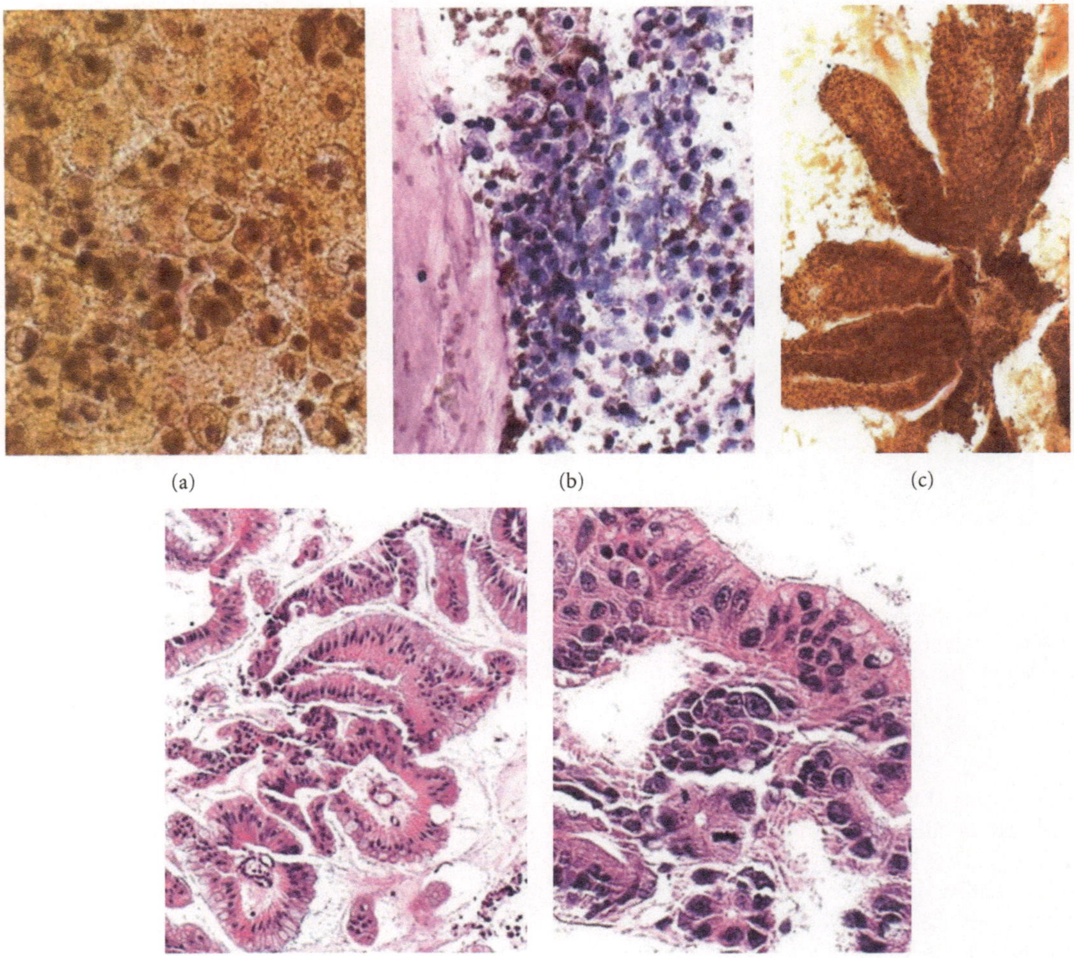

(a) (b) (c)

(d) (e)

Figure 9: Intraductal papillary mucinous neoplasm (IPMN): Muciphages in a necrotic and mucinous background in (a) Papanicolaou stain at 400x; (b) Diff-Quik stain at 200x; Papillary fronds in (c) Papanicolaou stain at 100x; (d) cell block H&E at 200x; (e) mitosis and cytologic atypia, cell block H&E at 400x.

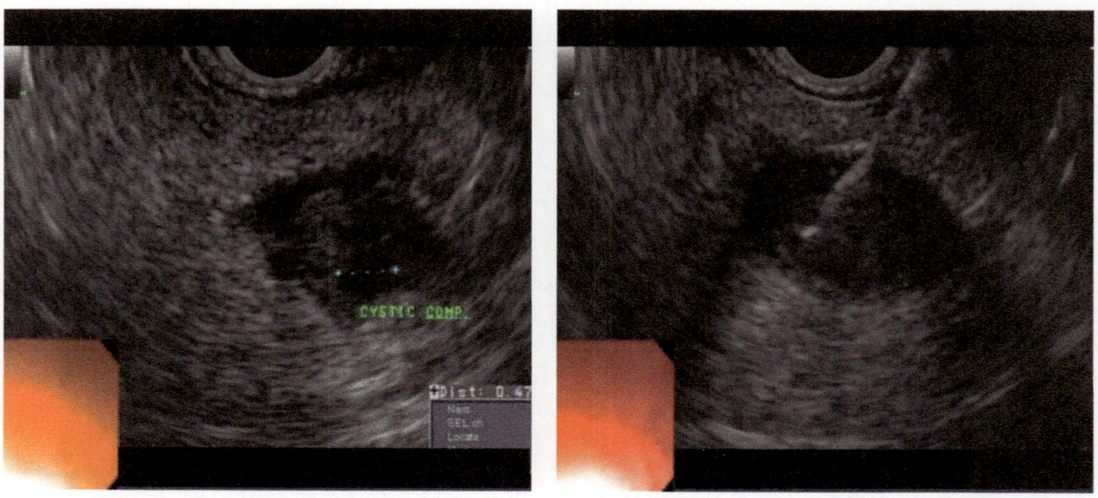

(a) (b)

Figure 10: Pancreatic neuroendocrine tumor. (a) EUS showed an 18.9 mm by 9.6 mm hypoechoic solid mass with anechoic microcystic (most likely necrotic) components in body/tail of the pancreas. (b) An FNA needle is passed into the solid component via transgastric approach.

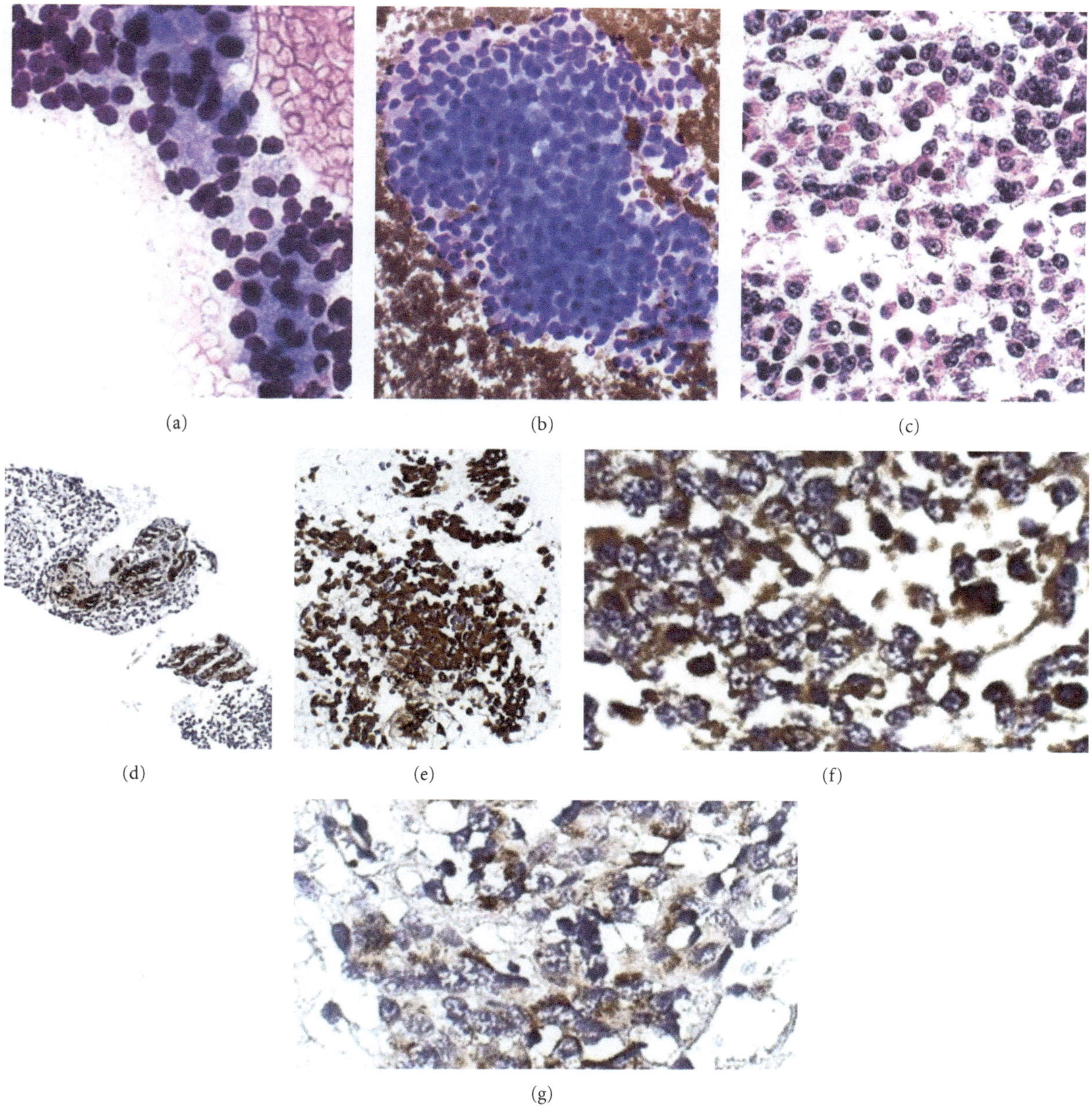

FIGURE 11: Pancreatic neuroendocrine tumor: (a) normal pancreatic acini, Diff-Quik stain at 400x; (b) cohesive 3-dimensional cluster in Diff-Quik stain at 200x; (c) discohesive cells with salt and pepper chromatin and rare pinpoint nucleolus in cell block H&E at 400x; Immunohistochemical profile of the tumor: (d) cytokeratin AE1/AE3 highlights residual ductal epithelium but not the tumor, at 100x; (e) synaptophysin, strong and diffuse positivity, at 400x; (f) positive cytokeratin Cam 5.2 at 200x; (g) positive chromogranin at 400x.

using 22- and 25-gauge needles via transgastric approach. The specimen was analyzed by onsite cytopathologist for adequate cellularity.

These tumors tend to be extremely cellular and dyscohesive on aspirate smears (Figure 15). Typically they have abundant cytoplasm and a prominent nucleolus, evident even on Diff-Quik-stained aspirate smears. Arriving at the correct final diagnosis is only possible after establishing the presence of zymogen granules by immunohistochemical stains for trypsin. Acinar cell carcinoma may mimic pancreatic neuroendocrine tumors on cytomorphology and immunohistochemistry because they may occasionally stain with neuroendocrine markers [47]. In a small sample such as a cell block preparation, it is often difficult to prove its true lineage and may be erroneously diagnosed as a neuroendocrine tumor.

(6) Autoimmune pancreatitis: a 44-year-old gentleman with new onset diabetes mellitus presented with obstructive jaundice and weight loss. ERCP showed common hepatic biliary stricture. Brushings were negative for malignancy. A plastic biliary stent was placed. CT abdomen showed mild intrahepatic biliary dilatation, stent in place, but no obvious mass lesion. EUS was then performed. The pancreas was diffusely enlarged lobulated, and hypoechoic in appearance

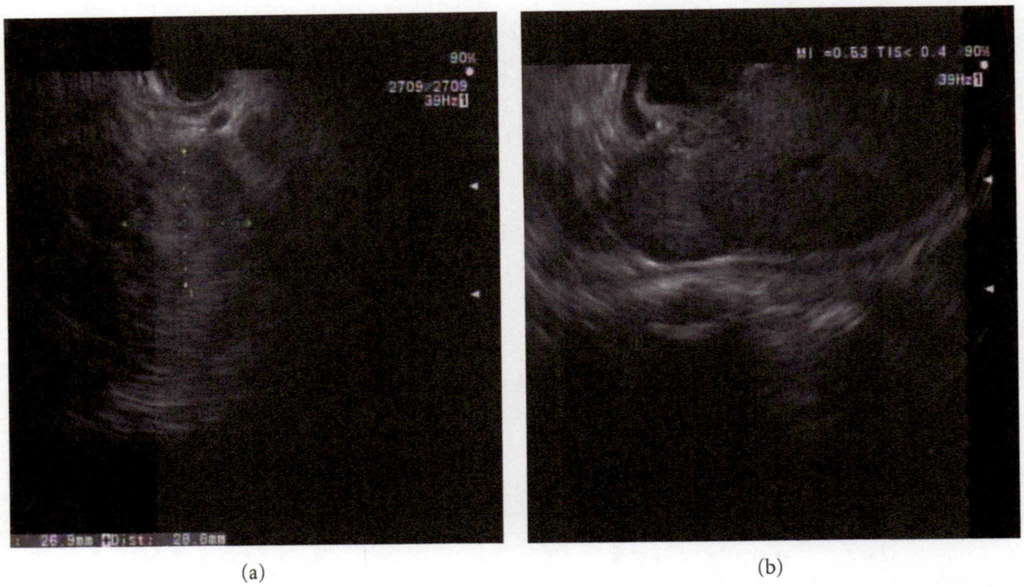

Figure 12: High-grade neuroendocrine carcinoma. (a) EUS showed a 29 mm by 27 mm pancreatic body hypoechoic and homogenous solid lesion. (b) Multiple solid liver lesions were also noted, consistent with metastases.

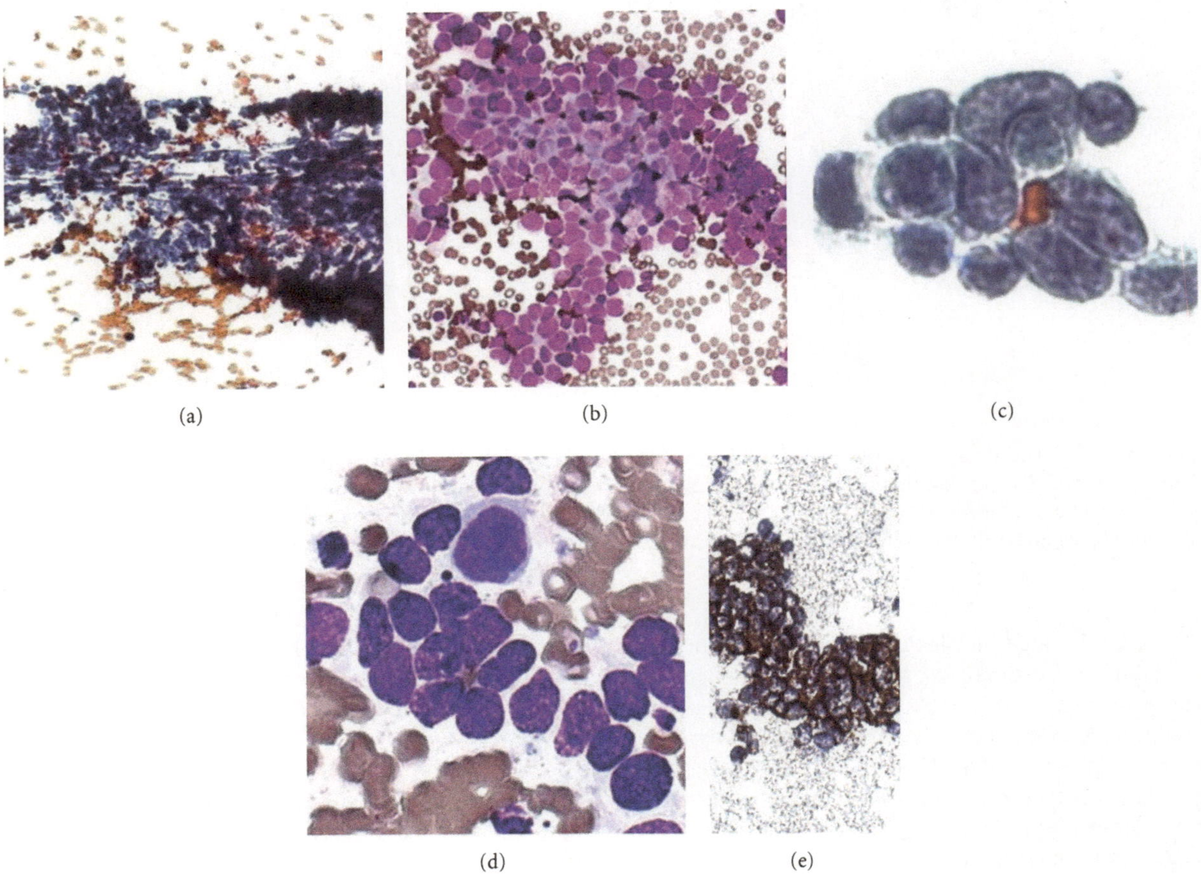

Figure 13: High-grade neuroendocrine carcinoma: (a) cellular smears with nuclear streaking artifact, Papanicolaou stain at 200x; (b) closely packed nuclei due to scant cytoplasm, Diff-Quik stain at 200x; (c) and (d) nuclear molding, Papanicolaou and Diff-Quik stains at 400x; (e) immunoperoxidase stain for cytokeratin Cam 5.2, at 200x.

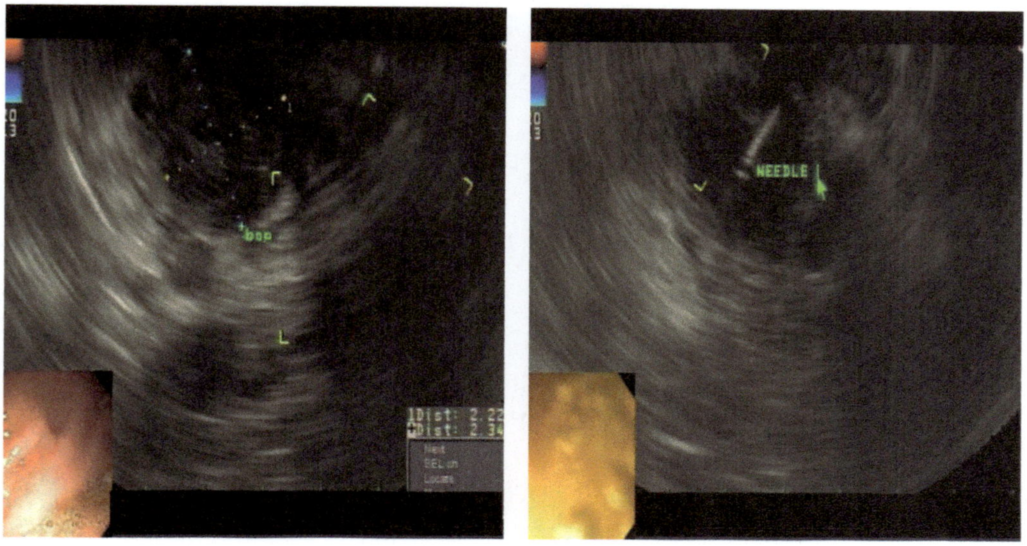

(a) (b)

FIGURE 14: Acinar cell carcinoma: EUS showed a 25 mm by 23 mm hypoechoic solid lesion with few anechoic cystic areas (most likely necrosis) in distal pancreatic body. (b) An FNA pass is being done using 22-gauge needle via transgastric approach.

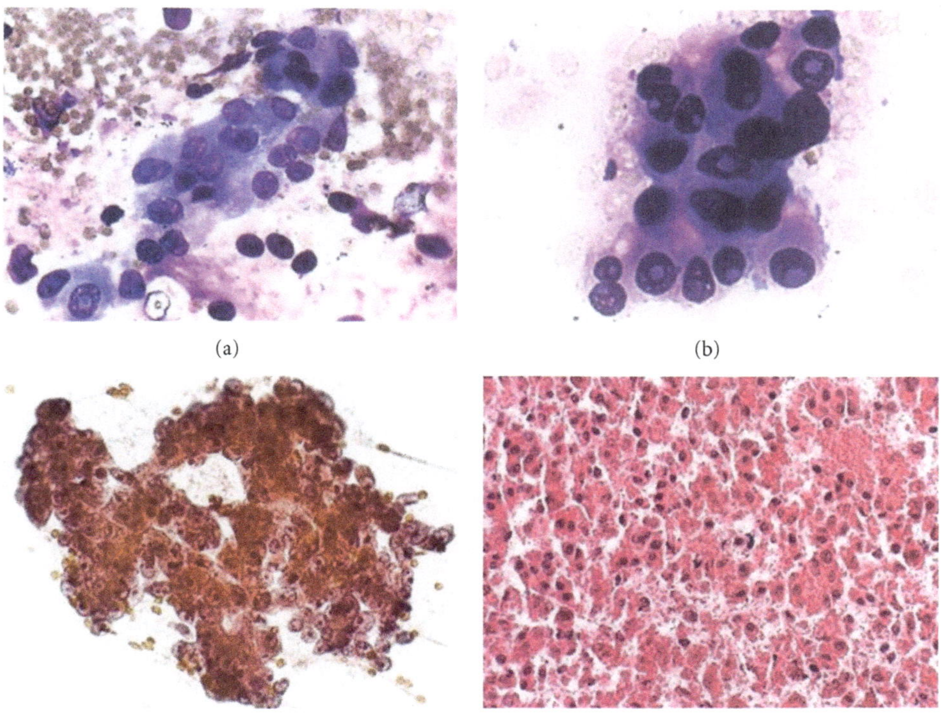

(a) (b) (c) (d)

FIGURE 15: Acinar cell carcinoma: (a) one cohesive group and scattered bare nuclei, Diff-Quik stain at 400x; (b) abundant cytoplasm and prominent nucleoli, Diff-Quik stain at 600x, (c) prominent nucleoli, Papanicolaou stain at 400x; (d) discohesive cells in cell block H&E at 400x.

with coarse echogenic foci. The main PD was small in size. The proximal superior mesenteric vein (SMV) was encased, and partially obstructed with portal collaterals (Figure 16). Four passes were done of the pancreatic neck with 19-gauge Quick core needle via transgastric approach. After confirmation of adequate cellularity, the specimen was submitted for cytologic and histologic analyses.

Aspirate smears from sclerotic areas in autoimmune pancreatitis (AIP) may yield no cells; conversely, identifying ductal epithelium during onsite evaluation does not

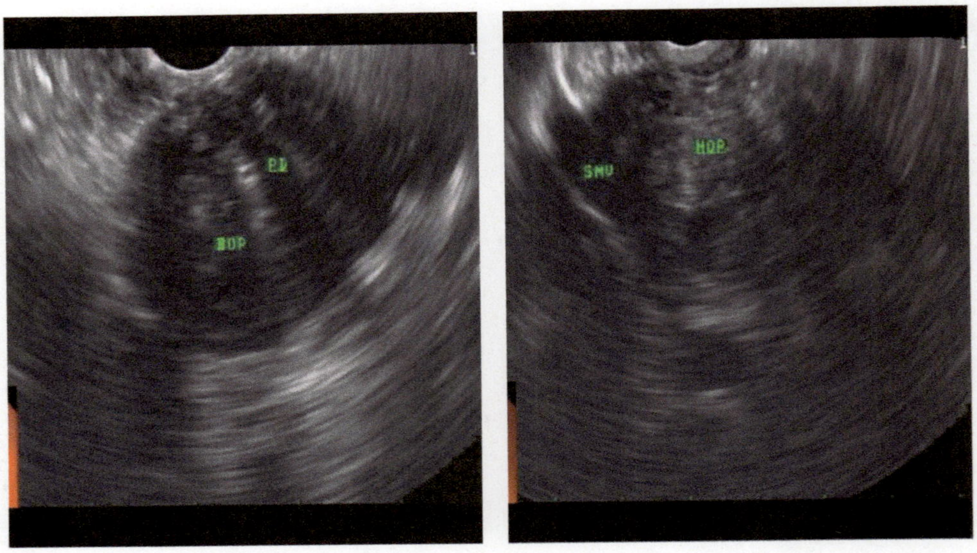

(a) (b)

FIGURE 16: Autoimmune pancreatitis: EUS showed the entire pancreas to be diffusely enlarged, lobulated, and hypoechoic in appearance with coarse echogenic foci. The main PD was small in size. (a) and (b) showed the changes in body and head of pancreas, respectively. The proximal SMV (superior mesenteric vein) was encased and partially obstructed.

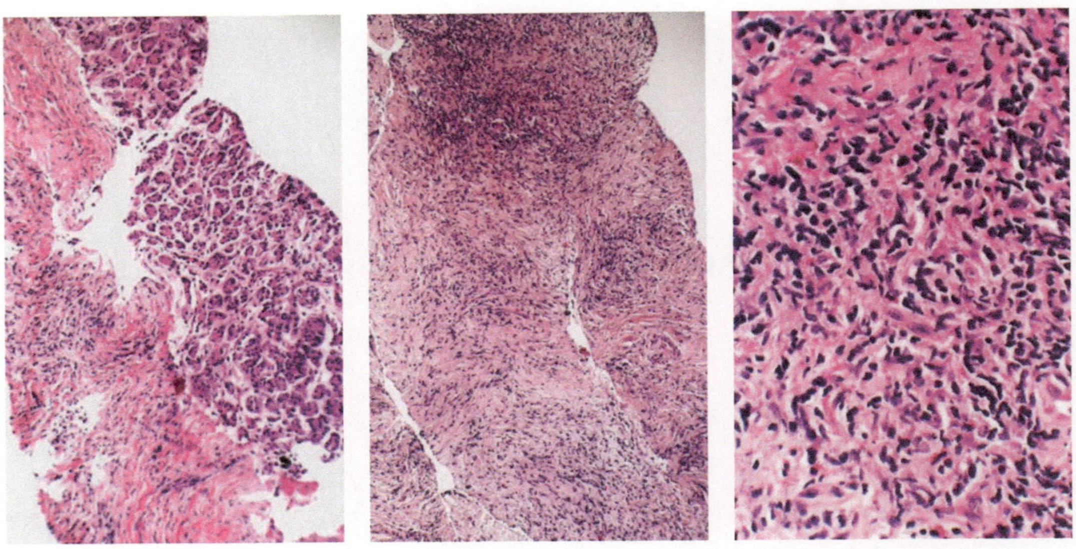

(a) (b) (c)

FIGURE 17: Autoimmune pancreatitis: sclerotic parenchyma compared to an intact acinar parenchyma, H&E cell block at 100x (a), infiltrated by inflammatory cells, H&E cell block at 100x (b), consisting predominantly of lymphocytes and rare eosinophils, H&E cell block at 100x (c).

guarantee diagnostic tissue in the cell block. Therefore, there is only a limited role for onsite evaluation if this diagnosis is already radiologically and serologically (elevated serum IgG4) established. Typically, the role for cytopathologist during the EUS-FNA procedure in patients with AIP is to rule out a pancreatic malignancy in a mass lesion. For suspected AIP lesions, instead of an FNA, a core biopsy with cutting needle is preferable [48] for documenting sclerosis, pancreatic atrophy, and lymphoplasmacytic inflammation in the sclerotic areas, by means of a cell block (Figure 17). Inflammation is usually patchy and includes predominantly lymphocytes [49]. If sufficient numbers of plasma cells are present, IgG4 stain may be attempted on the cell block by immunohistochemistry.

(7) Solid pseudopapillary tumor: a 43-year-old female with no significant past medical history presented with abdominal pain. CT abdomen showed a 3 cm cystic lesion in the head of pancreas. EUS showed a 36 mm anechoic irregular lesion with a hypoechoic thick irregular rim and a solid polypoid component in the pancreatic head/body

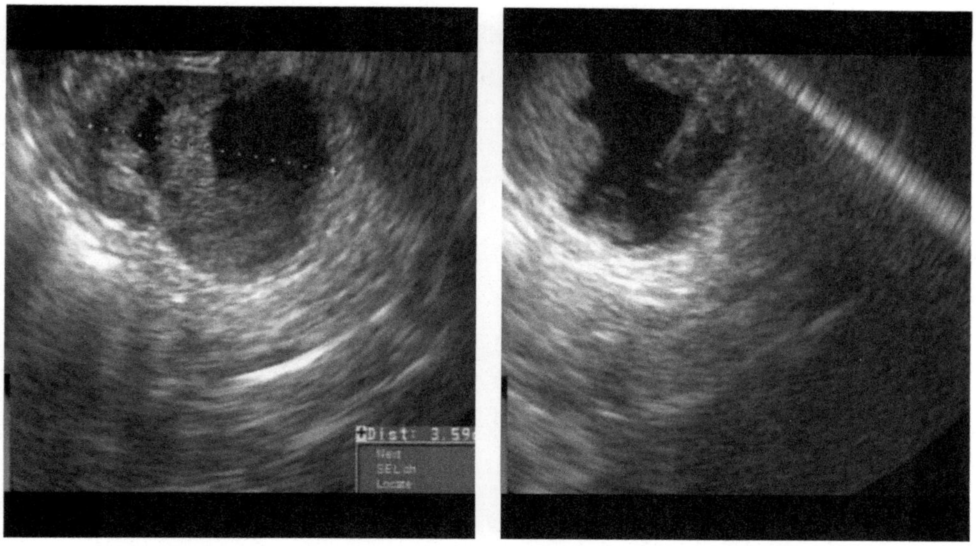

(a) (b)

FIGURE 18: Solid pseudopapillary tumor. (a) EUS showed a 36 mm anechoic cystic lesion with a hypoechoic thick irregular rim and a solid polypoid component in the pancreatic head/body junction. (b) The cystic and solid components were separately FNA using a 19-gauge needle via transgastric approach.

junction (Figure 18). The cystic and solid components were separately aspirated using a 19-gauge needle via transgastric approach. The specimen adequacy was confirmed by an onsite cytopathologist.

Onsite evaluation revealed markedly cellular aspirate smears with the cells arrayed along elongate papillary structures with central fibrovascular cores (Figure 19). Uniformly bland, dyscohesive cells were scattered between the papillae. There was no mucin or macrophages in the background. These two key features (papillae and bland dyscohesive cells) were the clues to a spot diagnosis of solid and cystic pseudopapillary tumor of pancreas [50]. Immunohistochemical profile of this tumor is interesting: mostly negative for cytokeratin, positive for vimentin and CD10 and nuclear staining for beta catenin [51].

(8) Metastatic lung cancer An 80-year-old female with history of bilateral lung adenocarcinoma, surgical lobectomy, chemotherapy, and radiation in the past presented with new onset jaundice. CT abdomen showed a large 38 mm by 31 mm mass located in the peripancreatic area that was causing distal CBD stenosis. PET scan showed an increasing hypermetabolic focus in the same area, suggestive of neoplastic process. EUS showed a 37 mm by 30 mm well-defined, hypoechoic, and heterogeneous peripancreatic mass at the level of pancreatic head causing distal CBD stenosis (Figure 20). Two FNA passes were done using 25-gauge needle via transduodenal approach. The specimen was analyzed by onsite cytopathologist for adequate cellularity.

The composite on Figure 21 shows adequate atypical clusters on immediate evaluation. It does not appear different from a pancreatic ductal adenocarcinoma. However, on immunohistochemistry, the tumor was CK7+/TTF1+/CK20−. This immunoprofile is consistent with the lung primary. A typical pancreatic primary would be CK7+/TTF1−/CK20+. Clinical history and cell block for immunohistochemistry are essential in arriving at the right diagnosis.

(9) Metastatic renal cell cancer: a 73-year-old woman was found to have multiple peripancreatic masses, left adrenal mass, and a left lower pole kidney mass on imaging studies. EUS showed multiple confluent, well-circumscribed hypoechoic, spherical masses, measuring up to 40 mm, in the peripancreatic (head) area compressing distal CBD. Multiple anechoic areas were noted within these mass, representing necroses (Figure 22). A single FNA pass was done using a 19-gauge needle via transduodenal approach. A 31 mm hypoechoic, well-circumscribed mass was noted in left adrenal. Its appearance was similar to other masses imaged. One FNA pass was done using 22-gauge needle via transgastric approach and submitted for cell block only. The peripancreatic mass was analyzed by onsite cytopathologist for adequate cellularity.

Onsite evaluation of the peripancreatic mass showed an extremely cellular aspirate on Diff Quick stain and was deemed adequate for evaluation. The clear cell morphology of the metastatic tumor is best appreciated on routine H&E stain of the cell block (Figure 23), least evident on air-dried smears for onsite evaluation, moderately so on alcohol fixed, Papanicolaou-stained smears. Cell blocks from both lesions (peripancreatic and left adrenal) showed identical morphology with clear cells. Immunoperoxidase stains are mandatory to differentiate the following: normal left adrenal cortical parenchyma/adrenal cortical adenoma versus a left clear cell renal carcinoma (RCC) in the upper pole. Normal adrenal cortical parenchyma cannot be distinguished from an adrenal cortical adenoma by immunoperoxidase stains but they can both be distinguished from an RCC. Synaptophysin, Melan 1, and inhibin are positive in adrenal cortical cells while CD10, vimentin, and RCC antigen highlight RCC

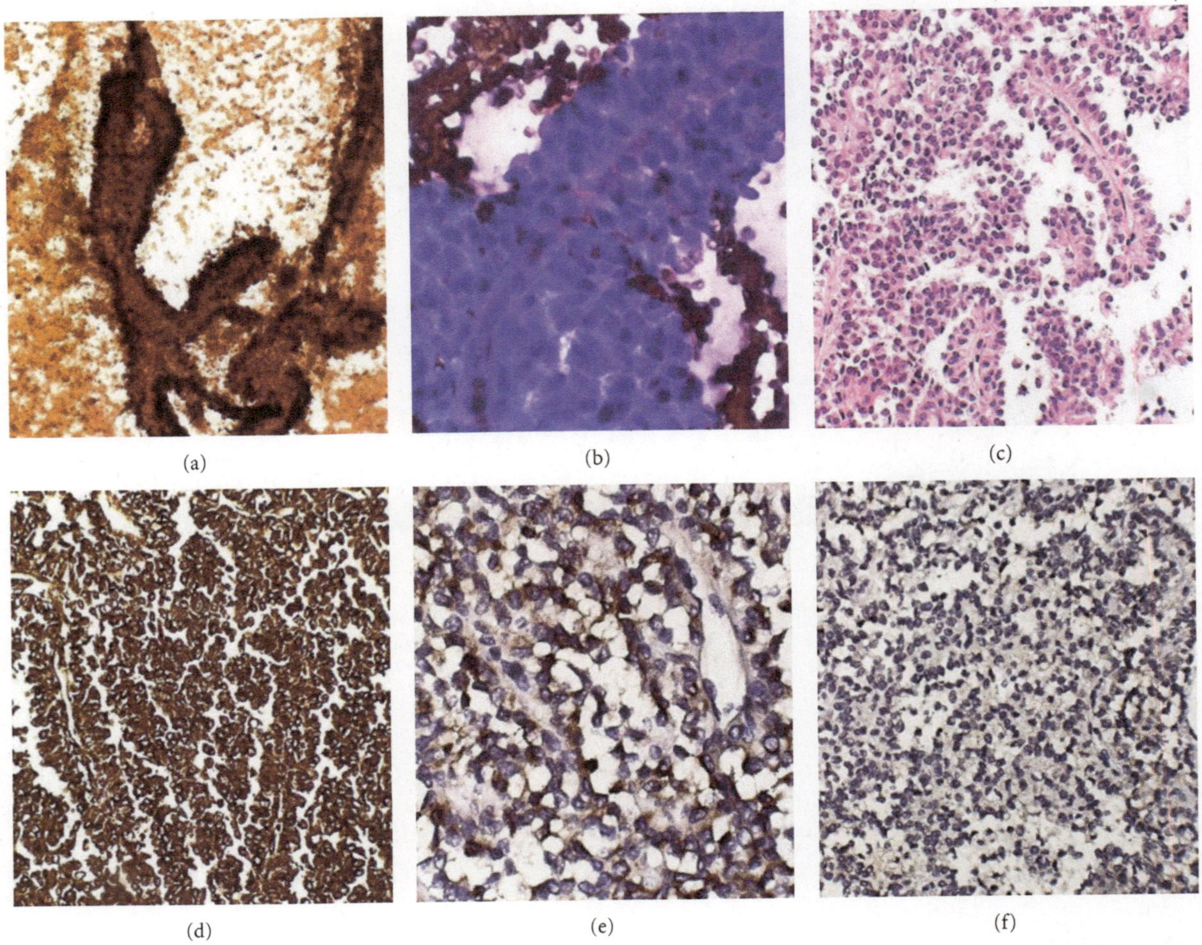

Figure 19: Solid pseudopapillary tumor: (a) slender pseudopapillary structures, Papanicolaou stain at 200x; (b) central fibrovascular cores, Diff-Quik stain at 400x; (c) cell block, H&E at 200x; immunoperoxidase stains (d) positive vimentin, 200x; (e) positive CD10, 400x; (f). negative cytokeratin Cam 5.2, 200x.

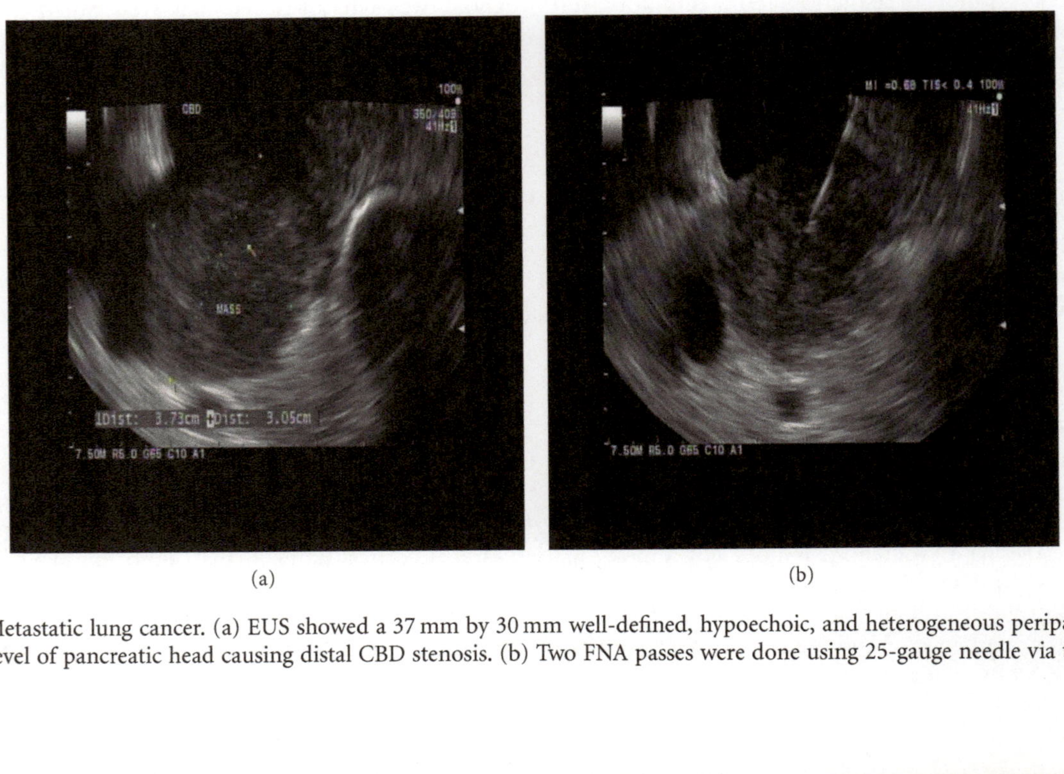

Figure 20: Metastatic lung cancer. (a) EUS showed a 37 mm by 30 mm well-defined, hypoechoic, and heterogeneous peripancreatic solid mass at the level of pancreatic head causing distal CBD stenosis. (b) Two FNA passes were done using 25-gauge needle via transduodenal approach.

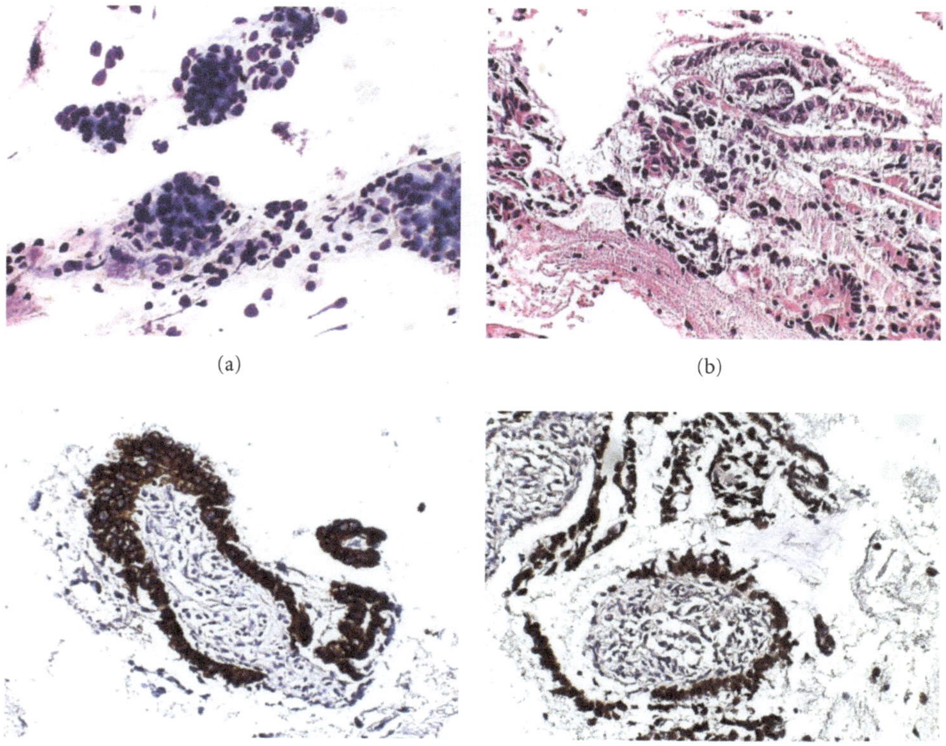

(a) (b) (c) (d)

Figure 21: Lung metastasis to pancreas: (a) tumor cell clusters, Diff-Quik stain at 200x; (b) strips of tumor epithelium, H&E cell block at 200x; (c) cytoplasmic staining of cytokeratin CK7, immunoperoxidase stain, 400x; (d) nuclear staining of TTF1, immunoperoxidase stain, 200x.

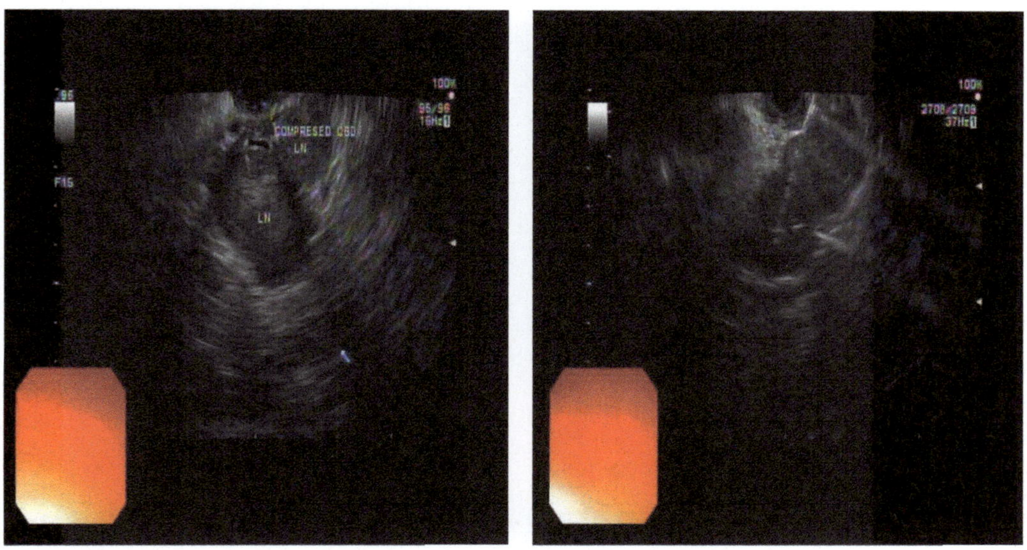

(a) (b)

Figure 22: Renal metastasis to pancreas. (a) EUS showed multiple confluent, well-circumscribed hypoechoic, spherical masses measuring up to 40 mm in the peripancreatic (head) area compressing distal CBD. Multiple anechoic areas of necrosis were seen inside the lesions. (b) A single FNA pass was done using a 19-gauge needle via transduodenal approach.

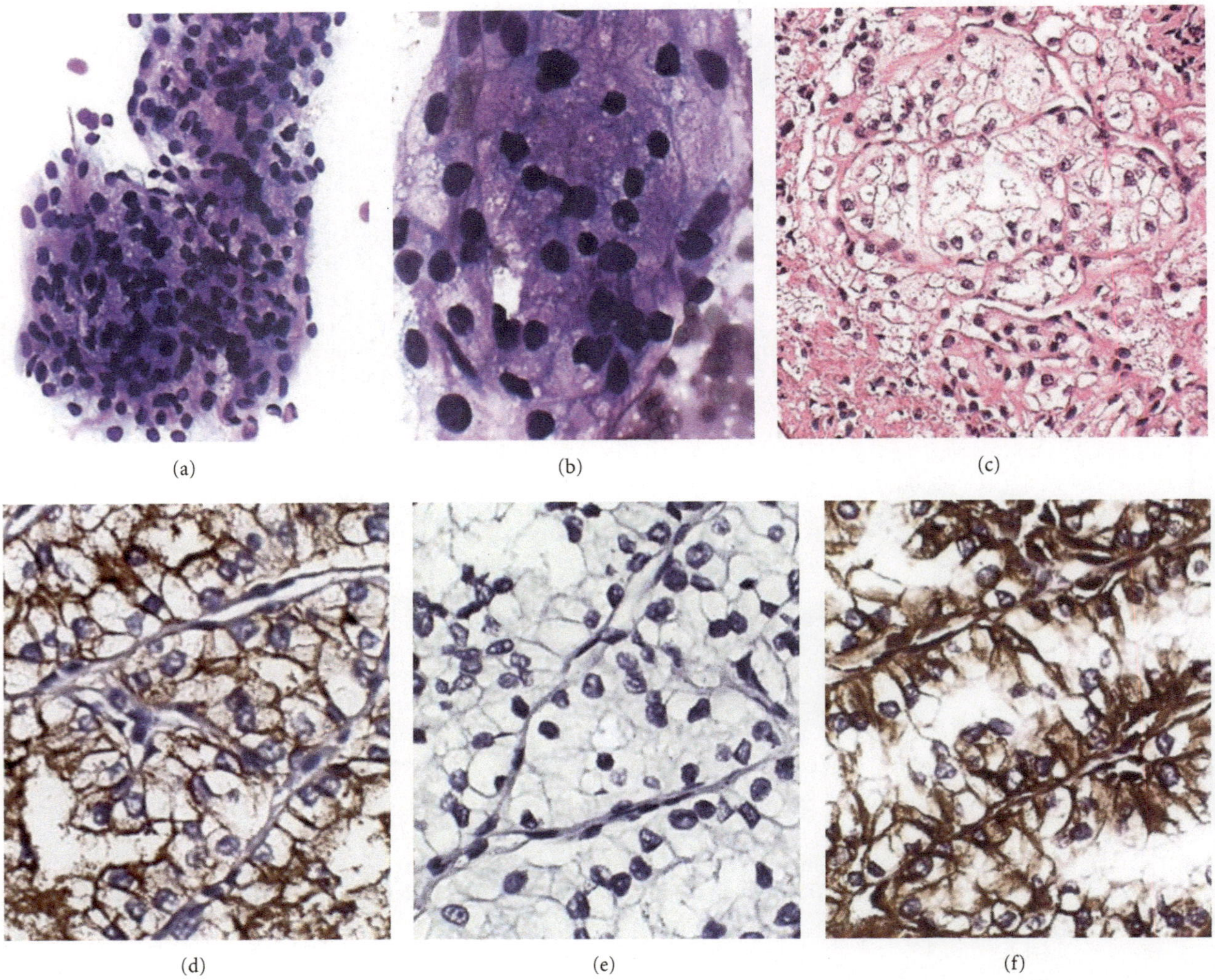

Figure 23: Renal metastasis to pancreas: (a) and (b) abundant, bubbly cytoplasm, Diff-Quik stain at 200x and 400x; (c) clear cytoplasm, outlined by sharp cell membrane, cell block H&E at 200x; (d) positive CD10 immunoperoxidase stain, at 400x; (e) negative cytokeratin CK7, at 400x; (f) positive vimentin immunoperoxidase stain, at 400x.

and do not crossreact with adrenal cortex [52]. Based on the immunohistochemical profile, both masses were diagnosed as metastatic renal cell carcinoma to peripancreatic tissue and left adrenal.

7. Conclusion

In summary, endoscopic ultrasound is the most sensitive imaging modality for solid pancreatic lesions. It is an outpatient safe procedure, with high accuracy of 78–94% for T (local tumor) stage and 64–82% for N (lymph node) stage. The specificity is low (about 75%), but can be increased to 100% with an accuracy of 95% with the addition of fine needle aspiration. The diagnostic yield of EUS-FNA for solid pancreatic lesion is 86.8–98.5% for cytologic and 68.9–89% for histologic examinations, while 65–100% for lymph nodes. Factors related to either endoscopist or cytopathologist affect the diagnostic yield of EUS-FNA. A close interaction with cytopathologist is vital in improving the diagnostic yield. The final diagnosis is based upon correlation of clinical, EUS, and cytologic features.

References

[1] E. P. DiMagno, J. L. Buxton, and P. T. Regan, "Ultrasonic endoscope," *Lancet*, vol. 1, no. 8169, pp. 629–631, 1980.

[2] F. G. Gress, R. H. Hawes, T. J. Savides et al., "Role of EUS in the preoperative staging of pancreatic cancer: a large single-center experience," *Gastrointestinal Endoscopy*, vol. 50, no. 6, pp. 786–791, 1999.

[3] L. Palazzo, G. Roseau, B. Gayet et al., "Endoscopic ultrasonography in the diagnosis and staging of pancreatic adenocarcinoma. Results of a prospective study with comparison to ultrasonography and CT scan," *Endoscopy*, vol. 1993, no. 25, pp. 2–143, 150.

[4] K. Yasuda, H. Mukai, M. Nakajima, and K. Kawai, "Staging of pancreatic carcinoma by endoscopic ultrasonography," *Endoscopy*, vol. 25, no. 2, pp. 151–155, 1993.

[5] D. O'Toole, L. Palazzo, R. Arotçarena et al., "Assessment of complications of EUS-guided fine-needle aspiration," *Gastrointestinal Endoscopy*, vol. 53, no. 4, pp. 470–474, 2001.

[6] M. J. Wiersema, P. Vilmann, M. Giovannini, K. J. Chang, and L. M. Wiersema, "Endosonography-guided fine-needle aspiration biopsy: diagnostic accuracy and complication assessment," *Gastroenterology*, vol. 112, no. 4, pp. 1087–1095, 1997.

[7] A. Affi, E. Vazquez-Sequeiros, I. D. Norton, J. E. Clain, and M. J. Wiersema, "Acute extraluminal hemorrhage associated with EUS-guided fine needle aspiration: frequency and clinical significance," *Gastrointestinal Endoscopy*, vol. 53, no. 2, pp. 221–225, 2001.

[8] ASGE Standards of Practice Committee, S. Banerjee, B. Shen, T. H. Baron et al., "Antibiotic prophylaxis for GI endoscopy," *Gastrointestinal Endoscopy*, vol. 67, no. 6, pp. 791–798, 2008.

[9] C. Micames, P. S. Jowell, R. White et al., "Lower frequency of peritoneal carcinomatosis in patients with pancreatic cancer diagnosed by EUS-guided FNA vs. percutaneous FNA," *Gastrointestinal Endoscopy*, vol. 58, no. 5, pp. 690–695, 2003.

[10] T. Rosch, R. Lorenz, C. Braig et al., "Endoscopic ultrasound in pancreatic tumor diagnosis," *Gastrointestinal Endoscopy*, vol. 37, no. 3, pp. 347–352, 1991.

[11] K. J. Chang, P. Nguyen, R. A. Erickson, T. E. Durbin, and K. D. Katz, "The clinical utility of endoscopic ultrasound-guided fine-needle aspiration in the diagnosis and staging of pancreatic carcinoma," *Gastrointestinal Endoscopy*, vol. 45, no. 5, pp. 387–393, 1997.

[12] B. Agarwal, E. Abu-Hamda, K. L. Molke, A. M. Correa, and L. Ho, "Endoscopic ultrasound-guided fine needle aspiration and multidetector spiral CT in the diagnosis of pancreatic cacer," *American Journal of Gastroenterology*, vol. 99, no. 5, pp. 844–850, 2004.

[13] M. B. Wallace, T. Woodward, and M. Raimondo, "Endoscopic ultrasound and fine-needle aspiration for pancreatic cancer," *Digestive Endoscopy*, vol. 16, no. 2, pp. S193–S196, 2004.

[14] S. Varadarajulu and M. A. Eloubeidi, "The role of endoscopic ultrasonography in the evaluation of pancreatico-biliary cancer," *Gastrointestinal Endoscopy Clinics of North America*, vol. 15, no. 3, pp. 497–511, 2005.

[15] A. Irisawa, T. Hikichi, M. S. Bhuttani et al., "Basic technique of FNA," *Gastrointestinal Endoscopy*, vol. 69, no. 2, pp. S125–S129, 2009.

[16] A. Ginès, M. Solé, and G. Fernández-Esparrach, "What I need to know and what I need to do if I do not have a cytopathologist present for the procedure," *Gastrointestinal Endoscopy*, vol. 69, no. 2, pp. S142–S145, 2009.

[17] A. Ribeiro, E. Vazquez-Sequeiros, L. M. Wiersema et al., "EUS-guided fine-needle aspiration combined with flow cytometry and immunocytochemistry in the diagnosis of lymphoma," *Gastrointestinal Endoscopy*, vol. 52, no. 4, pp. 485–491, 2004.

[18] C. F. Dietrich, "Endoscopic ultrasound: an introductory manual and atlas," in *EUS-Guided Biopsy- Indications, Problems, Pitfalls, Troubleshooting, and Clinical Impact*, C. Jenssen, K. Moeller, and M. Sarbia, Eds., pp. 91–167, Thieme, New York, NY, USA, 2011.

[19] G. M. Eisen, J. A. Dominitz, D. O. Faigel et al., "Guidelines for credentialing and granting privileges for endoscopic ultrasound.," *Gastrointestinal Endoscopy*, vol. 54, no. 6, pp. 811–814, 2001.

[20] T. J. Savides, "Tricks for improving EUS-FNA accuracy and maximizing cellular yield," *Gastrointestinal Endoscopy*, vol. 69, no. 2, pp. S130–S133, 2009.

[21] T. E. Yusuf, S. Ho, D. A. Pavey, H. Michael, and F. G. Gress, "Retrospective analysis of the utility of endoscopic ultrasound-guided fine-needle aspiration (EUS-FNA) in pancreatic masses, using a 22-gauge or 25-gauge needle system: a multicenter experience.," *Endoscopy*, vol. 41, no. 5, pp. 445–448, 2009.

[22] H. Imazu, Y. Uchiyama, H. Kakutani et al., "A prospective comparison of EUS-guided FNA using 25-gauge and 22-gauge needles," *Gastroenterology Research and Practice*, vol. 2009, Article ID 546390, 6 pages, 2009.

[23] J. H. Lee, J. Stewart, W. A. Ross, S. Anandasabapathy, L. Xiao, and G. Staerkel, "Blinded prospective comparison of the performance of 22-gauge and 25-gauge needles in endoscopic ultrasound-guided fine needle aspiration of the pancreas and peri-pancreatic lesions," *Digestive Diseases and Sciences*, vol. 54, no. 10, pp. 2274–2281, 2009.

[24] U. D. Siddiqui, F. Rossi, L. S. Rosenthal, M. S. Padda, V. Murali-Dharan, and H. R. Aslanian, "EUS-guided FNA of solid pancreatic masses: a prospective, randomized trial comparing 22-gauge and 25-gauge needles," *Gastrointestinal Endoscopy*, vol. 70, no. 6, pp. 1093–1097, 2009.

[25] H. Sakamoto, M. Kitano, T. Komaki et al., "Prospective comparative study of the EUS guided 25-gauge FNA needle with the 19-gauge Trucut needle and 22-gauge FNA needle in patients with solid pancreatic masses," *Journal of Gastroenterology and Hepatology*, vol. 24, no. 3, pp. 384–390, 2009.

[26] T. T. H. Nguyen, C. E. Lee, C. S. Whang et al., "A Comparison of the Diagnostic Yield and Specimen Adequacy between 22 and 25 Gauge Needles for Endoscopic Ultrasound Guided Fine-Needle Aspiration (EUS-FNA) of Solid Pancreatic Lesions (SPL): Is Bigger Better?" *Gastrointestinal Endoscopy*, vol. 67, no. 5: AB100, 2008.

[27] K. Takahashi, K. Yamao, K. Okubo et al., "Differential diagnosis of pancreatic cancer and focal pancreatitis by using EUS-guided FNA," *Gastrointestinal Endoscopy*, vol. 61, no. 1, pp. 76–79, 2005.

[28] T. Thomas, P. V. Kaye, K. Ragunath, and G. Aithal, "Efficacy, safety, and predictive factors for a positive yield of EUS-guided trucut biopsy: a large tertiary referral center experience," *American Journal of Gastroenterology*, vol. 104, no. 3, pp. 584–591, 2009.

[29] E. B. Stelow, R. H. Bardales, and M. W. Stanley, "Pitfalls in endoscopic ultrasound-guided fine-needle aspiration and how to avoid them," *Advances in Anatomic Pathology*, vol. 12, no. 2, pp. 62–73, 2005.

[30] C. Jenssen, K. Möller, S. Wagner, and M. Sarbia, "Endoscopic ultrasound-guided biopsy: diagnostic yield, pitfalls, quality management—part 1: optimizing specimen collection and diagnostic efficiency," *Zeitschrift fur Gastroenterologie*, vol. 46, no. 6, pp. 590–600, 2008.

[31] B. G. Skov, U. Baandrup, G. K. Jakobsen et al., "Cytopathologic diagnoses of fine-needle aspirations from endoscopic ultrasound of the mediastinum: reproducibility of the diagnoses and representativeness of aspirates from lymph nodes," *Cancer*, vol. 111, no. 4, pp. 234–241, 2007.

[32] I. A. Eltoum, D. C. Chhieng, D. Jhala et al., "Cumulative sum procedure in evaluation of EUS-guided FNA cytology: the learning curve and diagnostic performance beyond sensitivity and specificity," *Cytopathology*, vol. 18, no. 3, pp. 143–150, 2007.

[33] J. B. Klapman, R. Logrono, C. E. Dye, and I. Waxman, "Clinical impact of on-site cytopathology interpretation on endoscopic ultrasound-guided fine needle aspiration," *American Journal of Gastroenterology*, vol. 98, no. 6, pp. 1289–1294, 2003.

[34] R. A. Erickson, L. Sayage-Rabie, and R. S. Beissner, "Factors predicting the number of EUS-guided fine-needle passes for

diagnosis of pancreatic malignancies," *Gastrointestinal Endoscopy*, vol. 51, no. 2, pp. 184–190, 2000.

[35] A. D. Savoy, M. Raimondo, T. A. Woodward et al., "Can endosonographers evaluate on-site cytologic adequacy? A comparison with cytotechnologists," *Gastrointestinal Endoscopy*, vol. 65, no. 7, pp. 953–957, 2007.

[36] J. K. LeBlanc, D. Ciaccia, M. T. Al-Assi et al., "Optimal number of EUS-guided fine needle passes needed to obtain a correct diagnosis," *Gastrointestinal Endoscopy*, vol. 59, no. 4, pp. 475–481, 2004.

[37] K. Möller, I. S. Papanicolaou, T. Toermer et al., "EUS-guided FNA of solid pancreatic masses: high yield of 2 passes with combined histologic-cytologic analysis," *Gastrointestinal Endoscopy*, vol. 70, no. 1, pp. 60–69, 2009.

[38] Y. P. Nguyen, J. T. Maple, Q. Zhang et al., "Reliability of gross visual assessment of specimen adequacy during EUS-guided FNA of pancreatic masses," *Gastrointestinal Endoscopy*, vol. 69, no. 7, pp. 1264–1270, 2009.

[39] B. Kim, D. C. Chhieng, D. R. Crowe et al., "Dynamic telecytopathology of on site rapid cytology diagnoses for pancreatic carcinoma," *CytoJournal*, vol. 3, article no. 27, 2006.

[40] H. J. C. Shin, S. Lahoti, and N. Sneige, "Endoscopic ultrasound-guided fine-needle aspiration in 179 cases: the M. D. Anderson cancer center experience," *Cancer*, vol. 96, no. 3, pp. 174–180, 2002.

[41] R. M. DeMay, *The Art and Science of Cytopathology*, ASCP Press, 1996.

[42] N. Volkan Adsay, K. C. Conlon, S. Y. Zee, M. F. Brennan, and D. S. Klimstra, "Intraductal papillary-mucinous neoplasms of the pancreas: an analysis of in situ and invasive carcinomas in 28 patients," *Cancer*, vol. 94, no. 1, pp. 62–77, 2002.

[43] R. A. DeLellis, R. V. Lloyd, P. U. Heitz et al., *World Health Classification of Tumors: Pathology and Genetics of Endocrine Organs*, IARC Press, 2004.

[44] D. S. Klimstra, I. R. Modlin, D. Coppola, R. V. Lloyd, and S. Suster, "The pathologic classification of neuroendocrine tumors: a review of nomenclature, grading, and staging systems," *Pancreas*, vol. 39, no. 6, pp. 707–712, 2010.

[45] I. D. Fleming et al., *AJCC Cancer Staging Manual*, Springer, 7th edition, 2010.

[46] L. Verset, M. Arvanitakis, P. Loi et al., "TTF1 positive small cell cancers: don't think they're always primary pulmonary!," *World Journal of Gastrointestinal Oncology*, vol. 3, no. 10, pp. 144–147, 2011.

[47] E. B. Stelow, R. H. Bardales, V. M. Shami et al., "Cytology of pancreatic acinar cell carcinoma," *Diagnostic Cytopathology*, vol. 34, no. 5, pp. 367–372, 2006.

[48] T. Iwashita, I. Yasuda, S. Doi et al., "Use of samples from endoscopic ultrasound guided 19 gauge fine needle aspiration in diagnosis of autoimmune pancreatitis," *Clinical Gastroenterology and Hepatology*, vol. 10, no. 3, pp. 316–322, 2012.

[49] V. Deshpande, M. Mino-Kenudson, W. R. Brugge et al., "Endoscopic ultrasound guided fine needle aspiration biopsy of autoimmune pancreatitis: diagnostic criteria and pitfalls," *American Journal of Surgical Pathology*, vol. 29, no. 11, pp. 1464–1471, 2005.

[50] P. Bhanot, W. H. Nealon, E. M. Walser, M. S. Bhutani, W. W. Tang, and R. Logroño, "Clinical, imaging, and cytopathological features of solid pseudopapillary tumor of the pancreas: a clinicopathologic study of three cases and review of the literature," *Diagnostic Cytopathology*, vol. 33, no. 6, pp. 421–428, 2005.

[51] H. Burford, Z. Baloch, X. Liu, D. Jhala, G. P. Siegal, and N. Jhala, "E-cadherin/β-catenin and CD10: a limited immunohistochemical panel to distinguish pancreatic endocrine neoplasm from solid pseudopapillary neoplasm of the pancreas on endoscopic ultrasound-guided fine-needle aspirates of the pancreas," *American Journal of Clinical Pathology*, vol. 132, no. 6, pp. 831–839, 2009.

[52] A. K. Avery, J. Beckstead, A. A. Renshaw, and C. L. Corless, "Use of antibodies to RCC and CD10 in the differential diagnosis of renal neoplasms," *American Journal of Surgical Pathology*, vol. 24, no. 2, pp. 203–210, 2000.

3

Evidences Suggesting Involvement of Viruses in Oral Squamous Cell Carcinoma

Kanupriya Gupta and Rashmi Metgud

Department of Oral and Maxillofacial Pathology, Pacific Dental College and Hospital, Udaipur, Rajasthan 313001, India

Correspondence should be addressed to Kanupriya Gupta; drkanupriya12@gmail.com

Academic Editor: Piero Tosi

Oral cancer is one of the most common cancers and it constitutes a major health problem particularly in developing countries. Oral squamous cell carcinoma (OSCC) represents the most frequent of all oral neoplasms. Several risk factors have been well characterized to be associated with OSCC with substantial evidences. The etiology of OSCC is complex and involves many factors. The most clearly defined potential factors are smoking and alcohol, which substantially increase the risk of OSCC. However, despite this clear association, a substantial proportion of patients develop OSCC without exposure to them, emphasizing the role of other risk factors such as genetic susceptibility and oncogenic viruses. Some viruses are strongly associated with OSCC while the association of others is less frequent and may depend on cofactors for their carcinogenic effects. Therefore, the exact role of viruses must be evaluated with care in order to improve the diagnosis and treatment of OSCC. Although a viral association within a subset of OSCC has been shown, the molecular and histopathological characteristics of these tumors have yet to be clearly defined.

1. Introduction

The significant role of viruses in cancer was acknowledged finally in the second half of the past century after various rodent tumorigenic viruses were discovered, and evidence had accumulated supporting an association between viruses and human cancer. Indeed, the Nobel Prize was awarded to Rous in 1966 in recognition of his seminal discovery of tumor-inducing viruses. In addition, almost at the same time, a Special Virus Cancer Program (VCP) was launched by the US Congress in 1964 providing enormous funds for intensive research into the supposed role of viruses in human cancer. This program, criticized by some investigators as being a political moonshot-style plan, failed to identify candidate human cancer-causing viruses yet generated fundamental information about the molecular biology and mechanisms underlying, in particular, virus-related animal cancer and cancer in general [1].

The strong cohort effect that accounted for the increased incidence of head and neck cancers after 1915 indicates that oral cancer is a disease largely attributable to behaviors that expose an individual to environmental carcinogens. The majority of oral cancers in individuals above and below the age of 45 can be attributed to the combined effects of alcohol and tobacco smoking. Other risk factors for oral cancers include diet, Body Mass Index, oral hygiene, and viral infections [2]. The most commonly implicated viruses in oral cancer transformation have been the human papillomavirus (HPV) [3, 4], herpes group viruses [5], adenoviruses [6], and the hepatitis C viruses [7, 8].

Of these, HPV and herpes have been the most thoroughly studied and are now considered to be the most likely "synergistic viruses" involved in human oral cancer. The herpes viruses most often linked to oral cancer are the Epstein-Barr virus (EBV), human herpes virus- (HHV-) 8, and cytomegalovirus (CMV) [9].

This review will attempt to focus on the approaches taken to discover human cancer viruses and promising methods for detecting new viruses. We also discuss how causal association is established and possible cofactors that influence development of virus-associated cancers.

2. Criteria for Defining Viral Carcinogenesis

Even though human oncogenic viruses belong to different virus families and utilize diverse strategies to contribute to

TABLE 1: Overview of HPV gene products (E) early and (L) late.

Gene product	Description
E1	Helicase function; essential for viral replication and control of gene transcription.
E2	Viral transcription factor; essential for viral replication and control of gene transcription.
E4	Interaction with cytoskeleton proteins; viral assembly.
E5	Growth stimulation by interaction with growth factor receptors; downregulation surface HLA class I molecules.
E6	Cell immortalization; p-53 degradation; telomerase activation; antiapoptotic effect; induction of genomic instability.
E7	Cell immortalization; interaction with pRb and pRb-associated pocket proteins; transactivation of E2F dependent promoters; induction of genomic instability.
L1	Major capsid proteins.
L2	Minor capsid protein; role in recruiting viral genomes for encapsidation; involvement in nuclear transport of viral DNA.

cancer development, they share many common features. One key feature is their ability to infect but not kill their host cell. In contrast to many other viruses that cause disease, oncogenic viruses have the tendency to establish long-term persistent infections [10]. Consequently, they have evolved strategies for evading the host immune response, which would otherwise clear the virus during these persistent infections. Additional cofactors, such as host immunity and chronic inflammation, as well as additional host cellular mutations, also play an important role in the transformation process [11]. Different guidelines have been proposed to aid in establishing a causal relationship between viruses and human cancers [12–15].

Evans and Mueller Guidelines [13].

Epidemiologic Guidelines

(1) Geographic distribution of viral infection corresponds with that of tumor, adjusting for the presence of known cofactors.

(2) Viral markers are higher in case subjects than in matched control subjects.

(3) Viral markers precede tumor development, with a higher incidence of tumors in persons with markers than those without.

(4) Tumor incidence is decreased by viral infection prevention.

Virologic Guidelines

(1) Virus can transform cells *in vitro*.

(2) Viral genome is present in tumor cells but not in normal cells.

(3) Virus induces the tumor in an experimental animal.

Hill Criteria for Causality [14, 15]

(1) Strength of association (how often is the virus associated with the tumor?).

(2) Consistency (has the association been observed repeatedly?).

(3) Specificity of association (is the virus uniquely associated with the tumor?).

(4) Temporal relationship (does virus infection precede tumorigenesis?).

(5) Biologic gradient (is there a dose response with viral load?).

(6) Biologic plausibility (is it biologically plausible that the virus could cause the tumor?).

(7) Coherence (does the association make sense with what is known about the tumor?).

(8) Experimental evidence (is there supporting laboratory data?).

3. Human Papillomavirus and OSCC

The human papillomavirus (HPV) family consists of more than 200 genotypes, classified in accordance with the ability to infect and transform epithelial cells. HPVs are DNA viruses that specifically target the basal cells of the epithelial mucosa [16]. Genotypes, such as HPV1, infect epidermal cells, whereas HPVs 6, 11, 16, and 18 infect epithelial cells of the oral cavity and other mucosal surfaces [17].

HPV belongs to the family Papovaviridae. These are small nonenveloped icosahedral viruses with an 8 kbp long double-stranded circular DNA genome. The papilloma virus genome comprises early and late genes that encode early proteins E1–E7 and late proteins L1-L2. The early proteins are nonstructural proteins involved in replication and transcription of the genome (E1–E5) or in host cell tumoral transformation (E6 and E7), whereas L1 and L2 are the structural capsid proteins of the virion. The late genes (L1-L2) code for the structural proteins of viral capsid and are activated during the final stages of the viral cycle. Up to six early genes and two late genes can be detected in HPV [18–23] (Table 1).

The ability of HPV to transform epithelial cells is divided into high-risk and low-risk types. Low-risk types are associated with development of benign lesions such as warts, while infections with high-risk types may progress to malignant lesions [17].

Both high-risk and low-risk types of HPV can cause the growth of abnormal cells, but only the high-risk types lead to cancer because only the E7 protein encoded by high-risk HPVs can immortalize human epithelial cells. Sexually transmitted, high-risk HPVs include types 16, 18, 31, 33, 35, 39, 45, 51, 52, 56, 58, 59, 66, 68, and 73 [24]. It is important to note, however, that in the genital tract the large majority of high-risk HPV infections regress on their own and do not cause cancer [25].

The HPV involvement in oral carcinogenesis was supported on the basis of the following evidences:

(1) the strongly established etiological role of HPV in cervical SCC [26, 27];

(2) the epithelial tropism of HPV;

(3) the similarity between oral and genital epithelia [28];

(4) the detection of HPV genotypes in samples of OSCC [29–33].

4. Genital HPV Infection and Risk of OSCC

Several studies examined the incidence of second cancers after an initial diagnosis of anogenital cancers [34, 35] and have showed that there is an increased risk of head and neck cancer as well as other HPV-associated anogenital cancers in the two major HPV 16 oncogenes E6- and E7-positive patients. This association between HPV-associated anogenital cancers and head and neck cancer was further strengthened by two larger studies [36, 37]. Additionally, the presence of antibodies to HPV E6 and E7 proteins was found to be more associated with tumors of the oropharynx than with these of the oral cavity.

A recent study has shown that besides the classical horizontal transmission during the sexual life, a vertical transmission occurs in approximately 20% of case HPV-positive people. In these individuals, HPV-DNA is detected in amniotic fluid, foetal membranes, blood, and placental trophoblastic cells, all suggesting HPV infection in utero, that is, prenatal transmission [38].

4.1. Human Papillomavirus- (HPV-) Induced Carcinogenesis. E6 and E7 oncoproteins can inactivate the genetic mechanisms that control both the cell cycle and apoptosis. The hallmark of high-risk HPV E6 oncogenic activity is degradation of the p53 tumour-suppressor gene [39, 40]. The functions of p53 in the cell cycle include controlling the G1 transition to the S phase of the cell cycle at the G1 checkpoint by inducing expression of cyclin inhibitors p16, p21, and p27 that block the activities of cyclin-CDKs (cyclin-dependent kinases) complexes, thus mediating arrest of the cell cycle by blocking the progression of the cell cycle at the G1/S transition. p53 activities mediate cell proliferation in response to mitogenic stimulation; mediate arrest of the cell cycle growth at the G1 checkpoint following DNA damage, hence permitting repair of the damaged DNA before the cell enters the DNA synthesis phase; and mediate induction of apoptosis of cells in which the DNA damage is beyond repair. Therefore, inactivation, degradation, or mutation of the p53 gene may dysregulate its functions resulting in increased cell proliferation, in accumulation of damaged DNA, in growth of cells harbouring DNA errors, and in prolonged cell survival. However, loss of p53 function alone is not sufficient for the development of cancer, and other cytogenetic alterations are required for complete malignant transformation [41].

In addition to these properties, E6 oncoprotein of high-risk HPV types can also mediate cell proliferation through the PDZ-ligand domain. The PDZ domain is located at areas of cell-to-cell contact, such as tight junctions of epithelial cells, and is associated with signal transduction pathways. The binding of high-risk HPV E6 oncoprotein to the PDZ family of proteins may result in degradation of the PDZ domain leading to dysregulation of organization, differentiation, and the chromosomal integrity of HPV infected epithelial cells [41]. This may contribute to morphological transformation of keratinocytes infected with high-risk HPV and to induction of epithelial hyperplasia. Telomerase is an enzyme that adds hexanucleotide repeats onto the end of the chromosome telomere. Telomerase activity is usually restricted to embryonic cells and is absent in normal somatic cells. When telomerase is absent, there is progressive shortening of telomeres as the cells repetitively divide, ultimately resulting in senescence of these cells [42].

HPV-induced activation of telomerase prevents the shortening of telomeres resulting in prolongation of the lifespan of HPV-infected cells. High-risk HPV E7 oncoprotein has the capacity to initiate DNA synthesis in differentiated epithelial cells mainly by binding and inactivating the Rb apoptosis/tumour suppressor gene. The Rb family of proteins plays an essential role in controlling the cell cycle by governing the checkpoint between the G1 and the S phase. Hypophosphorylated Rb binds to E2F transcription factor forming a Rb-E2F complex, making E2F unavailable for transcription of genes associated with DNA synthesis. Upon phosphorylation of Rb by cyclin-CDK complexes, E2F is released from the Rb-E2F transcription repressor complex, and it induces transcription of the S-phase genes. E7 oncoprotein of high-risk HPV types functionally inactivates the Rb family of proteins resulting in overexpression of E2F transcription factor with upregulation of cell cycle genes resulting in DNA replication, in the transition of the cell from the G1 to the S phase, and in increased cell proliferation [43–45].

E7 oncoprotein can also interact with other cellular factors that control the cell cycle including histone deacetylases, AP-1 transcription complex, and CDK inhibitors, p21 and p27. Furthermore, E7 of high-risk HPV 16 and HPV 18 can decrease the expression of major histocompatibility complex (MHC) class I molecules, thus interfering with MHC class I antigen presentation, resulting in downregulation of cellular immune responses, allowing HPV to persist in infected epithelial cells [46].

In addition to these properties, high-risk HPV E7 oncoprotein can induce chromosome duplication errors leading to dysregulation of mitotic spindle formation and function, contributing to the genomic instability of the cell. The separate pathological effects of high-risk HPV E6 and E7 on the cell cycle complement each other, and together E6 and

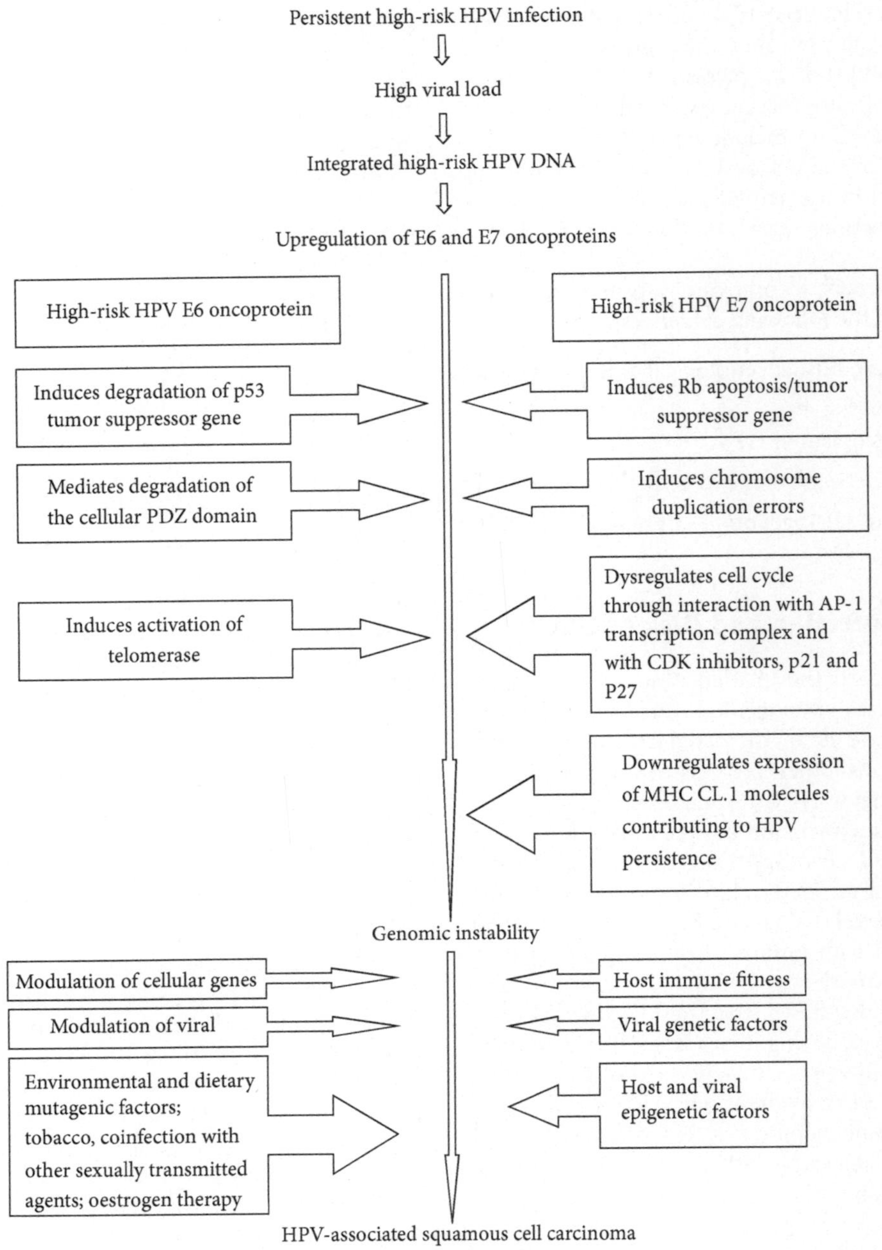

Figure 1

E7 mediate the HPV-associated epithelial cell transformation and promote cellular genomic instability that predisposes the infected cells to full malignant transformation. High-risk HPV E7 activates the DNA synthesis and cell replication mechanisms that are normally inactive in matured epithelial cells, thus initiating pathological cell growth. By inducing cell survival and delayed apoptosis of cells with DNA damage, E6 allows E7 to exert and sustain its pathological effect [47].

Typically, infected epithelial cells of HPV-associated benign lesions harbor low-risk HPV episomally in the nuclei. In HPV-associated malignancies, high-risk HPV DNA may either be integrated within the cellular genome or it may be maintained as an episome in the nuclei of the malignant cells. It is unclear how the HPV genome, whether episomal within the nucleus or integrated into the nuclear cellular genome, brings about the same end result of malignancy. The integration of HPV DNA favours the inactivation of tumour suppressor genes, p53 and Rb, contributing to increased cellular chromosomal instability and prolonging the life-span of the cell, which are essential steps in the multistep process of HPV-associated carcinogenesis. It is probable that following the initial HPV-induced cellular transformation, additional interactions with chemical carcinogens will provide the necessary additional impetus for the development of frank malignancy [47] (Figure 1).

The HPV involvement in oral and oropharyngeal carcinogenesis was first proposed in 1983 by Syrjänen et al. [121] (Table 2). Their results showed that 40% of the laryngeal

TABLE 2: Studies on HPV in oral squamous cell carcinoma.

Study/year	Geographic location	Tumour site(s)	No. of cases	HPV +ve N (%)	Genotype(s)	DNA method
Loning et al., 1985 [48]	Germany	Oscc	6	50%	16, 11	SB
Maitland et al., 1987 [49]	United Kingdom	Oscc	15	46.7%	16	SB
Gassenmaier and Hornstein, 1988 [50]	Germany	Oscc	68	23.5%	16	ISH
Syrjänen et al., 1988 [51]	Finland	Oscc	51	11.8%	16, 18	ISH
Chang et al., 1990 [52]	Finland	Oscc	40	2.5; 27.5%	16	ISH; PCR
Greer et al., 1990 [53]	USA	Oscc	100	6%	n.d	ISH
Kashima et al., 1990 [54]	USA	Oscc	26	19.2%		SB
Young and Min et al., 1991 [55]	USA	Oscc	27	0%	6, 11, 16, 18, 31, 33, 35	PCR
Zeuss et al., 1991 [56]	Spain	Oscc	15	0%	6, 11	ISH
Holladay and Gerald, 1993 [57]	USA	Oscc	39	17.9%	16	PCR
Cox et al., 1993 [58]	UK	Oscc	8	50%	16	SB
Brandwein et al., 1994 [59]	USA	Oscc	64	25%	16	PCR
González-Moles et al., 1994 [60]	Spain	Oscc	27	37%	6, 11	ISH
Ostwald et al., 1994 [61]	Germany	Oscc	26	61.5%	16, 18	PCR
Balaram et al., 1995 [62]	India	Oscc	91	73.6%	6, 11, 16, 18	PCR
Shindoh et al., 1995 [63]	Japan	Oscc	77	31.2%	16	PCR
Van Rensburg et al., 1995 [64]	South Africa	Oscc	66	1.5%	18	ISH
Cruz et al., 1996 [65]	The Netherlands	Oscc	35	54.3%	16	PCR
Mao et al., 1996 [66]	USA	Oscc	64	31%	n.d.	PCR
Van Rensburg et al., 1996 [67]	South Africa	Oscc	146	1.4%	11, 16	PCR
Chiba et al., 1996 [68]	Japan	Oscc	38	21%	16, 18, 33	PCR
Wen et al., 1997 [69]	Japan	Oscc	45	31.1%	16, 18	PCR
Gopalakrishnan et al., 1997 [70]	USA	Oscc	10	30%	16	PCR
Ibrahim et al., 1998 [71]	Sudan	Oscc	88	0; 0%	n.d.	ISH; PCR
Koh et al., 1998 [72]	Korea	Oscc	42	52%	n.d.	PCR
Premoli-De-Percoco et al., 1998 [73]	Venezuela	Oscc	50	70%	16, 18	ISH
D'Costa et al., 1998 [74]	India	Oscc	100	15%	16, 18	PCR
Schwartz et al., 1998 [33]	USA	Oscc	193	21.2%	16	PCR
Elamin et al., 1998 [75]	UK	Oscc	28	50%	6, 16	PCR
Aggelopoulou et al., 1999 [76]	Greece	Oscc	81	49%	n.d	PCR
Pillai et al., 1999 [77]	India	Oscc	61	16.8%	16	PCR
Pintos et al., 1999 [78]	Canada	Oral cavity	29	10%	n/s	PCR
Badaracco et al., 2000 [79]	Italy	Oscc	66	36.4%	16, 6	PCR
Bouda et al., 2000 [80]	Greece	Oscc	19	94.7%	16, 18, 33	PCR
Cao et al., 2000 [81]	China	Oscc	40	72.5%	16, 18	PCR
Patima Cao et al., 2000 [82]	China	Oscc	73	74%	16, 18	PCR
Sand et al., 2000 [83]	Sweden	Oscc	24	12.5%	16, 18, 6, 11	PCR
Tsuhako et al., 2000 [84]	Japan	Oscc	83	56.9%	n.d.	PCR
Gillison et al., 2000 [30]	USA	Oscc	84	11.9%	16	PCR & ISH & SB
Bouda et al., 2000 [80]	Greece	Oscc	19	89.5%	16, 18	PCR

Table 2: Continued.

Study/year	Geographic location	Tumour site(s)	No. of cases	HPV +ve N (%)	Genotype(s)	DNA method
Premoli-De-Percoco and Ramirez 2001 [85]	Venezuela	Oscc	50	60%	16, 18	PCR
Schwartz et al., 2001 [86]	USA	Oscc	254	24.4%	16	PCR
Chen et al., 2002 [87]	Taiwan	Oscc	29	82.7%	16, 18, 6	PCR
Kojima et al., 2002 [88]	Japan	Oscc	53	66%	38	PCR
Nagpal et al., 2002 [89]	India	Oscc	110	33.6%	16, 18	PCR
Chang et al., 2003 [90]	Japan	Oscc	103	49.5%	HR	PCR
Fregonesi et al., 2003 [91]	Brazil	Oscc	46	39%	16, 18, 6, 11	ISH
Kansky et al., 2003 [92]	Slovenia	Oscc	62	95%	16, 33, 58, 11, 31, 68	PCR
Ritchie et al., 2003 [93]	USA	Oscc	141	15%	16, 33	PCR
Sugiyama et al., 2003 [94]	Japan	Oscc	86	34.8%	16	PCR
Herrero et al., 2003 [95]	France	Oscc	58	5.17%	16	PCR
Ostwald et al., 2003 [96]	Germany	Oscc	118	43.2%	6, 11, 16, 18	PCR/SB
Correnti et al., 2004 [97]	Venezuela	Oscc	16	50%	HR	PCR
Dahlgren et al., 2004 [98]	Sweden	Oscc	110	10.9%	16	PCR
Smith et al., 2004 [99]	USA	Oscc	106	9.4%	16, 33	PCR
Zhang et al., 2004 [100]	Japan	Oscc	73	34%	16, 18	PCR
Yang et al., 2004 [101]	Taiwan	Oscc	37	10.8%	16, 18	PCR
Koppikar et al., 2005 [102]	India	Oscc	101	31.7%	16, 18	PCR
Lo Muzio et al., 2005 [103]	Italy	Oscc	18	50%	n.d.	PCR
Boy et al., 2006 [104]	South Africa	Oscc	59	11%	18	PCR; ISH
El-Mofty and Patil 2006 [105]	USA	Oscc	94	30%	16, 31, 33	PCR
Nemes et al., 2006 [106]	Hungary	Oscc	79	41.7%	16	PCR
Rivero and Nunes 2006 [107]	Brazil	Oscc	23	0%	n.d.	PCR
Campisi et al., 2006 [108]	Italy	Oscc	63	38.1%	n.d	PCR
Furrer et al., 2006 [109]	Argentina	Oscc	14	42.8%	16, 18	PCR/SB
Koyama et al., 2007 [110]	Japan	Oscc	20	100%	18, 22, 16, 70	PCR
Sugiyama et al., 2007 [111]	Japan	Oscc	66	100%	16	PCR
Luo et al., 2007 [112]	Taiwan	Oscc	51	73%	—	PCR
Khovidhunkit et al., 2008 [113]	Thailand	Oscc	65	1.54%	16, 18	PCR
Szarka et al., 2009 [114]	Hungary	Oscc	65	47.7%	16, 18	PCR
Zhao et al., 2009 [115]	China	Oscc	52	40.4%	16, 18, 11, 6	PCR
Attner et al., 2010 [116]	Sweden	Oscc	87	68 (78)%	16, 33	PCR
Elango et al., 2011 [117]	India	Oscc	60	48%	16	PCR/IHC
Kristoffersen et al., 2012 [118]	Norway	Oscc	50	30%	6, 11, 16	PCR
Chen et al., 2012 [119]	Taiwan	Oscc	64	39%	16	ISH/IHC
Lee et al., 2012 [120]	Taiwan	Oscc	173	22%	16, 18	PCR

PCR: polymerase chain reaction; SB: southern blotting; ISH: *in situ* hybridization; IHC: immunohistochemistry.

and oral cancers contained histological and morphological similarities with HPV-infected lesions, and 50% of the samples demonstrated HPV structural proteins by immunohistochemistry [122]. Since then, several studies have focused on HPV detection in oral cancer but results have been conflicting [65, 123, 124]. It was found that the prevalence of HPV detection varies broadly, depending on the population, on the location of the cancerous lesion, on type of specimen, and on detection method. By contrast, HPV was more frequently detected in OSCCs of the oropharynx and tonsil than at other head and neck sites [125–127]. However, in a systematic review that was performed by Syrjänen et al. [128] it was suggested that a potentially important causal association between HPV (specifically HPV 16) and OSCC exists. In a recent study the overall HPV prevalence was 10.5% in oral cavity carcinomas and was higher in female than in male cases. Ninety-five percent of HPV-positive cases were infected by a single HPV type. HPV 16 was the most prevalent type and was found in 95.5% of HPV-positive oral cavity carcinoma cases [129].

Furthermore, other studies have proved the existence of a synergistic effect between HPV and alcohol. The risk of head and neck cancer was statistically significantly increased in heavy alcohol users detected with the virus, compared to that of HPV-negative cancer drinkers. Therefore, it has been proposed that alcohol can biologically modify mucosal tissue, by increasing its permeability to viral infection or by influencing the immune response to HPV [99]. It is believed that one of the major events of HPV-induced carcinogenesis is the integration of the HPV genome into a host chromosome. HPV genome integration often occurs near fragile sites of the human genome, but there are no apparent sites for integration and no evidence for insertional mutagenesis [130].

Slightly modifying Koch's postulates, in order to establish a relationship between a causative virus and a disease, four criteria are needed: (1) viral genome ought to be present in tumor lesions or in tumor cells; (2) virus must be isolated from a pathologic lesion and grown in culture; (3) cultured virus should cause disease when inoculated into a healthy organism; and (4) virus must be reisolated from the inoculated host and identified as being identical to the original specific causative factor. However, the use of Koch's postulates to establish disease causation does not fully apply to these phenomena, since the etiology of cancer is multifactorial [131]. On the contrary, other authors suggest that the incidence of HPV infection in the oral cavities of healthy population is very low and therefore other risk factors are most likely responsible to promote oral carcinogenesis [132]. Hence, we have tried to collect the studies done on HPV in oral cancer.

5. HPV Testing

HPV testing is critical for the estimation of HPV prevalence in various oral diseases. HPV testing is usually based on PCR method. General or consensus primers targeting L1 gene are most frequently used for HPV detection because they are able to identify several HPV genotypes at the same time. Sampling techniques together with widely divergent PCR methods in different studies explain most of the variability in HPV prevalence among OSCC and control samples [133]. *In situ* hybridization and *in situ* oncogenic protein staining techniques have also increased sensitivity and specificity and are used for HPV testing. These techniques have allowed for not only the detection of HPV in cytological smears or histopathological immunesections but also the determination of the topographic site of the infection [134]. According to recent studies, HPV-positive squamous cell carcinomas have intact p16 gene and wild type p53 compared to HPV-negative ones [135]. Other authors have noted that a distinctive mark of the presence of HPV in oral cancer could be found in p16 nuclear or cytoplasmic overexpression [136, 137]. However, one goal of the scientific research is to find new biological markers able to identify the set(s) of genes involved in oral carcinogenesis.

6. HPV Serology

The immune response to HPV infection involves both the cell-mediated and humoral responses. However, serological evidence is circumstantial since it provides only data on prior exposure to HPV. Since not all patients with HPV-associated cancers have detectable HPV antibodies, serum antibody determination may be a limited biomarker for HPV infection and carcinogenesis. Serum antibodies to HPV capsid proteins (virus-like particles) are thought to be a marker of lifetime HPV infection [138, 139]. Antibodies against HPV E6 and E7 proteins are associated with increased risk of HPV-associated cancer [140, 141] but are rather linked more with tumors from the oropharynx than from the oral cavity. The use of HPV viral load in oral biopsies in conjunction with serological markers may serve to identify a subset of HPV-associated oral cancers in which HPV is biologically active.

7. Herpes Simplex Virus (HSV)

HSV is a double-stranded DNA virus that is enveloped. When it infects cells the series of events that takes place is very complex but can be analyzed logically since it follows a coordinated series of steps. The virus exists in two closely related forms, known as HSV 1 and HSV 2. HSV 1 causes mainly oral and ocular infections, while HSV 2 causes mainly genital infections. However, the overall behavior and structure of the two viruses are very similar. Each virus causes a severe primary infection followed by a latent infection that may be followed by recurrent infections. Cells that are infected by HSV are killed. Gene maps of HSV 1 and HSV 2 have been developed and show that the various functions of the two viruses are encoded by identical regions of the genome of each virus [142].

The only viral function that is not in a related location between the two types is the ability to transform cells, and the reason is unknown. The transforming region of HSV 1 (minimum transforming region 1, mtr-1) is located in the left third of the genome, while the equivalent two functions of HSV 2 (mtr-2 and mtr-3) are close to the center of the genome [143].

7.1. Transformation by HSV. Induction of cellular proteins has been studied as a possible mechanism for transformation by HSV. It is known that infection by HSV 1 induces the expression of "stress" or "heat shock" proteins. The mechanism of induction is not known but does depend on the expression of the immediate-early family of HSV proteins. Since HSV might transform cells by stimulating the expression of cellular proteins, some workers have started to study such proteins by isolating cDNA from cells that were transformed by HSV 2 [142–144].

However, the function of these cloned fragments is still not known. Host cell shutoff is recognized as being an important event during infection of cells by HSV. The infected cell ceases to synthesize cellular proteins, and cell RNA is degraded very quickly. Recently, it was found that the gene of HSV that mediates shutoff is located in the same region of the genome as the mtr-2 region of HSV 2, which mediates cell transformation [145]. This has raised the possibility that the mechanism of transformation might be related to the mechanism of shutoff. Shutoff is known to be a multistep process, depending on more than one viral activity [146].

The first phase of host cell shutoff is due to some activity by the virus particle itself. It happens very soon after infection and occurs even if virus gene expression is prevented by Actinomycin D or by irradiation of the virus [147].

The second phase of the host cell shutoff does require the expression of virus genes and eliminates any remaining host protein synthesis. It seems likely that these phenomena will be studied quite closely in the future to find which of them is most likely to be involved in cell transformation. Other activities of HSV that might be related to cell transformation include the fact that the virus can stimulate the replication of other viruses. This can also occur when cells are exposed to chemical carcinogens [148].

7.1.1. Induction of Cellular Proteins. Infection by HSV induces the expression of stress or heat shock proteins. According to Steele and Shillitoe, the exact mechanism is not known but it depends on the expression of the immediate early family of HSV proteins. It was, therefore, concluded that HSV might transform cells by stimulating the expression of cellular proteins [149].

7.1.2. Host Cell Shutoff Process. Infected cell ceases to synthesize cellular proteins and cell RNA would be very quickly degraded. A mediating gene was located in the same region of the genome as the mtr-2 region of HSV 2 that mediates cell transformation [145]. Steele and Shillitoe raised the possibility that the mechanism of cell transformation might be related to the mechanism of shutoff [149].

7.1.3. Stimulation of Other Viruses by HSV. This comes from the idea that at least in cervical carcinogenesis, HSV and HPV may act as cocarcinogens, with HSV as an initiator and HPV as a promoter. In oral lesions, however, Scully et al. in 1993 showed that very few premalignant or carcinoma specimens appeared to have both HPV 16 and HSV 1 DNA sequences. They, therefore, concluded that there is no evidence that these potentially oncogenic DNA viruses do play a synergistic role in oral cancer development, but the possibility cannot be discounted [150].

7.1.4. Chromosomes as Targets. Stich et al. [151], Mincheva et al. [152], and Peat and Stanley [153] suggested that when cells are infected by HSV there is chromosomal damage which is at first restricted to a site on chromosome 1q and to some extent on chromosomes 3, 9, and 16. Based on these studies, Steele and Shillitoe gave a plausible explanation for the possibility that HSV has specific chromosomal targets for rearrangement. Damage to a particular chromosomal site might be another possible mechanism of cell transformation by HSV [149].

El Sissy [154] attempted to search for possible presence of HSY-2 protein in 21 lesional tissues of oral squamous cell carcinoma, as well as in normal oral mucosa, using immunohistochemical peroxidase-antiperoxidase (PAP) technique. Specimens of normal oral mucosa revealed frequent positive staining for polyclonal HSY-2 protein marker, thus indicating that HSY-2 is not an uncommon inhabitant of the oral mucosa. Only highly differentiated grades of oral squamous cell carcinoma showed positive staining for HSY-2, while less differentiated carcinomas failed to reveal any immunoreactivity. This raised the suggestion of a possible causative role played by HSY-2 in the establishment of the neoplastic process in oral squamous cell carcinoma through a "hit and run" mechanism. The present results point to HSY-2 as a promoter or an initiator in early neoplastic changes in well-differentiated oral squamous cell carcinoma that becomes denatured and consequently not evident in less highly differentiated tumours.

Jalouli et al. [155], using PCR/DNA sequencing, investigated the prevalence of human papillomavirus (HPV), herpes simplex virus (HSV), and Epstein-Barr virus (EBV) DNA in brush biopsies obtained from 150 users of Sudanese snuff (toombak) and 25 nonusers of toombak in formalin-fixed paraffin-embedded tissue samples obtained from 31 patients with oral dysplasias (25 toombak users and 6 nonusers) and from 217 patients with oral cancers (145 toombak users and 72 nonusers). In the brush tissue samples from toombak users, HPV was detected in 60 (40%), HSV in 44 (29%), and EBV in 97 (65%) of the samples. The corresponding figures for the 25 samples from non-users were 17 (68%) positive for HPV, 6 (24%) positive for HSV and 21 (84%) for EBV. The formalin-fixed samples with oral dysplasias were all negative for HPV. In the 145 oral cancer samples from toombak users, HPV was detected in 39 (27%), HSV in 15 (10%), and EBV in 53 (37%) of the samples. The corresponding figures for the samples from nonusers were 15 (21%) positive for HPV, 5 (7%) for HSV and 16 (22%) for EBV. These findings illustrate that prevalence of HSV, HPV, and EBV infections is common and may influence oral health and cancer development.

Delavarian et al. [156] investigated the presence of viruses in oral squamous cell carcinoma (OSCC) in young patients (20–40 years old) attending Mashhad Dental Faculty from 1996 to 2009 for the first time in Iranian population. Twenty-one formalin-fixed, paraffin-embedded sections of patients under 40 years with clinical diagnosis of OSCC, who had been referred to Mashhad Dental Faculty from 1996 and 2009, were evaluated for DNA extraction. All specimens were tested for presence of human papillomavirus, Epstein-Barr virus, Herpes simplex virus type 1, and cytomegalovirus virus. From 21 specimens, viruses were detected only in three cases. Two samples were positive for EBV and the third one was coinfected with EBV and HSV 1. All specimens were negative for HPV and CMV. Authors concluded that viruses had no important role in OSCC in young patients. Further researches are needed to clarify this role and to identify other possible risk factors.

7.1.5. Epidemiological Studies. The herpes simplex viruses (HSVs), types 1 and 2, have been investigated in the past for possible associations with human cancers. Levels of antibody to HSV 1 have been reported to be higher in patients with oral cancer than in control subjects [157]. These antibodies were largely of the IgA and IgM classes, and patients with the highest levels of anti-HSV IgM had a shorter survival than other patients [158]. It has been reported that a combination of HSV seropositivity and a history of cigarette smoking is associated with a higher risk of oral cancer than would be expected from a purely additive effect [159]. Early studies attempted to find if DNA of HSV could be detected in oral cancers, and preliminary reports did indicate the presence of both viral DNA and RNA [58, 160]. However, the nature of the HSV genome makes it difficult to produce specific probes, and the possible sequences that were detected have not been identified [58].

7.2. Molecular Mechanisms of Carcinogenesis. The explanation for the association between oral cancer and HSV could well be that of a confounding variable, except for the fact that HSV can transform some animal cells to a malignant phenotype *in vitro* [161]. Indeed HSV has shown cocarcinogenic activity in combination with chemicals *in vivo* [162]. Unfortunately, the association is difficult to study, because cells that are transformed by HSV do not express specific virus antigens or retain any specific genes of the virus [163]. Instead it seems likely that the transformation is due to the virus acting as a mutagen, and a region of the viral genome has been isolated which raises the mutation frequency in cultured cells [164]. This results in some but not all of the features of malignancy [165]. Neither the mutations nor the phenotypic changes are sufficiently specific to act as markers by which a herpes-induced malignancy could be diagnosed [166]. Recent years have seen little or no progress in the study of HSV and its malignant potential.

8. Epstein-Barr Virus Infection (EBV)

EBV was named after Tony Epstein and Yvonne Barr who were the two scientists who first isolated and described the virus in 1964 from lymphoma samples collected by Denis Burkitt. The EBV genome is a double-stranded DNA molecular of approximately 172,000 base pairs; as in other herpes viruses, the molecule is divided into unique, internal repeat, and terminal repeat domains [167]. The genome encodes approximately 80 proteins. The function of many of the genes involved in viral replication has been inferred from their homology to herpes simplex virus genes; however, genes expressed during latent infection of B cells do not have recognized counterparts in other human herpes viruses.

All phases of the EBV life cycle are associated with human disease. In immunocompromised individuals, infected cells increase in number and eventually B cell growth control pathways are activated, inducing transformation and leading to malignancies such as nasopharyngeal carcinoma (NPC), Burkitt's lymphoma (BL), posttransplant lymphomas, and gastric carcinomas [168]. EBV encodes several viral proteins that have transforming potential, including EBV latent membrane proteins 1 and 2 (LMP1 and LMP2) and EBV nuclear antigens 2 and 3 (EBNA2 and EBNA3). LMP1 can transform a variety of cell types, including rodent fibroblasts [169], and is essential for the ability of EBV to immortalize B cells [170]. The multiple transmembrane-spanning domains and the carboxyl terminus of LMP1 can interact with several tumor necrosis factor receptor associated factors (TRAFs) [171, 172]; this interaction results in high levels of activity of NF-jB, Jun, and p38 in LMP1-expressing epithelial and B cells [173–175].

LMP1 also upregulates the expression of numerous anti-apoptotic and adhesion genes and activates the expression of IRF-7 [176], matrix metalloproteinase-9 (MMP-9), and fibroblast growth factor-2 (FGF-2) [177]. A second viral membrane protein, LMP2, is dispensable for transformation of naïve B cells but is required for transformation of post-germinal center B cells. LMP2 interacts with Lyn and Syk to mimic B cell receptor (BCR) signaling, including activation of the PI3 K/AKT survival pathway [178]. These pathways are constitutively active and drive proliferation through a normal cell cycle cascade.

Horiuchi et al. [179] carried out a study to determine the presence of EBV in various squamous cell proliferative lesions in the oral cavity. They made use of PCR and *in situ* hybridization for detecting the presence of EBV DNA and EBV encoded small messenger RNA. Nearly 60% of SCC was EBV genome positive, but none of papilloma demonstrated EBV genome. On the other hand, oral hairy leukoplakia lesion seen in patients with AIDS has been proved to be EBV associated. Horiuchi et al. concluded that EBV virus infection of oral squamous epithelium may be carcinogenic or, alternatively, the virus may merely exist in epithelial cells of squamous cell carcinoma, carcinoma *in situ,* and leukoplakia.

González-Moles et al. [180] showed a positive correlation between different grades of OSCC and EBV DNA positivity and also showed that percentage positivity of EBV DNA increases from well-differentiated OSCC to poorly differentiated OSCC. In a study by Higa et al. [181], fifty-four patients with oral squamous cell carcinoma reported from 1997 to 1999 in Okinawa were compared with 21 and 20 patients from Kitakyushu and Kumamoto in Kyushu, mainland Japan, respectively. 51 diagnoses were confirmed by conventional histological examination of paraffin wax sections. EBV was detected by nonisotopic *in situ* hybridization and PCR (Bam HI-F, EBV nuclear antigen 2 (EBNA2), and latent membrane protein 1 (LMP-1) regions). Sequence analysis of the PCR products was also carried out. In Okinawa, 25 patients were found to be infected with EBV type A by analyzing the 3-sequence divergence of the EBNA2 genes. Six patients were positive for EBV type B and 8 for both types A and B. Therefore, type A virus infection was demonstrated in 33 of 54 patients and type B in 14 of 54. In total, 39 of 54 patients were infected with EBV. Authors concluded that, in Okinawa, EBV infection was frequently demonstrated in oral squamous cell carcinoma ($P < 0.001$). However, in mainland Japan, there was no significant correlation between EBV and oral squamous cell carcinoma [181].

A study by Li et al. [182] to detect EBV infection and gene expression in oral cancer from patients in Taiwan by microarray analysis revealed that the majority of the specimens (82.5%) were EBV positive that probably expressed coincidently the genes for EBNAs, LMP2A, and 2B and certain structural proteins. Importantly, the genes fabricated at the spots 61 (BBRF1, BBRF2, and BBRF3) and 68 (BDLF4 and BDRF1) on EBV-chip were actively expressed in a significantly greater number of OSCC exhibiting exophytic morphology or ulceration than those tissues with deep invasive lesions.

In a study conducted by Sand et al. [183] examining 29 patients with OSCC, 23 with OLP, and 67 with clinically healthy oral mucosa, a nested polymerase chain reaction method for EBV DNA analysis was used. The overall EBV prevalence in patients with oral disease was 32.1%. Of the OSCC patients, 37.9% were EBV positive, and, of the OLP patients, 26.1% were EBV positive. Both percentages were statistically significant compared with that of control patients (7.3%). The difference in EBV prevalence between the smoking control group and the nonsmoking control group was without significance. Increased age did not enhance EBV prevalence. The authors were of the opinion that EBV is present in oral diseases such as OSCC and OLP. Smoking, alcohol use, or age does not seem to be a risk factor for EBV infection.

Jiang et al. [184] isolated epithelial cells by laser capture microdissection and levels of CD21, CK19, and EBV RNA were measured by quantitative reverse transcriptase PCR in oral dysplasia and squamous cell carcinoma. Results showed that expression of CD21 increased in frequency and intensity as oral epithelial cells become more dysplastic and that expression correlates with an increase in infection by EBV. Tumors or dysplastic lesions that carry EBV also generally express higher levels of CK19 than those that do not. Hence, the findings suggest that dysplasia may make cells more susceptible to infection by EBV and that infection by the virus may alter the phenotype of the infected cell in a manner which could affect prognosis.

9. Hepatitis C Virus

The worldwide prevalence of hepatitis C virus (HCV) is estimated to be around 3%, representing approximately 170 million infected individuals. Morbidity associated with HCV infection is due to not only the sequelae of chronic liver disease but also a variety of extra hepatic manifestations, including that involving the oral cavity [185].

Hepatitis C virus (HCV) is an enveloped, single-stranded positive-sense RNA virus that was isolated in 1989 from a chimpanzee chronically infected by contamination with a human factor VIII concentrate (Choo et al.) [186].

There are six HCV genotypes and more than 100 subtypes. Its envelope contains two glycoproteins, E1 and E2, which form heterodimers at the surface of the virion. The genomic RNA is translated into a viral polyprotein which is cleaved by cellular proteases to generate the capsid protein (C), the two glycoproteins E1 and E2, a small protein the role of which is unclear (p7), viral proteases NS2 and NS3, and nonstructural proteins NS4A and 4B and NS5A and 5B, which are required for viral RNA replication [187].

Although details of HCV replication are not known, it is thought to take place in the cytoplasm, where, among other products, negative-sense viral RNA (vRNA), replicative double-stranded forms, and nonstructural proteins are synthesized. Their presence can thus be used as evidence that virus multiplication, as opposed to passive transportation, is occurring (Negro et al.) [188]. Furthermore, sequence variants forming a quasispecies may circulate within an individual, possibly as a consequence of ongoing immune surveillance and viral mutations (Toyoda et al.) [189].

Johnson et al. suggested a possible involvement of HCV in diseases outside the liver and concluded that since oral cavity is frequently exposed to HCV viruses, this in turn increases the risk of genetic instability in these cells [185]. Nagao et al. studied a group of 100 patients including 88 SCC. Anti-HCV antibodies were detected in sera of 25 patients [190]. The exact mechanism is unclear. Gandolfo et al. found very high prevalence of anti-HCV antibodies in patients with oral lichen planus (OLP) [191]. Nagao et al. suggested that, since OLP is also histologically a disease of squamous cells, the squamous cells of oral region are continuously exposed to HCV from saliva as well as from serum in HCV-positive patients and that this may be involved in the development of SCC and OLP in these patients [190].

10. Conclusion

Oral cancer is an important cause of morbidity and mortality, especially in developing countries, and its prevalence may rise in the foreseeable future. The studies of virus-associated head and neck cancers have provided many critical insights into key mechanisms of carcinogenesis. The human tumor virus oncogenes play central roles in viral life cycles and their oncogenic potential is a manifestation of these activities.

Some viruses, most notably the high-risk HPVs, play essential roles in the initiation as well as progression of cancers and continued expression of their viral transforming activities is necessary for the maintenance of the transformed phenotype. Recent reviews establish the increased evidence of HPV-related oral cavity cancer in man.

Standardization of the methods for sample collection and analysis is mandatory to obtain reliable data and to compare the results obtained in different studies in the presence of HPV in variable proportions in oral squamous cell carcinoma tissues. Some tumors are associated with papillomaviruses and some with viruses of the herpes family; however, the exact role of these viruses must still be evaluated carefully. These viruses may provide targets for therapy and for diagnostic tests and may widen our understanding of the mechanisms by which the tumors develop.

Vaccines are designed strictly for prevention of such viral infections which may be involved in cancers of the head and neck. Few studies found sufficient evidence to support a global immunization program against HPV, irrespective of gender and geography, to help to achieve a reduction in HPV-related malignant diseases in the future. Clearly, large, prospective randomized trials are needed to document the clinical usefulness of these vaccines against oral cancer.

Conflict of Interests

The authors declare that there is no conflict of interests regarding the publication of this paper.

References

[1] R. T. Javier and J. S. Butel, "The history of tumor virology," *Cancer Research*, vol. 68, no. 19, pp. 7693–7706, 2008.

[2] M. E. McLaughlin-Drubin and K. Munger, "Viruses associated with human cancer," *Biochimica et Biophysica Acta*, vol. 1782, no. 3, pp. 127–150, 2008.

[3] S. M. Gondivkar, R. V. Parikh, A. R. Gadbail et al., "Involvement of viral factors with head and neck cancers," *Oral Oncology*, vol. 48, no. 3, pp. 195–199, 2012.

[4] R. O. Greer Jr., J. M. Douglas Jr., P. Breese, and L. K. Crosby, "Evaluation of oral and laryngeal specimens for human papillomavirus (HPV) DNA by dot blot hybridization," *Journal of Oral Pathology and Medicine*, vol. 19, no. 1, pp. 35–38, 1990.

[5] R. O. Greer, K. Shroyer, and L. Crosby, "Identification of human papillomavirus DNA in smokeless tobacco keratoses and premalignant and malignant oral lesions by PCR amplification with consensus sequence primers," NIH Publication No. 92-3461, US Department of Health and Human Services, Public Health Service, National Institutes of Health, Bethesda, Md, USA, 1992.

[6] N. H. Park, M. M. Byung, and L. L. Sheng, "Role of viruses in oral carcinogenesis," NIH Publication No. 92-3461, US Department of Health and Human Services, Public Health Service, National Institutes of Health, Bethesda, Md, USA, 1992.

[7] N. W. Johnson, *Risk Markers for Oral Disease, Oral Cancer Detection of Patients and Lesions at Risk*, Cambridge University Press, Cambridge, UK, 1991.

[8] Y. Nagao, M. Sata, K. Tanikawa, K. Itoh, and T. Kameyama, "High prevalence of hepatitis C virus antibody and RNA in patients with oral cancer," *Journal of Oral Pathology and Medicine*, vol. 24, no. 8, pp. 354–360, 1995.

[9] S. R. Porter, G. Lodi, K. Chandler, and N. Kumar, "Development of squamous cell carcinoma in hepatitis C virus-associated lichen planus," *Oral Oncology*, vol. 33, no. 1, pp. 58–59, 1997.

[10] Y. Chang, E. Cesarman, M. S. Pessin et al., "Identification of herpesvirus-like DNA sequences in AIDS-associated Kaposi's sarcoma," *Science*, vol. 266, no. 5192, pp. 1865–1869, 1994.

[11] S. M. Cohen, *Microbes and MAlignancy: Infection as a Cause of Human Cancers*, Oxford University Press, Oxford, UK, 1999, J. Parsonnet (Ed.).

[12] R. Koch, in *Vernhandlungen des X Internationalen Medicinischen Congresses*, vol. 1, pp. 35–47, Berlin, 1890.

[13] A. S. Evans and N. E. Mueller, "Viruses and cancer. Causal associations," *Annals of Epidemiology*, vol. 1, no. 1, pp. 71–92, 1990.

[14] A. B. HILL, "The environment and disease: association or causation?" *Proceedings of the Royal Society of Medicine*, vol. 58, pp. 295–300, 1965.

[15] A. B. Hill and I. D. Hill, *Bradford Hill's Principles of Medical Statistics*, Edward Arnold, London, UK, 12th edition, 1991.

[16] H. Z. Zur Hausen and E.-M. De Villiers, "Human papillomaviruses," *Annual Review of Microbiology*, vol. 48, pp. 427–447, 1994.

[17] C. C. R. Ragin, F. Modugno, and S. M. Gollin, "The epidemiology and risk factors of head and neck cancer: a focus on human papillomavirus," *Journal of Dental Research*, vol. 86, no. 2, pp. 104–114, 2007.

[18] Y. Yabe, H. Sadakane, and H. Isono, "Connection between capsomeres in human papilloma virus," *Virology*, vol. 96, no. 2, pp. 547–552, 1979.

[19] L. Gissmann, H. Pfister, and H. Zur Hausen, "Human papilloma viruses (HPV): characterization of four different isolates," *Virology*, vol. 76, no. 2, pp. 569–580, 1977.

[20] O. Danos, M. Katinka, and M. Yaniv, "Human papillomavirus 1a complete DNA sequence: a novel type of genome organization among papovaviridae," *The EMBO Journal*, vol. 1, no. 2, pp. 231–236, 1982.

[21] E. Schwarz, M. Dürst, C. Demankowski et al., "DNA sequence and genome organization of genital human papillomavirus type 6b," *The EMBO Journal*, vol. 2, no. 12, pp. 2341–2348, 1983.

[22] D. Kremsdorf, M. Favre, and S. Jablonska, "Molecular cloning and characterization of the genomes of nine newly recognized human papillomavirus types associated with epidermodysplasia verruciformis," *Journal of Virology*, vol. 52, no. 3, pp. 1013–1018, 1984.

[23] K. Seedorf, G. Krammer, and M. Durst, "Human papillomavirus type 16 DNA sequence," *Virology*, vol. 145, no. 1, pp. 181–185, 1985.

[24] N. Munoz, F. X. Bosch, and X. Castellsague, "Against which human papillomavirus types shall we vaccinate and screen? The international perspective," *International Journal of Cancer*, vol. 111, pp. 278–285, 2004.

[25] M. Schiffman, P. E. Castle, J. Jeronimo, A. C. Rodriguez, and S. Wacholder, "Human papillomavirus and cervical cancer," *The Lancet*, vol. 370, no. 9590, pp. 890–907, 2007.

[26] H. Zur Hausen, E. M. De Villiers, and L. Gissmann, "Papillomavirus infections and human genital cancer," *Gynecologic Oncology*, vol. 12, no. 2, pp. S124–S128, 1981.

[27] F. X. Bosch, A. Lorincz, N. Muñoz, C. J. L. M. Meijer, and K. V. Shah, "The causal relation between human papillomavirus and cervical cancer," *Journal of Clinical Pathology*, vol. 55, no. 4, pp. 244–265, 2002.

[28] I. O. C. Thompson, P. van der Bijl, C. W. van Wyk, and A. D. van Eyk, "A comparative light-microscopic, electron-microscopic and chemical study of human vaginal and buccal epithelium," *Archives of Oral Biology*, vol. 46, no. 12, pp. 1091–1098, 2001.

[29] K. J. Syrjänen, S. Pyrhönen, S. M. Syrjänen, and M. A. Lamberg, "Immunohistochemical demonstration of human Papilloma virus (HPV) antigens in oral squamous cell lesions," *British Journal of Oral Surgery*, vol. 21, no. 2, pp. 147–153, 1983.

[30] M. L. Gillison, W. M. Koch, R. B. Capone et al., "Evidence for a causal association between human papilloma virus and a subset of head and neck cancers," *Journal of the National Cancer Institute*, vol. 92, no. 9, pp. 709–720, 2000.

[31] E. M. Smith, H. T. Hoffman, K. S. Summersgill, H. L. Kirchner, L. P. Turek, and T. H. Haugen, "Human papillomavirus and risk of oral cancer," *Laryngoscope*, vol. 108, no. 7, pp. 1098–1103, 1998.

[32] C. S. Miller and B. M. Johnstone, "Human papillomavirus as a risk factor for oral squamous cell carcinoma: a meta-analysis, 1982–1997," *Oral Surgery, Oral Medicine, Oral Pathology, Oral Radiology, and Endodontics*, vol. 91, no. 6, pp. 622–635, 2001.

[33] S. M. Schwartz, J. R. Daling, D. R. Doody et al., "Oral cancer risk in relation to sexual history and evidence of human papillomavirus infection," *Journal of the National Cancer Institute*, vol. 90, no. 21, pp. 1626–1636, 1998.

[34] T. Bjorge, E. M. Hennig, G. B. Skare, O. Soreide, and S. O. Thoresen, "Second primary cancers in patients with carcinoma in situ of the uterine cervix. The Norwegian experience 1970–1992," *International Journal of Cancer*, vol. 62, no. 1, pp. 29–33, 1995.

[35] C. S. Rabkin, R. J. Biggar, M. Melbye, and R. E. Curtis, "Second primary cancers following anal and cervical carcinoma: evidence of shared etiologic factors," *American Journal of Epidemiology*, vol. 136, no. 1, pp. 54–58, 1992.

[36] M. Frisch and R. J. Biggar, "Aetiological parallel between tonsillar and anogenital squamous-cell carcinomas," *The Lancet*, vol. 354, no. 9188, pp. 1442–1443, 1999.

[37] K. Hemminki, C. Dong, and M. Frisch, "Tonsillar and other upper aerodigestive tract cancers among cervical cancer patients and their husbands," *European Journal of Cancer Prevention*, vol. 9, no. 6, pp. 433–437, 2000.

[38] S. Syrjänen, "Current concepts on human papillomavirus infections in children," *APMIS*, vol. 118, no. 6-7, pp. 494–509, 2010.

[39] M. Scheffner, J. M. Huibregtse, R. D. Vierstra, and P. M. Howley, "The HPV-16 E6 and E6-AP complex functions as a ubiquitin-protein ligase in the ubiquitination of p53," *Cell*, vol. 75, no. 3, pp. 495–505, 1993.

[40] M. Scheffner and N. J. Whitaker, "Human papillomavirus-induced carcinogenesis and the ubiquitin-proteasome system," *Seminars in Cancer Biology*, vol. 13, no. 1, pp. 59–67, 2003.

[41] M. Scheffner, B. A. Werness, J. M. Huibregtse, A. J. Levine, and P. M. Howley, "The E6 oncoprotein encoded by human papillomavirus types 16 and 18 promotes the degradation of p53," *Cell*, vol. 63, no. 6, pp. 1129–1136, 1990.

[42] R. R. Reddel, "Alternative lengthening of telomeres, telomerase, and cancer," *Cancer Letters*, vol. 194, no. 2, pp. 155–162, 2003.

[43] B. Damania, "DNA tumor viruses and human cancer," *Trends in Microbiology*, vol. 15, no. 1, pp. 38–44, 2007.

[44] R. H. Kim, M. K. Kang, K.-H. Shin et al., "Bmi-1 cooperates with human papillomavirus type 16 E6 to immortalize normal human oral keratinocytes," *Experimental Cell Research*, vol. 313, no. 3, pp. 462–472, 2007.

[45] X. Liu, G. L. Disbrow, H. Yuan, V. Tomaić, and R. Schlegel, "Myc and human papillomavirus type 16 E7 genes cooperate to immortalize human keratinocytes," *Journal of Virology*, vol. 81, no. 22, pp. 12689–12695, 2007.

[46] W.-M. Chien, F. Noya, H. M. Benedict-Hamilton, T. R. Broker, and L. T. Chow, "Alternative fates of keratinocytes transduced by human papillomavirus type 18 E7 during squamous differentiation," *Journal of Virology*, vol. 76, no. 6, pp. 2964–2972, 2002.

[47] S. G. Hwang, D. Lee, J. Kim, T. Seo, and J. Choe, "Human papillomavirus type 16 E7 binds to E2F1 and activates E2F1-driven transcription in a retinoblastoma protein-independent manner," *Journal of Biological Chemistry*, vol. 277, no. 4, pp. 2923–2930, 2002.

[48] T. Loning, H. Ikenberg, and J. Becker, "Analysis of oral papillomas, leukoplakias, and invasive carcinomas for human papillomavirus type related DNA," *Journal of Investigative Dermatology*, vol. 84, no. 5, pp. 417–420, 1985.

[49] N. J. Maitland, M. F. Cox, C. Lynas, S. S. Prime, C. A. Meanwell, and C. Scully, "Detection of human papillomavirus DNA in biopsies of human oral tissue," *British Journal of Cancer*, vol. 56, no. 3, pp. 245–250, 1987.

[50] A. Gassenmaier and O. P. Hornstein, "Presence of human papillomavirus DNA in benign and precancerous oral leukoplakias and squamous cell carcinomas," *Dermatologica*, vol. 176, no. 5, pp. 224–233, 1988.

[51] S. M. Syrjänen, K. J. Syrjänen, and R. P. Happonen, "Human papillomavirus (HPV) DNA sequences in oral precancerous lesions and squamous cell carcinoma demonstrated by in situ hybridization," *Journal of Oral Pathology*, vol. 17, no. 6, pp. 273–278, 1988.

[52] F. Chang, S. Syrjanen, J. Nuutinen, J. Karja, and K. Syrjanen, "Detection of human papillomavirus (HPV) DNA in oral squamous cell carcinomas by in sity hybridization and polymerase chain reaction," *Archives of Dermatological Research*, vol. 282, no. 8, pp. 493–497, 1990.

[53] R. O. Greer Jr., L. R. Eversole, and L. K. Crosby, "Detection of human papillomavirus-genomic DNA in oral epithelial dysplasias, oral smokeless tobacco-associated leukoplakias, and epithelial malignancies," *Journal of Oral and Maxillofacial Surgery*, vol. 48, no. 11, pp. 1201–1205, 1990.

[54] H. K. Kashima, L. S. Levin, M. Kutcher, E.-M. De Villiers, T. Kessis, and K. Shah, "Human papillomavirus in squamous cell carcinoma, leukoplakia, lichen planus, and clinically normal epithelium of the oral cavity," *Annals of Otology, Rhinology and Laryngology*, vol. 99, no. 1, pp. 55–61, 1990.

[55] S. K. Young and K. W. Min, "In situ DNA hybridization analysis of oral papillomas, leukoplakias, and carcinomas for human papillomavirus," *Oral Surgery Oral Medicine and Oral Pathology*, vol. 71, no. 6, pp. 726–9, 1991.

[56] M. S. Zeuss, C. S. Miller, and D. K. White, "In situ hybridization analysis of human papillomavirus DNA in oral mucosal lesions," *Oral Surgery Oral Medicine and Oral Pathology*, vol. 71, no. 6, pp. 714–720, 1991.

[57] E. B. Holladay and W. L. Gerald, "Viral gene detection in oral neoplasms using the polymerase chain reaction," *American Journal of Clinical Pathology*, vol. 100, no. 1, pp. 36–40, 1993.

[58] M. Cox, N. Maitland, and C. Scully, "Human herpes simplex-1 and papillomavirus type 16 homologous DNA sequences in normal, potentially malignant and malignant oral mucosa," *European Journal of Cancer B*, vol. 29, no. 3, pp. 215–219, 1993.

[59] M. Brandwein, J. Zeitlin, G. J. Nuovo et al., "HPV detection using "hot start" polymerase chain reaction in patients with oral cancer: a clinicopathological study of 64 patients," *Modern Pathology*, vol. 7, no. 7, pp. 720–727, 1994.

[60] M. A. González-Moles, I. Ruiz-Avila, S. González-Moles, I. Martinez, A. Ceballos, and F. Nogales, "Detection of HPV DNA by in situ hybridization in benign, premalignant and malignant lesions of the oral mucosa," *Bulletin du Groupement International pour la Recherche Scientifique en Stomatologie & Odontologie*, vol. 37, no. 3-4, pp. 79–85, 1994.

[61] C. Ostwald, P. Muller, M. Barten et al., "Human papillomavirus DNA in oral squamous cell carcinomas and normal mucosa," *Journal of Oral Pathology and Medicine*, vol. 23, no. 5, pp. 220–225, 1994.

[62] P. Balaram, K. R. Nalinakumari, E. Abraham et al., "Human papillomaviruses in 91 oral cancers from indican betel quid chewers—High prevalence and multiplicity of infections," *International Journal of Cancer*, vol. 61, no. 4, pp. 450–454, 1995.

[63] M. Shindoh, I. Chiba, M. Yasuda et al., "Detection of human papillomavirus DNA sequences in oral squamous cell carcinomas and their relation to p53 and proliferating cell nuclear antigen expression," *Cancer*, vol. 76, pp. 1513–1521, 1995.

[64] E. J. van Rensburg, W. F. P. van Heerden, E. H. Venter, and E. J. Raubenheimer, "Detection of human papillomavirus DNA with in situ hybridisation in oval squamous carcinoma in a rural black population," *South African Medical Journal*, vol. 85, no. 9, pp. 894–896, 1995.

[65] I. B. F. Cruz, P. J. F. Snijders, R. D. M. Steenbergen et al., "Age-dependence of human papillomavirus DNA presence in oral squamous cell carcinomas," *European Journal of Cancer B*, vol. 32, no. 1, pp. 55–62, 1996.

[66] E. J. Mao, S. M. Schwartz, J. R. Daling et al., "Human papilloma viruses and p53 mutations in normal pre-malignant and malignant oral epithelia," *International Journal of Cancer*, vol. 69, pp. 152–158, 1996.

[67] E. J. van Rensburg, S. Engelbrecht, W. F. P. van Heerden, E. J. Raubennheimer, and B. D. Schoub, "Human papillomavirus DNA in oral squamous cell carcinomas from an African population sample," *Anticancer Research*, vol. 16, no. 2, pp. 969–973, 1996.

[68] I. Chiba, M. Shindoh, M. Yasuda et al., "Mutations in the p53 gene and human papillomavirus infection as significant prognostic factors in squamous cell carcinomas of the oral cavity," *Oncogene*, vol. 12, no. 8, pp. 1663–1668, 1996.

[69] S. Wen, T. Tsuji, X. Li, Y. Mizugaki, Y. Hayatsu, and F. Shinozaki, "Detection and analysis of human papillomavirus 16 and 18 homologous DNA sequences in oral lesions," *Anticancer Research*, vol. 17, no. 1 A, pp. 307–311, 1997.

[70] R. Gopalakrishnan, C. M. Weghorst, T. A. Lehman et al., "Mutated and wild-type p53 expression and HPV integration in proliferative verrucous leukoplakia and oral squamous cell carcinoma," *Oral Surgery, Oral Medicine, Oral Pathology, Oral Radiology, and Endodontics*, vol. 83, no. 4, pp. 471–477, 1997.

[71] S. O. Ibrahim, B. Bertelsen, M. B. Kalvenes et al., "Expression of keratin 13, 14 and 19 in oral squamous cell carcinomas from Sudanese snuff dippers: lack of association with human papillomavirus infection," *APMIS*, vol. 106, no. 10, pp. 959–969, 1998.

[72] J. Y. Koh, N. P. Cho, G. Kong, J. D. Lee, and K. Yoon, "p53 mutations and human papillomavirus DNA in oral squamous cell carcinoma: correlation with apoptosis," *British Journal of Cancer*, vol. 78, no. 3, pp. 354–359, 1998.

[73] G. Premoli-De-Percoco, J. L. Ramírez, and I. Galindo, "Correlation between HPV types associated with oral squamous cell carcinoma and cervicovaginal cytology: an in situ hybridization study," *Oral Surgery, Oral Medicine, Oral Pathology, Oral Radiology, and Endodontics*, vol. 86, no. 1, pp. 77–81, 1998.

[74] J. D'Costa, D. Saranath, P. Dedhia, V. Sanghvi, and A. R. Mehta, "Detection of HPV-16 genome in human oral cancers and potentially malignant lesions from India," *Oral Oncology*, vol. 34, no. 5, pp. 413–420, 1998.

[75] F. Elamin, H. Steingrimsdottir, S. Wanakulasuriya, N. Johnson, and M. Tavassoli, "Prevalence of human papillomavirus infection in premalignant and malignant lesions of the oral cavity in U.K. subjects: a novel method of detection," *Oral Oncology*, vol. 34, no. 3, pp. 191–197, 1998.

[76] E. P. Aggelopoulou, D. Skarlos, C. Papadimitriou, C. Kittas, and C. Troungos, "Human papilloma virus DNA detection in oral lesions in the Greek population," *Anticancer Research*, vol. 19, no. 2B, pp. 1391–1395, 1999.

[77] M. R. Pillai, A. Phanidhara, A. L. Kesari et al., "Cellular manifestations of human papillomavirus infection in the oral mucosa," *Journal of Surgical Oncology*, vol. 71, pp. 10–15, 1999.

[78] J. Pintos, E. L. Franco, M. J. Black, J. Bergeron, and M. Arella, "Human papillomavirus and prognoses of patients with cancers of the upper aerodigestive tract," *Cancer*, vol. 85, pp. 1903–1909, 1999.

[79] G. Badaracco, A. Venuti, R. Morello, A. Muller, and M. L. Marcante, "Human papillomavirus in head and neck carcinomas: prevalence, physical status and relationship with clinical/pathological parameters," *Anticancer Research*, vol. 20, no. 2 B, pp. 1301–1305, 2000.

[80] M. Bouda, V. G. Gorgoulis, N. G. Kastrinakis et al., "'High risk' HPV types are frequently detected in potentially malignant and malignant oral lesions, but not in normal oral mucosa," *Modern Pathology*, vol. 13, no. 6, pp. 644–653, 2000.

[81] J. Cao, Z. Y. Zhang, P. Patima, Y. X. Zhang, and W. T. Chen, "Human papillomavirus infection and p53 alteration in oral squamous cell carcinoma," *The Chinese Journal of Dental Research*, vol. 3, no. 3, pp. 44–49, 2000.

[82] J. Patima Cao, W. T. Chen, and Z. Y. Zhang, "Detection of high risk human papillomavirus DNA in oral squamous cell carcinoma," *Shanghai Kou Qiang Yi Xue*, vol. 9, pp. 212–215, 2000.

[83] L. Sand, J. Jalouli, P.-A. Larsson, and J.-M. Hirsch, "Human papilloma viruses in oral lesions," *Anticancer Research*, vol. 20, no. 2B, pp. 1183–1188, 2000.

[84] K. Tsuhako, I. Nakazato, J. Miyagi et al., "Comparative study of oral squamous cell carcinoma in Okinawa, Southern Japan and Sapporo in Hokkaido, Northern Japan; with special reference to human papillomavirus and Epstein-Barr virus infection," *Journal of Oral Pathology and Medicine*, vol. 29, no. 2, pp. 70–79, 2000.

[85] G. Premoli-De-Percoco and J. L. Ramirez, "High risk human papillomavirus in oral squamous carcinoma: evidence of risk factors in a Venezuelan rural population. Preliminary report," *Journal of Oral Pathology and Medicine*, vol. 30, no. 6, pp. 355–361, 2001.

[86] S. R. Schwartz, B. Yueh, J. K. McDougall, J. R. Daling, and S. M. Schwartz, "Human papillomavirus infection and survival in oral squamous cell cancer: a population-based study," *Otolaryngology*, vol. 125, no. 1, pp. 1–9, 2001.

[87] P. C.-H. Chen, C. Kuo, C.-C. Pan, and M.-Y. Chou, "Risk of oral cancer associated with human papillomavirus infection, betel quid chewing, and cigarette smoking in Taiwan—an integrated molecular and epidemiological study of 58 cases," *Journal of Oral Pathology and Medicine*, vol. 31, no. 6, pp. 317–322, 2002.

[88] A. Kojima, H. Maeda, Y. Sugita, S. Tanaka, and Y. Kameyama, "Human papillomavirus type 38 infection in oral squamous cell carcinomas," *Oral Oncology*, vol. 38, no. 6, pp. 591–596, 2002.

[89] J. K. Nagpal, S. Patnaik, and B. R. Das, "Prevalence of high-risk human papilloma virus types and its association with p53 codon 72 polymorphism in tobacco addicted oral squamous cell carcimona (OSCC) patients of Eastern India," *International Journal of Cancer*, vol. 97, no. 5, pp. 649–653, 2002.

[90] J. Y.-F. Chang, M.-C. Lin, and C.-P. Chiang, "High-risk human papillomaviruses may have an important role in non-oral habits-associated oral squamous cell Carcinomas in Taiwan," *American Journal of Clinical Pathology*, vol. 120, no. 6, pp. 909–916, 2003.

[91] P. A. G. Fregonesi, D. B. Teresa, R. A. Duarte, C. B. Neto, M. R. B. De Oliveira, and C. P. Soares, "p16INK4A immunohistochemical overexpression in premalignant and malignant oral lesions infected with human papillomavirus," *Journal of Histochemistry and Cytochemistry*, vol. 51, no. 10, pp. 1291–1297, 2003.

[92] A. A. Kansky, M. Poljak, K. Seme et al., "Human papillomavirus DNA in oral squamous cell carcinomas and normal oral mucosa," *Acta Virologica*, vol. 47, no. 1, pp. 11–16, 2003.

[93] J. M. Ritchie, E. M. Smith, K. F. Summersgill et al., "Human papillomavirus infection as a prognostic factor in carcinomas of the oral cavity and oropharynx," *International Journal of Cancer*, vol. 104, no. 3, pp. 336–344, 2003.

[94] M. Sugiyama, U. K. Bhawal, T. Dohmen, S. Ono, M. Miyauchi, and T. Ishikawa, "Detection of human papillomavirus-16 and HPV-18 DNA in normal, dysplastic, and malignant oral epithelium," *Oral Surgery, Oral Medicine, Oral Pathology, Oral Radiology, and Endodontics*, vol. 95, no. 5, pp. 594–600, 2003.

[95] R. Herrero, X. Castellsagué, M. Pawlita et al., "Human papillomavirus and oral cancer: the international agency for research on cancer multicenter study," *Journal of the National Cancer Institute*, vol. 95, no. 23, pp. 1772–1783, 2003.

[96] C. Ostwald, K. Rutsatz, J. Schweder, W. Schmidt, K. Gundlach, and M. Barten, "Human papillomavirus 6/11, 16 and 18 in oral carcinomas and benign oral lesions," *Medical Microbiology and Immunology*, vol. 192, no. 3, pp. 145–148, 2003.

[97] M. Correnti, H. Rivera, and M. E. Cavazza, "Detection of human papillomaviruses of high oncogenic potential in oral squamous cell carcinoma in a Venezuelan population," *Oral Diseases*, vol. 10, no. 3, pp. 163–166, 2004.

[98] L. Dahlgren, H. Dahlstrand, D. Lindquist et al., "Human papillomavirus is more common in base of tongue than in mobile tongue cancer and is a favorable prognostic factor in base of tongue cancer patients," *International Journal of Cancer*, vol. 112, no. 6, pp. 1015–1019, 2004.

[99] E. M. Smith, J. M. Ritche, K. F. Summersgill et al., "Human papillomavirus in oral exfoliated cells and risk of head and neck cancer," *Journal of the National Cancer Institute*, vol. 96, no. 6, pp. 449–455, 2004.

[100] Z.-Y. Zhang, P. Sdek, J. Cao, and W.-T. Chen, "Human papillomavirus type 16 and 18 DNA in oral squamous cell carcinoma and normal mucosa," *International Journal of Oral and Maxillofacial Surgery*, vol. 33, no. 1, pp. 71–74, 2004.

[101] Y.-Y. Yang, L.-W. Koh, J.-H. Tsai et al., "Involvement of viral and chemical factors with oral cancer in Taiwan," *Japanese Journal of Clinical Oncology*, vol. 34, no. 4, pp. 176–183, 2004.

[102] P. Koppikar, E.-M. De Villiers, and R. Mulherkar, "Identification of human papillomaviruses in tumors of the oral cavity in an Indian community," *International Journal of Cancer*, vol. 113, no. 6, pp. 946–950, 2005.

[103] L. Lo Muzio, M. D'Angelo, M. Procaccini et al., "Expression of cell cycle markers and human papillomavirus infection in oral squamous cell carcinoma: Use of fuzzy neural networks," *International Journal of Cancer*, vol. 115, no. 5, pp. 717–723, 2005.

[104] S. Boy, E. J. V. Rensburg, S. Engelbrecht, L. Dreyer, M. van Heerden, and W. van Heerden, "HPV detection in primary intra-oral squamous cell carcinomas—commensal, aetiological agent or contamination?" *Journal of Oral Pathology and Medicine*, vol. 35, no. 2, pp. 86–90, 2006.

[105] S. K. El-Mofty and S. Patil, "Human papillomavirus (HPV)-related oropharyngeal nonkeratinizing squamous cell carcinoma: characterization of a distinct phenotype," *Oral Surgery, Oral Medicine, Oral Pathology, Oral Radiology and Endodontology*, vol. 101, no. 3, pp. 339–345, 2006.

[106] J. A. Nemes, L. Deli, Z. Nemes, and I. J. Márton, "Expression of p16INK4A, p53, and Rb proteins are independent from the presence of human papillomavirus genes in oral squamous cell carcinoma," *Oral Surgery, Oral Medicine, Oral Pathology, Oral Radiology and Endodontology*, vol. 102, no. 3, pp. 344–352, 2006.

[107] E. R. C. Rivero and F. D. Nunes, "HPV in oral squamous cell carcinomas of a Brazilian population: amplification by PCR," *Brazilian Oral Research*, vol. 20, no. 1, pp. 21–24, 2006.

[108] G. Campisi, L. Giovannelli, F. Calvino et al., "HPV infection in relation to OSCC histological grading and TNM stage. Evaluation by traditional statistics and fuzzy logic model," *Oral Oncology*, vol. 42, no. 6, pp. 638–645, 2006.

[109] V. E. Furrer, M. B. Benitez, M. Furnes, H. E. Lanfranchi, and N. M. Modesti, "Biopsy versus superficial scraping: detection of human papillomavirus 6, 11, 16, and 18 in potentially malignant and malignant oral lesions," *Journal of Oral Pathology and Medicine*, vol. 35, no. 6, pp. 338–344, 2006.

[110] K. Koyama, K. Uobe, and A. Tanaka, "Highly sensitive detection of HPV-DNA in paraffin sections of human oral carcinomas," *Journal of Oral Pathology and Medicine*, vol. 36, no. 1, pp. 18–24, 2007.

[111] M. Sugiyama, U. K. Bhawal, M. Kawamura et al., "Human papillomavirus-16 in oral squamous cell carcinoma: clinical correlates and 5-year survival," *British Journal of Oral and Maxillofacial Surgery*, vol. 45, no. 2, pp. 116–122, 2007.

[112] C.-W. Luo, C.-H. Roan, and C.-J. Liu, "Human papillomaviruses in oral squamous cell carcinoma and pre-cancerous lesions detected by PCR-based gene-chip array," *International Journal of Oral and Maxillofacial Surgery*, vol. 36, no. 2, pp. 153–158, 2007.

[113] S.-O. P. Khovidhunkit, W. Buajeeb, S. Sanguansin, S. Poomsawat, and W. Weerapradist, "Detection of human papillomavirus in oral squamous cell carcinoma, leukoplakia and lichen planus in Thai patients," *Asian Pacific Journal of Cancer Prevention*, vol. 9, no. 4, pp. 771–775, 2008.

[114] K. Szarka, I. Tar, E. Feher et al., "Progressive increase of human papillomavirus carriage rates in potentially malignant and malignant oral disorders with increasing malignant potential," *Oral Microbiology and Immunology*, vol. 24, no. 4, pp. 314–318, 2009.

[115] D. Zhao, Q.-G. Xu, X.-M. Chen, and M.-W. Fan, "Human papillomavirus as an independent predictor in oral squamous cell cancer," *International journal of oral science*, vol. 1, no. 3, pp. 119–125, 2009.

[116] P. Attner, J. Du, A. Näsman et al., "The role of human papillomavirus in the increased incidence of base of tongue cancer," *International Journal of Cancer*, vol. 126, no. 12, pp. 2879–2884, 2010.

[117] K. J. Elango, A. Suresh, E. M. Erode et al., "Role of human papilloma virus in oral tongue squamous cell carcinoma," *Asian Pacific Journal of Cancer Prevention*, vol. 12, no. 4, pp. 889–896, 2011.

[118] A. K. Kristoffersen, M. Enersen, E. Kverndokk et al., "Human papillomavirus subtypes in oral lesions compared to healthy oral mucosa," *Journal of Clinical Virology*, vol. 53, no. 4, pp. 364–366, 2012.

[119] S.-F. Chen, F.-S. Yu, Y.-C. Chang, E. Fu, S. Nieh, and Y.-S. Lin, "Role of human papillomavirus infection in carcinogenesis of oral squamous cell carcinoma with evidences of prognostic

association," *Journal of Oral Pathology and Medicine*, vol. 41, no. 1, pp. 9–15, 2012.

[120] L.-A. Lee, C.-G. Huang, C.-T. Liao et al., "Human papillomavirus-16 infection in advanced oral cavity cancer patients is related to an increased risk of distant metastases and poor survival," *PLoS ONE*, vol. 7, no. 7, Article ID e40767, 2012.

[121] K. J. Syrjänen, S. Pyrhönen, S. M. Syrjänen, and M. A. Lamberg, "Immunohistochemical demonstration of Human papilloma virus (HPV) antigens in oral squamous cell lesions," *British Journal of Oral Surgery*, vol. 21, no. 2, pp. 147–153, 1983.

[122] K. Syrjänen, S. Syrjänen, and M. Lamberg, "Morphological and immunohistochemical evidence suggesting human papillomavirus (HPV) involvement in oral squamous cell carcinogenesis," *International Journal of Oral Surgery*, vol. 12, no. 6, pp. 418–424, 1983.

[123] C. S. Miller and D. K. White, "Human papillomavirus expression in oral mucosa, premalignant conditions, and squamous cell carcinoma a retrospective review of the literature," *Oral Surgery, Oral Medicine, Oral Pathology, Oral Radiology, and Endodontics*, vol. 82, no. 1, pp. 57–68, 1996.

[124] S. M. Syrjänen and K. J. Syrjänen, "HPV infections of the oral mucosa," in *Papillomavirus Infections in Human Pathology*, K. J. Syrjänen and S. M. Syrjänen, Eds., pp. 379–412, John Wiley & Sons, New York, NY, USA, 2000.

[125] H. Mellin, S. Friesland, R. Lewensohn, T. Dalianis, and E. MunckWikland, "Human papillomavirus (HPV) DNA in tonsillar cancer: clinical correlates, risk of relapse, and survival," *International Journal of Cancer*, vol. 89, pp. 300–304, 2000.

[126] G. D'Souza, A. R. Kreimer, R. Viscidi et al., "Case-control study of human papillomavirus and oropharyngeal cancer," *The New England Journal of Medicine*, vol. 356, no. 19, pp. 1944–1956, 2007.

[127] K. K. Ang, J. Harris, R. Wheeler et al., "Human papillomavirus and survival of patients with oropharyngeal cancer," *The New England Journal of Medicine*, vol. 363, no. 1, pp. 24–35, 2010.

[128] S. Syrjänen, G. Lodi, I. von Bültzingslöwen et al., "Human papillomaviruses in oral carcinoma and oral potentially malignant disorders: a systematic review," *Oral Diseases*, vol. 17, no. 1, pp. 58–72, 2011.

[129] J. L. St Guily, A.-C. Jacquard, J.-L. Prétet et al., "Human papillomavirus genotype distribution in oropharynx and oral cavity cancer in France–the EDiTH VI study," *Journal of Clinical Virology*, vol. 51, no. 2, pp. 100–104, 2011.

[130] C. Ziegert, N. Wentzensen, S. Vinokurova et al., "A comprehensive analysis of HPV integration loci in anogenital lesions combining transcript and genome-based amplification techniques," *Oncogene*, vol. 22, no. 25, pp. 3977–3984, 2003.

[131] H. W. Haverkos, "Viruses, chemicals and co-carcinogenesis," *Oncogene*, vol. 23, no. 38, pp. 6492–6499, 2004.

[132] M. Migaldi, M. Pecorari, G. Forbicini et al., "Low prevalence of human papillomavirus infection in the healthy oral mucosa of a Northern Italian population," *Journal of Oral Pathology and Medicine*, vol. 41, no. 1, pp. 16–20, 2012.

[133] G. Pannone, A. Santoro, S. Papagerakis, L. Lo Muzio, G. De Rosa, and P. Bufo, "The role of human papillomavirus in the pathogenesis of head & neck squamous cell carcinoma: an overview," *Infectious Agents and Cancer*, vol. 6, no. 1, article 4, 2011.

[134] J. E. Burns, M. C. Baird, L. J. Clark et al., "Gene mutations and increased levels of p53 protein in human squamous cell carcinomas and their cell lines," *British Journal of Cancer*, vol. 67, no. 6, pp. 1274–1284, 1993.

[135] M. B. Gillespie, S. Rubinchik, B. Hoel, and N. Sutkowski, "Human papillomavirus and oropharyngeal cancer: what you need to know in 2009," *Current Treatment Options in Oncology*, vol. 10, no. 5-6, pp. 296–307, 2009.

[136] P. K. C. Goon, M. A. Stanley, J. Ebmeyer et al., "HPV & head and neck cancer: a descriptive update," *Head & Neck Oncology*, vol. 1, article 36, 2009.

[137] R. Kirnbauer, N. L. Hubbert, C. M. Wheeler, T. M. Becker, D. R. Lowy, and J. T. Schiller, "A virus-like particle enzyme-linked immunosorbent assay detects serum antibodies in a majority of women infected with human papillomavirus type 16," *Journal of the National Cancer Institute*, vol. 86, no. 7, pp. 494–499, 1994.

[138] J. J. Carter, L. A. Koutsky, G. C. Wipf et al., "The natural history of human papillomavirus type 16 capsid antibodies among a cohort of university women," *Journal of Infectious Diseases*, vol. 174, no. 5, pp. 927–936, 1996.

[139] W. Meschede, K. Zumbach, J. Braspenning et al., "Antibodies against early proteins of human papillomaviruses as diagnostic markers for invasive cervical cancer," *Journal of Clinical Microbiology*, vol. 36, no. 2, pp. 475–480, 1998.

[140] M. Stanley, "Antibody reactivity to HPV E6 and E7 oncoproteins and early diagnosis of invasive cervical cancer," *American Journal of Obstetrics and Gynecology*, vol. 188, no. 1, pp. 3–4, 2003.

[141] A. K. Markopoulos, "Role of human papillomavirus in the pathogenesis of oral squamous cell carcinoma," *The World Journal of Experimental Medicine*, vol. 2, no. 4, pp. 65–69, 2012.

[142] M. Filion, D. Skup, and M. Suh, "Specific induction of cellular gene transcription in herpes simplex virus type -2-transformed cells," *Journal of General Virology*, vol. 69, no. 8, pp. 2011–2019, 1988.

[143] N. B. La Thangue and D. S. Latchman, "A cellular protein related to heat-shock protein 90 accumulates during herpes simplex virus infection and is overexpressed in transformed cells," *Experimental Cell Research*, vol. 178, no. 1, pp. 169–179, 1988.

[144] E. L. Notarianni and C. M. Preston, "Activation of cellular stress protein genes by herpes simplex virus temperature-sensitive mutants which overproduce immediate early polypeptides," *Virology*, vol. 123, no. 1, pp. 113–122, 1982.

[145] A. D. Kwong, J. A. Kruper, and N. Frenkel, "Herpes simplex virus virion host shutoff function," *Journal of Virology*, vol. 62, no. 3, pp. 912–921, 1988.

[146] M. Fenwick, "The effects of herpes viruses on cellular macromolecular synthesis," in *Comprehensive Virology*, H. Fraenkel-Conrat and R. R. Wagner, Eds., vol. 19, pp. 359–390, Plenum, New York, NY, USA, 1984.

[147] A. D. Kwong and N. Frenkel, "Herpes simplex virus-infected cells contain a function(s) that destabilizes both host and viral mRNAs," *Proceedings of the National Academy of Sciences of the United States of America*, vol. 84, no. 7, pp. 1926–1930, 1987.

[148] G. S. Read and N. Frenkel, "Herpes simplex virus mutants defective in the virion-associated shutoff of host polypeptide synthesis and exhibiting abnormal synthesis of α (immediate early) viral polypeptides," *Journal of Virology*, vol. 46, no. 2, pp. 498–512, 1983.

[149] C. Steele and E. J. Shillitoe, "Viruses and oral cancer," *Critical Reviews in Oral Biology and Medicine*, vol. 2, no. 2, pp. 153–175, 1991.

[150] A. L. Boyd, L. Enquist, G. F. Vande Woude, and B. Hampar, "Activation of mouse retrovirus by herpes simplex virus type 1

cloned DNA fragments," *Virology*, vol. 103, no. 1, pp. 228–231, 1980.

[151] H. F. Stich, T. C. Hsu, and F. Rapp, "Viruses and mammalian chromosomes. I. Localization of chromosome aberrations after infection with herpes simplex virus," *Virology*, vol. 22, no. 4, pp. 439–445, 1964.

[152] A. Mincheva, S. Dundarov, and I. Bradvarova, "Effects of herpes simplex virus strains on human fibroblast and lymphocyte chromosomes and the localization of chromosomal aberrations," *Acta Virologica*, vol. 28, no. 2, pp. 97–106, 1984.

[153] D. S. Peat and M. A. Stanley, "Chromosome damage induced by herpes simplex virus type 1 in early infection," *Journal of General Virology*, vol. 67, no. 10, pp. 2273–2277, 1986.

[154] A. A. I. El Sissy, "Herpes simplex virus type 2 (HSV-2) proteins in oral squamous cell carcinoma—in situ detection," *Cairo Dental Journal*, vol. 13, no. 2, pp. 265–270, 1997.

[155] J. Jalouli, S. O. Ibrahim, D. Sapkota et al., "Presence of human papilloma virus, herpes simplex virus and Epstein-Barr virus DNA in oral biopsies from Sudanese patients with regard to toombak use," *Journal of Oral Pathology and Medicine*, vol. 39, no. 8, pp. 599–604, 2010.

[156] Z. Delavarian, A. Pakfetrat, F. Falaki, and M. Pazouki, "The role of viruses in oral squamous cell carcinoma in young patients in Khorasan (Northeast of Iran)," *Journal of Applied Sciences*, vol. 10, no. 11, pp. 981–985, 2010.

[157] E. J. Shillitoe, D. Greenspan, J. S. Greenspan, and S. Silverman Jr., "Immunogloblin class of antibody to herpes simplex virus in patients with oral cancer," *Cancer*, vol. 51, no. 1, pp. 65–71, 1983.

[158] S. P. Schantz, E. J. Shillitoe, B. Brown, and B. Campbell, "Natural killer cell activity and head and neck cancer: a clinical assessment," *Journal of the National Cancer Institute*, vol. 77, no. 4, pp. 869–875, 1986.

[159] J. R. Starr, J. R. Daling, E. D. Fitzgibbons et al., "Serologic evidence of herpes simplex virus 1 infection and oropharyngeal cancer risk," *Cancer Research*, vol. 61, no. 23, pp. 8459–8464, 2001.

[160] R. P. Eglin, C. Scully, and T. Lehner, "Detection of RNA complementary to herpes simplex virus in human oral squamous cell carcinoma," *The Lancet*, vol. 2, no. 8353, pp. 766–767, 1983.

[161] F. Rapp and R. Duff, "Transformation of hamster embryo fibroblasts by herpes simplex viruses type I and type II," *Cancer Research*, vol. 33, no. 6, pp. 1527–1534, 1973.

[162] J. M. Hirsch, S. L. Johansson, and A. Vahlne, "Effect of snuff and herpes simplex virus-1 on rat oral mucosa: possible associations with the development of squamous cell carcinoma," *Journal of oral pathology*, vol. 13, no. 1, pp. 52–62, 1984.

[163] D. A. Galloway and J. K. McDougall, "The oncogenic potential of herpes simplex viruses: evidence for a 'hit-and-run' mechanism," *Nature*, vol. 302, no. 5903, pp. 21–24, 1983.

[164] E. J. Shillitoe, S. Zhang, G. Wang, and C. B. C. Hwang, "Functions and proteins of herpes simplex virus type-1 that are involved in raising the mutation frequency of infected cells," *Virus Research*, vol. 27, no. 3, pp. 239–251, 1993.

[165] H. Mikola, M. Waris, and J. Tenovuo, "Inhibition of herpes simplex virus type 1, respiratory syncytial virus and echovirus type 11 by peroxidase-generated hypothiocyanite," *Antiviral Research*, vol. 26, no. 2, pp. 161–171, 1995.

[166] C. B. C. Hwang and E. J. Shillitoe, "DNA sequence of mutations induced in cells by herpes simplex virus type-1," *Virology*, vol. 178, no. 1, pp. 180–188, 1990.

[167] R. Baer, A. T. Bankier, and M. D. Biggin, "DNA sequence and expression of the B95-8 Epstein-Barr virus genome," *Nature*, vol. 310, no. 5974, pp. 207–211, 1984.

[168] D. M. Parkin, "The global health burden of infection-associated cancers in the year 2002," *International Journal of Cancer*, vol. 118, no. 12, pp. 3030–3044, 2006.

[169] D. Wang, D. Liebowitz, and E. Kieff, "An EBV membrane protein expressed in immortalized lymphocytes transforms established rodent cells," *Cell*, vol. 43, no. 3, pp. 831–840, 1985.

[170] A. Rickinson and E. Kieff, in *Fields Virology*, D. M. Knipe and P. M. Howley, Eds., pp. 2575–2627, Lippincott Williams and Wilkins, Philadelphia, Pa, USA, 2001.

[171] G. Mosialos, M. Birkenbach, R. Yalamanchili, T. VanArsdale, C. Ware, and E. Kieff, "The Epstein-Barr virus transforming protein LMP1 engages signaling proteins for the tumor necrosis factor receptor family," *Cell*, vol. 80, no. 3, pp. 389–399, 1995.

[172] E. Kieff and A. Rickinson, in *Fields Virology*, D. M. Knipe and P. M. Howley, Eds., pp. 2511–2573, Lippincott Williams and Wilkins, Philadelphia, Pa, USA, 2001.

[173] W. E. Miller, J. L. Cheshire, A. S. Baldwin Jr., and N. Raab-Traub, "The NPC derived C15 LMP1 protein confers enhanced activation of NF-κB and induction of the EGFR in epithelial cells," *Oncogene*, vol. 16, no. 14, pp. 1869–1877, 1998.

[174] A. G. Eliopoulos and L. S. Young, "Activation of the cJun N-terminal kinase (JNK) pathway by the Epstein-Barr virus-encoded latent membrane protein 1 (LMP1)," *Oncogene*, vol. 16, no. 13, pp. 1731–1742, 1998.

[175] A. G. Eliopoulos, N. J. Gallagher, S. M. S. Blake, C. W. Dawson, and L. S. Young, "Activation of the p38 mitogen-activated protein kinase pathway by Epstein-Barr virus-encoded latent membrane protein 1 coregulates interleukin- 6 and interleukin-8 production," *Journal of Biological Chemistry*, vol. 274, no. 23, pp. 16085–16096, 1999.

[176] L. Zhang and J. S. Pagano, "Interferon regulatory factor 7 is induced by Epstein-Barr virus latent membrane protein 1," *Journal of Virology*, vol. 74, no. 3, pp. 1061–1068, 2000.

[177] N. Wakisaka, S. Murono, T. Yoshizaki, M. Furukawa, and J. S. Pagano, "Epstein-Barr virus latent membrane protein 1 induces and causes release of fibroblast growth factor-2," *Cancer Research*, vol. 62, no. 21, pp. 6337–6344, 2002.

[178] R. G. Caldwell, J. B. Wilson, S. J. Anderson, and R. Longnecker, "Epstein-Barr virus LMP2A drives B cell development and survival in the absence of normal B cell receptor signals," *Immunity*, vol. 9, no. 3, pp. 405–411, 1998.

[179] K. Horiuchi, K. Mishima, K. Ichijima, M. Sugimura, T. Ishida, and T. Kirita, "Epstein-Barr virus in the proliferative diseases of squamous epithelium in the oral cavity," *Oral Surgery, Oral Medicine, Oral Pathology, Oral Radiology and*, vol. 79, no. 1, pp. 57–63, 1995.

[180] M. González-Moles, J. Gutiérrez, I. Ruiz, J. A. Fernández, M. Rodriguez, and J. Aneiros, "Epstein-Barr virus and oral squamous cell carcinoma in patients without HIV infection: viral detection by polymerase chain reaction," *Microbios*, vol. 96, no. 383, pp. 23–31, 1998.

[181] M. Higa, T. Kinio, K. Kamiyama, T. Iwamasa, T. Hamada, and K. Iyama, "Epstein-Barr virus (EBV) subtype in EBV related oral squamous cell carcinoma in Okinawa, a subtropical island in southern Japan, compared with Kitakyushu and Kumamoto in mainland Japan," *Journal of Clinical Pathology*, vol. 55, no. 6, pp. 414–423, 2002.

[182] C. Li, C.-Y. Yen, M.-C. Lu et al., "Detection of EBV infection and gene expression in oral cancer from patients in taiwan by

microarray analysis," *Journal of Biomedicine and Biotechnology*, vol. 2009, Article ID 904589, 15 pages, 2009.

[183] L. P. Sand, J. Jalouli, P.-A. Larsson, and J.-M. Hirsch, "Prevalence of Epstein-Barr virus in oral squamous cell carcinoma, oral lichen planus, and normal oral mucosa," *Oral Surgery, Oral Medicine, Oral Pathology, Oral Radiology, and Endodontics*, vol. 93, no. 5, pp. 586–592, 2002.

[184] R. Jiang, X. Gu, T. N. Moore-Medlin, C.-A. Nathan, and L. M. Hutt-Fletcher, "Oral dysplasia and squamous cell carcinoma: correlation between increased expression of CD21, Epstein-Barr virus and CK19," *Oral Oncology*, vol. 48, no. 9, pp. 836–841, 2012.

[185] R. J. Johnson, D. R. Gretch, H. Yamabe et al., "Membranoproliferative glomerulonephritis associated with hepatitis C virus infection," *The New England Journal of Medicine*, vol. 328, no. 7, pp. 465–470, 1993.

[186] Q.-L. Choo, G. Kuo, A. J. Weiner, L. R. Overby, D. W. Bradley, and M. Houghton, "Isolation of a cDNA clone derived from a blood-borne non-A, non-B viral hepatitis genome," *Science*, vol. 244, no. 4902, pp. 359–362, 1989.

[187] M. Carrozzo, R. Quadri, P. Latorre et al., "Molecular evidence that the hepatitis C virus replicates in the oral mucosa," *Journal of Hepatology*, vol. 37, no. 3, pp. 364–369, 2002.

[188] F. Negro, K. Krawczynski, R. Quadri et al., "Detection of genomic- and minus-strand of hepatitis C virus RNA in the liver of chronic hepatitis C patients by strand-specific semi-quantitative reverse-transcriptase polymerase chain reaction," *Hepatology*, vol. 29, no. 2, pp. 536–542, 1999.

[189] H. Toyoda, Y. Fukuda, I. Nakano et al., "Quasispecies nature of hepatitis C virus (HCV) in patients with chronic hepatitis C with mixed HCV subtypes," in *Journal of Medical Virology*, vol. 54, pp. 80–85, 1998.

[190] Y. Nagao, M. Sata, K. Itoh, K. Tanikawa, and T. Kameyama, "Quantitative analysis of HCV RNA and genotype in patients with chronic hepatitis C accompanied by oral lichen planus," *European Journal of Clinical Investigation*, vol. 26, no. 6, pp. 495–498, 1996.

[191] S. Gandolfo, M. Carbone, M. Carrozzo, and V. Gallo, "Oral lichen planus and hepatitis C virus (HCV) infection: is there a relationship? A report of 10 cases," *Journal of Oral Pathology & Medicine*, vol. 23, no. 3, pp. 119–122, 1994.

4

Predictive Response Value of Pre- and Postchemoradiotherapy Variables in Rectal Cancer: An Analysis of Histological Data

Marisa D. Santos,[1] Cristina Silva,[1] Anabela Rocha,[1] Carlos Nogueira,[1] Eduarda Matos,[2] and Carlos Lopes[3,4]

[1] *Department of Surgery, Digestive Surgery Service, Hospital de Santo António, Centro Hospitalar do Porto, Largo Abel Salazar, 4099-003 Porto, Portugal*
[2] *Department of Community Health, Instituto de Ciências Biomédicas Abel Salazar, Rua Jorge Viterbo Ferreira, No. 228, 4050-313 Porto, Portugal*
[3] *Department of Pathology, Pathological Anatomy Service, Hospital de Santo António, Centro Hospitalar do Porto, Largo Professor Abel Salazar, 4099-003 Porto, Portugal*
[4] *Department of Pathology and Molecular Immunology, Instituto de Ciências Biomédicas Abel Salazar, Rua Jorge Viterbo Ferreira, No. 228, 4050-313 Porto, Portugal*

Correspondence should be addressed to Marisa D. Santos; marisadsantos@gmail.com

Academic Editor: Shahid Pervez

Background. Neoadjuvant chemoradiotherapy (nCRT) followed by curative surgery in locally advanced rectal cancer (LARC) improves pelvic disease control. Survival improvement is achieved only if pathological response occurs. Mandard tumor regression grade (TRG) proved to be a valid system to measure nCRT response. Potential predictive factors for Mandard response are analyzed. *Materials and Methods.* 167 patients with LARC were treated with nCRT and curative surgery. Tumor biopsies and surgical specimens were reviewed and analyzed regarding mitotic count, necrosis, desmoplastic reaction, and inflammatory infiltration grade. Surgical specimens were classified according to Mandard TRG. The patients were divided as "good responders" (Mandard TRG1-2) and "bad responders" (Mandard TRG3-5). According to results from our previous data, good responders have better prognosis than bad responders. We examined predictive factors for Mandard response and performed statistical analysis. *Results.* In univariate analysis, distance from anal verge and ten other postoperative variables related with nCRT tumor response had predictive value for Mandard response. In multivariable analysis only mitotic count, necrosis, and differentiation grade in surgical specimen had predictive value. *Conclusions.* There is a lack of clinical and pathological preoperative variables able to predict Mandard response. Only postoperative pathological parameters related with nCRT response have predictive value.

1. Introduction

Neoadjuvant chemoradiotherapy (CRT) followed by total mesorectum excision (TME) surgery and systemic chemotherapy remains the standard of care for locally advanced rectal cancer (LARC), but only a few patients benefit from this treatment modality. Sauer et al. [1] reported a persistent significant improvement of preoperative CRT versus postoperative CRT on local control, although without overall survival improvement, which is only achieved in situations of good or complete pathological response to CRT [2, 3]. Chemoradiation induces tumor downstaging effect, which increases the probability of a complete resection and a sphincter- preserving surgery, benefiting local control. However, some patients still develop distant and/or local recurrence that compromise survival, particularly those with poor pathological tumor response. The histological response to preoperative CRT has been reported in several studies to be closely related to oncologic outcomes [2, 4–7]. A complete pathologic response (pCR), which is characterized by sterilization of all tumor cells, leads to excellent prognosis and is observed in approximately 10% to 30% of cases [8].

The remaining patients exhibit a spectrum of residual disease, ranging from microscopic tumor cell foci on a background of radiation-induced fibrosis to no response at all [9]. The prognostic relevance of pathological tumor response according to several standard grading criteria has been studied extensively [4, 10–13]. In our previous study, the Mandard system proved to be a good determinant of outcome, when cases were grouped into TRG1+2 (good responders) and TRG3+4+5 (bad responders). This methodology proved superior compared to division in groups of ypCR (TRG1) versus all other (TRG2–5) regarding disease-free survival (DFS) and overall survival (OS) [14]. For this reason it would be of great value to predict nCRT-induced histologic regression and tumor shrinkage. The ability to predict the response, either before treatment or during its early stages, could spare "bad responders" patients the expense and stress of undergoing treatment from which they will derive no benefit. Instead, these patients would be candidates for more intensive treatment strategies. Identifying "bad responders" only in posttreatment may also be an indicator for a different and more intensive adjuvant therapy. Nowadays, individualizing the treatment approach in LARC is a demanding goal to achieve.

The present study aims to analyze predictive factors of Mandard tumor response, trying to identify and characterize the "good" and the "bad responders," comparing classic histological data obtained from diagnostic biopsies with histological alterations from surgical specimens after treatment.

2. Materials and Methods

2.1. Patient Population. A single-institution database was queried for consecutive patients with LARC, biopsy-proven rectal adenocarcinoma, who underwent nCRT followed by elective radical surgery with TME with curative intent between January 1, 2003, and December 31, 2013.

Admission Criteria. Patients with rectal cancers located at less than 12 cm of distance from the anal verge and clinical stages cT2N+M0 or cT3/4 N0/+M0 are included.

Exclusion Criteria. Patients with other diagnosed neoplasia, short course RT, yp stage IV, R1/R2 surgery, and death within 60-day postoperative time are excluded.

All patients receiving nCRT who were operated within 8 weeks after radiotherapy conclusion were included in this analysis. Patients receiving short-course radiation were excluded since no downstaging occurs when immediate surgery is carried out.

Staging included rigid proctoscopy, total colonoscopy, chest, abdominal, and pelvic CT scan, endorectal ultrasound (ERUS), pelvic magnetic resonance image (MRI) (since 2008), and carcinoembryonic antigen (CEA) serum levels.

Diagnostic pretreatment paraffin-embedded biopsies of 152 patients (91%) were available and reviewed by an independent element. All of them were characterized in terms of grade, mitotic index (for 10 fields), necrosis grade (scarce/moderate/marked), inflammatory reaction (scarce/moderate/marked), and desmoplastic infiltration (scarce, moderate, and marked). Tumor biopsy samples classification, including grade, were obtained on worst areas whenever available material contained several areas with neoplasia.

Neoadjuvant CRT protocol included total irradiation of 50.4 Gy in 28 fractions and 5-fluorouracil by infusion pump.

Radical surgery consisted mainly in sphincter saving rectal resection (SSRE) or abdominoperineal resection (APR) both with TME. Regarding operative procedure selection, we considered the distance of the lesion to the anus, the comorbidities of the patient, and the condition of the anal sphincter.

The number of samples taken from the resected specimens was variable, with a mean of 6 paraffin blocks per case. The methodology used was the following:

(1) Five samples were from the area with macroscopic lesion (assuming it exists), that is, the same as dealing with a specimen from a patient who has not received neoadjuvant therapy. These included the closest macroscopic approach of the macroscopic lesion to the peritoneal surface and/or the mesorectal excision plane, as appropriate.

(2) If no viable tumour was identified within the initial 5 blocks, the whole of the remainder of any macroscopic lesion in additional blocks was included.

(3) If no viable tumour was identified within the initial or extra blocks, another three further levels from all of these blocks were taken. If no viable tumour was identified in these sections then complete histological tumour regression was assumed.

All obtained slides were seen and reviewed by the same pathologist. Items observed and registered in the biopsies were subsequently analyzed in the resected specimen and the same criteria adopted.

Standard pathologic tumor staging of the resected specimen was performed in accordance with the guidelines of the American Joint Committee on Cancer (AJCC). Circumferential resection margin (CRM) was scored as positive when cancer cells were within 1 mm of the margin. Evidence of ypCR was defined as an absence of viable adenocarcinoma in the surgical specimen or the presence of lakes of mucus without tumor cells.

The histology of all surgical specimens was reviewed and confirmed by an independent element and were classified based on Mandard tumor regression grading system.

Patients were divided in two groups according to Mandard TRG system: good responders were defined as Mandard TRG1 or TRG2; bad responders were defined as Mandard TRG3, TRG4, or TRG5 (Figure 1).

Both groups (good responders *versus* bad responders) were used to evaluate outcome results. Operated patients were subjected to adjuvant chemotherapy protocol for 6 months performed preferably with 5-fluorouracil (5-FU) or a combination 5-FU and oxaliplatinum.

Disease recurrence was evaluated according to location: locoregional (LR), systemic (DR), or mixed.

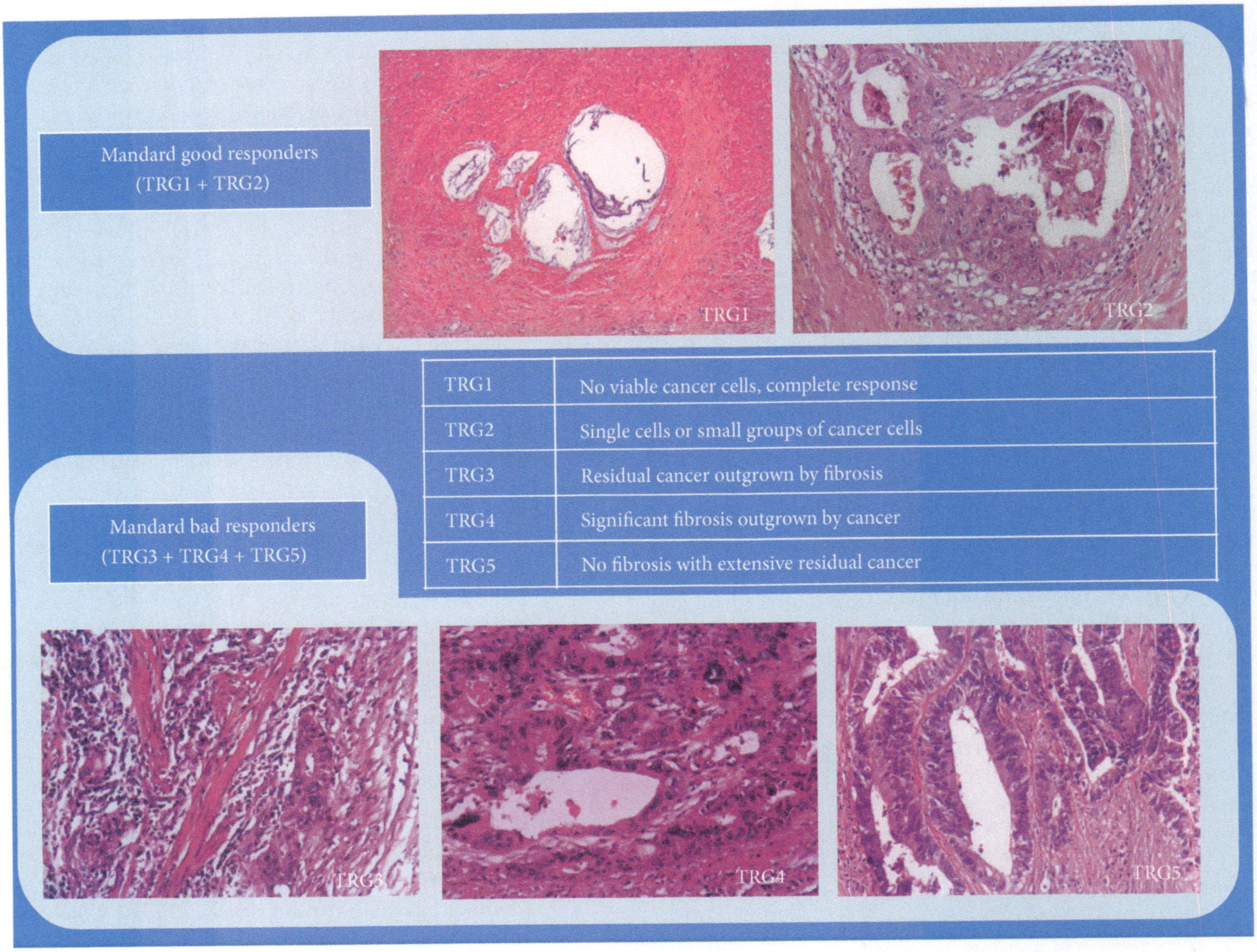

FIGURE 1: Mandard system.

None of the patients were lost for follow-up.

All surviving patients were observed and their current status was confirmed.

Clinical nodal staging may present some inaccuracies; consequently, downstaging evaluation including N stage may introduce some bias, so the term "downstaging" used to describe the efficacy of treatment was defined specifically as T stage downstaging.

Disease-free survival (DFS) was calculated from the date of surgery to the date of progression (local and/or distant), and overall survival (OS) was calculated from the first date of treatment to the date of death or last follow-up.

2.2. Statistical Analysis. The survival function was estimated using the Kaplan-Meier method. The difference in survival rates between groups was tested for significance using the log rank test. The significance of differences in proportions was calculated with Chi-square test and the differences in means with Student's *t*-test. A logistic regression analysis was used to assess the independent significance of factors predictive of response, defined as "good" or "bad" responders (TRG1-2/TRG3–5): age; gender; clinical stage; anal–tumor distance; pretreatment CEA; biopsy specimen characteristics: mitotic index, desmoplastic infiltration, inflammatory reaction, and necrosis; CEA post-CRT; surgical procedure; surgical morbidity; pathological stage; circumferential involvement; tumor grade; tumor mitosis number; tumor desmoplastic infiltration; tumor inflammatory reaction; and tumor necrosis in resected specimen were studied.

The statistical analysis was made with SPSS statistical software (version 21.0 for Windows; SPSS Inc., Chicago, IL). All statistical tests were conducted at a two-sided level of significance of 0.05.

3. Results

3.1. Patient Population. Between January 2003 and December 2013, 186 consecutive patients with LARC were treated with neoadjuvant CRT followed by TME surgery at one single university hospital. We excluded 11 patients with positive radial margin (R1 surgery), 4 patients with yp stage IV, and four deaths within 60 days of postoperative period. In the end, 167 patients were included in the present analysis. Male : female ratio was 1.69 : 1. Median age was 64.6 years (range, 29–83 years). Clinical parameters are summarized in Table 1.

TABLE 1: Clinical parameters.

Variable	N (%)
Age	
Mean	64.62
Range	(29–83)
Gender	
Male	105 (62.9)
Female	62 (37.1)
Tumor length	
<4 cm	41 (24.6)
≥4 cm and <6 cm	85 (50.8)
≥6 cm	41 (24.6)
Tumor circumference	
≤1/3	27 (16.2)
>1/3 and ≤1/2	59 (35.3)
>1/2 and ≤2/3	39 (23.4)
>2/3 and ≤3/3	42 (25.1)
Distance from anal verge	
>6 cm	81 (48.5)
≤6 cm	86 (51.5)
CEA pre-CRT	
<5	116 (69.5)
≥5	44 (26.3)
Missing	7 (4.2)
cT stage	
2-3	152 (91.0)
4	15 (9.0)
Clinical stage	
II	76 (45.5)
III	91 (54.5)
CEA post-CRT	
<5	141 (84.4)
≥5	14 (8.4)
Missing	12 (7.2)
Surgery procedure	
AAR/SSO	107 (64.1)
AAP/others	60 (35.9)
Surgery	
Open	129 (77.2)
Laparoscopic	38 (22.8)
Perioperative complications	42 (25.1)
Morbidity	
Abdominal or pelvic abscess	16 (9.5)
Anastomose leak	3 (1.7)
Reoperation	6 (3.5)
Readmission	3 (1.7)

3.2. Biopsy Characteristics. The biopsy results are shown in Table 2.

The mitotic index is the number of mitoses for 10 high-powered fields and the cut-off was chosen taking into account the best ratio of sensitivity : specificity. If no 10 high-power fields were present with neoplasia, the number of mitoses was counted in the number of observed fields, reducing the final result to 10 fields.

TABLE 2: Biopsies characteristics.

Variable	N (%)
Biopsy	
Grade	
1	46 (27.5)
2	98 (58.7)
3	8 (4.8)
Missing	15 (9.0)
Mucinous presence	
No	145 (86.8)
Yes	7 (4.2)
Missing/not applied	15 (9.0)
Mitosis number	
≤9.5	34 (20.4)
≥9.6	117 (70.0)
Missing/not applied	16 (9.6)
Inflammatory infiltrate	
Scarce	33 (19.8)
Moderated	66 (39.5)
Marked	52 (31.1)
Missing/not applied	16 (9.6)
Desmoplastic reaction	
Scarce	44 (26.3)
Moderated	80 (47.9)
Marked	27 (16.2)
Missing/not applied	16 (9.6)
Necrosis degree	
Scarce	79 (47.3)
Moderated	40 (23.9)
Marked	32 (19.2)
Missing/not applied	16 (9.6)

3.3. Surgery. Sphincter saving rectal resection with anastomosis (with or without protective ileostomy) was performed on 107 patients (64.1%). Abdominoperineal resection was performed on 53 patients, and seven patients were subjected to proctectomy with definitive stoma. The perioperative morbidity of the series was of 25,1% with 16 abdominal or pelvic abscesses, 3 anastomotic leaks, 6 reoperations, and 3 readmissions.

3.4. Pathology. Stage distribution is shown in Table 3.

The average number of dissected lymph nodes in the surgical specimen was 8.2 (range 0–22).

Circumferential resection margin >1 mm was confirmed in all 167 patients. Response to neoadjuvant therapy is characterized in Table 3.

Downstaging and Final Pathologic Stage Classification. T stage downstaging was observed in 67 patients (40.1%). Reduction in T stage by one level was observed in 29 patients (17.4%) and

Table 3: Pathological parameters.

Variable	N (%)
ypT stage	
pT0-1	38 (22.8)
pT2–4	129 (77.2)
ypN stage	
pN0	110 (65.9)
pN1-2	57 (34.1)
Pathological stage	
0	58 (34.7)
II	58 (34.7)
III	51 (30.5)
T downstaging	
Yes	67 (40.1)
No	100 (59.9)
Pathological TNM downstaging	
Yes	95 (56.9)
No	72 (43.1)
CRM distance	
>2 mm	159 (95.2)
≤2 and >1 mm	8 (4.8)
Mandard TRG	
TRG1-2 (good responders)	85 (50.9)
TRG3–5 (bad responders)	82 (49.1)
Other characteristics of resected specimen	
Grade	
0	32 (19.2)
1	31 (18.6)
2	98 (58.7)
3	6 (3.6)
Mucinous presence	
Yes	41 (24.5)
No	126 (75.4)
Inflammatory infiltrate	
Scarce	60 (35.9)
Moderated	75 (44.9)
Marked	28 (16.8)
Missing	4 (2.4)
Desmoplastic reaction	
Scarce	45 (26.9)
Moderated	64 (38.3)
Marked	51 (30.5)
Missing	7 (4.2)
Necrosis grade	
Scarce	27 (16.2)
Moderated	38 (22.8)
Marked	99 (59.3)
Missing	3 (1.8)
Mitosis number	
≤9.5	73 (43.7)
>9.5	68 (40.7)
Missing	26 (15.6)

Table 3: Continued.

Variable	N (%)
Lymphatic permeation	
No	100 (59.9)
Yes	67 (40.1)
Vascular permeation	
No	142 (85)
Yes	25 (15)
Perineural permeation	
No	96 (57.5)
Yes	71 (42.5)
Distal margin	
≥2 cm	108 (65.7)
<2 cm and ≥1 cm	59 (35.3)

by two or more levels in 38 patients (22.8%). Observations indicating pathologic downstaging are given in Table 3. Ninety-five (56.8%) patients presented pathologic stage one or lower pathologic stage than initial clinical tumor stage. Pathologic complete response (ypCR or Mandard TRG1) was confirmed in 31 patients (18.5%).

TRG Classification. The use of Mandard system allowed us to define two groups as previously mentioned: good responders (Mandard TRG1-2) and bad responders (Mandard TRG3–5). Using Mandard system a good response to nCRT was attributed to 85 patients (50.9%) and a bad response was attributed to 82 patients (49.1%).

3.5. Clinical Outcome. Table 4 shows long term clinical outcome, relapse of disease, and survival.

With a median follow-up of 59 months (range, 6–139 months), five-year overall survival was 74.6% and pelvic control was 95.8%. Seven patients (4.2%) developed pelvic recurrence (5 isolated and 2 with synchronous metastatic disease) and 22 (12.6%) distant metastases alone. Mandard TRG3–5 (bad responders) is associated with adverse prognosis.

3.6. Predictive Factors of Mandard Response. A logistic regression analysis was used to assess the independent significance of pre- and on-treatment variables as predictive factors of Mandard good responders (TRG1-2). Table 5 shows the 11 variables with predictive value for Mandard response in univariate analysis.

All were related with tumor downstaging and/or with tumor CRT response except the tumor anal distance. The other variables of Tables 1, 2, and 3 have no significant predictive value.

The eleven variables were entered into the Cox-stepwise likelihood ratio. The selection was based upon their statistical significance in univariate analysis and their potential clinical interaction. In the multivariate analysis, after adjustment for the effects of the other variables, tumor with moderated or poor differentiation grade, scarce or moderated necrosis, and >9.5 mitosis number for 10 high-powered fields were more likely to present a bad response (Table 6).

TABLE 4: Clinical long term outcome (follow-up median: 59 months; range 6–139).

Variable	
Overall disease recurrence	29 (17.3%)
Local	5 (3%)
Distant	22 (13.2%)
Local and distant	2 (1.1%)
Five-year overall survival	74.6% (se = 3.8%)
Five-year overall survival for "good responders"*	88.3% (se = 3.9%)
Five-year overall survival for "bad responders"*	58.3% (se = 6.5%)

*$p < 0.001$ (log rank test).

4. Discussion

Neoadjuvant CRT followed by curative surgery and adjuvant chemotherapy is used in advanced rectal cancer and the prognosis depends essentially on tumor response. This kind of treatment allows a better pelvic disease control, but better prognosis is achieved only in good responders [2].

The variety of tumor responses has increased the need to find a useful predictive model for the response to CRT in order to identify patients who will really benefit from this multimodal treatment.

In our previous studies Mandard TRG system proved to be fairly accurate, and patients division in good (TRG1-2) and bad responders (TRG3-5) proved effective [10, 14]. These results have been confirmed by other groups [2, 12, 15, 16]. Based on those results it would be important to analyze potential clinical and pathological factors that influence Mandard response.

The influence of clinical parameters in tumor response has been widely studied. In some studies, tumor size, tumor circumferential extent, poor differentiation, mucinous tumor, distance from anal verge, clinical T stage, nodal clinical stage, pretreatment carcinoembryonic antigen (CEA) level, and/or interval of time between surgery and radiotherapy completion were associated with CRT tumor response [17–26]. Magnetic resonance imaging (MRI) and positron emission tomography-computed tomography (PET-CT) also may be useful to predict the response at early stages [27–33]. However, no clinical parameters with prediction value of CRT response have been consistently identified. The results are often different [19, 23, 29, 34, 35]. In our series, distance from anal verge is the only clinical parameter in univariate analysis with predictive value for Mandard response: distal tumors (≤6 cm from anal verge) show a better response according to Mandard. This result is concordant with that described by Das et al. [18]. The opposite is described by Restivo et al. [36]. The delay of surgery after radiotherapy completion from 8 to 12 weeks seems to increase tumor necrosis grade and pathological complete response (ypCR) rate up to 30 to 40% [37–40]. We have 18.5% of ypCR but we cannot study this variable because our patients were operated on average within 8 weeks after radiotherapy conclusion. Pretreatment CEA level is probably the most cited clinical parameter as having tumor response predictive value [18, 20, 21, 41–44]. On our study CEA level, other clinical parameters and the biopsy characteristics analyzed did not predict tumor response to nCRT. Biopsy obtained data, namely, differentiation grade, mitotic index, necrosis, inflammatory, and desmoplastic reaction amount, had no utility to recognize or predict tumor behavior. Tumor hypoxia and proliferative cell activity reduce the effectiveness of both radiation therapy and chemotherapy and are a well-known risk factor for tumor radioresistance. So, it was expected that necrosis, grade, and mitotic number in 10 high-power fields could give any indication of CRT tumor response. However in our series it did not occur with a statistically significant correlation. This may be due to several reasons. The amount of tumor in the biopsy is a very small percentage of the total volume of the whole tumor and, as tumors are heterogeneous, biopsy may not be representative of tumor biology. On the other hand, it suggests that other biologic indicators of response must be investigated, because the ones included in this study are not important for this purpose. Finally it must be remembered that tumor is not the unique actor in the process; local and systemic response of the host, immune, and inflammatory factors also need to be considered.

In our data, all predictive factors found are one way or another related with tumor downstaging and/or nCRT tumor response pathological variables found after treatment. This is an expected result. Pathological TNM stage, tumor downstaging, and CMR of surgical specimen are reflected on nCRT tumor response and are considered in many studies prognostic factors of survival [45–49]. In our study the posttreatment differentiation, feasibility, and proliferative activity of tumor cells show greater impact as predictors of Mandard response (more than pathological TNM stage or tumor downstaging). The presence of accentuated necrosis, mitosis number >9.5 for 10 high-powered fields, and moderate or poorly differentiated grade in resected specimen had a predictive value for Mandard response of 85%. Those variables had a significant predictive value of Mandard response in multivariate analysis.

Thus, the only process for assessing nCRT response is obtained from posttreatment variables. The absence of reliable clinical predictors of response to CRT emphasizes the need to find other factors able to predict response and thus individualize the treatment approach in LARC. On this series the Mandard grade response proved useful to modify the adjuvant treatment plan in patients who were "bad responders" into a more aggressive treatment.

5. Conclusions

Mandard system provides an important tool for survival analysis. None of the clinical or the biopsy characteristics assessed had a predictive value of Mandard response, except the distance from anal verge. Only postoperative pathological parameters related with tumor response to chemoradiotherapy have predictive value for Mandard response.

TABLE 5: Predictive value of clinical and pathological characteristics to Mandard response (univariate analysis).

Variables	n	Bad responders % (Mandard TRG 3–5)	Odds ratio	p
Distance from anal verge				
≤6 cm	86	58.0	1.00	0.017
>6 cm	81	39.5	2.11 (1.14–3.92)	
Mitosis number in resected specimen				
≤9.5	73	32.9	1.00	<0.001
≥9.6	68	77.9	7.21 (3.40–15.32)	
Necrosis grade in resected specimen				
Scarce	27	77.8	10.36 (3.76–28.57)	<0.001
Moderate	38	92.1	34.53 (9.76–122.41)	<0.001
Marked	99	25.3	1.00	<0.001
CRM distance				
≥2 mm	159	45.9	1.00	0.003
<2 and >1 mm	8	100	2.18 (1.84–2.58)	
ypT stage				
0-1	38	7.9	1.00	<0.001
2–4	129	60.5	17.84 (5.21–61.09)	
ypN stage				
0	110	32.7	1.00	
1-2	57	78.9	7.71 (3.64–16.34)	<0.001
Pathological stage				
0-I	58	15.5	1.00	<0.001
II	58	55.2	6.70 (2.78–16.14)	<0.001
III	51	78.4	19.80 (7.47–52.48)	<0.001
T downstaging				
Yes	67	23.9	1.00	<0.001
No	100	65.0	5.92	
Pathological TNM downstaging				
Yes	96	34.4	1.00	<0.001
No	70	67.1	3.90	
Reduction of mitosis number				
Yes	83	41.0	1.00	<0.001
No	52	73.1	3.91 (1.84–8.30)	
Differentiation grade in resected specimen				
0 + 1	52	15.4	1.00	<0.001
2 + 3	115	63.5	9.56	

TABLE 6: Multivariate stepwise model-dependent variable Mandard response: "0" good response and "1" bad response.

Variable	Odds ratio	Confidence interval 95%	p
Differentiation grade in resected specimen			
0 + 1	1.00	3.38–32.30	<0.001
2 + 3	10.45		
Necrosis grade in resected specimen			
Marked	1.00	3.04–25.54	<0.001
Scarce/moderate	8.82		
Mitosis number in resected specimen			
≤9.5	1.00	1.52–10.90	0.005
≥9.6	4.07		

Based on these results it is not yet possible to identify the group of patients who truly benefits from neoadjuvant CRT, but we can identify the group of patients (the Mandard bad responders) that will benefit with a more aggressive adjuvant treatment.

Conflict of Interests

The authors of the paper do not have any financial relation or any financial interest with the subject matter or materials discussed in this paper.

References

[1] R. Sauer, T. Liersch, S. Merkel et al., "Preoperativeversus postoperative chemoradiotherapy for locally advanced rectal cancer: results of the German CAO/ARO/AIO -94 randomized phase III trial afteramedian follow-up of 11 years," *Journal of Clinical Oncology*, vol. 30, no. 16, pp. 1926–1933, 2012.

[2] Y.-C. Lee, C.-C. Hsieh, and J.-P. Chuang, "Prognostic significance of partial tumor regression after preoperative chemoradiotherapy for rectal cancer: a meta-analysis," *Diseases of the Colon & Rectum*, vol. 56, no. 9, pp. 1093–1101, 2013.

[3] S. T. Martin, H. M. Heneghan, and D. C. Winter, "Systematic review and meta-analysis of outcomes following pathological complete response to neoadjuvant chemoradiotherapy for rectal cancer," *British Journal of Surgery*, vol. 99, no. 7, pp. 918–928, 2012.

[4] C. Rodel, P. Martus, and T. Papadoupolos, "Prognostic significance of tumor regression after preoperative chemoradiotherapy for rectal cancer," *Journal of Clinical Oncology*, vol. 23, no. 34, pp. 8688–8696, 2005.

[5] P. Roy, S. Serra, E. Kennedy, and R. Chetty, "The prognostic value of grade of regression and oncocytic change in rectal adenocarcinoma treated with neo-adjuvant chemoradiotherapy," *Journal of Surgical Oncology*, vol. 105, no. 2, pp. 130–134, 2012.

[6] L. Topova, G. Hellmich, E. Puffer et al., "Prognostic value of tumor response to neoadjuvant therapy in rectal carcinoma," *Diseases of the Colon and Rectum*, vol. 54, no. 4, pp. 401–411, 2011.

[7] F. M. Vecchio, V. Valentini, B. D. Minsky et al., "The relationship of pathologic tumor regression grade (TRG) and outcomes after preoperative therapy in rectal cancer," *International Journal of Radiation Oncology, Biology, Physics*, vol. 62, pp. 752–760, 2005.

[8] J. M. D. Wheeler, E. Dodds, B. F. Warren et al., "Preoperative chemoradiotherapy and total mesorectal excision surgery for locally advanced rectal cancer: correlation with rectal cancer regression grade," *Diseases of the Colon & Rectum*, vol. 47, no. 12, pp. 2025–2031, 2004.

[9] A.-M. Mandard, F. Dalibard, J.-C. Mandard et al., "Pathologic assessment of tumor regression after preoperative chemoradiotherapy of esophageal carcinoma: clinicopathologic correlations," *Cancer*, vol. 73, no. 11, pp. 2680–2686, 1994.

[10] M. D. Santos, C. Silva, A. Rocha, E. Matos, C. Nogueira, and C. Lopes, "Prognostic value of Mandard and Dworak tumor regression grading in rectal cancer: study of a single tertiary center," *ISRN Surgery*, vol. 2014, Article ID 310542, 8 pages, 2014.

[11] A. C. Bateman, E. Jaynes, and A. R. Bateman, "Rectal cancer staging post neoadjuvant therapy—how should the changes be assessed?" *Histopathology*, vol. 54, no. 6, pp. 713–721, 2009.

[12] D. Beddy, J. M. P. Hyland, D. C. Winter et al., "A simplified tumor regression grade correlates with survival in locally advanced rectal carcinoma treated with neoadjuvant chemoradiotherapy," *Annals of Surgical Oncology*, vol. 15, no. 12, pp. 3471–3477, 2008.

[13] T. P. MacGregor, T. S. Maughan, and R. A. Sharma, "Pathological grading of regression following neoadjuvant chemoradiation therapy: the clinical need is now," *Journal of Clinical Pathology*, vol. 65, no. 10, pp. 867–871, 2012.

[14] M. D. Santos, C. Silva, A. Rocha, E. Matos, C. Nogueira, and C. Lopes, "Tumor regression grades: can they influence rectal cancer therapy decision tree?" *International Journal of Surgical Oncology*, vol. 2013, Article ID 572149, 8 pages, 2013.

[15] J. Suárez, R. Vera, E. Balén et al., "Pathologic response assessed by Mandard grade is a better prognostic factor than down staging for disease-free survival after preoperative radiochemotherapy for advanced rectal cancer," *Colorectal Disease*, vol. 10, no. 6, pp. 563–568, 2008.

[16] M. Huebner, B. G. Wolff, T. C. Smyrk, J. Aakre, and D. W. Larson, "Partial pathologic response and nodal status as most significant prognostic factors for advanced rectal cancer treated with preoperative chemoradiotherapy," *World Journal of Surgery*, vol. 36, no. 3, pp. 675–683, 2012.

[17] B. Farnault, L. Moureau-Zabotto, C. de Chaisemartin et al., "Predictive factors of tumour response after neoadjuvant chemoradiation for locally advanced rectal cancer and correlation of these factors with survival," *Cancer/Radiothérapie*, vol. 15, no. 4, pp. 279–286, 2011.

[18] P. Das, J. M. Skibber, M. A. Rodrigues-Bigas et al., "Predictors of tumor response and downstaging in patients who receive preoperative chemoradiation for rectal cancer," *Cancer*, vol. 109, no. 9, pp. 1750–1755, 2007.

[19] K.-L. Yang, S.-H. Yang, W.-Y. Liang et al., "Carcinoembryonic antigen (CEA) level, CEA ratio, and treatment outcome of rectal cancer patients receiving pre-operative chemoradiation and surgery," *Radiation Oncology*, vol. 8, article 43, 2013.

[20] H. Yan, R. Wang, K. Zhu et al., "Predictors of sensitivity to preoperative chemoradiotherapy of rectal adenocarcinoma," *Tumori*, vol. 97, no. 6, pp. 717–723, 2011.

[21] S.-G. Yeo, D. Y. Kim, H. J. Chang et al., "Reappraisal of pretreatment carcinoembryonic antigen in patients with rectal cancer receiving preoperative chemoradiotherapy," *Tumori*, vol. 99, no. 1, pp. 93–99, 2013.

[22] D. Tural, F. Selcukbiricik, M. A. Özturk et al., "The relation between pathological complete response and clinical outcome in patients with rectal cancer," *Hepatogastroenterology*, vol. 60, no. 126, pp. 1365–1370, 2013.

[23] H.-Z. Qiu, B. Wu, Y. Xiao, and G.-L. Lin, "Combination of differentiation and T stage can predict unresponsiveness to neoadjuvant therapy for rectal cancer," *Colorectal Disease*, vol. 13, no. 12, pp. 1353–1360, 2011.

[24] K. Oberholzer, M. Menig, A. Kreft et al., "Rectal cancer: mucinous carcinoma on magnetic resonance imaging indicates poor response to neoadjuvant chemoradiation," *International Journal of Radiation Oncology, Biology, Physics*, vol. 82, no. 2, pp. 842–848, 2012.

[25] H. Tulchinsky, E. Shmueli, A. Figer, J. M. Klausner, and M. Rabau, "An interval >7 weeks between neoadjuvant therapy and surgery improves pathologic complete response and disease-free survival in patients with locally advanced rectal cancer," *Annals of Surgical Oncology*, vol. 15, no. 10, pp. 2661–2667, 2008.

[26] J. W. Huh, H. R. Kim, and Y. J. Kim, "Clinical prediction of pathological complete response after preoperative chemoradiotherapy for rectal cancer," *Diseases of the Colon and Rectum*, vol. 56, no. 6, pp. 698–703, 2013.

[27] D. W. Dietz, F. Dehdashti, P. W. Grigsby et al., "Tumor hypoxia detected by positron emission tomography with 60Cu-ATSM as a predictor of response and survival in patients undergoing neoadjuvant chemoradiotherapy for rectal carcinoma: a pilot study," *Diseases of the Colon & Rectum*, vol. 51, no. 11, pp. 1641–1648, 2008.

[28] X. Meng, Z. Huang, R. Wang, and J. Yu, "Prediction of response to preoperative chemoradiotherapy in patients with locally advanced rectal cancer," *BioScience Trends*, vol. 8, no. 1, pp. 11–23, 2014.

[29] J. W. Kim, H. C. Kim, J. W. Park et al., "Predictive value of ^{18}FDG PET-CT for tumour response in patients with locally advanced rectal cancer treated by preoperative chemoradiotherapy," *International Journal of Colorectal Disease*, vol. 28, no. 9, pp. 1217–1224, 2013.

[30] H. Everaert, A. Hoorens, C. Vanhove et al., "Prediction of response to neoadjuvant radiotherapy in patients with locally advanced rectal cancer by means of sequential 18FDG-PET," *International Journal of Radiation Oncology Biology Physics*, vol. 80, no. 1, pp. 91–96, 2011.

[31] D. Ippolito, L. Monguzzi, L. Guerra et al., "Response to neoadjuvant therapy in locally advanced rectal cancer: assessment with diffusion-weighted MR imaging and 18FDG PET/CT," *Abdominal Imaging*, vol. 37, no. 6, pp. 1032–1040, 2012.

[32] S. H. Jung, S. H. Heo, J. W. Kim et al., "Predicting response to neoadjuvant chemoradiation therapy in locally advanced rectal cancer: diffusion-weighted 3 tesla MR imaging," *Journal of Magnetic Resonance Imaging*, vol. 35, no. 1, pp. 110–116, 2012.

[33] S. Shanmugan, R. Arrangoiz, J. R. Nitzkorski et al., "Predicting pathological response to neoadjuvant chemoradiotherapy in locally advanced rectal cancer using ^{18}FDG-PET/CT," *Annals of Surgical Oncology*, vol. 19, no. 7, pp. 2178–2185, 2012.

[34] D. J. Kim, J. H. Kim, J. S. Lim et al., "Restaging of rectal cancer with MR imaging after concurrent chemotherapy and radiation therapy," *Radiographics*, vol. 30, no. 2, pp. 503–516, 2010.

[35] C. H. Choi, W. D. Kim, S. J. Lee, and W. Y. Park, "Clinical predictive factors of pathologic tumor response after preoperative chemoradiotherapy in rectal cancer," *Radiation Oncology Journal*, vol. 30, no. 3, pp. 99–107, 2012.

[36] A. Restivo, L. Zorcolo, I. M. F. Cocco et al., "Elevated CEA levels and low distance of the tumor from the anal verge are predictors of incomplete response to chemoradiation in patients with rectal cancer," *Annals of Surgical Oncology*, vol. 20, no. 3, pp. 864–871, 2013.

[37] L. F. de Campos-Lobato, D. P. Geisler, A. da Luz Moreira, L. Stocchi, D. Dietz, and M. F. Kalady, "Neoadjuvant therapy for rectal cancer: the impact of longer interval between chemoradiation and surgery," *Journal of Gastrointestinal Surgery*, vol. 15, no. 3, pp. 444–450, 2011.

[38] A. Habr-Gama, R. O. Perez, I. Proscurshim et al., "Interval between surgery and neoadjuvant chemoradiation therapy for distal rectal cancer: does delayed surgery have an impact on outcome?" *International Journal of Radiation Oncology, Biology, Physics*, vol. 71, no. 4, pp. 1181–1188, 2008.

[39] J. Garcia-Aguilar, D. D. Smith, K. Avila, E. K. Bergsland, P. Chu, and R. M. Krieg, "Optimal timing of surgery after chemoradiation for advanced rectal cancer: preliminary results of a multicenter, nonrandomized phase II prospective trial," *Annals of Surgery*, vol. 254, no. 1, pp. 97–102, 2011.

[40] C. G. Willett and B. G. Czito, "Impact of time duration after neoadjuvant therapy to surgery on response and outcome in rectal cancer patients," *Annals of Surgical Oncology*, vol. 15, no. 10, pp. 2636–2638, 2008.

[41] Y.-J. Kim, S. C. Park, D. Y. Kim et al., "No correlation between pretreatment serum CEA levels and tumor volume in locally advanced rectal cancer patients," *Clinica Chimica Acta*, vol. 413, no. 3-4, pp. 511–515, 2012.

[42] L. Moureau-Zabotto, B. Farnault, C. de Chaisemartin et al., "Predictive factors of tumor response after neoadjuvant chemoradiation for locally advanced rectal cancer," *International Journal of Radiation Oncology Biology Physics*, vol. 80, no. 2, pp. 483–491, 2011.

[43] D. Tural, F. Selcukbiricik, M. A. Özturk et al., "The relation between pathological complete response and clinical outcome in patients with rectal cancer," *Hepato-Gastroenterology*, vol. 60, no. 126, pp. 1365–1370, 2013.

[44] U. Wallin, D. Rothenberger, A. Lowry, R. Luepker, and A. Mellgren, "CEA—a predictor for pathologic complete response after neoadjuvant therapy for rectal cancer," *Diseases of the Colon & Rectum*, vol. 56, no. 7, pp. 859–868, 2013.

[45] S.-G. Yeo, D. Y. Kim, T. H. Kim et al., "Pathologic complete response of primary tumor following preoperative chemoradiotherapy for locally advanced rectal cancer: long-term outcomes and prognostic significance of pathologic nodal status (KROG 09-01)," *Annals of Surgery*, vol. 252, no. 6, pp. 998–1004, 2010.

[46] S.-G. Yeo, D. Y. Kim, J. W. Park et al., "Stage-to-stage comparison of preoperative and postoperative chemoradiotherapy for T3 mid or distal rectal cancer," *International Journal of Radiation Oncology Biology Physics*, vol. 82, no. 2, pp. 856–862, 2012.

[47] A. K. P. Chan, A. Wong, D. Jenken, J. Heine, D. Buie, and D. Johnson, "Posttreatment TNM staging is a prognostic indicator of survival and recurrence in tethered or fixed rectal carcinoma after preoperative chemotherapy and radiotherapy," *International Journal of Radiation Oncology, Biology, Physics*, vol. 61, no. 3, pp. 665–677, 2005.

[48] H. M. Quah, J. F. Chou, M. Gonen et al., "Pathologic stage is most prognostic of disease-free survival in locally advanced rectal cancer patients after preoperative chemoradiation," *Cancer*, vol. 113, pp. 57–64, 2008.

[49] P. Luna-Pérez, E. Bustos-Cholico, I. Alvarado et al., "Prognostic significance of circumferential margin involvement in rectal adenocarcinoma treated with preoperative chemoradiotherapy and low anterior resection," *Journal of Surgical Oncology*, vol. 90, no. 1, pp. 20–25, 2005.

5

Immunohistochemical Investigation of HER/AKT/mTOR Pathway and Cellular Adhesion Molecules in Urothelial Carcinomas

Nikolaos Koletsas,[1] Triantafyllia Koletsa,[2] Spyros Choidas,[1] Konstantinos Anagnostopoulos,[3] Stavros Touloupidis,[4] Thomas Zaramboukas,[2] Georgia Raptou,[2] Nikolaos Papadopoulos,[5] and Maria Lambropoulou[5]

[1] *Urology Department, Interbalkan Medical Center, Thessaloniki, Greece*
[2] *Pathology Department, Medical School, Aristotle University of Thessaloniki, Thessaloniki, Greece*
[3] *Laboratory of Biochemistry, School of Medicine, Democritus University of Thrace, Alexandroupolis, Greece*
[4] *Urology Department, School of Medicine, Democritus University of Thrace, Alexandroupolis, Greece*
[5] *Laboratory of Histology-Embryology, School of Medicine, Democritus University of Thrace, Alexandroupolis, Greece*

Correspondence should be addressed to Triantafyllia Koletsa; koletsa@med.auth.gr

Academic Editor: Marco Volante

Background. Several investigators have suggested the possibility that the expression of both EGFR and HER2 could be utilized for molecularly targeted therapy in urinary bladder cancer. We tried to evaluate the expression of HER2 and EGFR and activation of the AKT/PTEN/mTOR pathway in urothelial carcinomas and if there is any association between them and cellular adhesion molecules (CAMs). *Materials and Methods.* Forty-one paraffin-embedded urothelial cancer tissue blocks were collected. Immunostains for HER2, EGFR, MIB1, phospho-AKT, PTEN, phospho-mTOR, e-cadherin, p-cadherin, and b-catenin were performed on tissue microarrays sections. The immunohistochemical results were correlated with clinicopathological parameters. *Results.* The overexpression of HER2 was found in 19.6% of the cases and it was associated with high grade tumors with a high mitotic index and phosphorylation of AKT and mTOR. Muscle-invasive tumors presented both cytoplasmic and nuclear losses of PTEN expression. There was no association between HER/AKT/mTOR pathway activation and CAM expression. Although cadherins were often coexpressed, only p-cadherin immunoreactivity was associated with tumor grade and high proliferative index. *Conclusions.* HER2 overexpression is found in a respective proportion of urothelial carcinomas. P-cadherin expression is associated with high grade UCs but it is not affected by HER2 overexpression or by activation of HER/AKT/mTOR pathway.

1. Background

The human epidermal growth factor receptors (HER) protein family consists of four different transmembrane receptors (HER1–HER4). HER1/EGFR and HER2/c-erb-B2 are the most thoroughly investigated family members and have been documented to be involved in the pathogenesis of several types of cancers. In urothelial carcinomas HER1 and HER2 expression has been implicated in tumor aggressiveness, poor outcome, or even pathogenesis [1–4]. In recent years, their importance has been emphasized due to the development of targeted anti-HER therapy.

The dimerization of HER members leads to the activation of intracellular RAS/MEK/ERK [5] and PI3K/AKT/PTEN/mTOR [6, 7] pathways which plays an important role in cell proliferation, angiogenesis, invasion, and metastasis. The PI3K/AKT/PTEN/mTOR pathway is considered to be essential for cell growth, survival, cell motility, and angiogenesis [8–11]. The activation of this pathway has been implicated in carcinogenesis or malignant potential of several cancers, including urothelial ones [12, 13].

The categorization of urothelial carcinomas is based on grading and muscle invasion. The majority of urothelial carcinomas are noninvasive tumors of low grade [14]. Muscle invasion carcinomas are characterized by mutations in TP53, RB1, and PIK3CA genes and deletions in PTEN gene [4, 15] and loss of e-cadherin [16]. Cell adhesion molecules (CAMs) are required for maintaining a normal epithelial phenotype and abnormalities in their expression have been related to cancer progression [16].

The present study was conducted to investigate the expression of EGFR and HER2 proteins, as well as intracellular signaling molecules in sections of urothelial carcinomas by immunohistochemistry, to analyze e-cadherin, p-cadherin, and b-catenin expression in low and high grade urothelial carcinomas, and to correlate the immunohistochemical results with clinicopathologic parameters.

2. Materials and Methods

A total of 41 archived cases of urothelial bladder carcinomas were included in this study. Clinical data and complete follow-up were known in 23 patients. The pertinent hematoxylin and eosin (HE) stained sections were retrieved and reevaluated by pathologist and the representative neoplastic areas corresponding to tumor classification and grading were marked for tissue microarrays formation.

2.1. Construction of Tissue Microarrays (TMAs). Formalin-fixed paraffin-embedded (FFPE) tissue samples from urothelial tumors (paraffin blocks) were collected retrospectively. TMA blocks were constructed with the Alphelys Minicore 3 Tissue Microarray system (Plaisir, France). Each tumor was represented by 3 tissue cores, 1 mm in diameter, which were obtained from the marked representative areas of neoplasms and reembedded in recipient paraffin blocks. TMAs also contained cores from placenta, tonsil and normal thyroid, breast, and renal and colon tissue, used as control markers and for section orientation. Four-micrometer-thick sections were obtained and stained by immunohistochemical (IHC) method.

2.2. Immunohistochemistry. IHC staining was performed on freshly cut sections. Primary antibodies against HER2 (polyclonal, Dako, Glostrup, Denmark), EGFR (clone 31G7, Invitrogen, Carlsbad, CA, USA), phospho-AKT 1/2/3 (Thr308)-R (polyclonal, Santa Cruz Biotechnology, Santa Cruz, CA, USA), PTEN (clone 6h2.1, Dako, Denmark), phospho-mTOR (Ser2448) (clone 49F9, Cell Signaling Technology, Danvers, MA, USA), Ki67 (clone MIB1, Dako, Denmark), E-cadherin (#610181, BD Transduction Laboratories, San Jose, CA, USA), and beta-catenin (#610153, BD Transduction Laboratories, San Jose, CA, USA) were used. IHC stains were performed on a Bond automated stainer (Dako).

2.3. Immunohistochemical Evaluation. There is no standard protocol or guidelines for the estimation of HER2 expression in urothelial carcinomas or what the most appropriate cutoff value is. The HER2 immunostain scoring was performed based on the guidelines of the American Society of Clinical Oncology/College of American Pathologist (0: no staining, 1+: incomplete membranous staining, 2+: complete but weak or moderate membranous staining in >10% of cells, and 3+: strong membranous staining in more than 10% of the cells) [17]. There is no standard protocol for EGFR evaluation. EGFR expression was considered as positive when complete membrane positivity was observed in a percentage of >10% of the cells, as it was used before [18]. For phospho-AKT (pAKT) and PTEN both percentage of positive cells and intensity for nuclear and cytoplasmic immunoreaction were evaluated. The percentage of positive tumor cells (0–100%) was multiplied by dominant staining intensity (1: weak, 2: medium, and 3: intense) and a cutoff value based on the median tumor H-score was used, as described by Gonzalez-Roibon et al. [19]. phospho-mTOR (pmTOR) immunostaining was considered negative when expression was observed in <10% of cells and positive if immunoreactivity was found in ≥10% of cells [20]. A tumor was considered to have a high mitotic index when there were positive cells to Ki67/MIB1 antibody in a percentage of >20%.

TABLE 1: Clinicopathologic characteristics of the tumors.

	N	%
pTa	22	53.6
pT1	6	14.7
pT2	9	21.9
pT3	2	4.9
pT4	2	4.9
Low grade	19	46.3
High grade	22	53.7
<3 cm	24	58.5
≥3 cm	17	41.5
One lesion	20	48.8
Multifocal	17	41.4
Missing data	4	9.8

In 35 cases with adequate specimen immunohistochemistry for CAM expression was also applied. Eighteen out of 35 tumors were of high grade while only ten were invasive. Tumors with positive cells in a percentage >10% was considered positive for e-cadherin, p-cadherin, and b-catenin. According to the intensity of staining tumors were categorized as weak, moderate, and strong [21].

2.4. Statistical Analysis. The statistical software package SPSS v. 21 was used for statistical analyses. Chi-square test was employed to test the dependence between different parameters. Values of 0.05 or less were considered to be statistically significant.

3. Results

3.1. Clinicopathological Characteristics of Patients. Forty-one patients were included in the study, 32 males and 9 females. Their mean age was 68 years (range 47–87). Tumor characteristics are presented in Table 1. Nineteen of the carcinomas were low grade (46.3%) while 22 (53.7%) were of high grade. All tumors with advanced stage were of high grade. Almost one-third of the cases were muscle-invasive tumors. Patients with stages pTa and pT1 were treated either with epirubicin or BCG depending on histological grade, tumor size, and multiplicity. Radical cystectomy was followed for those patients with invasive tumors. Chemotherapy was added in two cases with metastatic disease. A third patient underwent only radiotherapy due to the small size of a solitary lesion located on the frontal bladder wall.

3.2. Immunohistochemical Distribution of the Markers. The immunohistochemical results are summarized in Table 2. HER2 overexpression (3+) was found in 8 cases (19.6%), seven of which were of high grade ($p = 0.032$). HER2 2+ and 3+ immunoscores accounted for almost 46.4% and were mainly found in high grade tumors ($p = 0.179$). Sixty percent of HER2 3+ tumors measured more than 3 cm ($p = 0.039$). HER2 expression exhibited positive correlation with pAKT cytoplasmic and nuclear immunoreactivity ($p = 0.049$ and $p = 0.021$, resp.) (Figure 1). Moreover, in 12 out of 19 HER2 positive cases, pmTOR was coexpressed ($p = 0.021$). The majority of the HER2 positive cases had high mitotic index ($p = 0.021$), defined as >20% positive cells to Ki67/MIB1 antibody.

HER2/EGFR coexpression was observed in four cases (9.75%). There was no association between EGFR expression (14/41, 34.14%) or HER2/EGFR coexpression (4/41, 9.75%) and the examined clinicopathologic parameters (x^2, $p > 0.05$).

Fifteen out of eighteen high grade cases (83.3%) presented high mitotic indices ($p = 0.001$). MIB1 positivity was associated with HER2 positivity ($p = 0.021$) and pmTOR cytoplasmic ($p = 0.035$) expression ($p < 0.001$).

Loss of PTEN cytoplasmic expression was found mainly in muscle-invasive tumors ($p = 0.001$) (Table 3). A loss of PTEN expression was defined as simultaneous lack of nuclear and cytoplasmic immunoreactivity. Muscle-invasive tumors presented commonly a loss of PTEN expression ($p = 0.023$). None of the cases without cytoplasmic PTEN staining exhibited cytoplasmic expression of pAKT ($p = 0.032$). PTEN cytoplasmic expression was positively associated with the cytoplasmic expression of pmTOR protein ($p = 0.01$). However, lack of PTEN nuclear immunoreactivity was not associated with any of the other studied markers, apart from a trend of negative association observed with pAKT nuclear expression ($p = 0.09$). In three cases PTEN was immunoreactive in membranes, as well.

The majority of the muscle-invasive tumors (pT2–pT4) (9/13, 69.2%) expressed pmTOR protein compared to pTa-pT1 urothelial carcinomas ($p = 0.045$) (Table 3). Cytoplasmic pmTOR expression was associated with high MIB1 labeling index ($p = 0.035$) and neoplastic invasion ($p = 0.045$). Notably, membranous immunoreactivity to pmTOR was found in seven cases.

In this cohort, HER2 overexpression along with pAKT nuclear expression, both nuclear and cytoplasmic PTEN deletion and pmTOR expression, was found in three of the patients. Two of them coexpressed the EGFR protein, and they had the worst prognosis.

Expression of e-cadherin and p-cadherin was observed in 54.3% (19/35) and 41.2% (14/34) of the cases, respectively (Table 2). There was no association between CAM expression and tumor size (Table 3) or aggressive behavior (x^2, $p > 0.05$).

Table 2: Immunohistochemical distribution of the examined markers.

	N	%
HER2		
0	8	19.5
1+	14	34.1
2+	11	26.8
3+	8	19.6
EGFR		
Negative	27	65.9
Positive	14	34.1
pAKT nuclear		
Negative	17	41.5
Positive	24	58.5
pAKT cytoplasmic		
Negative	29	70.7
Positive	12	29.3
PTEN cytoplasmic		
Negative	19	47.5
Positive	21	52.5
Missing data	1	—
PTEN nuclear		
Negative	31	77.5
Positive	9	22.5
Missing data	1	—
PTEN nuclear/cytoplasmic		
Negative	10	25
Positive	30	75
Missing data	1	—
pmTOR		
Negative	19	46.3
Positive	22	53.7
MIB1		
≤20	23	56.1
>20	18	43.9
e-cadherin		
Negative	16	45.7
Positive	19	54.3
Missing data	6	—
p-cadherin		
Negative	20	58.8
Positive	14	41.2
Missing data	7	—
b-catenin		
Negative	10	28.6
Positive	25	71.4
Missing data	6	—

Fifteen out of 19 tumors with stage pTa were negative to p-cadherin antibody, reflecting a trend of association between stage and protein expression of this marker (x^2, $p = 0.07$). A positive association was observed between e-cadherin and p-cadherin expression ($p = 0.002$) (Figure 2). The majority

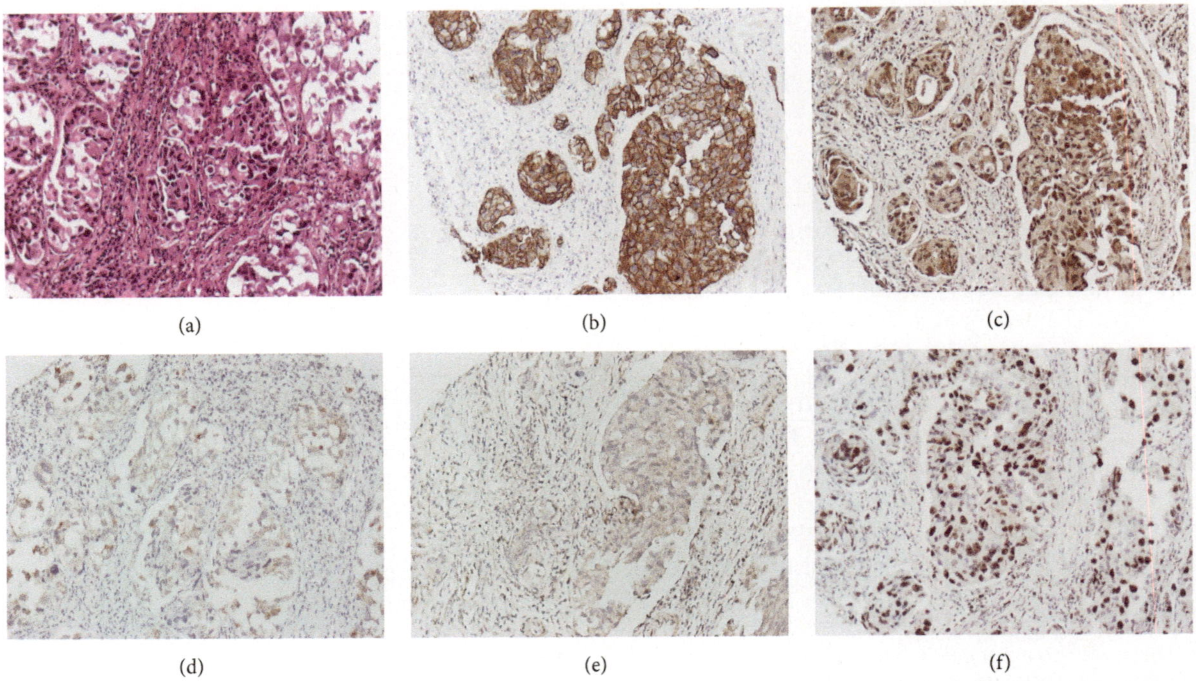

Figure 1: A case of high grade infiltrative urothelial carcinoma (a) presenting HER2 overexpression (b), pAKT (c) and pmTOR (d) expression, loss of PTEN expression (e), and high MIB1 labeling index (f). ((a) HE ×200; (b–f) IHC ×200).

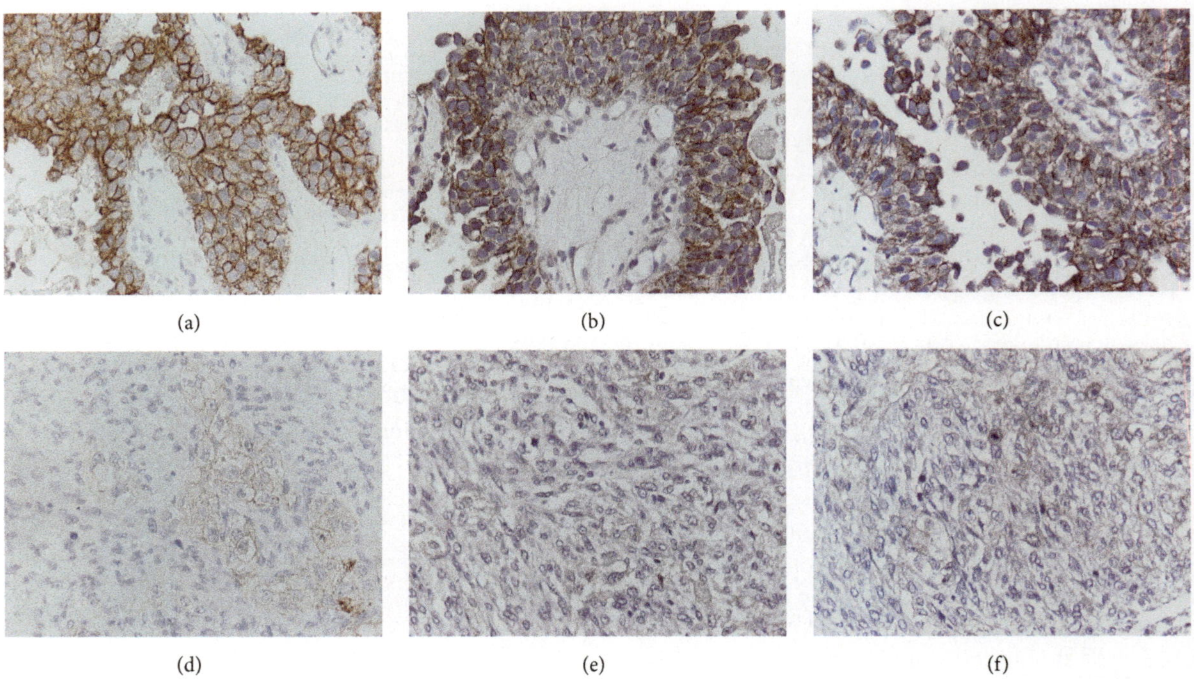

Figure 2: CAM expression in different urothelial tumors. A case of noninfiltrative high grade urothelial carcinoma positive for e-cadherin (a), p-cadherin (b), and b-catenin (c) markers, in contrast to high grade infiltrative urothelial carcinoma with sarcomatoid features, exhibited no or weak expression in few cells to e-cadherin (d), p-cadherin (e), and b-catenin (f) antibodies ((a–f) IHC ×400).

of the cases (25/35, 71.4%) expressed b-catenin. E-cadherin and p-cadherin positive tumors were mainly of high grade (x^2, $p = 0.037$ and $p = 0.002$, resp.). P-cadherin expression was mostly found in tumors with high mitotic indices (MIB1 > 20%) (x^2, $p = 0.007$). There was no association between CAM expression and muscle-invasive tumors (x^2, $p > 0.05$), pointing out the small sample of the tumors examined for these adhesion molecules. Of note, a case of sarcomatoid carcinoma included in the study exhibited no immunoreactivity to antibodies for CAMs (Figure 2).

TABLE 3: Immunoexpression of the markers according to tumors invasiveness.

	Muscle-invasive UC (pT2–pT4)	Non-muscle-invasive UC (pTa-pT1)	p value
HER2			
0	4	4	
1	3	11	0.252
2	2	9	
3	4	4	
EGFR			
Negative	10	17	0.308
Positive	3	11	
pAKT			
Nuclear positive	16	8	0.790
Nuclear negative	5	12	
pAKT			
Cytopl positive	2	9	0.315
Cytopl negative	11	19	
pmTOR			
Negative	9	10	**0.045**
Positive	4	18	
PTEN			
Nuclear positive	1	8	
Nuclear negative	12	19	0.120
Missing data	0	1	
PTEN			
Cytopl positive	3	18	
Cytopl negative	10	9	**0.01**
Missing data	0	1	
e-cadherin			
Negative	4	12	
Positive	6	13	0.668
Missing data	3	3	
p-cadherin			
Negative	4	16	
Positive	5	9	0.307
Missing data	4	3	
b-catenin			
Negative	2	8	
Positive	8	17	0.518
Missing data	3	3	

Cytopl: cytoplasmic; UC: urothelial carcinomas.

4. Discussion

Over the last decade, two of the HER family members, HER1/EGFR and HER2, have been researched extensively in the context of various types of cancer. Apart from their role in tumor proliferation, infiltration, and metastatic potential [22], the increasing interest in them derives from being targets of newly developed and FDA approved therapies. HER2 expression in urothelial carcinomas has been reported in several percentages ranging from 9% to 74.8% [23–25]. This discrepancy is mainly attributed to the differences in the used cutoffs and the constitution of cohorts, that is, the aggressiveness of the cases included in a study.

Notably, many studies defined HER2 overexpression as both HER2 2+ and 3+ immunoscores in urothelial carcinomas [25], as opposed to breast carcinomas. Scoring of the HercepTest corresponds to the number of extracellular domains located in the membrane [26]. In several types of cancer, such as breast carcinomas or gastric/gastroesophageal carcinomas, there are guidelines for protein expression evaluation and criteria for determining overexpression [17, 27, 28]. In urothelial carcinomas there are varying methods and cutoffs used by several studies. However, in a large cohort, Laé et al. [25] found that a true HER2 overexpression in bladder carcinomas corresponded to HER2 gene amplification, being defined in the same way as in breast cancer.

In the present study, HER2 3+ was observed in 19.6% of the cases, while HER2 2+ and 3+ account for 46.4%. The observed association between tumor grade and HER2 expression has been previously well documented [29, 30]. In addition, the aforementioned associations between HER2 expression and tumor size, pAKT, and pmTOR expression indicate that the PI3K/AKT/mTOR pathway could be activated by HER dimerization. Indeed, cases with HER2 overexpression (HER2 3+) were of high grade and they were usually characterized by pAKT and pmTOR protein overexpression and PTEN nuclear deletion. This was the immunophenotypic profile of the tumors of the two patients that presented the worst prognosis in this study. In one of these tumors, EGFR coexpression was also observed, which suggests that both AKT/PTEN/TOR and RAS/MEK/ERK pathways were activated. The increased interest to personalize therapy leads to a thorough investigation of patients who will benefit the most from a particular treatment. Hence, these patients could be the most appropriate candidates for targeted therapy, when conventional therapy fails, taking into account the side effects of these therapeutic options [31].

PTEN deletion affected more often the nucleus than the cytoplasm, a finding in line with those of previous reported studies [32, 33], and it could be found in noninfiltrating tumors but it occurs more often in muscle-invasive ones [34–36]. PTEN deletion is also observed in tumors without HER/AKT/mTOR pathway activation [35, 37], as found in our study, suggesting that PTEN loss is not always responsible for AKT activation, adding that it may be involved in other pathways [37], as it is known that different intracellular pathways are linked through cross-talking [38] or that synergistic action of different pathways is essential for carcinogenesis or aggressive biological behavior [39].

It has been reported that inactivation of p53 and inactivation of PTEN are the principal adverse prognostic markers [40]. In addition, PTEN deletion in combination with altered p53 leads to deregulation of the mTOR pathway and, consequently, reinforces the use of newly therapeutic agents, such as rapamycin [41], everolimus (RAD001) [42], or a combination of mTOR and PI3K inhibitors [43–45].

The cadherins are a group of membrane glycoprotein and the mediators of cell to cell adhesion. E-cadherin, which is an epithelial-specific cadherin, plays a major role in the selective adhesion of cells in epithelial tissue and is necessary for the maintenance of normal epithelial cells integrity. Abnormal expression of p-cadherin has been associated with an invasive and aggressive phenotype of UCs and it has been hypothesized that it may act as a key effector of muscle invasion [46]. CAMs in this study was generally coexpressed, especially in high grade tumors, but they were not associated with infiltration status, a finding that may be biased due to small sample of infiltrative tumors. As previously mentioned [46], and confirmed by this study, p-cadherin seems to be commonly expressed in high grade tumors exhibiting high mitotic index. HER pathway does not appear to affect CAM expression.

In conclusion, HER2 overexpression is found in a respective proportion of urothelial carcinomas and it seems to characterize an aggressive tumor behavior. The combination of pAKT and pmTOR expression along with a loss of PTEN expression is associated with adverse clinicopathological characteristics. P-cadherin is associated with high grade UCs but its expression is not affected by HER2 overexpression or by activation of HER/AKT/mTOR pathway.

Competing Interests

The authors declare that they have no competing interests.

References

[1] C. Bolenz, S. F. Shariat, P. I. Karakiewicz et al., "Human epidermal growth factor receptor 2 expression status provides independent prognostic information in patients with urothelial carcinoma of the urinary bladder," *BJU International*, vol. 106, no. 8, pp. 1216–1222, 2010.

[2] N.-H. Chow, H.-S. Liu, E. I. C. Lee et al., "Significance of urinary epidermal growth factor and its receptor expression in human bladder cancer," *Anticancer Research*, vol. 17, no. 2B, pp. 1293–1296, 1997.

[3] M. Enache, C. E. Simionescu, and A. Stepan, "EGFR and Her2/neu immunoexpression in papillary urothelial bladder carcinomas," *Romanian Journal of Morphology and Embryology*, vol. 54, no. 1, pp. 137–141, 2013.

[4] P. Korkolopoulou, G. Levidou, E.-A. Trigka et al., "A comprehensive immunohistochemical and molecular approach to the PI3K/AKT/mTOR (phosphoinositide 3-kinase/v-akt murine thymoma viral oncogene/mammalian target of rapamycin) pathway in bladder urothelial carcinoma," *BJU International*, vol. 110, no. 11, pp. E1237–E1348, 2012.

[5] M. Campiglio, S. Ali, P. G. Knyazev, and A. Ullrich, "Characteristics of EGFR family-mediated HRG signals in human ovarian cancer," *Journal of Cellular Biochemistry*, vol. 73, no. 4, pp. 522–532, 1999.

[6] N. V. Sergina, M. Rausch, D. Wang et al., "Escape from HER-family tyrosine kinase inhibitor therapy by the kinase-inactive HER3," *Nature*, vol. 445, no. 7126, pp. 437–441, 2007.

[7] S. P. Soltoff, K. L. Carraway III, S. A. Prigent, W. G. Gullick, and L. C. Cantley, "ErbB3 is involved in activation of phosphatidylinositol 3-kinase by epidermal growth factor," *Molecular and Cellular Biology*, vol. 14, no. 6, pp. 3550–3558, 1994.

[8] R. J. Shaw and L. C. Cantley, "Ras, PI(3)K and mTOR signalling controls tumour cell growth," *Nature*, vol. 441, no. 7092, pp. 424–430, 2006.

[9] K. D. Courtney, R. B. Corcoran, and J. A. Engelman, "The PI3K pathway as drug target in human cancer," *Journal of Clinical Oncology*, vol. 28, no. 6, pp. 1075–1083, 2010.

[10] C. Bartholomeusz and A. M. Gonzalez-Angulo, "Targeting the PI3K signaling pathway in cancer therapy," *Expert Opinion on Therapeutic Targets*, vol. 16, no. 1, pp. 121–130, 2012.

[11] H. Pópulo, J. M. Lopes, and P. Soares, "The mTOR signalling pathway in human cancer," *International Journal of Molecular Sciences*, vol. 13, no. 2, pp. 1886–1918, 2012.

[12] M. A. Knowles, F. M. Platt, R. L. Ross, and C. D. Hurst, "Phosphatidylinositol 3-kinase (PI3K) pathway activation in bladder cancer," *Cancer and Metastasis Reviews*, vol. 28, no. 3-4, pp. 305–316, 2009.

[13] J. M. Askham, F. Platt, P. A. Chambers, H. Snowden, C. F. Taylor, and M. A. Knowles, "AKT1 mutations in bladder cancer: identification of a novel oncogenic mutation that can co-operate with E17K," *Oncogene*, vol. 29, no. 1, pp. 150–155, 2010.

[14] M. Burger, W. Oosterlinck, B. Konety et al., "ICUD-EAU international consultation on bladder cancer 2012: non-muscle-invasive urothelial carcinoma of the bladder," *European Urology*, vol. 63, no. 1, pp. 36–44, 2013.

[15] S. Z. Millis, D. Bryant, G. Basu et al., "Molecular profiling of infiltrating urothelial carcinoma of bladder and nonbladder origin," *Clinical Genitourinary Cancer*, vol. 13, no. 1, pp. e37–e49, 2015.

[16] W. Sun and G. A. Herrera, "E-cadherin expression in invasive urothelial carcinoma," *Annals of Diagnostic Pathology*, vol. 8, no. 1, pp. 17–22, 2004.

[17] A. C. Wolff, M. E. Hammond, D. G. Hicks et al., "American Society of Clinical Oncology; College of American Pathologists. Recommendations for human epidermal growth factor receptor 2 testing in breast cancer: American Society of Clinical Oncology/College of American Pathologists clinical practice guideline update," *Journal of Clinical Oncology*, vol. 31, no. 31, pp. 3997–4013, 2013.

[18] S. Leibl, R. Zigeuner, G. Hutterer, T. Chromecki, P. Rehak, and C. Langner, "EGFR expression in urothelial carcinoma of the upper urinary tract is associated with disease progression and metaplastic morphology," *Acta Pathologica, Microbiologica, et Immunologica Scandinavica*, vol. 116, no. 1, pp. 27–32, 2008.

[19] N. D. Gonzalez-Roibon, A. Chaux, T. Al-Hussain et al., "Dysregulation of mammalian target of rapamycin pathway in plasmacytoid variant of urothelial carcinoma of the urinary bladder," *Human Pathology*, vol. 44, no. 4, pp. 612–622, 2013.

[20] J. Afonso, A. Longatto-Filho, V. M. Da Silva, T. Amaro, and L. L. Santos, "Phospho-mTOR in non-tumour and tumour bladder urothelium: pattern of expression and impact on urothelial bladder cancer patients," *Oncology Letters*, vol. 8, no. 4, pp. 1447–1454, 2014.

[21] S. T. dos Reis, K. R. M. Leite, A. M. Neto et al., "Immune expression of E-cadherin and α, β and γ-catenin adhesion molecules and prognosis for upper urinary tract urothelial carcinomas," *International Braz J Urol*, vol. 38, no. 4, pp. 466–473, 2012.

[22] S. Kaptain, L. K. Tan, and B. Chen, "Her-2/neu and breast cancer," *Diagnostic Molecular Pathology*, vol. 10, no. 3, pp. 139–152, 2001.

[23] D. A. Pigott, A. J. Proctor, M. E. Eydmann et al., "Amplification and over-expression of c-erbB-2 in transitional cell carcinoma

of the urinary bladder," *British Journal of Cancer*, vol. 63, no. 4, pp. 601–608, 1991.

[24] C. Wülfing, D. Von Struensee, S. Bierer, M. Bögemann, L. Hertle, and E. Eltze, "ExpressIon of her2/neu in locally advanced bladder cancer: implication for a molecular targeted therapy," *Aktuelle Urologie*, vol. 36, no. 5, pp. 423–429, 2005.

[25] M. Laé, J. Couturier, S. Oudard, F. Radvanyi, P. Beuzeboc, and A. Vieillefond, "Assessing HER2 gene amplification as a potential target for therapy in invasive urothelial bladder cancer with a standardized methodology: results in 1005 patients," *Annals of Oncology*, vol. 21, no. 4, pp. 815–819, 2009.

[26] J. S. Ross, J. A. Fletcher, K. J. Bloom et al., "Targeted therapy in breast cancer: the HER-2/neu gene and protein," *Molecular & Cellular Proteomics*, vol. 3, no. 4, pp. 379–398, 2004.

[27] L. Albarello, L. Pecciarini, and C. Doglioni, "HER2 testing in gastric cancer," *Advances in Anatomic Pathology*, vol. 18, no. 1, pp. 53–59, 2011.

[28] F. De Vita, F. Giuliani, N. Silvestris, G. Catalano, F. Ciardiello, and M. Orditura, "Human epidermal growth factor receptor 2 (HER2) in gastric cancer: a new therapeutic target," *Cancer Treatment Reviews*, vol. 36, no. 3, pp. S11–S15, 2010.

[29] S. Krüger, G. Weitsch, H. Büttner et al., "HER2 overexpression in muscle-invasive urothelial carcinoma of the bladder: prognostic implications," *International Journal of Cancer*, vol. 102, no. 5, pp. 514–518, 2002.

[30] A. Alexa, F. Baderca, D. E. Zăhoi, R. Lighezan, D. Izvernariu, and M. Raica, "Clinical significance of Her2/neu overexpression in urothelial carcinomas," *Romanian Journal of Morphology and Embryology*, vol. 51, no. 2, pp. 277–282, 2010.

[31] P. H. Abbosh, D. J. McConkey, and E. R. Plimack, "Targeting signaling transduction pathways in bladder cancer," *Current Oncology Reports*, vol. 17, no. 12, article 58, 2015.

[32] H. Tsuruta, H. Kishimoto, T. Sasaki et al., "Hyperplasia and carcinomas in Pten-deficient mice and reduced PTEN protein in human bladder cancer patients," *Cancer Research*, vol. 66, no. 17, pp. 8389–8396, 2006.

[33] F. M. Platt, C. D. Hurst, C. F. Taylor, W. M. Gregory, P. Harnden, and M. A. Knowles, "Spectrum of phosphatidylinositol 3-kinase pathway gene alterations in bladder cancer," *Clinical Cancer Research*, vol. 15, no. 19, pp. 6008–6017, 2009.

[34] L. Schultz, R. Albadine, J. Hicks et al., "Expression status and prognostic significance of mammalian target of rapamycin pathway members in urothelial carcinoma of urinary bladder after cystectomy," *Cancer*, vol. 116, no. 23, pp. 5517–5526, 2010.

[35] C. Cordon-Cardo, "Molecular alterations associated with bladder cancer initiation and progression," *Scandinavian Journal of Urology and Nephrology*, vol. 42, no. 218, pp. 154–165, 2008.

[36] W. Tian and J. I. Epstein, "Invasive low-grade papillary urothelial carcinoma: an immunohistochemical study of 26 cases," *Human Pathology*, vol. 46, no. 12, pp. 1836–1841, 2015.

[37] M. Castillo-Martin, J. Domingo-Domenech, O. Karni-Schmidt, T. Matos, and C. Cordon-Cardo, "Molecular pathways of urothelial development and bladder tumorigenesis," *Urologic Oncology: Seminars and Original Investigations*, vol. 28, no. 4, pp. 401–408, 2010.

[38] N. Houédé and P. Pourquier, "Targeting the genetic alterations of the PI3K-AKT-mTOR pathway: its potential use in the treatment of bladder cancers," *Pharmacology & Therapeutics*, vol. 145, pp. 1–18, 2015.

[39] I. Ahmad, J. P. Morton, L. B. Singh et al., "β-Catenin activation synergizes with PTEN loss to cause bladder cancer formation," *Oncogene*, vol. 30, no. 2, pp. 178–189, 2011.

[40] A. M. Puzio-Kuter, M. Castillo-Martin, C. W. Kinkade et al., "Inactivation of p53 and Pten promotes invasive bladder cancer," *Genes & Development*, vol. 23, no. 6, pp. 675–680, 2009.

[41] G. Fechner, K. Claßen, D. Schmidt, S. Hauser, and S. C. Müller, "apamycin inhibits in vitro growth and release of angiogenetic factors in human bladder cancer," *Urology*, vol. 73, no. 3, pp. 665–668, 2009.

[42] J. J. Mansure, R. Nassim, S. Chevalier, J. Rocha, E. Scarlata, and W. Kassouf, "Inhibition of mammalian target of rapamycin as a therapeutic strategy in the management of bladder cancer," *Cancer Biology and Therapy*, vol. 8, no. 24, pp. 2339–2347, 2009.

[43] B. Markman, R. Dienstmann, and J. Tabernero, "Targeting the PI3K/Akt/mTOR pathway–beyond rapalogs," *Oncotarget*, vol. 1, no. 7, pp. 530–543, 2010.

[44] E. Seront, A. Pinto, C. Bouzin, L. Bertrand, J.-P. Machiels, and O. Feron, "PTEN deficiency is associated with reduced sensitivity to mTOR inhibitor in human bladder cancer through the unhampered feedback loop driving PI3K/Akt activation," *British Journal of Cancer*, vol. 109, no. 6, pp. 1586–1592, 2013.

[45] A. Bagrodia, L.-M. Krabbe, B. A. Gayed et al., "Evaluation of the prognostic significance of altered mammalian target of rapamycin pathway biomarkers in upper tract urothelial carcinoma," *Urology*, vol. 84, no. 5, pp. 1134–1140, 2014.

[46] R. T. Bryan, "Cell adhesion and urothelial bladder cancer: the role of cadherin switching and related phenomena," *Philosophical Transactions of the Royal Society of London, Series B: Biological Sciences*, vol. 370, no. 1661, Article ID 20140042, 2015.

6

Cervical Cytology and Human Papillomavirus Testing in Adolescent Women: Implications in Management of a Positive HPV Test

Marilin Rosa[1,2] and Amir Mohammadi[1]

[1] *Department of Pathology and Laboratory Medicine, College of Medicine, University of Florida, Jacksonville, FL 32209, USA*
[2] *Anatomic Pathology and Women's Oncology, Moffitt Cancer Center and Research Institute, 12902 Magnolia Drive, Tampa, FL 33612, USA*

Correspondence should be addressed to Marilin Rosa; marilin.rosa@moffitt.org

Academic Editor: Hanlin L. Wang

Objectives. Consensus guidelines establish that HPV testing should not be used to manage adolescents with atypical squamous cells of undetermined significance (ASC-US). This study aimed to estimate the impact on follow-up of HPV testing after the first-time ASC-US diagnosis. *Methods.* From January 2009 to December 2010, all ASC-US diagnoses in adolescents were retrieved. *Results.* 1950 cervical cytologies were received from this population and 335 cases (17.1%) were reported as ASC-US. A total of 287 cases were included in the study. Cases were divided into control group (no HPV test; 46 cases) and case group (HPV test performed; 241 cases). On follow-up, in the control group, 43.4% patients had cytology, and 56.6% patients had no follow-up. The case group was divided into negative HPV (60 cases) and positive HPV (181 cases). In the negative-HPV group, 41.7% had cytology and 58.3% had no follow-up. In the positive-HPV group, 41% had cytology, 22% underwent colposcopy, and 37% had no follow-up. Patients with positive-HPV results were more likely to have follow-up than patients in the control and negative-HPV groups (63% versus 43.4% versus 41.7%, resp.). *Conclusions.* HPV infections are common in adolescents. A positive HPV test cannot predict which women will develop carcinoma. Adherence to current guidelines is recommended in this population.

1. Introduction

Human papillomavirus is one of the most common sexually transmitted infections in young women with prevalence rates as high as 82% in some populations [1]. The majority of HPV infections are cleared by the immune system in a period of 2 to 3 years [1]. Only persistent infections with oncogenic (high-risk) types have the potential to progress to invasive carcinoma [2].

Cervical cancer is extremely rare in adolescents with only approximately 0.2% of cases of cervical cancer diagnosed under the age of 20 [2]. Therefore, cervical cytology screening and HPV testing are not recommended in this population. Albeit screening guidelines published in 2006 established that HPV test should not be used in women under 21 years of age [3]; in our setting routine cervical cytology screening and HPV testing are commonly performed in this population. The aim of this study was to evaluate the frequency of testing and how a positive HPV test result impacted initial clinical management of patients with first time ASC-US diagnosis.

2. Methods

The study was approved by the University of Florida (UF) Institutional Review Board (IRB). Our laboratory receives cervical cytology from community based primary care clinics run by family practice specialized physicians as well as UF-based gynecologists. All gynecologic cytology is processed using ThinPrep (Hologic, Marlborough, MA) liquid based preparation and HPV test is performed on site using the Digene Hybrid Capture II (HCII) method on residual cytologic material.

From January 2009 to December 2010, all cases diagnosed as ASC-US in adolescent patients were retrieved. The inclusion criterion was patients under 20 years of age and first time ASC-US diagnosis. Follow-up data of these cases were collected until 1 year after the initial diagnosis of ASC-US. The one-year period of follow-up was chosen because, according to 2006 screening guidelines (in effect in 2009-2010), adolescents with ASC-US should have repeat cytology at 1 year, and additional tests, including HPV testing, were not expected before that time [3]. The purpose was to prove that those adolescents with HPV test were more prone to additional testing beyond what is recommended for this population. Patients with known previously diagnosed cervical abnormalities were excluded from the study since clinical history of dysplasia may influence clinician's decision. HPV test was performed upon physician's request (test requested as reflex if ASC-US).

Enrolled patients were divided into two groups: (1) control group (HPV test was not performed/requested); (2) HPV group (HPV test was performed). This latter group was further divided into positive-HPV group and negative-HPV group. Follow-up within 1 year was classified into three possibilities as follows: (1) repeat cytology, (2) colposcopy with biopsy, and (3) no follow-up.

3. Results

During the study period, 1950 Papanicolaou tests (Pap test) were received from this patient population. Three hundred thirty-five cases (17%) were reported as ASC-US. Two hundred eighty-seven cases (287) met the inclusion criteria, meaning that the patient did not have history of previous abnormal cytology in our electronic medical record system and no history of dysplasia was provided on the pathology requisition. One hundred fifty-nine (55%) of the patients had at least one follow-up within one year. One hundred fourteen (71%) of these patients belong to the positive-HPV group. Seventy-five percent (75%) of patients with ASC-US in which the high-risk HPV test was performed had a positive result (181/241 cases).

3.1. Control Group. The control group included 46 cases with ASC-US. As a follow-up, in the control group, 20 patients had repeated cytology (43.4%), 26 patients had no follow-up (56.6%), and no patient underwent colposcopy. One patient was diagnosed with high grade squamous intraepithelial lesion (HSIL) on follow-up cervical cytology. This patient did not undergo colposcopy during the study period. A subsequent Pap test performed one year later revealed ASC-US. HPV test was negative.

3.2. HPV Group. The positive-HPV and negative-HPV groups included 181 and 60 patients, respectively.

In the positive-HPV group, a total of 114 (63%) patients had follow-up. Seventy-four patients had repeated cytology (41%), 40 patients underwent colposcopy (22%), and 67 had no follow-up (37%). Four patients were diagnosed with cervical intraepithelial neoplasia 2 (CIN-2) on follow-up biopsy during colposcopy. Of these patients, one underwent cone biopsy (conization) with the diagnosis of cervical intraepithelial neoplasia 3 (CIN-3), one patient underwent loop electrosurgical excision procedure (LEEP) with the diagnosis of CIN-2, one patient did not received surgical treatment and had a subsequent negative Pap test, and one patient was lost to follow-up.

In the negative-HPV group, 25 patients had cytology follow-up (41.7%), 35 patients had no follow-up (58.3%), and no patient underwent colposcopy. No cases of HSIL were found in this group.

Invasive carcinoma was not seen in our study during the follow-up period.

Data are summarized on Tables 1 and 2.

4. Discussion

Risky behavior is a major cause of morbidity and mortality among adolescents [1, 3]. According to the CDC's "Youth Risk Behavior Surveillance—United States, 2011," nationwide, 6.2% of students had had sexual intercourse for the first time before the age of 13 and 15.3% of high school students had had sexual intercourse with four or more persons during their life [4]. In addition, the presence of more active squamous metaplasia and a more exposed transformation zone towards the ectocervix in adolescents are factors that favor HPV infection and replication [1].

Screening guidelines published in 2006 established that adolescents with ASC-US should be followed up with annual cytology. In addition, HPV testing should not be used under the age of 21 years and if it is inadvertently performed, a positive result should not influence management [3, 5]. Furthermore, it is recommended that adolescents with a histological diagnosis of CIN 1, CIN 2, and CIN 2,3 (meaning cases where the pathologist equivocated between CIN 2 and CIN 3) may be followed with observation rather than invasive interventions. For biopsy confirmed CIN 3, treatment is indicated [5].

In 2012, updated guidelines for screening and management of cervical dysplasia were published. These recent guidelines recommend no screening in adolescents. Additionally, since cervical cancer risk remains low through age 25 years, HPV infections are common, and lesions often regress; a less intensive management for young women with abnormal cytology was advised [6].

Some of the reasons behind these recommendations included the current knowledge that HPV infection, ASC-US, and even LSIL are common in adolescents. There is currently good evidence that in adolescents more than 90% of HPV infections, LSIL cytology, and CIN 1 lesions regress within 3 years [5]. Therefore, observation over intervention for adolescents with LSIL and CIN 1 is strongly recommended. Additionally, more than 70% of adolescents with ASC-US are HPV positive (75% in our study); thus HPV testing is not useful for triage in adolescent populations. Many adolescents experience multiple sequential HPV infections, and a repetitively positive HPV test may represent repeated transient infections rather than a persistent infection [5, 7–15]. Certainly, in the era of HPV vaccination, guidelines and role of testing will significantly change.

TABLE 1: Follow-up data by group.

Follow-up	Control group	Positive HPV	Negative HPV
Cervical cytology	20 (43.4%)	74 (41%)	25 (41.7%)
Colposcopy with biopsy	0	40 (22%)	0
No follow-up	26 (56.6%)	67 (37%)	35 (58.3%)
Total	20/46	114/181	25/60

TABLE 2: Follow-up diagnoses by group.

Follow-up diagnosis	Control group	Negative-HPV	Positive-HPV
Negative	11	19	41
ASC-US	3	4	26
LSIL/CIN-1	5	2	43
HSIL/CIN-2/3	1	0	4
Total	20 patients	25 patients	114 patients

ASC-US: atypical cells of undetermined significance; LSIL: low grade squamous intraepithelial lesion; CIN: cervical intraepithelial neoplasia; HSIL: high-grade squamous intraepithelial lesion.

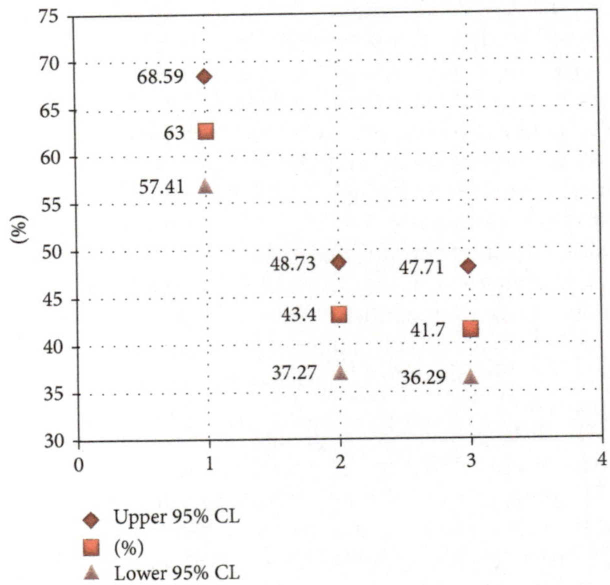

FIGURE 1: Comparison of HPV-positive group (1), control group (2), and HPV-negative group (3) using 95% confidential intervals (CL) indicates a significant difference in follow-up between the HPV-positive group and the other two groups, while no difference was detected between the control and the HPV-negative groups.

After 2006 guidelines publication and dissemination, we expected the use of HPV test in adolescents with ASC-US to be totally discontinued or at least gradually decreased. However, in our study, the majority of ASC-US girls (83.9%) had HPV test performed after first known ASC-US diagnosis. Patients with positive-HPV results were more likely to have follow-up in comparison with the control group and the negative-HPV group (63% versus 43.4% versus 41.7%, resp.). Only patients with a positive-HPV result underwent colposcopy.

Based on the results from the case group (HPV tested patients) on follow-up, the positive predictive value (PPV) of a positive-HPV test for significant dysplasia (moderate or severe dysplasia) in our population was only 3.5% and 0% for invasive carcinoma. For statistical analysis, the three groups were compared using 95% confidence intervals calculated using SPSS 17.0 (SPSS. Chicago, IL). Results showed that there was a significant difference in follow-up between the HPV-positive group and the other two groups. No difference was detected between the control and the HPV-negative groups (Figure 1). This may indicate that clinicians, at least in our setting, strongly rely on HPV results for clinical decisions in this population.

Although five patients were detected with HSIL, CIN 2, and CIN 3 during the study period (Table 2), there is no data to support that screening under the age of 21 years prevents invasive cervical cancer [3, 5]. These patients probably had previous abnormal cytology not recorded in our system or were infected with high-risk HPV virus long before being enrolled in the study. On follow-up, two of these patients had subsequent negative results. These findings might support the recent notion that even high-grade lesions (at this age) can be carefully observed since they may regress if given the opportunity. Also, although these patients should be carefully observed, other modalities and not HPV testing should be used since HPV test results do not provide significant information about the real risk for developing or having CIN 3 or carcinoma. Given that HPV test has very low PPV in adolescents, annual cytology would suffice for the detection of these rare high-grade lesions before they become invasive. Taken into consideration that the cost of HPV testing is near 300 dollars (280 dollars at our institution), unnecessary testing will also increase healthcare cost.

In spite of the discussion, it is valid to mention here that although HPV testing and cervical screening are currently not recommended in adolescents, guidelines are developed to assist clinicians in patient management; however they may not apply to all clinical scenarios [6], meaning that clinical history such as early onset of sexual activity and previous dysplasia is important in screening and follow-up determinations.

Due to the results of the study and after the 2012 guidelines were published, our department joined efforts with the Department of Obstetrics and Gynecology (OB-GYN) and started an educational campaign targeted to educate community physicians about the adequate use of cytology and HPV and promote the use of current guidelines while treating adolescents. Additionally, our cytology requisition form was changed to modify the HPV options and accommodate current accepted guidelines. A prospective study is currently undergoing to evaluate the impact of 2012 guidelines and our efforts to disseminate them (data not available).

5. Conclusions

Since low- and high-risk HPV infections are highly prevalent in adolescents and are commonly transitory, HPV testing is of little predictive value and should not be used to decide the management of adolescent with ASC-US cytology. An abnormal result cannot determine which patients currently may have or will develop cancer in the future and can result in more harm than benefit for the patient. Overuse of diagnostic and therapeutic procedures at this young age may increase morbidity and compromise reproduction in the future due to cervical incontinence. Our experience highlights a significant health care problem that is probably not limited to our setting. Education and adherence to guidelines will help reduce health care costs and emotional and physical patient harm without compromising early cervical cancer detection and treatment.

Conflict of Interests

The authors declare that there is no conflict of interests regarding the publication of this paper. No financial support was received for this study.

References

[1] A. B. Moscicki, "Management of adolescents who have abnormal cytology and histology," *Obstetrics and Gynecology Clinics of North America*, vol. 35, no. 4, pp. 633–643, 2008.

[2] S. F. Altekruse, C. L. Kosary, M. Krapcho et al., *SEER Cancer Statistics Review, 1975–2007*, National Cancer Institute, Bethesda, Md, USA, 2009, http://seer.cancer.gov/archive/csr/1975_2007/.

[3] T. C. Wright Jr., L. S. Massad, C. J. Dunton, M. Spitzer, E. J. Wilkinson, and D. Solomon, "2006 Consensus guidelines for the management of women with abnormal cervical screening tests," *Journal of Lower Genital Tract Disease*, vol. 11, no. 4, pp. 201–222, 2007.

[4] D. K. Eaton, L. Kann, S. Kinchen et al., "Youth risk behavior surveillance—United States, 2011," *Morbidity and Mortality Weekly Report*, vol. 61, no. 4, pp. 1–162, 2012.

[5] A. B. Moscicki and J. T. Cox, "Practice improvement in cervical screening and management (PICSM): symposium on management of cervical abnormalities in adolescents and young women," *Journal of Lower Genital Tract Disease*, vol. 14, no. 1, pp. 73–80, 2010.

[6] L. S. Massad, M. H. Einstein, W. K. Huh et al., "2012 updated consensus guidelines for the management of abnormal cervical cancer screening tests and cancer precursors," *Journal of Lower Genital Tract Disease*, vol. 17, supplement 1, pp. S1–S27, 2013.

[7] R. L. Winer, S. K. Lee, J. P. Hughes, D. E. Adam, N. B. Kiviat, and L. A. Koutsky, "Genital human papillomavirus infection: incidence and risk factors in a cohort of female university students," *American Journal of Epidemiology*, vol. 157, no. 3, pp. 218–226, 2003.

[8] A. B. Moscicki, N. Hills, S. Shiboski et al., "Risks for incident human papillomavirus infection and low-grade squamous intraepithelial lesion development in young females," *The Journal of the American Medical Association*, vol. 285, no. 23, pp. 2995–3002, 2001.

[9] R. L. Winer, Q. Feng, J. P. Hughes, S. O'Reilly, N. B. Kiviat, and L. A. Koutsky, "Risk of female human papillomavirus acquisition associated with first male sex partner," *Journal of Infectious Diseases*, vol. 197, no. 2, pp. 279–282, 2008.

[10] A. N. Burchell, R. L. Winer, S. de Sanjosé, and E. L. Franco, "Chapter 6: epidemiology and transmission dynamics of genital HPV infection," *Vaccine*, vol. 24, supplement 3, pp. S52–S61, 2006.

[11] N. Muñoz, F. Méndez, H. Posso et al., "Incidence, duration, and determinants of cervical human papillomavirus infection in a cohort of Colombian women with normal cytological results," *Journal of Infectious Diseases*, vol. 190, no. 12, pp. 2077–2087, 2004.

[12] A. B. Moscicki, J. Palefsky, G. Smith, S. Siboshski, and G. Schoolnik, "Variability of human papillomavirus DNA testing in a longitudinal cohort of young women," *Obstetrics & Gynecology*, vol. 82, no. 4, part 1, pp. 578–585, 1993.

[13] A. B. Moscicki, S. Shiboski, N. K. Hills et al., "Regression of low-grade squamous intra-epithelial lesions in young women," *The Lancet*, vol. 364, no. 9446, pp. 1678–1683, 2004.

[14] G. Y. Ho, R. Bierman, L. Beardsley, C. J. Chang, and R. D. Burk, "Natural history of cervicovaginal papillomavirus infection in young women," *The New England Journal of Medicine*, vol. 338, no. 7, pp. 423–428, 1998.

[15] L. A. Boardman, C. Stanko, S. Weitzen, and C. J. Sung, "Atypical squamous cells of undetermined significance: human papillomavirus testing in adolescents," *Obstetrics & Gynecology*, vol. 105, no. 4, pp. 741–746, 2005.

7

Study Assessing the Quality of Quantification of Estrogen Receptor Protein Expression by Immunohistochemistry and Gene Expression in Breast Cancer

Sas Leen,[1,2] Van Laere Steven,[1,3] Dierick Anne Marie,[4] Duwel Valérie,[4] De Pauw Annemie,[5] Van Den Eynden Gert,[1] Van Dam Peter,[2] Dirix Luc,[1] Vermeulen Peter,[1] and Lardon Filip[2]

[1] *Translational Cancer Research Unit, GZA Hospitals Sint-Augustinus, Oosterveldlaan 24, 2610 Antwerp, Belgium*
[2] *Department of Medical Oncology, University of Antwerp, Universiteitsplein 1, 2610 Antwerp, Belgium*
[3] *Department of Oncology, KU Leuven, Herestraat 49, 3000 Leuven, Belgium*
[4] *Department of Pathology, AZ Klina Hospital, Augustijnslei 100, 2930 Brasschaat, Belgium*
[5] *Department of Pathology, AZ Nikolaas Hospital, Moerlandstraat 1, 9100 Sint-Niklaas, Belgium*

Correspondence should be addressed to Sas Leen; leen.sas@uantwerpen.be

Academic Editor: Paul J. Van Diest

Although immunohistochemistry (IHC) is a widely used technique to classify tumors in ER-positive versus ER-negative ones, interlab variabilities can occur. This study aims to investigate the influences of preanalytical and analytical factors on IHC results. For this purpose, the different steps of the preparation of IHC sections and scoring procedures were compared between two participating laboratories and a central lab. There was a significant positive correlation between the IHC results of the participating laboratories and those of the central lab (correlation coefficient > 0.600; $P < 0.05$). Nevertheless, some discordant cases for immunostaining (5.3% for ER and 5.6% for PR) and for scoring (10.5% for PR) occur at site 1. Comparing IHC results with ESR1 gene expression results revealed a significant positive correlation (correlation coefficients > 0.769; $P < 0.05$). PCR results of ER target genes showed some heterogeneity in the ER-signalling pathway. These results suggest that differences in the IHC procedure between these laboratories did not have a big influence on the end result. Nevertheless, discordant cases caused by preanalytical and analytical lab-specific procedures have been identified.

1. Introduction

Breast cancer is one of the most important causes of mortality in women. Intensive research has revealed the existence of 2 nuclear receptors, the estrogen receptor (ER) and progesterone receptor (PR), which play a role in normal development of the breast as well as breast cancer. Generally, ER-positive tumors are treated with endocrine therapy, such as antiestrogens and aromatase inhibitors [1–3]. ER-negative tumors are usually treated with cytotoxic chemotherapy. The first goal in the treatment of patients with breast cancer is to select the most appropriate therapy. For this purpose, patients are screened for the presence of ER and PR in the tumor tissue. In general, ER-positive/PR-positive tumors have the best outcome, while the prognosis of patients with ER-positive/PR-negative tumors is less favorable. Patients with ER-negative/PR-negative tumors have the least favorable prognosis [4]. At the moment, the common technique to determine the status of ER and PR is by immunohistochemistry (IHC) on sections of formalin-fixed and paraffin-embedded tissues (FFPET) followed by scoring of nuclear immunostaining. However, variability between different laboratories occurs, leading to different interpretations and results, with misclassification as a consequence [5]. This variability can be caused by preanalytic differences, such as fixation and protocol variants, as well as analytic differences, such as inter-/intraobserver variability, different scoring systems, and related cut-off values for ER-positivity.

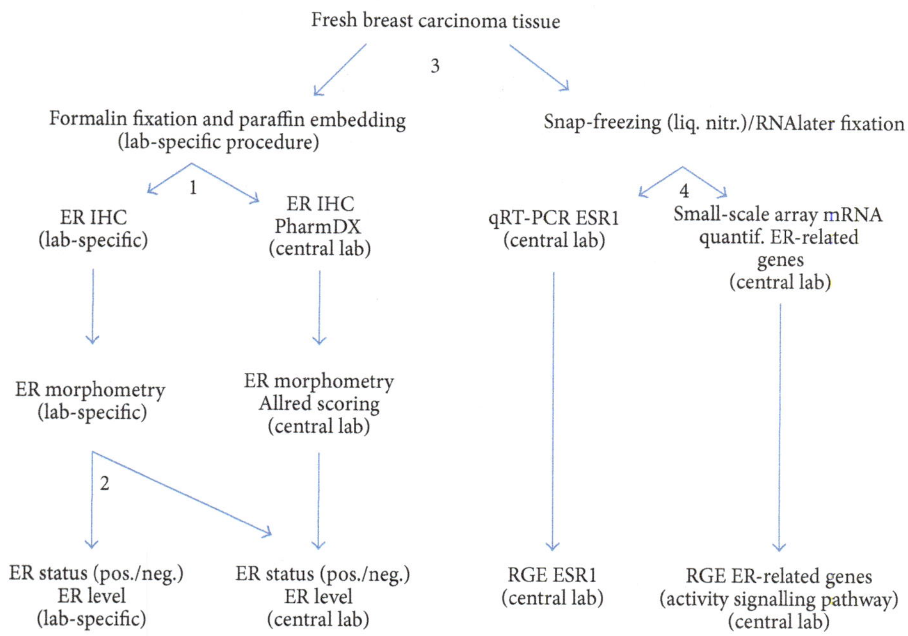

Figure 1: Schematic representation of the study: the scheme indicates the different steps of the study to evaluate the influence of (1) immunostaining; (2) scoring; (3) tissue fixation; and (4) heterogeneity within groups of carcinomas with comparable immunohistochemical receptor status.

The purpose of this study is to assess the quality of (semi) quantification of the ERα- and PR-protein expression by IHC on breast adenocarcinoma tissue sections (FFPET) in different pathology laboratories.

2. Material and Methods

The study is a multicenter study wherein 2 clinical sites and translational cancer research unit, the central lab, participate. A schematic representation of the study is given in Figure 1.

2.1. Patient Inclusion Criteria. Samples used in this experiment are of patients who gave written approval. The samples include histologically proven breast adenocarcinoma (primary or metastatic, with or without prior treatment), which were at least 1 cm (T1c or higher). The tumors had to be large enough to be able to collect RNAlater fixed carcinoma tissue without influence on the standard diagnostic procedure.

2.2. Sample Preparation. After mastectomy or tumorectomy the specimens were transported without delay to the pathology lab. The pathologist took a representative part of the carcinoma (peripheral, viable, and without adjacent normal tissue) immediately upon arrival of the specimen in the lab. The carcinoma tissue was divided into small parts of $5 \times 5 \times 5$ mm or smaller and was submerged in RNAlater solution and incubated at −80°C. Total warm ischemia time did not exceed 20 minutes. Each participating center collected 20 breast cancer samples and sent a referral of each tissue sample and an immunostained section to the central lab.

2.3. Immunohistochemistry. Each of the participating laboratories performed an immunohistochemical staining for ER and PR on 20 FFPE tissue sections using their own staining procedure. Next, the IHC coupes were scored by the laboratories themselves using their proper scoring system and rescored by the central lab. At the central lab scoring of the stained FFPE was performed using the Allred histomorphometrical scoring system for ER and PR, resulting in scores (intensity + proportion) from 0 to 8. Scores higher than 2 indicate a positive status [6, 7].

Besides the 20 stained tissue sections, each lab also provided 20 unstained sections that were stained at the central lab using the ER/PR pharmDx kit (DAKO). This kit consists of a cocktail of two mouse monoclonal antibodies for ER, 1D5, and ER-2-123, which bind to different regions of the protein. Finally the stained sections were scored by the researcher and a trained pathologist.

2.4. Polymerase Chain Reaction (PCR). RNA was isolated from the 40 fixed (RNAlater) breast carcinoma tissues received from the participating labs using the RNeasy mini kit (Qiagen, Venlo, Belgium). The amount of RNA was measured by means of the Nanodrop ND3300 Fluorospectrometer (Isogen, Temse, Belgium). Next, 1 μg of RNA was converted to cDNA using the high capacity RNA-to-cDNA kit (Applied Biosystems, Ghent, Belgium). Further, qRT-PCR was done for the ER-coding gene, ESR1 and 11 ER target genes, ESR2, PGR, TGFβ3, HSD17β4, RAB31, STARD10, XBP1, GATA3, MYB, MUC1, and BTG2 (Assays-On-Demand, Applied Biosystems, Ghent, Belgium). 18S and beta-actin (Applied Biosystems, Ghent, Belgium) and Universal Human

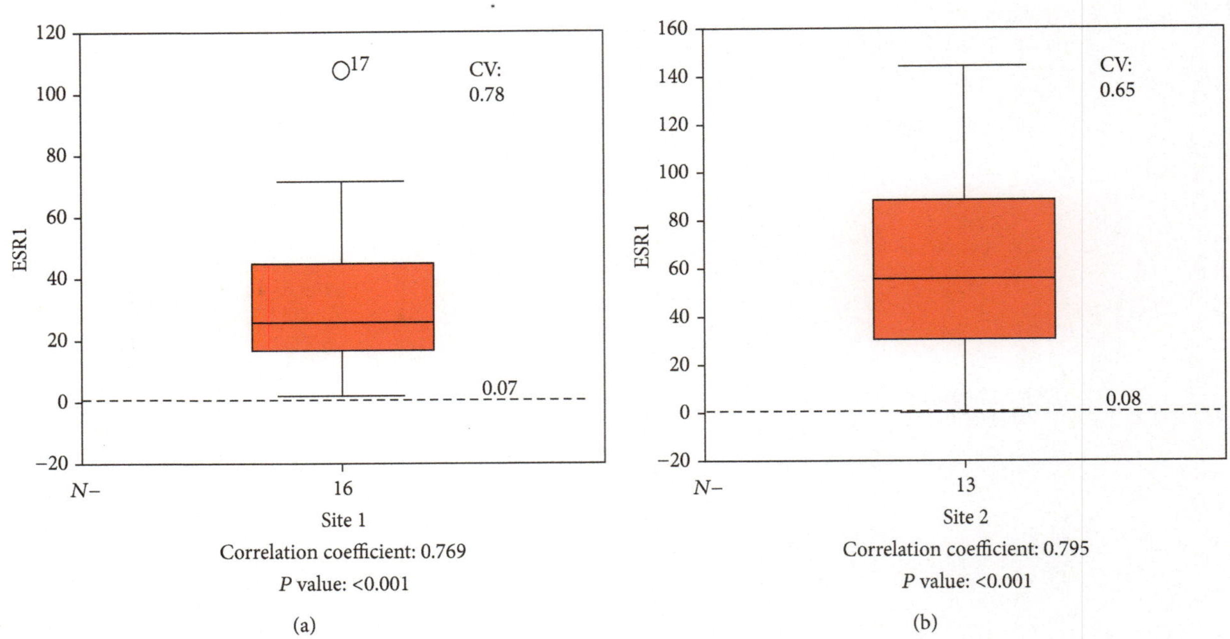

FIGURE 2: Comparison of the fixation and paraffin embedding procedure.

reference RNA (Stratagene) were used as housekeeping genes and calibrator. The results obtained from qRT-PCR were compared with those of IHC.

2.5. Statistical Analysis. The Spearman rank test was used to evaluate correlations between results. Statistical significance was defined at the level of $P < 0.05$. Per participating site, a principal component analysis was performed on the ER target gene expression data to evaluate heterogeneity within the tumors.

3. Results

3.1. Formalin Fixation and Paraffin Embedding Did Not Influence IHC Results. To establish the influence of tissue fixation and paraffin embedding, we evaluated the correlation between the IHC results with ER gene expression results. For this purpose, we used 35 samples of another study of which IHC results and gene expression results for ESR1 were provided. Of these samples, the ER-positive samples with an Allred score of more than 5 were selected and were used to calculate the coefficients of variation (CV), which was 0.85. Next, the CV-values of the ESR1 gene expression for site 1 and site 2 were calculated, which were 0.78 and 0.65, respectively (Figure 2). ESR1 gene expression of samples with low Allred scores (i.e., 0: dashed line) was significantly lower (i.e., 0.07 and 0.08 for site 1 and site 2, resp.) than those with high (i.e., >5) scores. Statistical analysis showed a significant positive correlation between the scoring results and qRT-PCR results ($P < 0.05$). The correlation coefficients of site 1 and site 2 were 0.769 and 0.795, respectively. These results suggest that formalin fixation and paraffin embedding did not influence the results between different laboratories.

3.2. Immunostaining in the Different Laboratories Showed Similar Results. In the next step, variability in immunostaining between the peripheral labs and the central lab was evaluated. Slides of 20 tissue samples were stained at the participating laboratories by their proper staining method. Unstained tissue sections from the same tissue block were stained at the central lab using the ER/PR PharmDX kit. All tissue sections were scored blind at the central lab using the Allred scoring system. IHC results between the participating laboratories and the central lab were significantly correlated with a correlation coefficient of higher than 0.600 ($P < 0.05$) (Figure 3). Nevertheless, discordant cases for ER (5.3%) and PR (5.6%) were found for site 1. There were no discordant results between the central lab and site 2.

3.3. Scoring Systems of the Different Laboratories Gave Similar Results. Slides stained by the participating laboratories were scored by trained pathologists on site and at the central lab. Comparison of the results of both sites revealed a significant positive correlation of 0.918 and more ($P < 0.001$) (Figure 4). Classifying samples in ER-positive versus ER-negative tumors showed no discordant results. PR scores revealed a discordance of 10.5% for site 1, but no discordant cases for site 2.

3.4. ER Pathway Heterogeneity Can Occur in ER-Positive Samples. To determine ER pathway activity we performed qRT-PCR for 11 ER target genes on all tissue samples obtained from the participating sites ($N = 40$). The correlations in gene expression between ESR1 and those of the different ER target genes were examined. There was no significant correlation between ESR1 and the following genes: MUC1,

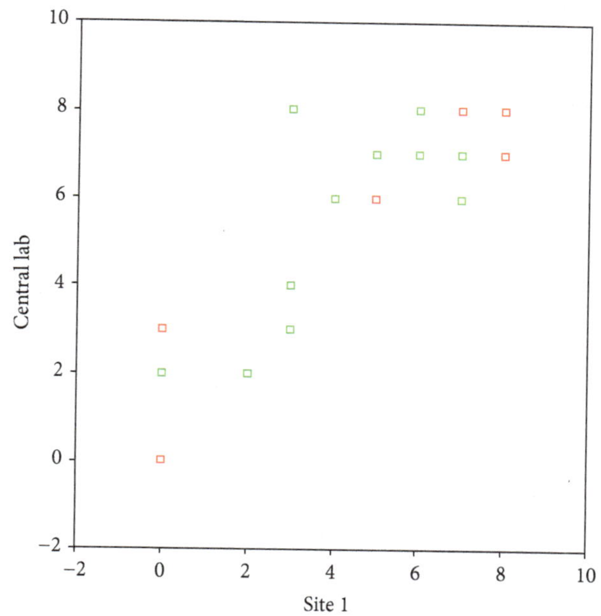

	Correlation coefficient	*P* value
□ ER	0.600	= 0.007
□ PR	0.816	<0.001

Discordance:
ER: 5.3%; PR: 5.6%

(a)

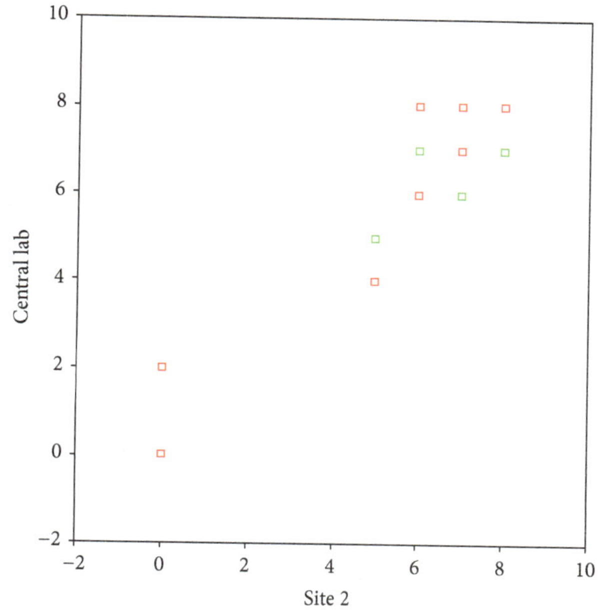

	Correlation coefficient	*P* value
□ ER	0.899	<0.001
□ PR	0.915	<0.001

Discordance:
No discordant cases

(b)

FIGURE 3: Comparison of the immunostaining method.

TGFb3, RAB31, and ESR2 (Figure 5; Table 1). So the majority of the target genes of ESR1 were correlated with ER-activity.

Next, a principal component analysis was performed on the ER target gene expression data for each participating site (Figure 6). As principal component 1 (i.e., the x-axis) defines the largest variation in ER target gene expression, the samples were dichotomized relative to the median expression of principal component 1 (green dashed line). Next we investigated if ER target genes were differentially expressed between samples segregated along the x-axis. For site 1 no ER target genes were differentially expressed indicating no difference in ER pathway activation between the samples to the left and the right of the green dashed line. These results were corroborated when analyzing ER protein expression data. For site 2, ~60% of the ER target genes were differentially expressed between the samples to the left and the right of the green dashed line, indicating ER pathway heterogeneity. Again, these results were corroborated by ER protein expression, as the Allred scores to the left of dashed line were significantly lower as compared to their counterparts ($P < 0.05$).

4. Discussion

IHC is a common technique to determine ER and PR status in tumors. In their review, Brouckaert and colleagues describe the importance of (semi)quantification of steroid hormone receptor expression in estimating the benefits of different treatments as chemotherapy and endocrine therapy [8]. As IHC on sections of FFPE tissue is a routine technique used to classify breast cancer in ER-positive versus -negative tumors, it is important to consider that intra- and interlaboratory variabilities exist. Quality assessment studies in the UK and EU showed significant interlaboratory variability, especially for tumors with low ER levels [5, 9]. In our study we saw a positive correlation between the IHC results of the participating laboratories and those of the central lab. But comparing the results awarded to immunostaining and scoring showed some discordant cases.

Fixation, the first step of IHC procedure, could already influence the IHC results. Delay in fixation, pH, underfixation, and overfixation could reduce immunostaining [10–16]. Williams et al. showed that a low pH could affect the morphology of the tissue but may result in a good immunoreactivity [11]. Also the fixation time is important. A minimal fixation time of 6 to 8 hrs was necessary to receive reliable results [12]. Overfixation was shown to be less important as tissue blocks fixed up to 72 hrs and 96 hrs did not show a reduction in ER, PR, and HER2 status [13, 14]. Fixation for more than 57 days could reduce immunostaining [15, 16]. As such long fixation times are not clinically relevant, overfixation would not be a concern in routine pathology

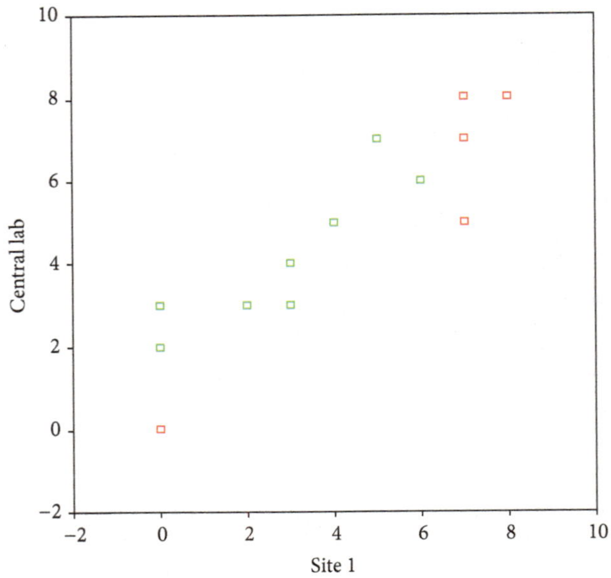

	Correlation coefficient	*P* value
□ ER	0.928	<0.001
□ PR	0.918	<0.001

Discordance:
ER: 0%; PR: 10.5%

(a)

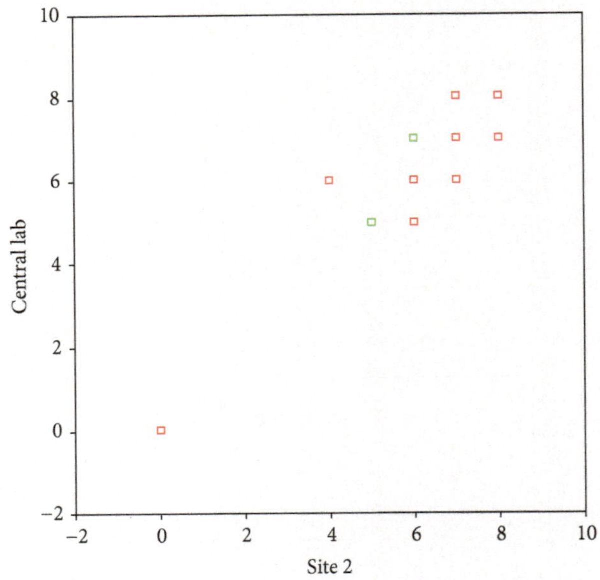

	Correlation coefficient	*P* value
□ ER	0.945	<0.001
□ PR	0.948	<0.001

Discordance:
No discordant cases

(b)

FIGURE 4: The influence of the scoring system.

TABLE 1: Determination of the pathway activity of ER.

Gene	Site 1		Site 2	
	Correlation with ESR1	*P* value	Correlation with ESR1	*P* value
PGR	0.588	0.006	0.693	0.001
GATA3	0.582	0.007	0.798	0.000
XBP1	0.561	0.010	0.773	0.000
MYB	0.573	0.008	0.901	0.000
MUC1	0.186	0.431	0.819	0.424
BTG2	0.472	0.036	0.701	0.001
TGFb3	0.072	0.762	0.329	0.156
RAB31	0.206	0.384	0.302	0.195
HSD17b4	0.498	0.026	0.668	0.001
ESR2	−0.137	0.565	−0.203	0.391
STARD10	0.447	0.048	0.714	0.000

labs. In our study, we found no influence of fixation on the results of IHC, as the results of ER-status obtained by IHC were significantly correlated with the qRT-PCR results of the ESR1 gene.

A second step that can differ between laboratories is the immunostaining procedure. The sensitivity of the antigen can have an impact on the results [17–20]. In a study by Cheang and colleagues two ER antibodies, the monoclonal rabbit antibody SP1 and the mouse monoclonal antibody 1D5, were compared. Of the 4105 samples SP1 detected ER positivity in 69.5% of the samples, while 1D5 detected ER positivity in 63.1% of the cases. SP1 showed to be more sensitive than 1D5 [18]. Similar results were found in a study by Huang showing an 8 times higher affinity of SP1 compared to 1D5 [20]. For this reason, it is plausible to use a cocktail of different antibodies to increase the sensitivity [21]. In our study, we used a cocktail of two mouse monoclonal antibodies to ER, 1D5, and ER-2-123, which bind to different regions of the protein.

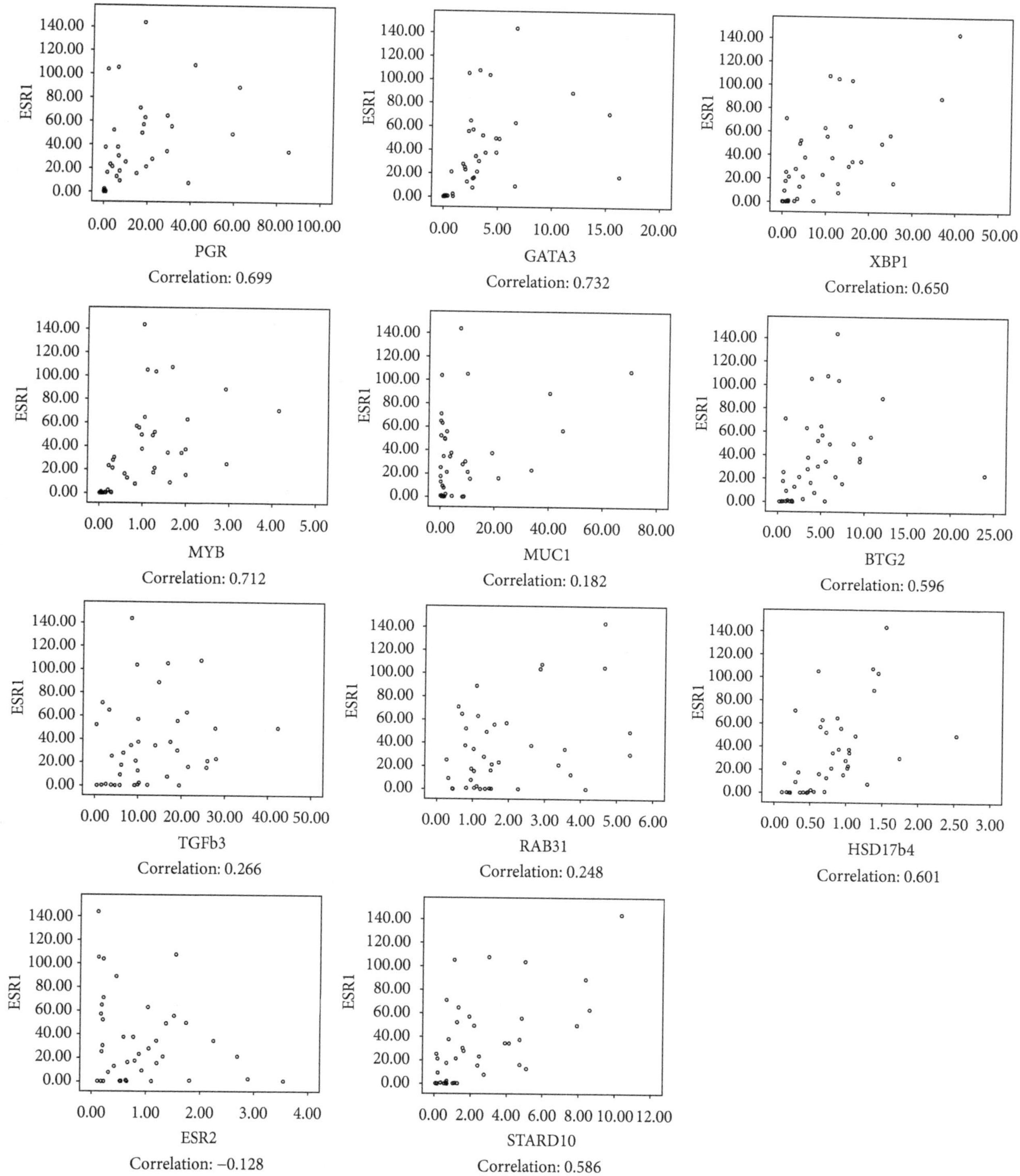

Figure 5: Determination of the pathway activity.

There was a significant positive correlation between the IHC results of tumor slides stained at the central lab and those stained at the participating laboratories. Nevertheless, the correlation for ER was much lower for site 1 in comparison to site 2. Classifying ER-positive versus ER-negative tumors revealed approximately 5% discordant results for ER and PR for site 1, but not for site 2.

Finally, different scoring systems can result in discordant cases between laboratories [22]. Some scoring procedures are based on the evaluation of the proportion of stained cells, while other scoring systems, like the Allred scoring procedure, rely on the evaluation of the proportion of stained cells and the intensity of the staining [23]. Discordant results obtained by one scoring system could result in concordant

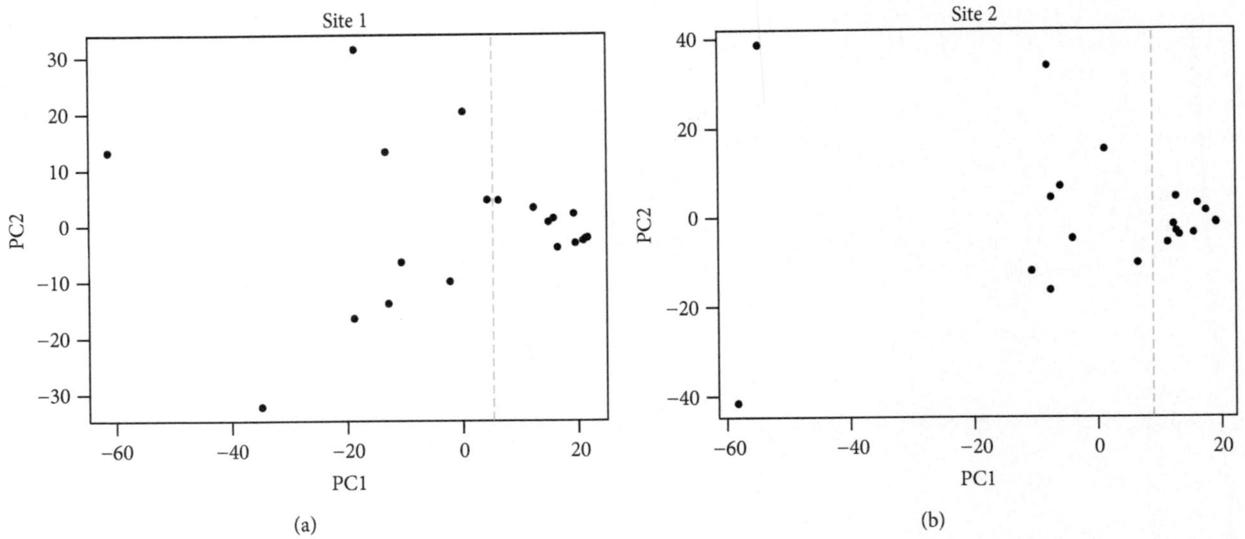

FIGURE 6: Principal component analysis. Samples were dichotomized relative to the median expression of principal component 1 (green dashed line). For site 1 all samples had comparable ER pathway activation. For site 2, the ER pathway was differential activated in the different samples.

cases when using the other scoring system [23]. Beside different scoring systems interobserver variability can also occur. Tumors with low levels of ER expression are often difficult to classify and can lead to observer discordance [24]. In our study the scoring results of the central lab using the Allred scoring method and those of the participating lab using their proper scoring system were significantly positive correlated for ER and PR. Again, despite the high concordance, discordant cases occurred.

As there were some discordant cases between different labs using IHC, it may be interesting to use a more robust, observer-independent technique. Quantitative mRNA-based measurements could be a suitable method to analyze the expression of ESR1 and PR. Studies comparing microarray mRNA quantification and qRT-PCR with IHC revealed a high concordance [25–30].

These results confirm that qRT-PCR could be an additional method for determining the status of hormonal receptors. Besides the advantage of being observer independent, qRT-PCR also allows to detect heterogeneity in the activity of the ER-signalling pathway of the different tumors as shown in our study. The assessment of ER-activity is of importance because not all patients with ER-positive breast cancer do respond to endocrine therapy [31].

5. Conclusions

IHC is a routinely used procedure to classify breast cancer in ER-positive and -negative tumors. Despite good overall concordance, discordant cases determined by preanalytical and analytical lab-specific procedures have been identified. These discordant cases lead to misclassification of tumors. qRT-PCR could be an additional observer-independent technique to determine hormone receptor status and activity. The weakness of the study is the low number of samples. It would also be interesting to use more samples with low ER and PR expression in the study.

Conflict of Interests

The authors of the paper do not have any conflict of interests.

Acknowledgments

The authors thank the participating labs, AZ klina and AZ Nikolaas hospital, for their cooperation by processing tissue slides and delivering slides and tissue blocks to TCRU.

References

[1] E. V. Jensen, V. C. Jordan, S. E. Hankinson, G. A. Colditz, and W. C. Willett, "The estrogen receptor: a model for molecular medicine," *Cancer Research*, vol. 9, pp. 1980–1989, 2003.

[2] A. Goldhirsch, M. Colleoni, and R. D. Gelber, "Endocrine therapy of breast cancer," *Annals of Oncology*, vol. 13, no. 4, pp. 61–68, 2002.

[3] A. Goldhirsch, J. H. Glick, R. D. Gelber, A. S. Coates, B. Thürlimann, and H. J. Senn, "Meeting highlights: international expert consensus in the primary therapy of early breast cancer," *Annals of Oncology*, vol. 16, pp. 1569–1583, 2005.

[4] V.-J. Bardou, G. Arpino, and R. M. Elledge, "Progesterone receptor status significantly improves outcome prediction over estrogen receptor status alone for adjuvant endocrine therapy in two large breast cancer databases," *Journal of Clinical Oncology*, vol. 21, no. 10, pp. 1973–1979, 2003.

[5] A. Rhodes, B. Jasani, D. M. Barnes, L. G. Bobrow, and K. D. Miller, "Reliability of immunohistochemical demonstration of oestrogen receptors in routine practice: interlaboratory variance in the sensitivity of detection and evaluation of scoring systems," *Journal of Clinical Pathology*, vol. 53, no. 2, pp. 125–130, 2000.

[6] D. C. Allred, J. M. Harvey, M. Berardo, and G. M. Clark, "Prognostic and predictive factors in breast cancer by immunohistochemical analysis," *Modern Pathology*, vol. 11, no. 2, pp. 155–168, 1998.

[7] J. M. Harvey, G. M. Clark, C. K. Osborne, and D. C. Allred, "Estrogen receptor status by immunohistochemistry is superior to the ligand-binding assay for predicting response to adjuvant endocrine therapy in breast cancer," *Journal of Clinical Oncology*, vol. 17, no. 5, pp. 1474–1481, 1999.

[8] O. Brouckaert, R. Paridaens, G. Floris, E. Rakha, K. Osborne, and P. A. Neven, "critical review why assessment of steroid hormone receptors in breast cancer should be quantitative," *Annals of Oncology*, vol. 24, pp. 47–53, 2013.

[9] C. A. Wells, J. P. Sloane, D. Coleman et al., "Consistency of staining and reporting of oestrogen receptor immunocytochemistry within the European Union—an inter-laboratory study," *Virchows Archiv*, vol. 445, no. 2, pp. 119–128, 2004.

[10] R. von Wasielewski, M. Mengel, M. Nolte, and M. Werner, "Influence of fixation, antibody clones, and signal amplification on steroid receptor analysis," *The Breast Journal*, vol. 4, no. 1, pp. 33–40, 1998.

[11] J. H. Williams, B. L. Mepham, and D. H. Wright, "Tissue preparation for immunocytochemistry," *Journal of Clinical Pathology*, vol. 50, no. 5, pp. 422–428, 1997.

[12] N. S. Goldstein, M. Ferkowicz, E. Odish, A. Mani, and F. Hastah, "Minimum formalin fixation time for consistent estrogen receptor immunohistochemical staining of invasive breast carcinoma," *American Journal of Clinical Pathology*, vol. 120, no. 1, pp. 86–92, 2003.

[13] T. Oyama, Y. Ishikawa, M. Hayashi, K. Arihiro, and J. Horiguchi, "The effects of fixation, processing and evaluation criteria on immunohistochemical detection of hormone receptors in breast cancer," *Breast Cancer*, vol. 14, no. 2, pp. 182–188, 2007.

[14] D. A. Arber, "Effect of prolonged formalin fixation on the immunohistochemical reactivity of breast markers," *Applied Immunohistochemistry and Molecular Morphology*, vol. 10, no. 2, pp. 183–186, 2002.

[15] L. C. Tong, N. Nelson, J. Tsourigiannis, and A. M. Mulligan, "The effect of prolonged fixation on the immunohistochemical evaluation of estrogen receptor, progesterone receptor, and her2 expression in invasive breast cancer: a prospective study," *American Journal of Surgical Pathology*, vol. 35, no. 4, pp. 545–552, 2011.

[16] I. Z. Yldriz-Aktas, D. J. Dabbs, K. L. Cooper, M. Chivukula, K. McManus, and R. Bhargava, "The effect of 96-hour formalin fixation on the immunohistochemical evaluation of estrogen receptor, progesterone receptor, and HER2 expression in invasive breast carcinoma," *American Journal of Clinical Pathology*, vol. 137, pp. 691–698, 2012.

[17] F. T. Bosman, A. F. P. M. de Goeij, and M. Rousch, "Quality control in immunocytochemistry: experiences with the oestrogen receptor assay," *Journal of Clinical Pathology*, vol. 45, no. 2, pp. 120–124, 1992.

[18] M. C. U. Cheang, D. O. Treaba, C. H. Speers et al., "Immunohistochemical detection using the new rabbit monoclonal antibody SP1 of estrogen receptor in breast cancer is superior to mouse monoclonal antibody 1D5 in predicting survival," *Journal of Clinical Oncology*, vol. 24, no. 36, pp. 5637–5644, 2006.

[19] S. Rossi, L. Laurino, A. Furlanetto et al., "A comparative study between a novel category of immunoreagents and the corresponding mouse monoclonal antibodies," *American Journal of Clinical Pathology*, vol. 124, no. 2, pp. 295–302, 2005.

[20] Z. Huang, W. Zhu, G. Szekeres, and H. Xia, "Development of new rabbit monoclonal antibody to estrogen receptor: Immunohistochemical assessment on formalin-fixed, paraffin-embedded tissue sections," *Applied Immunohistochemistry and Molecular Morphology*, vol. 13, no. 1, pp. 91–95, 2005.

[21] G. Santeusanio, A. Mauriello, L. Ventura et al., "Immunohistochemical analysis of estrogen receptors in breast carcinomas using monoclonal antibodies that recognize different domains of the receptor molecule," *Applied Immunohistochemistry and Molecular Morphology*, vol. 8, no. 4, pp. 275–284, 2000.

[22] A. M. Gown, "Current issues in ER and HER2 testing by IHC in breast cancer," *Modern Pathology*, vol. 21, no. 2, pp. S8–S15, 2008.

[23] K. Arihiro, S. Umemura, M. Kurosumi et al., "Comparison of evaluations for hormone receptors in breast carcinoma using two manual and three automated immunohistochemical assays," *American Journal of Clinical Pathology*, vol. 127, no. 3, pp. 356–365, 2007.

[24] E. S. Reisenbichler, S. C. Lester, A. Richardson, D. A. Dillon, A. Ly, and J. E. Brock, "Interobserver concordance in implementing the 2010 ASCO/CAP recommendations for reporting ER in breast carcinoma," *American Journal of Clinical Pathology*, vol. 140, pp. 487–494, 2013.

[25] P. Roepman, H. M. Horlings, O. Krijgsman et al., "Microarray-based determination of estrogen receptor, progesterone receptor, and HER2 receptor status in breast cancer," *Clinical Cancer Research*, vol. 15, no. 22, pp. 7003–7011, 2009.

[26] S. S. Badve, F. L. Baehner, R. P. Gray et al., "Estrogen- and progesterone-receptor status in ECOG 2197: comparison of immunohistochemistry by local and central laboratories and quantitative reverse transcription polymerase chain reaction by central laboratory," *Journal of Clinical Oncology*, vol. 26, no. 15, pp. 2473–2481, 2008.

[27] P. B. Vermeulen, S. L. van Laere, and L. Y. Dirix, "How to measure and report the estrogen (and progesterone) receptor in breast cancer," *International Journal of Gynecological Cancer*, vol. 16, no. 2, pp. 529–532, 2006.

[28] M. Cronin, M. Pho, D. Dutta et al., "Measurement of gene expression in archival paraffin-embedded tissues: development and performance of a 92-gene reverse transcriptase-polymerase chain reaction assay," *American Journal of Pathology*, vol. 164, no. 1, pp. 35–42, 2004.

[29] S. M. O'Connor, S. Beriwal, D. J. Dabbs, and R. Bhargava, "Concordance between semiquantitative immunohistochemical assay and oncotype DX RT-PCR assay for estrogen and progesterone receptors," *Applied Immunohistochemistry and Molecular Morphology*, vol. 18, no. 3, pp. 268–272, 2010.

[30] J. A. Kraus, D. J. Dabbs, S. Beriwal, and R. Bhargava, "Semi-quantitative immunohistochemical assay versus oncotype DX qRT-PCR assay for estrogen and progesterone receptors: an independent quality assurance study," *Modern Pathology*, vol. 25, pp. 869–876, 2012.

[31] F. J. Esteva, A. A. Sahin, M. Cristofanilli et al., "Prognostic role of a multigene reverse transcriptase-PCR assay in patients with node-negative breast cancer not receiving adjuvant systemic therapy," *Clinical Cancer Research*, vol. 11, no. 9, pp. 3315–3319, 2005.

8

Immunohistochemical Expression of Ki67 and p53 in Wilms Tumor and Its Relationship with Tumor Histology and Stage at Presentation

O. H. Radhika Krishna,[1] Geetha Kayla,[1] Mohammed Abdul Aleem,[1] Ramani Malleboyina,[1] and Ramesh Reddy Kota[2]

[1]*Department of Pathology, Niloufer Hospital for Women and Children, Red Hills, Hyderabad, Telangana 500004, India*
[2]*Department of Pediatric Surgery, Niloufer Hospital for Women and Children, Red Hills, Hyderabad, Telangana 500004, India*

Correspondence should be addressed to O. H. Radhika Krishna; othulururadhika@yahoo.co.in

Academic Editor: Maria M. Picken

Aim. Evaluate tumor proliferation marker (Ki67) and p53 tumor suppressor marker in Wilms tumor and correlate with histology, anaplasia, and staging. *Design*. Prospective, hospital based study conducted at a tertiary pediatric referral centre in south India. *Setting*. Wilms tumor is the most common childhood renal malignancy worldwide. Anaplasia on histology is associated with treatment resistance but not with aggressiveness clinical presentation. Chemotherapy for Wilms tumor is based on histology and staging. Most patients respond to current chemotherapy protocol. However, a small fraction relapses or metastasizes. Affordable prognostic markers are needed for histopathological evaluation of this tumor. *Subjects*. Cases of histologically confirmed Wilms tumor over five years. Cases after chemotherapy were excluded as the immunostaining was inconsistent in necrotic areas. *Methods*. The clinical and radiological findings of 31 cases of Wilms tumor were documented at a tertiary pediatric referral hospital over five years. In addition to Hematoxylin and Eosin staining, Ki67 proliferation index and p53 expression were correlated with tumor histology and staging. *Results*. Age incidence was 3–8 years with female preponderance. Significant correlation was noted between Ki67 proliferation index and tumor staging. p53 expression was not useful in stratification of Wilms tumor. *Conclusion*. Ki67 was cost-effective immunohistochemical marker for prognostication of pediatric Wilms tumor.

1. Introduction

Wilms tumor, the most common renal tumor of children, is known to be associated with chromosomal abnormalities [1]. It arises from the metanephric blastemal cells and recapitulates embryogenesis.

Chemotherapy protocol for Wilms tumor is based on tumor histology and tumor staging. Favourable or unfavourable histology has an impact on tumor prognosis. Stage I or low risk nephroblastoma receives no postoperative treatment while high risk tumors with diffuse anaplasia and blastemal types are treated with aggressive chemotherapy. Most patients respond to current chemotherapy protocol. However a small fraction relapses or metastasizes. There is therefore a need to identify ideal cost-effective prognostic markers for this very common tumor.

A large number of prognostic markers in nephroblastoma have been reviewed [2, 3]. Our study aims to evaluate the efficacy of two cost-effective immunohistochemical markers, tumor proliferation marker (Ki67) and tumor suppressor immunohistochemical marker p53. Their expression was correlated with tumor histology and staging.

2. Material and Methods

Case records of 31 cases of Wilms tumor were collected over a period of five years at a tertiary pediatric referral hospital. The clinical history and radiological investigations

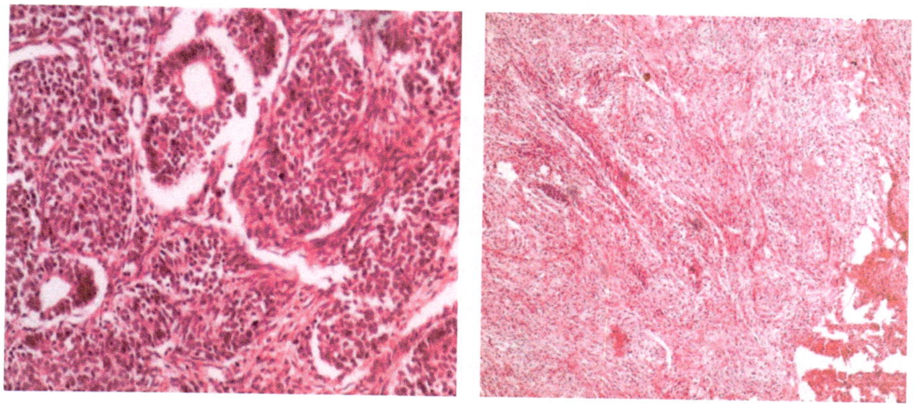

Figure 1: Photomicrograph showing a triphasic Wilms tumor and one with predominant mesenchymal component.

were documented in all the cases. Cases which had received prior chemotherapy were excluded from the study, since they contained large areas of necrosis and haemorrhage and were not amenable for immunohistochemistry.

All the specimens were received in formalin. A detailed macroscopic examination of the tumor was performed and adrenal glands, lymph nodes, renal vessels, renal sinus, capsule, and pelvic ureter wherever removed along with the kidney tumor were examined and sections were taken to make a pathological staging according to NWTS-5 staging [4].

Hematoxylin and Eosin stained sections were used for tumor diagnosis, histological and tumor staging. Further 3 μm sections were taken on positively charged slides for IHC with Ki67 and p53.

IHC was performed for Ki67 and p53 using standard IHC protocol. Ki67 antigen is a cell proliferation related nonhistone nuclear protein that can be labelled with monoclonal antibody MIB-1. The antigen is expressed in the active phases of the cell cycle. The Ki67 proliferation index is an excellent marker to recognize rapidly proliferating cells. A proliferative index was estimated and defined as percentage of positive Ki67 cells over 5 high power fields. It was semiquantitatively graded as low, moderate, or high and correlated with histological staging.

p53 is a 53 kDa nuclear protein product of tumor suppressor gene p53, located on short arm of chromosome 17. Mutations of p53 are common in human malignancies leading to tumor growth; detectable immunostaining for p53 differentiates malignant cells. p53 was semiquantitatively assessed as mild, moderate, or marked.

3. Results

A total of 31 cases of Wilms tumor were studied. Peak age of incidence was 3–8 years. There was significant female preponderance with a male to female ratio of 1 : 1.8.

Based on the NWTS-5 classification, of the 31 cases, 16 cases were in stage I, 11 cases were in stage II, two cases were in stage III, and one case was in stage IV and there was no case in stage V (Table 1).

Table 1: Staging of the tumor.

Stage of the tumor	Number of cases (n = 31)
Stage I	16 (51.6%)
Stage II	12 (39%)
Stage III	2 (6%)
Stage IV	1 (3%)
Stage V	0

Table 2: Ki67 proliferation index versus NWTS staging.

Stage of tumor	Epithelial	Mean	Blastema	Mean	Average
I (n = 16)	14–46	30	24–68	46	38
II (n = 12)	32–40	36	66–82	74	55
III (n = 2)	60		78		69
IV (n = 1)	76		82		79
V	0				

29 cases were triphasic Wilms tumor and three were biphasic. 22 cases showed favourable histology and remaining cases showed unfavourable histology (Figure 1).

Ki67 proliferation index was calculated and correlated with histology and with tumor staging. It ranged from 38 in stage I, 50 in stage II, 69 in stage III, and 79 in stage IV (Table 2). In all the stages the blastemal component showed higher Ki67 proliferation index as compared to the epithelial component (Figure 2).

The expression of p53 was expressed as mild, moderate, or marked. No difference was noted in the degree of expression in epithelial and blastemal components (Figure 3). Two cases in stage III and one case in stage IV showed moderate positivity while stages I and II cases were almost negative (Table 3).

4. Discussion

31 cases of Wilms tumor were studied over a period of 5 years. Median age incidence was 3 years, slightly lesser than worldwide incidence. An Indian study by Mishra et al. found

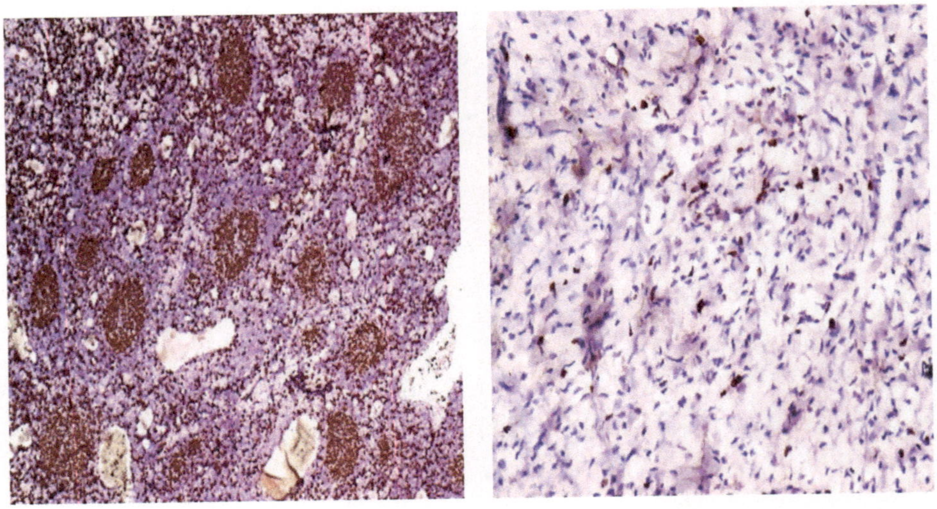

(a) (b)

FIGURE 2: Blastemal component (a) shows higher Ki67 proliferation index as compared to mesenchymal component (b).

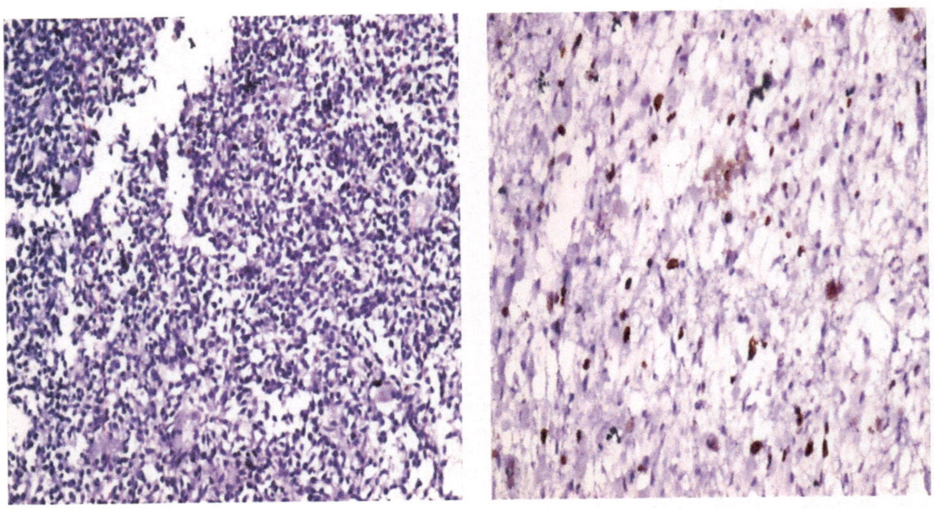

(a) (b)

FIGURE 3: Photomicrograph of stage I Wilms tumor (a) showing nil p53 positivity and a case in stage III (b) showing moderate positivity.

TABLE 3: p53 expression in Wilms tumor.

Stage of the tumor	Number of cases (n = 31)
Stage I	Low
Stage II	Low
Stage III	Moderate
Stage IV	Moderate

a median age incidence of 2.5 years [5]. Other Asian studies showed similar age incidence [6]. Sex incidence showed female preponderance, while other Asian studies showed a male preponderance [6]. A NWTS study done over a large population group however showed a female preponderance [7]. This might be a reflection of our social system where more female children are brought to the government hospitals. Tumors with favorable histology may present with aggressive behavior and therefore a need for prognostic evaluation of Wilms tumor.

Most of the cases, 16 out of 31, presented in stage I and 12 in stage II, 2 in stage III, and 1 in stage IV. Staging corresponds to other studies [6].

Dominant histological pattern was triphasic. Unfavourable histology was seen in 15 percent of cases as against western studies which showed only 5 percent [8]. This may be due to delayed presentation of the cases. Indicators of poor prognosis are anaplasia and tumor staging, and anaplasia on histology is subjective.

An attempt was made to characterize the cases through IHC in resource constrained government health centre. Two easily available markers Ki67 and p53 were evaluated. Ki67, tumor proliferation marker, is an important prognostic factor in a variety of cancers [9].

Ki67 is a nuclear antigen associated with cell proliferation, is present throughout the cell cycle, and is absent in resting cells. High Ki67 proliferation index (PI) is associated with a more aggressive clinical behaviour and is found to be a significant determinant of distant metastasis and tumor related deaths [9]. The study found higher Ki67 proliferative index in higher stages of Wilms tumor. Higher stage being associated with a higher index is well known as proven by Juric, Khine, Ghanem, and Juszkiewicz [8, 10–12]. This fact is once again reiterated. However, unlike the previous studies, proliferative index of the blastemal component was significantly high in our study; this can be explained based on the fact that the poorly differentiated blastema expresses higher PI than the well differentiated mesenchymal component. Juszkiewicz found similar results [12]. Das et al. in their study found higher index in the mesenchymal component. PI was higher in the anaplastic areas of the tumor. These findings show that greater proliferation is seen in advancing stage. Juric et al. in their study involving 48 cases of Wilms tumor supported the conclusion that Ki67 is a relevant marker for assessing the proliferative activity and tumor cell dynamics of nephroblastoma and that it may not be a good clinical prognostic marker [8]. Ghanem et al. observed higher PI indicative of clinical progression and poor survival [2]. The role of Ki67 as a proliferative marker in Wilms tumor stands reinforced again.

The role of p53 in the pathogenesis and progression of Wilms tumors is only partly understood [13]. Significance of p53 expression in Wilms tumor is conflicting. Wilms tumor has been associated with chromosomal abnormalities at the 11p13, 11p15, and 16q regions. A study into the possibility of mutations occurring within p53, the ubiquitous adult tumor suppressor gene, was made [14]. Several studies including one by Malkin et al. found the p53 mutations in Wilms tumor [15]. Cheah et al. in their Asian study mentioned that the immunohistochemical expression of p53 protein in Wilms tumor was presumably a result of mutation in the p53 tumor suppressor gene and correlates with histological classification [14]. The accumulation of p53 in these tumors may not only be due to mutations but also involve stabilization of normal p53 with other proteins, histological categorization being one of the useful features in the prognostic assessment of Wilms tumor [13].

However we found low to nil expression of p53 immunostaining in lower stages and moderate expression in higher stages. Similar findings were noted by Das and Zabolinezad in their study [1, 6]. This study does not find immunohistochemical expression of p53 utility in stratification of Wilms tumor. Skotnicka-Klonowicz et al. in their study found significant correlation between p53 expression and tumor staging [16]. All the relevant clinical and histopathological findings of our study including immunostaining are comparable with a similar north Indian study by Das et al. [6].

Therefore, these biological predictors may potentially provide the clinical oncologist with a biological rationale in identifying patients at high risk of tumor recurrence and to guide the adjuvant chemotherapy and/or radiotherapy [17].

Key Messages

Patients with favourable histology show aggressive clinical course. A need for objective assessment of tumor grade by prognostic markers is needed for better judgement of patient prognosis. Ki67 labelling index was found useful in prognostication of Wilms tumor by our study. However we did not find p53 immunostaining of any utility in Wilms tumor.

We advocate the routine use of Ki67 proliferative index in assessment of Wilms tumor histology.

Conflict of Interests

The authors declare that there is no conflict of interests regarding the publication of this paper.

References

[1] N. Zabolinezad, N. Sharifi, A. Tabatabaee et al., "Immunohistochemical expression of p53 protein in histologically favorable Wilms tumor and its relationship to tumor stage at presentation," *Iranian Journal of Basic Medical Sciences*, vol. 9, pp. 70–73, 2006.

[2] M. A. Ghanem, G. J. van Steenbrugge, R. J. M. Nijman, and T. H. van der Kwast, "Prognostic markers in nephroblastoma (Wilms' tumor)," *Urology*, vol. 65, no. 6, pp. 1047–1054, 2005.

[3] S. Wittmann, C. Wunder, B. Zirn et al., "New prognostic markers revealed by evaluation of genes correlated with clinical parameters in Wilms tumors," *Genes Chromosomes and Cancer*, vol. 47, no. 5, pp. 386–395, 2008.

[4] J. B. Beckwith, "Wilms' tumor and other renal tumors of childhood: a selective review from the National Wilms' Tumor Study Pathology Center," *Human Pathology*, vol. 14, no. 6, pp. 481–492, 1983.

[5] K. Mishra, M. Mathur, K. B. Logani, N. Kakkar, and A. Krishna, "Precursor lesions of Wilms' tumor in Indian children: a multiinstitutional study," *Cancer*, vol. 83, no. 10, pp. 2228–2232, 1998.

[6] R. N. Das, U. Chatterjee, S. K. Sinha, A. K. Ray, K. Saha, and S. Banerjee, "Study of histopathological features and proliferation markers in cases of Wilms' tumor," *Indian Journal of Medical and Paediatric Oncology*, vol. 33, no. 2, pp. 102–106, 2012.

[7] N. E. Breslow, R. Norris, P. A. Norkool et al., "Characteristics and outcomes of children with the Wilms tumor-aniridia syndrome: a report from the National Wilms Tumor Study Group," *Journal of Clinical Oncology*, vol. 21, no. 24, pp. 4579–4585, 2003.

[8] I. Juric, Z. Pogorelić, I. Kuzmić-Prusac et al., "Expression and prognostic value of the Ki-67 in Wilms' tumor: experience with 48 cases," *Pediatric Surgery International*, vol. 26, no. 5, pp. 487–493, 2010.

[9] D. Berrebi, J. Leclerc, G. Schleiermacher et al., "High cyclin E staining index in blastemal, stromal or epithelial cells is correlated with tumor aggressiveness in patients with nephroblastoma," *PLoS ONE*, vol. 3, no. 5, Article ID e2216, 2008.

[10] M. M. Khine, W. Aung, P. D. Sibbons et al., "Analysis of relative proliferation rates of Wilms' tumor components using proliferating cell nuclear antigen and MIB-1 (Ki-67 equivalent antigen) immunostaining and assessment of mitotic index," *Laboratory Investigation*, vol. 70, no. 1, pp. 125–129, 1994.

[11] M. A. Ghanem, T. H. Van der Kwast, M. K. Sudaryo et al., "MIB-1 (KI-67) proliferation index and cyclin-dependent kinase inhibitor $p27^{Kip1}$ protein expression in nephroblastoma," *Clinical Cancer Research*, vol. 10, no. 2, pp. 591–597, 2004.

[12] P. Juszkiewicz, "Immunohistochemical evaluation of the percentage of proliferating neoplastic cells of Wilms' tumor in children by means of the MIB-1 monoclonal antibody," *Annales Academiae Medicae Stetinensis*, vol. 43, pp. 113–127, 1997.

[13] C. Lahoti, P. Thorner, D. Malkin, and H. Yeger, "Immunohistochemical detection of p53 in Wilms' tumors correlates with unfavorable outcome," *The American Journal of Pathology*, vol. 148, no. 5, pp. 1577–1589, 1996.

[14] P. L. Cheah, L. M. Looi, and L. L. Chan, "Immunohistochemical expression of p53 proteins in Wilms' tumour: a possible association with the histological prognostic parameter of anaplasia," *Histopathology*, vol. 28, no. 1, pp. 49–54, 1996.

[15] D. Malkin, E. Sexsmith, H. Yeger, B. R. G. Williams, and M. J. Coppes, "Mutations of the p53 tumor suppressor gene occur infrequently in Wilms' tumor," *Cancer Research*, vol. 54, no. 8, pp. 2077–2079, 1994.

[16] G. Skotnicka-Klonowicz, J. Kobos, E. Łoś, E. Trejster, S. Szymik-Kantorowicz, and P. Daszkiewicz, "Prognostic value of p53 expression in Wilms' tumor in children," *Medical Science Monitor*, vol. 7, no. 6, pp. 1224–1229, 2001.

[17] A. G. Beniers, T. Effeth, L. Füzesi, B. Granzen, R. Mertens, and G. Jakse, "p53 expression in Wilms' tumor: a possible role as prognostic factor," *International Journal of Oncology*, vol. 18, no. 1, pp. 133–139, 2001.

A Cytological Study of Palpable Superficial Nodules of Parasitic Origin: A Study of 41 Cases

Prashant Goyal, Shelly Sehgal, Soumyesh Ghosh, Deepti Mittal, Awanindra Kumar, and Sompal Singh

Department of Pathology, Swami Dayanand Hospital, Dilshad Garden, Delhi 110095, India

Correspondence should be addressed to Prashant Goyal; drprashant549@yahoo.co.in

Academic Editor: Maria M. Picken

Background. Few parasitic infestations present as only superficial palpable subcutaneous or intramuscular nodule. The current study highlights the role of FNAC in the diagnosis of superficial palpable parasitic lesions. *Methods.* This was a retrospective study in which we reviewed the FNAC record of all patients over a period of two years from September 2011 to August 2013. During this period, FNA was performed on 5954 cases which presented as superficial palpable lump at various sites of body. There were 41 cases diagnosed as parasitic lesion or suspicious of parasitic lesion on cytology which were included in the study. *Results.* In the present study, most of the patients were children and young adults. The lesions were located over trunk in 18 (43.9%) cases, extremities in 12 (29.3%) cases, and head and neck region in 11 (26.8%) cases. Out of 41 cases, 27 (65.8%) cases were confirmed on cytology and/or histopathology as parasitic lesions, including 21 (51.2%) cases of cysticercosis, 5 (12.2%) cases of filariasis, and one (2.4%) case of hydatid cyst. Cytological findings of remaining cases were suggestive of parasitic lesion. *Conclusion.* Careful assessment of cytological material is helpful to detect parasite or inflammatory response to parasite even in asymptomatic patients.

1. Introduction

Parasitic infestation is a serious health problem in developing countries. Some parasitic infestations do not present with any other symptoms except single or multiple superficial palpable nodules. Subcutaneous or intramuscular palpable parasitic nodules are most commonly due to cysticercosis [1]. Most of these cases are clinically misdiagnosed as benign or malignant soft-tissue tumor or lymphadenitis depending on the site [2]. So, most of the time, diagnosis of parasitic lesion on cytology is an incidental finding. Fine needle aspiration cytology (FNAC) is simple, sensitive, cost-effective, and rapid diagnostic tool for evaluation of any superficial palpable lump over various sites of the body [3]. The diagnostic role of FNAC in cysticercosis was first emphasized by Kung et al. in 1989 [4]. Since then FNAC has become a pivotal tool in evaluating subcutaneous and muscle nodules caused by parasites [2]. FNAC also obviates the need for a subsequent histopathological examination, as the parasites may not be demonstrated even on biopsy examination [3].

In our study, the relevant clinical data, gross findings, cytomorphological findings, histopathological findings, and treatment response, wherever available, were evaluated. This study illustrates the value of careful screening of aspirated cytological material which can render definitive diagnosis of clinically unsuspected cases of parasitic infestation.

2. Material and Methods

This was a retrospective study in which we reviewed the FNAC record of all patients over a period of two years from September 2011 to August 2013 at the Department of Pathology of our hospital, a multispecialty Government Hospital catering low to middle class population. 5954 patients, who had superficial palpable lump, underwent FNAC during this period. Out of these, 41 cases (0.68%) were diagnosed as parasitic lesion or suspicious of parasitic lesion. FNAC was performed by pathologist with a 22 or 23 gauge needle attached to a 20 mL disposable syringe by free hand

TABLE 1: Clinical data and cytological features of all the cases included in present study.

Cytological diagnosis	No. of cases	Age range (mean) year	Sex	Size range (median) cm	Distribution of different cytological findings							
					N (%)	L (%)	E (%)	H (%)	PH (%)	GC (%)	G (%)	DGB (%)
Cysticercosis	19	4–34 (16.8)	M: 9 F: 10	0.5–3.0 (1.5)	10 (53)	16 (84)	7 (37)	14 (73)	6 (31)	9 (47)	6 (31)	6 (31)
Filariasis	5	10–32 (20.8)	M: 2 F: 3	1.0–2.5 (1.0)	2 (40)	4 (80)	2 (40)	3 (60)	0 (0)	1 (20)	1 (20)	0 (0)
Hydatid cyst	1	35	M: 1 F: 0	11	0	0	0	0	0	0	0	1 (100)
Suspicious parasitic lesion	16	5–38 (19.7)	M: 7 F: 9	0.5–4.5 (1.5)	8 (50)	12 (75)	4 (25)	11 (69)	5 (31)	6 (37)	2 (13)	5 (31)
Total	41	4–38 (18.9)	M: 19 F: 22	0.5–11 (1.5)	20 (49)	32 (78)	13 (32)	28 (68)	11 (27)	16 (39)	9 (22)	12 (29)

M: male; F: female; N: neutrophil; L: lymphocytes; E: eosinophil; H: histiocytes; PH: palisading histiocytes; GC: giant cells; G: granuloma; DGB: dirty granular background.

conventional method of aspiration. The aspirated cytological material was smeared on the glass slides. In cases of fluid aspirate from cystic lesion, smears were prepared from cystic fluid after cytocentrifugation. The air-dried smears were stained with May-Grunewald-Giemsa (MGG) stain after fixation in methanol. All cytological slides were reviewed by two independent pathologists. The evidence of parasite or fragment of parasite was noted along with other cytomorphological features. Subsequent excision biopsy and response to medical treatment was also evaluated whenever possible and findings were correlated with the cytological findings. The age and sex of patient, size, site, clinical diagnosis of nodule, and nature of aspirate were also noted (Table 1).

3. Results

We performed a total 5954 FNA of superficial palpable lumps from various sites during the study period and 41 cases (0.68%) were diagnosed as parasitic lesion or suspicious of parasitic lesion on cytology. Among 41 patients, 19 (46%) were males and 22 (56%) were females and presenting age ranged from 4 years to 38 years (mean age 18.9 years). All patients except two patients, presented with single, painless, superficial, slow-growing nodule of variable sizes while two patients presented with multiple nodules. On local examination, all the swellings were soft to firm, nontender, and nodular. In all the cases except one case of hydatid cyst, the diameter of swellings ranged from 0.5 to 4.5 cm (median 1.5 cm) while that of hydatid cyst was 11 cm. The lesions were located over trunk (including abdominal wall, chest, and back) in 18 (43.9%) cases, extremities in 12 (29.3%) cases, and head and neck in 11 (26.8%) cases (Figure 1). Provisional clinical diagnosis of parasitic lesion was made in only 2 (4.9%) cases, while the majority were clinically misdiagnosed as lipoma, neurofibroma, lymphadenitis, cold abscess, epidermal inclusion cyst, fibroadenoma, inflammatory lesion, and soft-tissue tumor. The aspirated material consisted of few drops to 5 mL fluid of variable consistency including clear fluid with or without granular deposit in 28 (68.3%) cases, purulent fluid in 10 (24.4%) cases, and blood-mixed fluid in 3 (7.3%) cases. No allergic reaction or any other complication was observed after the procedure. Out of 41 cases, 27 (65.8%) cases were confirmed on cytology and/or histopathology as parasitic lesions, included 21 (51.2%) cases of cysticercosis, 5 (12.2%) cases of filariasis, and one (2.4%) case of hydatid cyst (Figure 2).

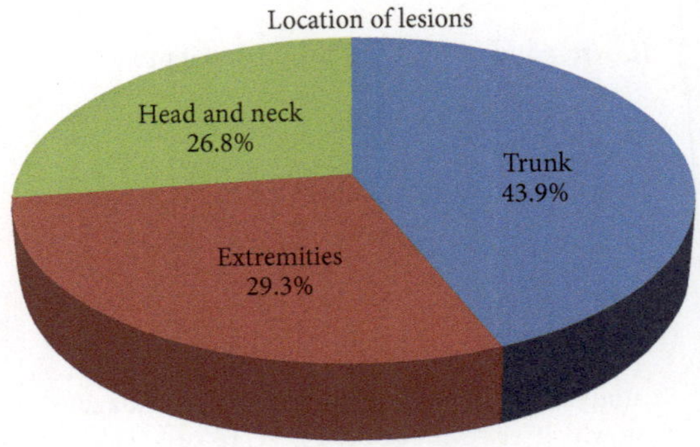

FIGURE 1: Distribution of lesions according to location.

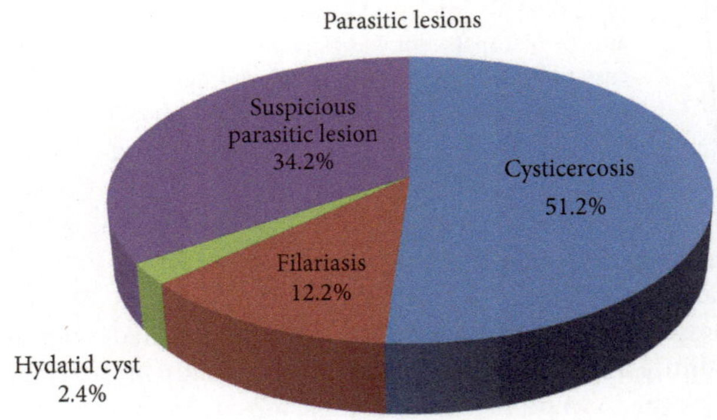

FIGURE 2: Distribution of parasitic lesions according to etiology.

3.1. Pathological Findings. In 19 (46.3%) cases, a definite evidence of cysticercosis was observed in form of fragments

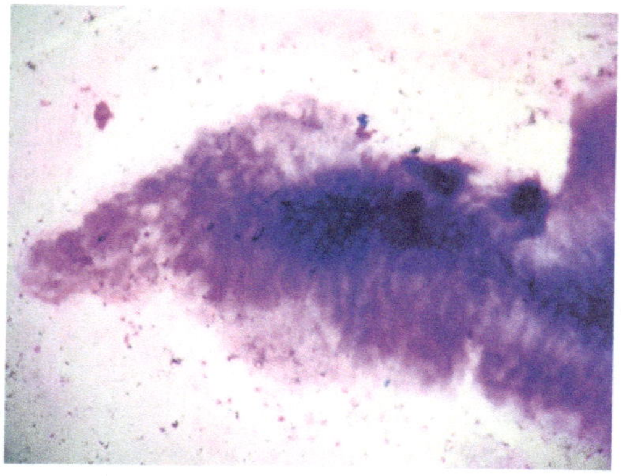

FIGURE 3: Cytological smear showing bladder wall of cysticercus cellulosae surrounded with mild inflammatory response (MGG stain, 60x).

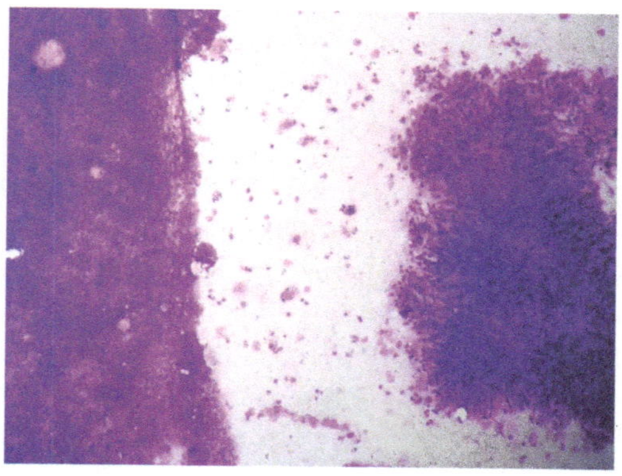

FIGURE 4: Cytological smear showing bladder wall of cysticercus cellulosae and epithelioid cell granuloma with palisading histiocytes (MGG stain, 40x).

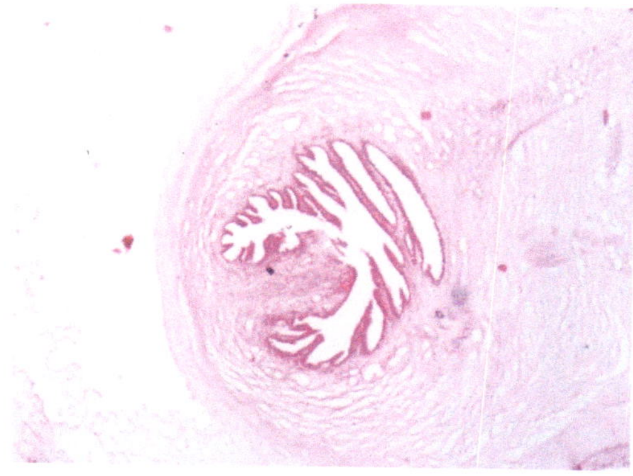

FIGURE 5: Histopathological section showing cysticercus cellulosae (H&E stain, 10x).

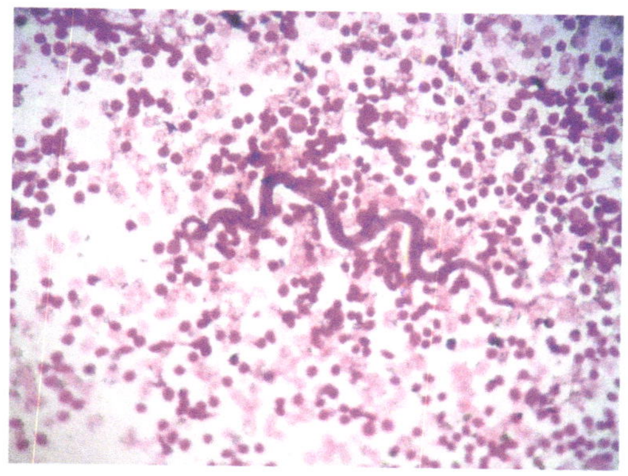

FIGURE 6: Cytological smear showing microfilaria surrounded with inflammatory cells and absence of eosinophil (MGG stain, 100x).

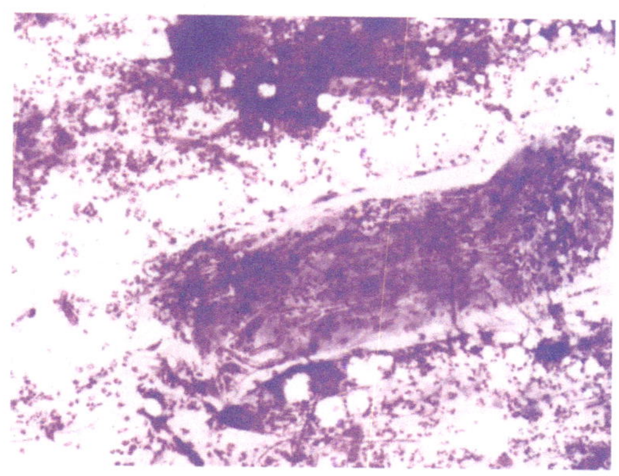

FIGURE 7: Cytological smear showing adult gravid filarial containing many microfilariae and surrounded with marked inflammatory cells (MGG Stain, 10x).

of cysticercus bladder wall on cytology (Figure 3) while none of them showed hooklets or scolex. All these cases showed varying proportion of inflammatory response with or without giant cells and granuloma (Figure 4). Out of these 19 cases, histopathological correlation was available only in 2 cases which correlated with cytodiagnosis (Figure 5). The rest of the cases responded to medical treatment for cysticercosis. All 5 cases of filariasis showed microfilaria along with mild to severe mixed inflammatory response (Figure 6) while one case also showed gravid adult filarial worm in cytology (Figure 7). Thick and thin blood smear examination of nocturnal venous blood revealed no microfilariae in all 5 cases. One case which was diagnosed as hydatid cyst showed acellular lamellated membrane on cytology and was confirmed on histopathology (Figure 8).

No parasite or fragment of parasite could be seen on cytology in 16 (39%) cases, but in these cases, the cytological findings were highly suggestive of a parasitic lesion. The cytology of these cases showed mild to moderate mixed inflammatory infiltrate, histiocytes, multinucleated giant cells, and epithelioid noncaseous granuloma in a dirty granular background. None of these cases showed hooklets or scolex on cytology. In 3 of these cases, a histopathological correlation was available, which revealed definite parasitic element of cysticercosis in 2 cases and the remaining case was reported as suggestive of parasitic lesion in view of absence of any parasitic element.

In this study, all cases of parasitic lesions or suspicious of parasitic lesion were associated with varying degree of mixed inflammatory response ranging from few histiocytes to marked mixed inflammatory cell infiltrate. Eosinophil was

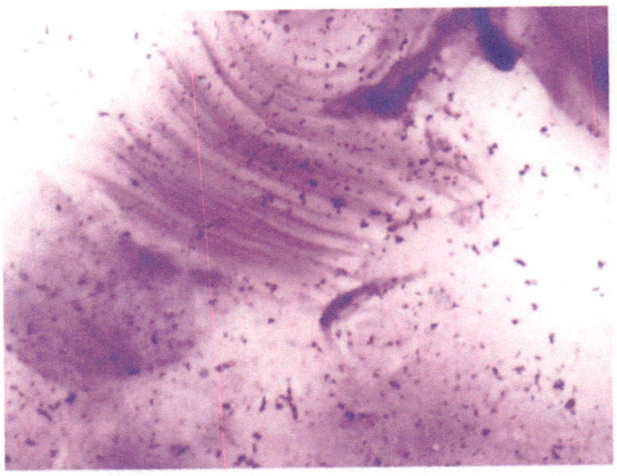

Figure 8: Cytological smear showing fragment of acellular lamellate membrane (MGG stain, 40x).

seen in only 13 (32%) out of the 41 cases while lymphocytes, histiocytes including palisading histiocytes, neutrophil, foreign body giant cells, and epithelioid granuloma were seen in 32 (78%), 28 (68%), 20 (49%), 16 (39%), and 9 (22%) cases, respectively. Dirty granular background was seen in 12 (29%) cases (Table 1).

4. Discussion

The palpable superficial parasitic nodules are often clinically misinterpreted as benign or malignant mesenchymal tumors or as lymphadenopathy. FNAC has emerged as a widely acceptable method for the diagnosis of parasitic lesion. In the present study, most of the patients were children and young adults with almost equal sex distribution. Cysticercosis was found to be the most common cause of superficial palpable parasitic nodules in previous studies as in our study [1, 5]. Other parasites identified were filaria and *Echinococcus*.

Cysticercosis in humans is an ancient disease and has even been detected in Egyptian mummies by paleoparasitologists [6]. Cysticercosis is the larval stage infection of the cestode *Taenia solium*. Humans are the only definitive host and can also act as intermediate hosts by ingestion of raw or poorly cooked vegetables or water contaminated with eggs or pork infested with larvae [7]. Cysticercosis is also common in vegetarians due to lack of basic sanitation facilities in developing countries [8]. Though cysticercus can be found in any organ, it commonly manifests as subcutaneous and intramuscular nodules which often are clinically misdiagnosed as inflammatory or mesenchymal lesions like in our study [8]. Essential for the cytodiagnosis of cysticercosis is identification of the parasitic fragments including its bladder wall and hooklets. Parasitic fragments may comprise bluish, fibrillary structures, sometimes with honeycombing, calcospherules, tegument thrown into rounded wavy folds, scolex with hooklets, and hyaline membrane surrounding it [9–11]. The physical factors such as the firm nonexpansile nature of the host tissue may limit the growth of the parasite and initiate the host inflammatory response. The presence of eosinophils, neutrophils, palisading histiocytes, giant cells, and atypical granular dirty background in an aspirate from a subcutaneous nodule should alert the cytopathologist of a parasitic infestation. Nonetheless, still in some cases of cysticercosis, none of these features may be present, and the inflammatory infiltrate may also be variable [2]. Finding an entire scolex in FNA is a rare event [12]. None of our cases showed hooklets or scolex on cytology.

Filariasis is a major public health problem in many tropical and subtropical countries and is prevalent in India, China, Indonesia, Africa, and the Far East. It is transmitted by the Culex mosquito and is caused by two closely related nematodes: *Wuchereria bancrofti* and *Brugia malayi*. *W. bancrofti* is responsible for 90% cases of filariasis [13]. All 5 cases of filariasis in our study were also caused by *W. bancrofti*. The majority of patients with filariasis are asymptomatic and diagnosed incidentally. Microfilaremia and eosinophilia are common in the acute phase. The various sites where microfilaria can be detected are thyroid, breast, skin and soft tissue swellings, epididymis, salivary glands, lymph nodes, urine, endoscopic brushings, and effusion fluids [14, 15]. In the present study, none of the patients was clinically suspected of filariasis; clinically they presented with breast lump (2 cases) and lymphadenopathy (3 cases). All cases showed mild to severe inflammatory reaction. In our study, only two cases had eosinophil in the aspirate; hence, eosinophils are not necessarily seen in lesions of filariasis.

Hydatid disease, also known as hydatosis or echinococcosis, is most frequently caused by *E. granulosus* and the commonly affected organs are liver and lung. This disease is endemic in cattle and sheep rearing regions of the world. The majority of cases of HCs are asymptomatic although clinical signs and symptoms depend on the anatomic location, size, and pressure effect of growing cysts. Therefore, the signs and symptoms are variable and never pathognomonic of HC [16]. So the majority of HC in subcutaneous or rare locations are misdiagnosed on clinical examination. Superficial HC usually presents as slow growing, fluctuant, and painless mass [16]. HC is usually not included in the differential diagnosis of subcutaneous or superficial palpable mass due to its rarity, even in endemic areas. The presence of a laminated membrane with parallel striations, dispersed retractile hooklets, granular debris, and multinucleated giant cells is consistent with the diagnosis of a HC [17]. FNAC is not recommended in suspected case of HC because of possibility of acute anaphylactic reaction due to spillage of hydatidfluid. However, some authors have reported that no complications were encountered during FNAC procedure as in our study [18].

In our study, the nature of aspirate was clear fluid with or without granular deposits in majority of cases. Hence, such clear fluid aspirate should alert the cytopathologist towards the possibility of parasitic etiology. In the majority of cytosmears, we found varying degree of inflammatory response comprising of histiocytes including palisading histiocytes and mixed inflammation including eosinophil, giant cells, and granulomas. Similar cytological features have been reported by other series also, although presence of eosinophils was relatively more common associated cytological feature as compared to our study [19].

5. Conclusion

Parasitic etiology is an important differential diagnosis of soft tissue nodule and FNAC is rapid, safe, cheap, and reliable diagnostic tool for such lesions. Careful assessment of cytological material is helpful to detect parasite or inflammatory response to parasite even in asymptomatic patients. The spectrum of host response may vary from no reaction to a marked inflammatory response. The entire spectrum of changes should be kept in mind while practicing cytopathology in an endemic area. In such situations, a high index of suspicion and careful screening of cytology smears are keys to a correct diagnosis.

Conflict of Interests

The authors declare that there is no conflict of interests regarding the publication of this paper.

References

[1] S. Suchitha, K. Vani, R. Sunila, and G. V. Manjunath, "Fine needle aspiration cytology of cysticercosis—a case report," *Case Reports in Infectious Diseases*, vol. 2012, Article ID 854704, 2 pages, 2012.

[2] M. Sawhney and S. Agarwal, "Cysticercosis: hooked by a hooklet on fine needle aspiration cytology—a case report," *Case Reports in Infectious Diseases*, vol. 2013, Article ID 315834, 2 pages, 2013.

[3] U. Handa, S. Garg, and H. Mohan, "Fine needle aspiration in the diagnosis of subcutaneous cysticercosis," *Diagnostic Cytopathology*, vol. 36, no. 3, pp. 183–187, 2008.

[4] I. T. M. Kung, D. Lee, and H. C. Yu, "Soft tissue cysticercosis. Diagnosis by fine-needle aspiration," *American Journal of Clinical Pathology*, vol. 92, no. 6, pp. 834–835, 1989.

[5] K. Verma and K. Kapila, "Fine needle aspiration diagnosis of cysticercosis in soft tissue swellings," *Acta Cytologica*, vol. 33, no. 5, pp. 663–666, 1989.

[6] F. Bruschi, M. Masetti, M. T. Locci, R. Ciranni, and G. Fornaciari, "Short report: cysticercosis in an Egyptian mummy of the late ptolemaic period," *American Journal of Tropical Medicine and Hygiene*, vol. 74, no. 4, pp. 598–599, 2006.

[7] R. Kraft, "Cysticercosis: an emerging parasitic disease," *American Family Physician*, vol. 76, no. 1, pp. 91–98, 2007.

[8] K. N. Prasad, A. Prasad, A. Verma, and A. K. Singh, "Human cysticercosis and Indian scenario: a review," *Journal of Biosciences*, vol. 33, no. 4, pp. 571–582, 2008.

[9] S. Nigam, T. Singh, A. Mishra, and K. U. Chaturvedi, "Oral cysticercosis—report of six cases," *Head and Neck*, vol. 23, no. 6, pp. 497–499, 2001.

[10] M. M. Kamal and S. V. Grover, "Cytomorphology of subcutaneous cysticercosis: a report of 10 cases," *Acta Cytologica*, vol. 39, no. 4, pp. 809–812, 1995.

[11] V. K. Arora, K. Gupta, N. Singh, and A. Bhatia, "Cytomorphologic panorama of cysticercosis on fine needle aspiration: a review of 298 cases," *Acta Cytologica*, vol. 38, no. 3, pp. 377–380, 1994.

[12] N. Singh, V. K. Arora, and A. Bhatia, "Are all subcutaneous parasitic cysts cysticercosis?" *Acta Cytologica*, vol. 50, no. 1, pp. 114–115, 2006.

[13] T. V. Katti, V. S. Athanikar, A. S. Ananthrao, and C. V. Rathod, "Cytodiagnosis of microfilarial lymphadenitis coexistent with metastatic squamous cell carcinoma in a left cervical lymph node: an unusual presentation," *Annals of Nigerian Medicine*, vol. 6, pp. 47–49, 2012.

[14] P. N. Kadam, K. G. Rathod, Y. H. Chavan, A. C. Panchamhalkar, and D. H. Bagre, "Isolated left supraclavicular lymphadenopathy—a rare presentation of lymphatic filariasis in children," *Journal of Evolution of Medical and Dental Sciences*, vol. 29, pp. 5426–5430, 2013.

[15] P. N. Yenkeshwar, D. T. Kumbhalkar, and S. K. Bobhate, "Microfilariae in fine needle aspirates: a report of 22 cases," *Indian Journal of Pathology and Microbiology*, vol. 49, no. 3, pp. 365–369, 2006.

[16] N. Sultana, T. K. Hashim, S. Y. Jan, Z. Khan, T. Malik, and W. Shah, "Primary cervical hydatid cyst: a rare occurrence," *Diagnostic Pathology*, vol. 7, article 157, 2012.

[17] M. J. Cancelo, M. Martín, and N. Mendoza, "Preoperative diagnosis of a breast hydatid cyst using fine-needle aspiration cytology: a case report and review of the literature," *Journal of Medical Case Reports*, vol. 6, article 293, 2012.

[18] M. Tekin, U. Osma, M. Yaldiz, and I. Topcu, "Preauricular hydatid cyst: an unusual location for echinoccosis," *European Archives of Oto-Rhino-Laryngology*, vol. 261, no. 2, pp. 87–89, 2004.

[19] K. Kapila, K. Sahai, and K. Verma, "Semi-quantitative analysis of soft-tissue reactions in fine needle aspirates from tissue cysticercosis," *Cytopathology*, vol. 14, no. 4, pp. 208–211, 2003.

10

Cytological and Pathological Correlation of FNAC in Assessing Breast Lumps and Axillary Lymph Node Swellings in a Public Sector Hospital

Vasu Reddy Challa,[1] Basavanna Goud Yale Guru,[1] Poornima Rangappa,[1] Vijayalakshmi Deshmane,[1] and Devi. M. Gayathri[2]

[1] *Department of Surgical Oncology, Kidwai Memorial Institute of Oncology, Bangalore, Karnataka 560029, India*
[2] *Department of Pathology, Kidwai Memorial Institute of Oncology, Bangalore, Karnataka 560029, India*

Correspondence should be addressed to Vasu Reddy Challa; vasureddyc@gmail.com

Academic Editor: Shahid Pervez

Background. Breast lumps have varied pathology, and there are different techniques to prove the diagnosis. The aim of the present study is to analyze the role of fine needle aspiration cytology (FNAC) of the breast lesions at our center. *Methods.* We had retrospectively analysed 854 patients who underwent FNAC for primary breast lumps and 190 patients who underwent FNAC for an axillary lymph node in the year 2010. *Results.* Of 854 patients, histological correlation was available in 723 patients. The analysis was done for 812 patients as medical records were not available for 42 patients. FNAC was false negative in seven cases; 2 cases of phyllodes were reported as fibroadenoma, and 5 cases of carcinoma were diagnosed as atypical hyperplasia. The sensitivity, specificity, and false negative value of FNAC in diagnosing breast lumps were 99% (715/723), 100%, and 1%, respectively. Of 190 patients for whom FNAC was performed for axilla, 170 had proven to have axillary lymph node metastases, and the rest had reactive hyperplasia or inflammatory cells. *Conclusions.* FNAC is rapid, accurate, outpatient based, and less complicated procedure and helps in diagnosis of breast cancer, benign diseases, and axillary involvement in experienced hands with less chance of false results.

1. Introduction

Breast cancer is one of the most common cancers in women in India and is a leading cause for mortality and morbidity. Breast tissue contains various tissue components, and there is change in composition of breast tissue with hormonal changes. So, it has varied pathology, and there are various modalities to prove the diagnosis. It is important for the clinician to examine properly and take proper decision during evaluation of a patient with palpable breast mass.

Triple assessment of breast mass had decreased the false negative rate to less than 1% [1]. But FNAC can be done as an outpatient procedure and helps in rapid diagnosis. The limitations of FNAC include difficulty to differentiate ductal carcinoma in situ (DCIS), atypical ductal hyperplasia from low grade DCIS, and fibroadenoma from phyllodes tumor [2, 3]. Core biopsy is an effective means to diagnose breast lumps, but it is expensive, time consuming, and associated with complications like haematoma and rarely pneumothorax [4, 5].

Many institutes in the United States, Canada, and the United Kingdom have given up FANC for diagnosing breast lesions, and they routinely perform core biopsy. But in many developing countries and in some European countries, FNAC is still routinely performed for diagnosing breast lesions [6]. FNAC is a rapid, less invasive, and less traumatic procedure but needs an experienced pathologist for better results.

The purpose of our study is to evaluate the efficacy of FNAC in diagnosing breast lumps in our setting, and it is one of the largest studies reported in India [6].

2. Materials and Methods

A retrospective analysis of medical records of the patients with detected breast mass (palpable and nonpalpable) and

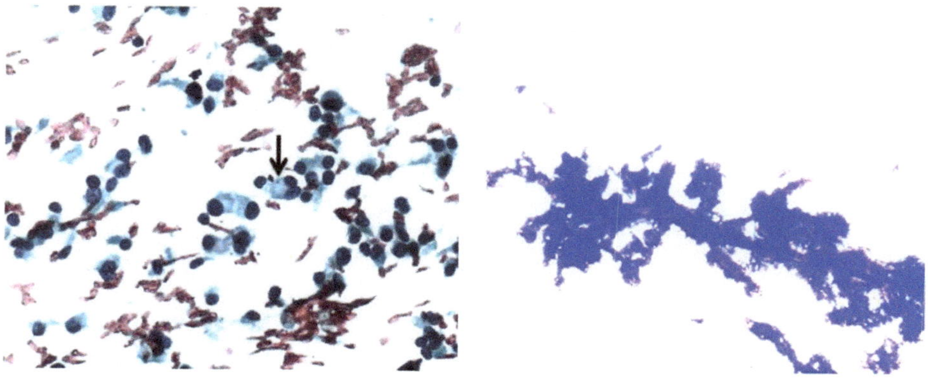

FIGURE 1: (a) FNAC breast lump showing PAP staining (20x) showing dispersed mildly pleomorphic plasmacytoid cells with azurophilic granules (arrow). Nucleus is irregular with some showing prominent nucleoli suggestive of neuroendocrine carcinoma. (b) FNAC breast lump with MGG staining (4x) showing papillary fragment with branching fibrovascular core suggestive of papillary neoplasm.

palpable axillary lymph node who were evaluated by FNAC at our centre in the year 2010 was valuated. Histopathological correlation was done wherever available. The procedure was performed by a pathologist using 21-22 Gauge needle with 2–4 aspirations and it was repeated if the sample was inadequate. For impalpable, and deeply located small lumps, ultrasound guided FNAC was performed. FNAC was done only for palpable lymph nodes. Sensitivity, specificity, and false negative and false positive values of FNAC for both breast lump and axilla were calculated. Statistical software SPSS 15.0 and MedCalc 9.0.1 were used to perform descriptive statistics.

3. Results

In a period of one year, 854 patients underwent FNAC of the primary breast lumps. As records of 42 patients were not available, they were excluded from the study. Hence, for 812 cases, histological correlation was available in 727 patients. The mean age of patients who underwent FNAC was 37.2 years (range 16–82 years). Ten male patients had undergone FNAC, two had gynaecomastia, and 8 had malignancy. Malignancy was the most common pathology of the patients who underwent fine needle aspiration cytology constituting 57% of all cases. The cytology reports were classified as benign, atypical, suspicious, malignancy, and unsatisfactory (Table 1).

Of the benign lesions, fibrocystic disease was the most common cytological diagnosis in 21% of patients (171 cases). Fibroadenoma was diagnosed in 98 patients with histology correlating with cytology in 96 cases. Two cases of phyllodes tumor were incorrectly reported as fibroadenoma on cytology. Of 27 cases who were diagnosed to have atypical lesions, (12 cases were papillary neoplasm, and 15 cases were atypical ductal hyperplasia) the final histopathology showed 12 cases of papillary carcinoma, 10 cases of papilloma, 10 had atypical ductal hyperplasia, 3 cases had ductal carcinoma in situ, and 2 cases had DCIS with a foci of invasive carcinoma. Cytology was useful in diagnosing various malignancies like neuroendocrine cancer, papillary neoplasms, and metastatic neoplasm from stomach (Figures 1 and 2).

TABLE 1: Cytology impression of the patients who underwent FNAC of breast lumps.

Report	Total number of patients (812)
Benign	314 (38.6%)
Benign lesions with no risk of cancer	83 (10.2%)
Benign proliferative disease without atypia	231 (28.4%)
Atypical	27 (3.3%)
Suspicious	12 (1.4%)
Malignancy	451 (55.5%)
Unsatisfactory	8 (0.9%)

Ten patients underwent ultrasound guided FNAC for deeply seated small lesions, of which 2 had invasive cancer, one was a case of papillary lesion later confirmed as papilloma, 2 were inflammatory lesions, and 5 patients had fibrocystic disease.

Of 8 patients with unsatisfactory reports, 4 patients were less than 30 years of age and were kept under followup, and clinicoradiologically, the lump appeared benign. The other 4 patients, though the FNAC was unsatisfactory due to discordance with clinicoradiological findings, were considered for excision, and one of the four patients had invasive ductal carcinoma. Seven cases were incorrectly diagnosed by FNAC (2 cases of phyllodes reported as fibroadenoma and 5 cases of carcinoma diagnosed as atypical hyperplasia). The sensitivity, specificity, and false negative value of FNAC in diagnosing breast lumps were 99% (715/723), 100%, and 1%, respectively (excluding patients with unsatisfactory samples) (Table 2). A concordance correlation coefficient was 0.99 (95% CI—0.9996 to 1.0000), and the Pearson coefficient was 0.99 which showed very good agreement between FNAC and the final histology (Figure 4).

3.1. FNAC—Fine Needle Aspiration Cytology. FNAC for a palpable axillary node was done in 190 patients of whom 170 had

Table 2: Comparison of cytology and histopathology of breast lesions.

Type of lesion	No. of cases (812)	Patients with histological correlation (727)
(A) Benign lesions with no risk of cancer	**83 (10.2%)**	**12**
(1) Inflammatory breast lesions	**27 (3.3%)**	
(a) Breast abscess	5 (0.6%)	—
(b) Granulomatous mastitis	12 (1.4%)	2
(c) Fat necrosis	5 (0.6%)	—
(d) Periductal mastitis/duct ectasia	5 (0.6%)	—
(2) Nonproliferative breast disorder	**40 (4.9%)**	
(a) Simple cyst	10 (1.2%)	—
(b) Fibrocystic change	30 (3.6%)	10
(3) Miscellaneous breast lesions	**16 (1.9%)**	
(a) Galactocele	2	—
(b) Lipoma	3	—
(c) Gynaecomastia	2	—
(d) Axillary breast tissue	3	—
(e) Suture granuloma	2	—
(f) Hamartoma	2	—
(g) Diabetic mastopathy	1	—
(h) Radiotherapy induced mastitis	1	—
(B) Benign lesions with mild to moderate risk of cancer	**258 (31.7%)**	**248**
(1) Proliferative breast disease without atypia	**231 (28.4%)**	**221**
(a) Fibrocystic disease without atypia (Moderate epithelial hyperplasia and adenosis)	121 (14.9%)	111
(b) Fibroadenoma	98 (12%)	98 (2 cases turned as phyllodes)
(c) Phyllodes tumor Figure 3	12 (1.4%)	12
(2) Proliferative breast disorder with Atypia	**27 (3.3%)**	**27**
(a) Atypical ductal hyperplasia	15 (1.8%)	15 (5 cases turned as carcinoma)
(b) Papillary neoplasm	12 (1.4%)	12 (10 cases papilloma, 2 cases papillary carcinoma)
(C) Suspicious and malignant lesions	**463 (57%)**	463
(1) Suspicious	12 (1.4%)	12
(2) Carcinoma	449 (55.2%)	449
(3) Malignant myoepithelioma	1	1
(4) Metastatic adenocarcinoma	1	1
(D) Unsatisfactory	8	4 (1 case invasive ductal carcinoma)

proven axillary lymph node metastases; the rest had reactive hyperplasia or inflammatory cells in the final histology. The sensitivity, specificity, and false positive and false negative results to rule out axillary lymph node metastases in a palpable lymph node were 90% (153/170), 100%, 0%, and 10% (17/170) (Tables 3 and 4).

4. Discussion

FNAC was first described by Martin and Ellis in 1930 for sampling cervical lymph nodes [7]. FNAC is a simple rapid technique performed as an outpatient procedure with less chance of complications unlike core biopsy which has risk of bleeding and occasionally rare complications like pneumothorax. It does not require any anesthesia or hospitalization and is cost effective. Experience and expertise in sampling and interpretation of specimen decide the effectiveness of FNAC. The other limitation of FNAC is it cannot differentiate few lesions like fibroadenoma from phyllodes, phyllodes from metaplastic carcinoma breast, papilloma from papillary carcinoma, and atypical ductal hyperplasia from ductal carcinoma in situ. Though a triple assessment is advocated for all palpable breast lumps, it is not feasible in developing countries like India, where affordability and availability are an issue at all centers and clinical decision takes a major role.

The sensitivity and specificity varied in different studies based on whether the unsatisfactory samples were considered positive or negative [6]. If the unsatisfactory samples were

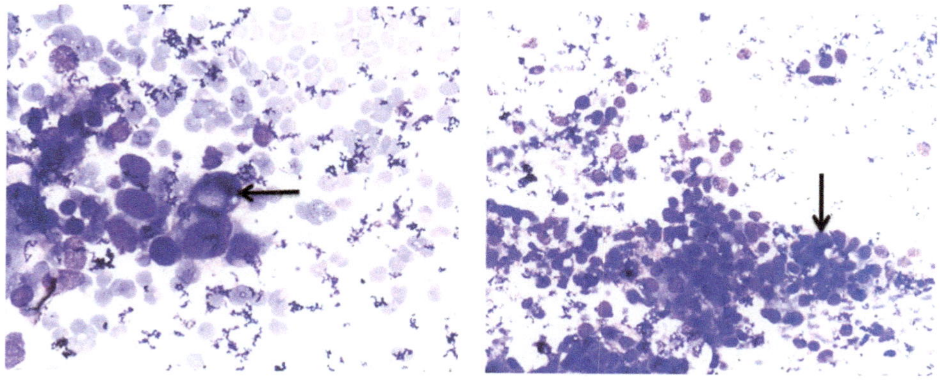

(a) (b)

FIGURE 2: (a) FNAC breast lump with MGG staining (20x) showing signet ring cell (arrow). (b) FNAC breast lump with MGG staining (20x) showing acinar formation (arrow). It was diagnosed as metastatic lesion and proved to be gastric cancer metastasizing to breast.

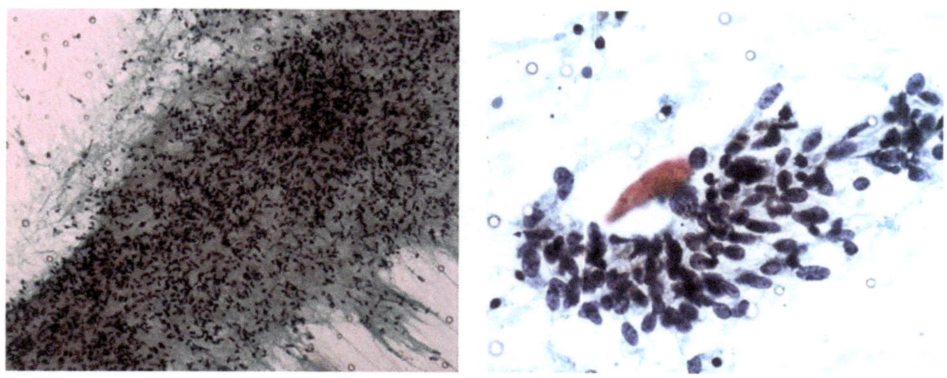

(a) (b)

FIGURE 3: (a) PAP staining (20x) showing hypercellular spindle cell stromal component. Moderate nuclear pleomorphism is evident. (b) PAP staining (40x) showing loose cohesive cluster of epithelial cells with moderate nuclear pleomorphism suggestive of phyllodes tumor.

TABLE 3: FNAC and histology correlation of axillary lymph node status.

	Axillary lymph node metastases present	Axillary lymph node metastases absent
FNAC positive	153	0
FNAC negative	17	20

TABLE 4: Diagnostic performance of FNAC axillary lymph node status ($N = 190$).

(i) Sensitivity	90% (153/170)
(ii) Specificity	100% (20/20)
(iii) False positive	0%
(iv) False negative	10% (17/170)

excluded from the study, the sensitivities and specificities varied from 58.3% to 100% and 55 to 100% [6]. Because an unsatisfactory sample needs further evaluation, few studies had considered them as a positive result and analysed there results. A meta-analysis of FNAC of breast lesions showed a sensitivity and specificity of 0.920 (95% CI, 0.906 to 0.933) and 0.768 (95% CI, 0.751 to 0.784) respectively (if the unsatisfactory samples were considered positive) [6]. If unsatisfactory samples were excluded from the study, the sensitivity was 0.927 (95% confidence interval [CI], 0.921 to 0.933); specificity 0.948 (95% CI, 0.943 to 0.952); positive likelihood ratio 25.72 (95% CI, 17.35 to 28.13); negative likelihood ratio 0.08 (95% CI, 0.06 to 0.11); diagnostic odds ratio 429.73 (95% CI, 241.75 to 763.87) (Table 5). Also, in these meta-analyses, when the pooled unsatisfactory samples were further analyzed, there was upgrading to cancer in 27.5% of cases. In our study, there was one of 8 cases (12.5%) who had been upgraded to cancer in unsatisfactory samples. We had 7 false negatives, 2 cases reported as fibroadenoma preoperatively turned out to be phyllodes, and 5 cases of carcinoma were diagnosed as atypical hyperplasia preoperatively.

The most common reason for a false negative result is failure to localize the lesion exactly. This can be overcome by performing the test under image guidance [8]. Also, tumors with extensive fibrosis like scirrhous carcinoma can give a false negative result because of low cellularity which can be avoided by performing FNAC in the periphery of the tumor with 27-gauge needle in this type of malignancies [9]. The false positive results occur because of some benign

TABLE 5: Summary of studies showing the results of FNAC (after excluding unsatisfactory samples).

Author (year)	Number of patients	Sensitivity	Specificity	False positive	False negative
Tao et al. (2004) [14]	2701	97.9%	99.8%	0.2%	2.1%
Yu et al. (2006) [15]	2128	98%	75.5%	24.5%	2%
Wang (1981) [16]	1024	88.1%	91.7%	8.3%	11.9%
Farshid et al. (2008) [17]	1093	97.8%	88%	12%	2.2%
Vasu et al. (present study)	723	99%	100%	0%	1%

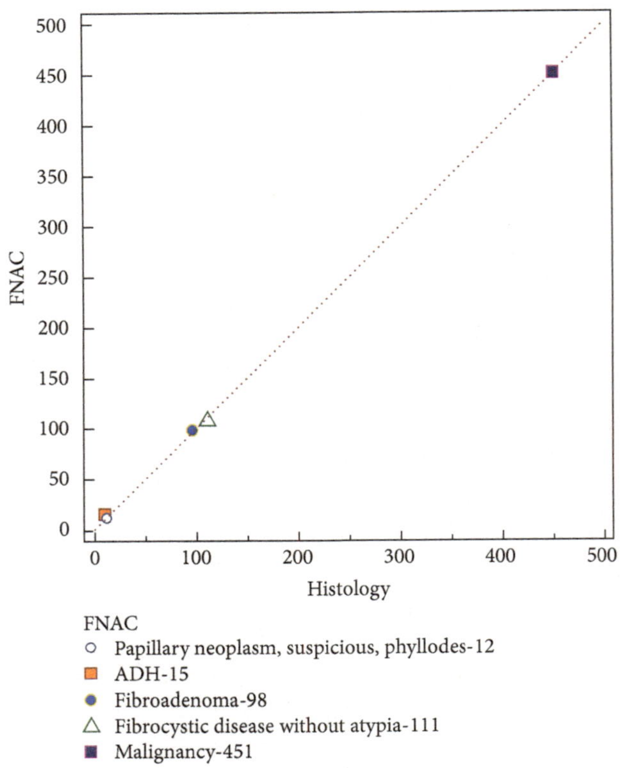

FIGURE 4: A concordance correlation coefficient scatter diagram of FNAC and histology showing the distribution of cases.

diseases with hypercellularity like cellular fibroadenoma, proliferative fibrocystic disease, phyllodes tumor, lactational changes, sclerosing adenosis, and so forth, and in lesions with atypia like postradiation, fat necrosis, and radial scar [9]. False positives can be reduced by considering for biopsy in patients fulfilling DeMay's criteria in cases with (a) poor cellular aspirate, (b) absent single intact cells, (c) presence of bare bipolar nuclei, and (d) absent/less amount of atypia [10].

For no palpable lymph nodes, ultrasonography with FNAC as a staging tool avoided sentinel lymph node biopsy in 68% of patients (upfront underwent axillary lymph node dissection) with positive axillary lymph nodes [11]. Roles of FNAC in palpable lymph nodes to rule out metastases were evaluated in a study which showed diagnostic accuracy for metastatic lymph nodes as 97.9%, sensitivity of 97.9%, and specificity of 100% [12]. Our study is in well correlation with literature with sensitivity of 90% in diagnosing axillary lymph node involvement. The cost effectiveness of FNAC of breast was studied in a study by Silverman et al. They demonstrated less costs with FNAC of breast and helped to triage the patients to either outpatient or inpatient setting [13]. This is important in poor resource setting like our hospital where most of the patients present in advanced stage and cannot afford expensive investigations. We would like to bring in light that FNAC is still an acceptable mode of diagnosis in experienced hands and where there is limitation of resources.

5. Conclusion

FNAC is a safe, rapid, and effective test for diagnosing breast lumps in experienced hands. Unsatisfactory samples should not be neglected and should be considered for excisional biopsy in presence of clinical suspicion.

List of Abbreviations

FNAC: Fine needle aspiration cytology
DCIS: Ductal carcinoma in situ
PAP: Papanicolaou
MGG: May-Grünwald Giemsa stain.

Conflict of Interests

The authors declare that they have no conflict of interests.

Authors' Contribution

Dr. Vasu Reddy was involved in design of study, literature search, and writing the paper. Dr. Basavanna Goud and Dr. Poornima were involved in data acquisition, data analysis, and literature search. Dr. Vijayalakshmi Deshmane and Dr. devi. M. Gayathri were the cytopathologist in reviewing the slides and collaborated for paper reviewing and editing.

References

[1] Z. Kaufman, B. Shpitz, M. Shapiro et al., "Triple approach in the diagnosis of dominant breast masses: combined physical examination, mammography, and fine-needle aspiration," *Journal of Surgical Oncology*, vol. 56, no. 4, pp. 254–257, 1994.

[2] P. Mendoza, M. Lacambra, P. H. Tan, and G. M. Tse, "Fine needle aspiration cytology of the breast: the nonmalignant categories," *Pathology Research International*, vol. 2011, Article ID 547580, 8 pages, 2011.

[3] "The uniform approach to breast fine-needle aspiration biopsy. NIH Consensus Development Conference," *The American Journal of Surgery*, vol. 174, pp. 371–385, 1997.

[4] K. Dowlatshahi, P. M. Jokich, R. Schmidt, M. Bibbo, and P. J. Dawson, "Cytologic diagnosis of occult breast lesions using

stereotaxic needle aspiration. A preliminary report," *Archives of Surgery*, vol. 122, no. 11, pp. 1343–1346, 1987.

[5] W. P. Evans and S. H. Cade, "Needle localization and fine-needle aspiration biopsy of nonpalpable breast lesions with use of standard and stereotactic equipment," *Radiology*, vol. 173, no. 1, pp. 53–56, 1989.

[6] Y.-H. Yu, W. Wei, and J.-L. Liu, "Diagnostic value of fine-needle aspiration biopsy for breast mass: a systematic review and meta-analysis," *BMC Cancer*, vol. 12, article 41, 2012.

[7] J. C. Litherland, "Should fine needle aspiration cytology in breast assessment be abandoned?" *Clinical Radiology*, vol. 57, no. 2, pp. 81–84, 2002.

[8] S. H. Parker, A. T. Stavros, and M. A. Dennis, "Needle biopsy techniques," *Radiologic Clinics of North America*, vol. 33, no. 6, pp. 1171–1186, 1995.

[9] M. F. Vazquez, "Needle biopsy diagnosis of breast cancer," in *Breast Cancer*, D. F. Roses, Ed., chapter 17, pp. 271–289, 2nd edition, 2008.

[10] R. M. Demay, "Diseases and conditions of the breast," in *The Art and Science of Cytopathology: Aspiration Cytology*, vol. 2, pp. 847–937, USA ASCP press, Chicago, Ill, USA, 1996.

[11] V. Altomare, G. Guerriero, R. Carino et al., "Axillary lymph node echo-guided fine-needle aspiration cytology enables breast cancer patients to avoid a sentinel lymph node biopsy. Preliminary experience and a review of the literature," *Surgery Today*, vol. 37, no. 9, pp. 735–739, 2007.

[12] K. Alam, V. Maheshwari, N. Haider, F. A. Siddiqui, A. Jain, and A. H. Khan, "Fine needle aspiration cytology (FNAC), a handy tool for metastatic lymphadenopathy," *The Internet Journal of Pathology*, vol. 10, no. 2, 2010.

[13] J. F. Silverman, D. R. Lannin, K. O'Brien, and H. T. Norris, "The triage role of fine needle aspiration biopsy of palpable breast masses: diagnostic accuracy and cost-effectiveness," *Acta Cytologica*, vol. 31, no. 6, pp. 731–736, 1987.

[14] G. H. Tao, Z. F. Liu, H. M. Liu, Y. Q. Liu, A. L. He, and T. Y. Guan, "A study of fine needle aspiration cytologic diagnosis for breast masses," *Henan Journal of Oncology*, vol. 17, pp. 350–351, 2004.

[15] K. Q. Yu, W. Q. Yang, and J. M. Yang, "The role of fine needle aspiration cytology in the diagnosis of breast tumor," *Shandong Medical Journal*, vol. 46, pp. 70–71, 2006.

[16] H.-F. Wang, "Cytologic examination of breast mass with fine needle aspiration technique in 1024 cases," *Oncology Supplement*, vol. 8, no. 3, pp. 139–140, 1981.

[17] G. Farshid, P. Downey, P. G. Gill, and S. Pieterse, "Assessment of 1183 screen-detected, category 3B, circumscribed masses by cytology and core biopsy with long-term follow up data," *British Journal of Cancer*, vol. 98, no. 7, pp. 1182–1190, 2008.

11

Prognostic Significance of N-Glycolyl GM3 Ganglioside Expression in Non-Small Cell Lung Carcinoma Patients: New Evidences

Rancés Blanco,[1] Elizabeth Domínguez,[2] Orlando Morales,[3] Damián Blanco,[4] Darel Martínez,[5] Charles E. Rengifo,[6] Carmen Viada,[7] Mercedes Cedeño,[1] Enrique Rengifo,[1] and Adriana Carr[8]

[1]*Laboratory of Recognition and Biological Activity Assays, Center of Molecular Immunology, 216 Street and 15th Avenue, Atabey, Playa, P.O. Box 16040, 11600 Havana, Cuba*
[2]*Laboratory of Biochemistry, Department of Quality Control, Center of Molecular Immunology, 216 Street and 15th Avenue, Atabey, Playa, P.O. Box 16040, 11600 Havana, Cuba*
[3]*Process Development Direction, Center of Molecular Immunology, 216 Street and 15th Avenue, Atabey, Playa, P.O. Box 16040, 11600 Havana, Cuba*
[4]*Department of Cell Biology and Tissues Banking, National Institute of Oncology and Radiobiology, 29 and F Street, Vedado, Plaza de la Revolución, 10400 Havana, Cuba*
[5]*Tumor Immunology Direction, Center of Molecular Immunology, 216 Street and 15th Avenue, Atabey, Playa, P.O. Box 16040, 11600 Havana, Cuba*
[6]*Department of Pathology, Manuel Fajardo General Hospital, Zapata and D Street, Vedado, Plaza de la Revolución, 10400 Havana, Cuba*
[7]*Clinical Trials Direction, Center of Molecular Immunology, 216 Street and 15th Avenue, Atabey, Playa, P.O. Box 16040, 11600 Havana, Cuba*
[8]*Research and Development Direction, Center of Molecular Immunology, 216 Street and 15th Avenue, Atabey, Playa, P.O. Box 16040, 11600 Havana, Cuba*

Correspondence should be addressed to Rancés Blanco; rances@cim.sld.cu

Academic Editor: Marco Volante

The prognostic role of N-glycolyl GM3 ganglioside (NeuGcGM3) expression in non-small cell lung carcinoma (NSCLC) still remains controversial. In this study, the NeuGcGM3 expression was reevaluated using an increased number of NSCLC cases and the 14F7 Mab (a highly specific IgG1 raised against NeuGcGM3). An immunohistochemical score integrating the percentage of 14F7-positive cells and the intensity of reaction was applied to reassess the relationship between NeuGcGM3 expression, some clinicopathological features, and the overall survival (OS) of NSCLC patients. The double and the triple expression of NeuGcGM3 with the epidermal growth factor receptor (EGFR) and/or its ligand, the epidermal growth factor (EGF), were also evaluated. NeuGcGM3 expression correlates with both S-Phase fraction ($p = 0.006$) and proliferation index ($p = 0.000$). Additionally, NeuGcGM3 expression was associated with a poor OS of patients in both univariate ($p = 0.020$) and multivariate ($p = 0.010$) analysis. Moreover, the double and/or the triple positivity of tumors to NeuGcGM3, EGFR, and/or EGF permitted us to identify phenotypes of NSCLC with a more aggressive biological behavior. Our results are in agreement with the negative prognostic significance of NeuGcGM3 expression in NSCLC patients. However, standardization of techniques to determine the expression of NeuGcGM3 in NSCLC as well as the implementation of a universal scoring system is recommended.

1. Introduction

Lung cancer is one of the most frequent cancers in the world and usually has a very poor prognosis. There are two main forms of the disease but non-small cell lung cancer (NSCLC) represents about 80–85% of these tumors [1, 2]. Consequently, numerous studies are currently focusing on the selection of newer biological and molecular prognostic factors as a potential complement of TNM (tumor, node, metastasis) staging system [3–5]. In line with this, unusual glycosylated gangliosides have been identified by immunohistochemistry (IHC) in NSCLC, also becoming attractive targets for immunotherapy [6, 7].

The aberrant expression of N-glycolyl GM3 ganglioside (NeuGcα2-3Galβ1-4Glcβ-Cer) (NeuGcGM3) in NSCLC, by mean of 14F7 Mab reactivity, using frozen [8] and formalin-fixed and paraffin-embedded (FFPE) [9, 10] tissues, was previously demonstrated. This Mab is a highly specific IgG1 raised against NeuGcGM3 that does not cross-react with other NeuGc-containing gangliosides [11]. In addition, the expression of NeuGcGM3 was also evidenced by immunohistochemistry and TLC-immunostaining in FFPE samples with GMR8 Mab [7]. GMR8 Mab is an IgM that reacts with an epitope shared by more than one of the NeuGc-containing gangliosides [12]. In line with this, at least another NeuGc-containing ganglioside, GD1a (NeuGc), was recognized by GMR8 Mab in NSCLC tissues, although NeuGcGM3 was the predominant ganglioside identified in these samples [7].

Additionally, the relevance of NeuGcGM3 in cancer progression and its capability of modulating CD4 expression on T cells have been published [13, 14]. Recently, the expression of NeuGcGM3, as shown as 14F7 Mab staining, has been associated with more aggressive disease in colon adenocarcinoma [15]. In NSCLC patients, the expression of NeuGcGM3 inhibits dendritic cells (DCs) differentiation, maturation, and migration leading to tumor-induced DCs suppression [9]. However, at present, the prognostic role of NeuGcGM3 expression in NSCLC still remains controversial [7, 9, 10].

For this reason, in this study the prognostic value of the 14F7 Mab reactivity was reevaluated using an increased number of Cuban NSCLC patients as well as an immunohistochemical score, which integrate the percentage of positive cells and the intensity of reaction. Additionally, the impact of the simultaneous expression of NeuGcGM3, epidermal growth factor receptor (EGFR), and/or epidermal growth factor (EGF) was assessed in the overall survival of these patients. A study of the antigen recognized by 14F7 Mab in FFPE tissues was also included.

2. Materials and Methods

2.1. Monoclonal Antibodies. We used the 14F7, a murine IgG1 highly specific against the N-glycosylated variant of GM3 ganglioside [11], the ior egf/r3 (anti-human EGFR) [16], and the CB-EGF1 (anti-human EGF) [17]. 14F7 and ior egf/r3 Mabs were produced by the Center for Molecular Immunology (Havana, Cuba), while CB-EGF1 was kindly provided by the Center for Genetic Engineering and Biotechnology (Havana, Cuba). Additionally, the anti-human EGFR Mab (Dako EGFR pharmDx kit, K1494), the negative control included in this kit, the P3 Mab, an IgM that recognize NeuGcGM3, and other NeuGc-containing gangliosides as well as sulfated glycolipids [6] were employed.

2.2. Tissue Specimens. A total of 90 formalin-fixed and paraffin-embedded (FFPE) tissues with diagnosis of NSCLC were received from the pathology department of both Hermanos Ameijeiras General Hospital and the National Institute of Oncology and Radiobiology, after approved consent by the institutional ethical committees. Specimens from patients with stages I–IIIA were surgically resected by means of wedge biopsy, lobectomy, or pneumonectomy before the standard radio-chemotherapeutic regimens, while samples from patients with stages IIIB–IV were obtained during the clinical autopsy.

2.3. Lipid Extraction. Paraffin blocks were melted by heating in a 70°C oven for 4 h. The tissue samples were maintained in xylene for 1 h at 70°C and then at room temperature (3 × 1 h). The tissues were rehydrated in graded ethanol series (100%, 100%, 90%, and 70%) for 1 h each. Finally, they were washed in tap and distilled water for 30 and 15 minutes, respectively. For the lipid extraction, the method as it was previously described by Bligh and Dyer (1959) with minor modifications was used [18]. Briefly, one of two fragments of NSCLC samples (1-2 g) was mechanically homogenized. Then, 3.75 mL of a mixture chloroform/methanol (1/2) was added and vortexed for 30 minutes. Afterward, 1.25 mL of chloroform and 1.25 mL of distilled water were added and the preparation was mixed during 1 minute in each step. The samples were centrifuged, the upper phase was discarded, and finally the lower phase was collected with a Pasteur pipette. After evaporation, the lipid extract (lower phase) was redissolved in 20 μL of chloroform/methanol (2/1).

2.4. Thin-Layer Chromatography. Glycolipids extracted from paraffin blocks were immunostained on a high-performance thin-layer chromatography (HPTLC) aluminium plates (Merck-Millipore, 105553) to determine the ganglioside fraction. The solvent system used for developing chromatograms was chloroform/methanol/0.25% ammonia (5 : 4 : 1, v/v/v). Afterward, the plates were air dried and carbohydrates were visualized with orcinol stain. For immunostaining, after chromatography, plates were soaked for 75 seconds on hexane (Sigma-Aldrich, 296090) containing 0.1% poly (isobutyl methacrylate) (Sigma-Aldrich, 445754). The plates were air dried, blocked with phosphate buffer saline (PBS) (Capricorn, PBS-1A) containing 1% bovine serum albumin (BSA) (Sigma-Aldrich, A2153) for 30 minutes, and incubated with 20 μg/mL of 14F7 Mab for 3 hours at room temperature. Afterward, the plates were washed with PBS/BSA 1% and incubated with peroxidase-conjugated goat anti-mouse IgG antibody (Sigma-Aldrich, A4416). The reaction was developed with 3,3-diaminobenzidine (Sigma-Aldrich, D800-1).

2.5. Mass Spectrometry. The gangliosides fractions extracted from FFPE tissues were analyzed by matrix-assisted laser desorption/ionization-time of flight (MALDI TOF) mass spectrometry. MALDI mass spectra were obtained using an AXIMA Performance MALDI TOF/TOF mass spectrometer (Shimadzu Biotech) with a 337 nm N_2 laser using delayed extraction, in positive reflectron mode. The glycolipid extracts were resuspended in 10 μL of 50% methanol, from which 1 μL was mixed with an equal volume of a saturated solution of 2,5-dihydroxybenzoic acid (DHB) (Sigma-Aldrich, 85707) in 50% acetonitrile (Sigma-Aldrich, 34851) on top of the MALDI target plate. Samples were allowed to dry off at room temperature and were recrystallized through the addition of 1 μL of ethanol. Two hundred laser shots were accumulated for each mass spectrum, with a 50 Hz laser repetition rate. In this analysis, signals between m/z 1.000 and 2.000 were collected. The data was processed using MALDI-MS software from Axima Biotech Launch pad software pack.

The spectra were externally calibrated against Proteo-MassTM peptide MALDI-MS calibration kit (Sigma-Aldrich, MSCAL2-1KT). The peaks corresponding to NeuAcGM3 and NeuGcGM3 were confirmed by comparison with purified samples of both gangliosides.

2.6. Immunohistochemical Staining. Five-micrometer serial sections from each block were obtained in a micrometer (Leitz, 1512) and they were mounted on plus slides (Dako, S2024). All sections were attached to the slide by heating in a 60°C oven for 1 h. Afterward, the slides were dewaxed in xylene and rehydrated in graded ethanol series in the usual way. The samples were maintained in tap water until they were stained.

The immunolocalization of NeuGcGM3 ganglioside was performed as it was previously described in [10] with some modifications. Briefly, the slides were incubated with 14F7 Mab in a humid chamber for 1 h at room temperature followed by the labeled streptavidin biotin (LSAB) two steps' system (Dako, K0690) both for 30 minutes at room temperature. The enzymatic activity was visualized with 3,3-diaminobenzidine (DAB) substrate chromogenic solution (Dako, K3465) and the tissues were counterstained with Mayer's Hematoxylin (Dako, S2020). Concerning the evaluation of both EGFR and EGF tissue antigens, the procedure as it was previously described in [19] was used.

2.7. Enzymatic Tissue Treatments. In essence, tissue treatments were performed as described by Kotani and Tai [20] with some variations to formalin-fixed and paraffin-embedded samples. After routine dewaxing and rehydration, tissue sections were treated with 4 U/mL of Neuraminidase *Clostridium perfringens* (Sigma-Aldrich, N2876) in PBS (Capricorn, PBS-1A) for 2 hours at 37°C. The enzyme from *Clostridium perfringens* cleaves terminal sialic acid residues which are α-2,3-, α-2,6-, or α-2,8-linked to Gal, GlcNac, GalNAc, AcNeu, GlcNeu, oligosaccharides, glycolipids, or glycoproteins. The relative rate of cleavage decreases in the order: α-2-3 > α-2-6, and α-2-8. As positive control, the antibody specific to the cell membrane glycoprotein EGFR (Dako, K1494) as well as the P3 Mab [6] was used. Slides incubated with the negative reactive (Dako, K1494) served as negative control.

2.8. Immunohistochemical Evaluation. The tissue expression of the NeuGcGM3, EGFR, and EGF in both cell membrane and cytoplasm of epithelial malignant cells was evaluated for percentage of positive cells and intensity of reaction. The most representative regions of each section were selected and the percentage of tumor cells showing immunostaining in them was estimated (0–100%) using the 10x objective lens. The intensity of reaction of each sample was judged as negative (0), weak (1), moderate (2), and strong (3). The final results were considered according to two observers' agreement (Charles E. Rengifo and Rancés Blanco).

2.9. Generation of Integrated IHC Scores. The percentage of positive cells and the intensity of reaction were multiplied for each specimen, resulting in a score ranging from 0 to 300. These scores ranges were grouped as follows: 0 (0), 1 (1 to 100), 2 (101–200), and 3 (>200) to generate an integrated score (H-score). Subsequently, the H-scores were grouped in this manner: low expression (scores < 150) and high expression (scores ≥ 150) to create the final score (F-score).

2.10. DNA Content, S and G_2/M Phases Measurements. The flow cytometry methodology using nuclei isolated from formalin-fixed and paraffin-embedded tissues was used as it was previously described in [5]. The percentage of cells in S and G_2/M phases of cell cycle was calculated for each sample based on DNA histograms. The S-Phase fraction (SPF) values were divided into two groups: a low-SPF group defined as having SPF less than 20% of proliferating cells and a high-SPF group with SPF greater than 20%. The proliferation index was calculated as the sum of cells in S and G_2/M phases of cell cycle and was scored as it was previously described for SPF.

2.11. Statistical Analysis. The relationships between 14F7Mab immunoreactivity and clinicopathological variables were analyzed using the Chi-square test. Correlations were assessed by Spearman ranks correlation coefficients. Survival distribution was estimated by the Kaplan-Meier method and compared with the log-rank test. For multivariate analysis, the Cox regression model was used to identify independent prognostic factors for overall survival (OS). The model included all variables and the backward stepwise elimination as the algorithm of selection was applied. OS was measured from the date of surgery to death for any cause or last follow-up (5 years) and was calculated for all patients. A p value < 0.05 was considered statistically significant. Statistical analysis was carried out using SPSS (version 15.0; SPSS Inc., Chicago, IL).

3. Results

3.1. Patient Description and Clinicopathological Features. Table 1 shows a summary of patient characteristics and some pathological features. The gender ratio was close to 2 : 1 in favor of males, with a mean age of 57.4 ± 10.6 years. In general,

TABLE 1: Clinicopathological characteristics of NSCLC patients.

Clinicopathological features	Number of cases (%) $n = 90$
Gender	
Female	31 (34.4)
Masculine	59 (65.6)
Age (years)	
<60	58 (64.4)
≥60	32 (35.6)
Tumor size (cm)	
<3	27 (30.0)
≥3	63 (70.0)
Lymph node metastasis	
Yes	30 (33.3)
No	60 (66.7)
Other sites metastasis	
Yes	7 (7.8)
No	83 (92.2)
Stage	
I-II	80 (88.9)
III-IV	10 (11.1)
Disease recurrence	
Yes	32 (35.6)
No	58 (64.4)
Histological type	
Epidermoid carcinoma	26 (28.9)
Adenocarcinoma	43 (47.8)
Large cell carcinoma	8 (8.9)
Carcinoid tumor	9 (10.0)
Others	4 (4.4)
Grade of differentiation	
Well/moderate	55 (61.1)
Poor	35 (38.9)

%, percentage.

TABLE 2: Tissue expression of NeuGcGM3 in NSCLC.

NeuGcGM3 expression	Number of cases (%) $n = 90$
Intensity of reaction	
Negative	6 (6.7)
Weak	15 (16.7)
Moderate	26 (28.9)
Intense	43 (47.8)
Percentage of positive cells (%)	
0–5	6 (6.7)
6–25	9 (10.0)
26–50	17 (18.9)
51–100	58 (64.4)
F-score	
Low (<150)	38 (42.2)
High (≥150)	52 (57.8)

%, percentage; *F*-score, final score.

the overall rate of NSCLC patients was 67.8% (61/90) and the median overall survival of this population at 5 years was 46.2 months (ranging from 0.7 to 67.1).

3.2. NeuGcGM3 Detection by Immunohistochemical and Biochemical Methods. Firstly, the specificity of the 14F7 Mab immunoreaction was confirmed with sialidase (*Clostridium perfringens*) treatment of NSCLC sections. The enzymatic digestion of tissues did not alter the level of EGFR expression, while the reactivity of P3 Mab was only reduced with this treatment (Figure 1). The staining with 14F7 Mab was significantly removed after sialidase digestion of tissue sections. No reaction was evidenced in NSCLC samples incubated with the negative control.

TLC-immunostaining of gangliosides fraction extracted from 3 different histological subtypes of NSCLC (epidermoid carcinoma, adenocarcinoma, and large cell carcinoma) that were positive for NeuGcGM3 in the immunohistochemistry study was performed. Both NeuAcGM3 and NeuGcGM3 gangliosides were evidenced in all NSCLC samples (Figure 2(a)). However, only NeuGcGM3 was recognized by 14F7 Mab, while no reaction was evidenced with NeuAcGM3 (Figure 2(b)). The expression of these gangliosides after formalin fixation and routine histological procedures was also confirmed by mass spectrometry (Figure 3). NeuAcGM3 was the major ganglioside detected in NSCLC samples using this technology, although a little amount of NeuGcGM3 was also evidenced.

3.3. Immunohistochemical Detection of NeuGcGM3. The tissue expression of NeuGcGM3 was observed in 84/90 (93.3%) cases, with variable intensity of reaction and percentage of positive cells. Most specimens had a moderate to intense staining (76.7%) and more than 50% of positive cells (64.4%) as shown in Table 2. A significant correlation was found between percentage of positive tumor cells and staining intensity ($p < 0.000$; Spearman's correlation coefficient = 0.725). According to the *F*-score, 58.9% of cases showed high level of NeuGcGM3 expression. The reactivity of 14F7 Mab was observed on both plasmatic membrane and cytoplasm of malignant cells with a homogeneous and finely granular pattern of staining as it was previously described in [8, 10].

3.4. Association of NeuGcGM3 Expression with Clinicopathological Features. The relation of 14F7 Mab immunostaining with clinicopathological variables is shown in Table 3. No significant differences were observed with gender, age, tumor size, occurrence of lymph node and other sites metastasis, stage, disease recurrence, grade of differentiation, and ploidy. However, a statistically significant difference was obtained when the reactivity of 14F7 Mab was compared in function of the histological subtype of tumors ($p = 0.008$; Chi-square test). Additionally, the level of NeuGcGM3 expression showed statistical correlation with both S-Phase fraction and

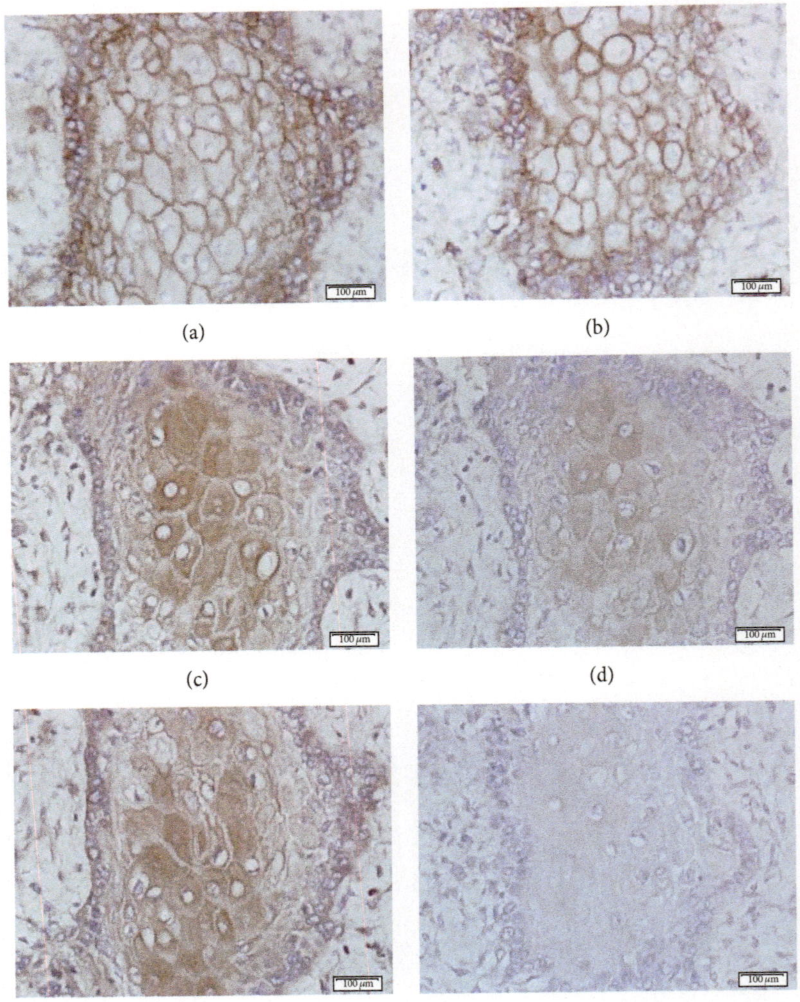

Figure 1: Microphotographs of formalin-fixed and paraffin-embedded NSCLC sections. Intense tissue reactivity of anti-EGFR (a), P3 (c), and 14F7 (e) Mabs without Neuraminidase (*Clostridium perfringens*) treatment. The expression of EGFR was not altered after enzymatic treatment (a), while the reactivity of P3 Mab was reduced but not completely eliminated (d) (brown color). Observe that the staining with 14F7 Mab was significantly removed after sialidase digestion (f) (brown color). Counterstaining with Mayer's Hematoxylin (blue color). White bar = 100 μm.

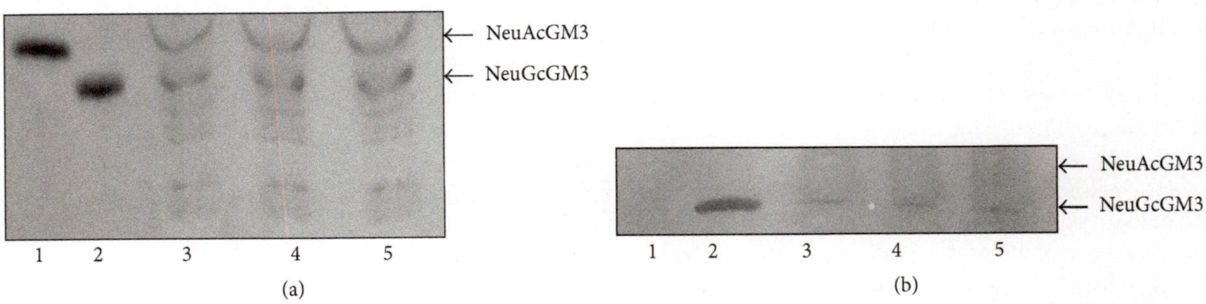

Figure 2: HP-TLC of glycolipids fraction isolated from FFPE samples of NSCLC. (a) Chemical staining with orcinol. 1 and 2: purified controls of NeuAcGM3 and NeuGcGM3, respectively. 3–5: glycolipids fraction extracted from NSCLC samples. Note the expression of both NeuAcGM3 and NeuGcGM3 gangliosides. (b) TLC-immunostaining using 14F7 Mab. Observe that the 14F7 Mab only reacted with the NeuGc-containing variant of GM3 ganglioside.

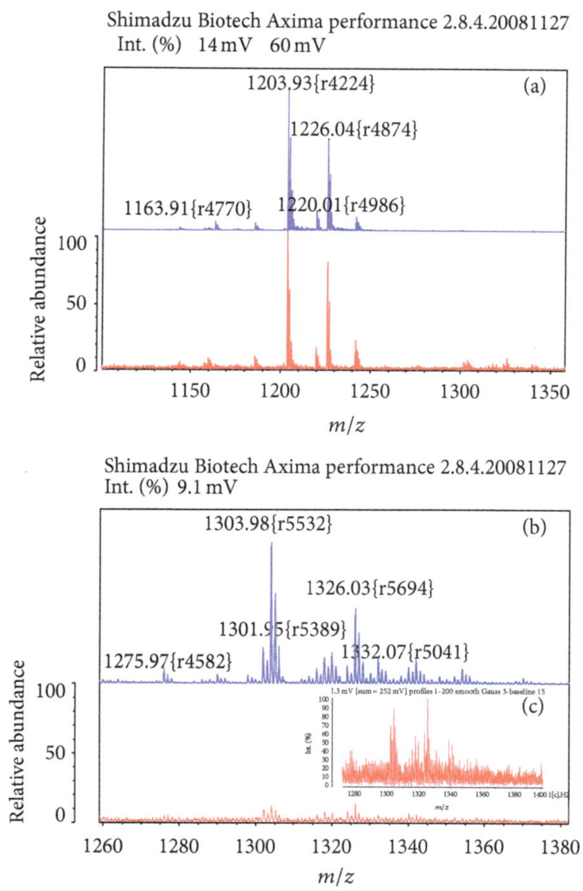

FIGURE 3: MALDI/TOF mass spectra of gangliosides extracted from NSCLC tissues. (a) and (b) (upper): purified controls of NeuAcGM3 and NeuGcGM3 gangliosides, respectively. Lower parts of panels (a) and (b) correspond to extracted fraction of NeuAcGM3 and NeuGcGM3 after the routine histological procedures. (c) Amplification of the lower part of panel (b).

index of cell proliferation (p = 0.006 and p = 0.000; Fisher exact test, resp.) (Table 4). When cases were analyzed independently, according to the intensity of reaction or the percentage of positive cells (data not shown), no significant associations with clinicopathological features were obtained. Nevertheless, higher levels of 14F7 Mab positive cells correlated with both S-Phase fraction and index of cell proliferation (p = 0.028 and p = 0.000; Fisher exact test, resp.), while for the intensity of reaction only a significant association (p = 0.037; Fisher exact test) was obtained with the proliferation index.

3.5. Survival Analysis. The results of univariate and multivariate survival analyses at 5 years are summarized in Table 5. Univariate analysis showed that lymph node metastasis (p = 0.000), other sites metastasis (p = 0.000), stage (p = 0.000), disease recurrence (p = 0.000), and the expression of NeuGcGM3 (p = 0.020) were significant prognostic factors for OS. Patients with high level of NeuGcGM3 expression had significantly impaired OS compared to those with low level by mean of the F-score (58.5% versus 81.1%; p = 0.001; Fisher's exact test). Five-year survival probabilities in

TABLE 3: Expression of NeuGcGM3 in relation to clinicopathological characteristics in NSCLC.

Clinicopathological features (n = 90)	NeuGcGM3 expression (F-score) Low	High	p value*
Gender			
Female	15	16	0.469
Masculine	23	36	
Age (years)			
<60	26	32	0.365
≥60	12	20	
Tumor size (cm)			
<3	12	15	0.832
≥3	26	37	
Lymph node metastasis			
Yes	9	21	0.403
No	29	31	
Other sites metastasis			
Yes	3	4	0.669
No	35	48	
Stage			
I-II	35	45	0.562
III-IV	3	7	
Disease recurrence			
Yes	11	21	0.632
No	27	31	
Histological type			
Epidermoid carcinoma	8	18	
Adenocarcinoma	15	28	**0.008****
Others	15	6	
Grade of differentiation			
Well/moderate	22	33	0.905
Poor	16	19	

*Fisher exact test; **Chi-square test.

NSCLC patients with higher levels of NeuGcGM3 expression were 3.4 times lower than those with reduced levels of this ganglioside. Kaplan-Meier curves according to 14F7 reactivity are represented in Figure 4(a). Among the studied variables, gender (p = 0.047), tumor size (p = 0.003), other sites metastasis (p = 0.029), disease recurrence (p = 0.001), and NeuGcGM3 expression (p = 0.010) were independent prognostic factors on multivariate analysis.

No association was obtained when the intensity of reaction or the percentages of positive cells were analyzed (p = 0.134 and p = 0.113; log-rank test, resp.).

3.6. Double and/or Triple Expression of NeuGcGM3, EGFR, and EGF Molecules. Higher levels of EGFR or EGF expression were observed in 58/80 (72.5%) and 67/80 (83.7%) of NSCLC samples, respectively. However, no correlation

TABLE 4: Expression of NeuGcGM3 in relation to ploidy and malignant cells proliferation.

Features	Number of cases (n = 51)	NeuGcGM3 expression		p value*
		Low	High	
Ploidy				
Diploid	25	8	17	1.000
Aneuploid	26	9	17	
S-Phase fraction				
<20%	21	12	9	**0.006**
≥20%	30	5	25	
Proliferation index				
<20%	15	11	4	**0.000**
≥20%	36	6	30	

S-Phase fraction, cells in S-Phase of cell cycle; proliferation index, sum of cells in both S and G_2/M phases of cell cycle; *Fisher exact test. Bold value indicates statistical significance.

TABLE 5: Univariate and multivariate analyses of overall survival in studied population.

Characteristics	Overall survival		
	Univariate	Multivariate	
	p value	p value	HR (CI 95%)
Gender	0.309	**0.047**	2.500 (1.014–6.164)
Age	0.739		
Tumor size	0.907	**0.003**	0.162 (0.049–0.528)
Lymph node metastasis	**0.000**		
Other sites metastasis	**0.000**	**0.029**	5.269 (1.190–23.323)
Stage	**0.000**		
Disease recurrence	**0.000**	**0.001**	7.412 (2.311–23.771)
Histological subtype	0.529		
Grade of differentiation	0.952		
NeuGcGM3 expression	**0.020**	**0.010**	3.394 (1.342–8.584)

HR: hazard ratio; CI: confidence interval. Bold value indicates statistical significance.

between the single expression of EGFR or EGF with the overall survival of NSCLC patients was obtained (data not shown). In addition, the dual expression of these molecules was only evidenced in 27/80 (33.7%) of cases. The patients with tumor displaying the phenotype $EGFR^+/EGF^+$ had a significantly impaired OS compared to those with $EGFR^+/EGF^-$ (48.1% versus 84.2%; $p < 0.000$; Fisher's exact test) (Table 6).

The double expression of NeuGcGM3 with EGFR or EGF was observed in 52/80 (65.0%) and 62/80 (77.5%) of cases, respectively. Patients with tumor $NeuGcGM3^+/EGFR^+$ had a significantly poorer OS than those with $NeuGcGM3^+/EGFR^-$ phenotype (40.0% versus 68.2%; $p < 0.000$; Fisher's exact test) (Figure 4(b)). But no association with the OS of patients was evidenced when $NeuGcGM3^+/EGF^+$ and $NeuGcGM3^+/EGF^-$ phenotypes of NSCLC were compared (Figure 4(c)).

Finally, the triple expression of NeuGcGM3, EGFR, and EGF was only detected in 16/80 (20.0%) of tumors (Figure 5). These patients displayed significantly reduced 5-year OS rates (p = 0.007; log-rank test) compared to those with $NeuGcGM3^+/EGFR^+/EGF^-$ or $NeuGcGM3^+/EGFR^-/EGF^+$

TABLE 6: Survival of NSCLC patients according to immunohistochemical profile.

Antigens expression	$EGFR^+$		$NeuGcGM3^+$			
	EGF		EGFR		EGF	
Negative/positive	−	+	−	+	−	+
% of cases	41.3	58.7	51.9	48.1	58.1	41.9
% 5-year survival rate	84.2	48.1	68.2	40.0	61.9	48.0
Median survival (months)	47.5	44.7	44.6	23.3	41.1	38.5
p value	**0.014**		**0.030**		0.256	

%, percentage; p value, log-rank test. Bold value indicates statistical significance.

(25.0% versus 66.7% versus 80.0%; $p < 0.000$, Chi-square test) (Figure 4(d)), respectively.

4. Discussion

Despite recent advances in the diagnosis and treatment, lung cancer still remains the leading cause of death from cancer worldwide and one of the 10 leading causes of death from all causes [21]. Usually patients with NSCLC have a poor prognosis because most of them present with advanced or metastatic disease at the time of diagnosis [22]. Even after early diagnosis and surgical resection with curative intent, in stages I–III NSCLC patients, recurrent disease or distant metastasis results in a 5-year survival rate of <50% [23–25]. It has been estimated that only 10–15% of NSCLC patients will ultimately be cured [22]. In this sense, a number of independent prognostic factors for survival in NSCLC patients have been evaluated, including disease stage, performance status, gender, age, histology, haemoglobin level, some primary tumor characteristics such as tumor size or local extension, and mediastinal neoplastic infiltration [22].

In this study, we showed the prognostic significance of gender, tumor size, the occurrence of lymph node and other sites metastasis, stage, and disease recurrence in NSCLC patients. However, only the existence of other sites metastasis and the disease recurrence were identified as prognostic

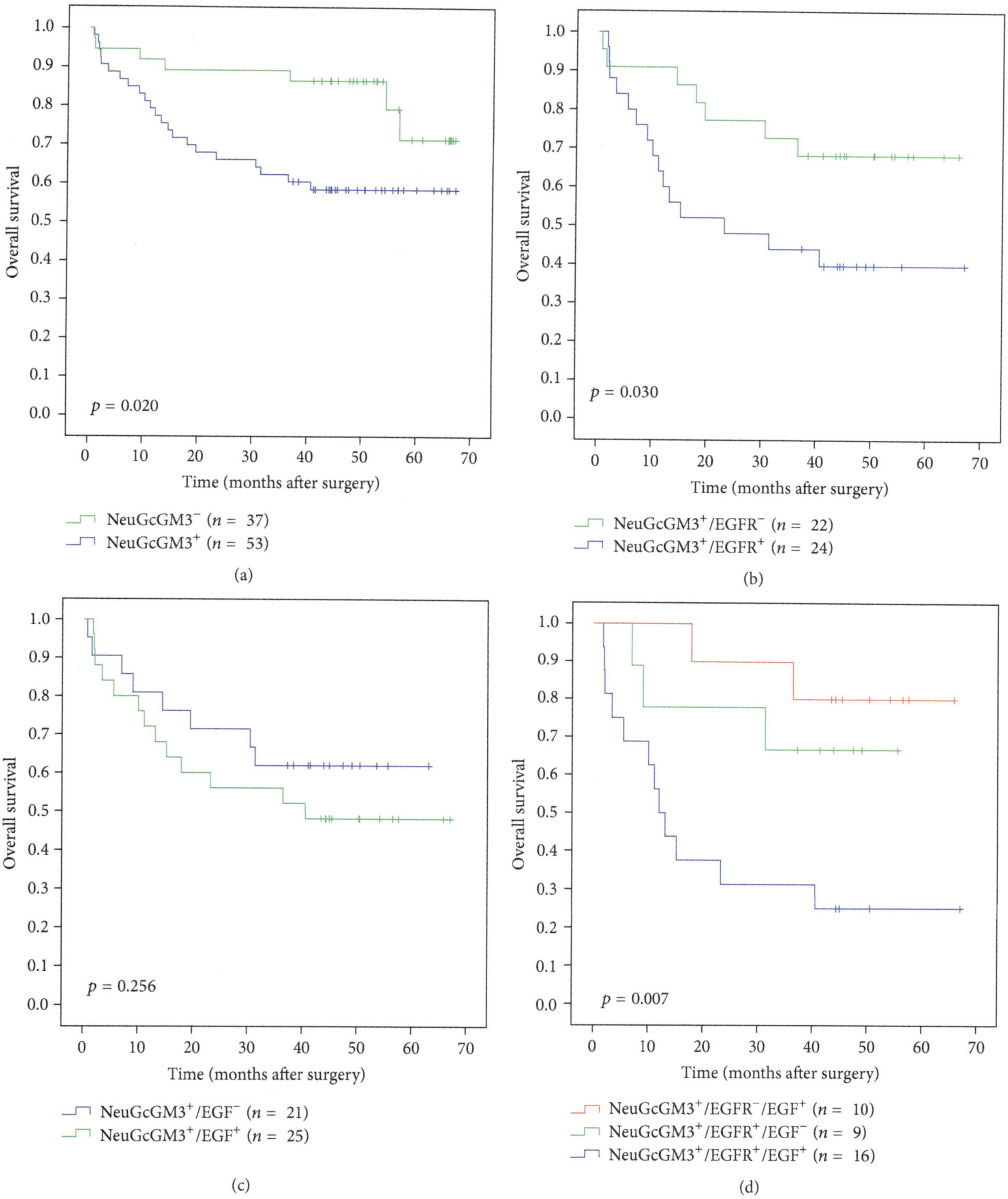

FIGURE 4: Kaplan-Meier curves for overall survival of NSCLC patients. (a) Expression of NeuGcGM3. (b) Dual expression of NeuGcGM3 and EGFR. (c) Double expression of NeuGcGM3 and EGF. (d) Triple expression of NeuGcGM3, EGFR, and EGF. Statistical analysis by log-rank test.

factor in both univariate and multivariate analyses. In previous reports, TNM (tumor, node, metastasis) staging system [26], disease stage, and performance status at time of diagnosis have been considered among most noticeable prognostic factors in these patients [22]. Nevertheless, the pathology-based TNM stage classification has been considered to provide imprecise information about the survival rates [27]. Since outcomes can be different even among patients with the same disease stage, numerous studies are currently focusing on the evaluation of other

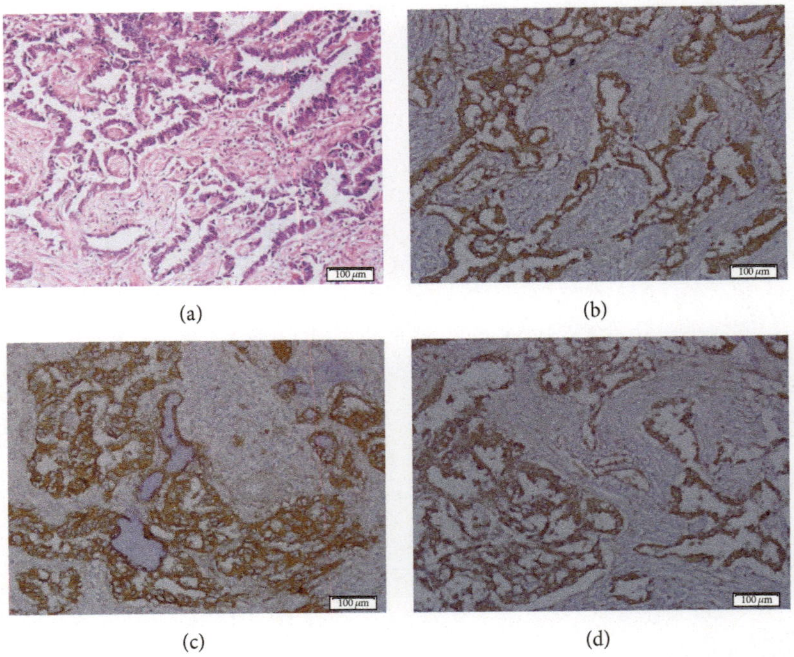

FIGURE 5: Triple expression of NeuGcGM3, EGFR, and EGF in lung adenocarcinoma. (a) Hematoxylin and eosin staining. ((b)–(d)) High levels of NeuGcGM3, EGFR, and EGF expression, respectively (brown color). Counterstaining with Mayer's Hematoxylin (blue color). White bar = 100 μm.

biological and molecular prognostic factors as a potential complement of TNM staging system [24, 25, 28].

GM3 is the major glycosphingolipid expressed in both tumor and nontumor tissues from human lung cancer patients [29]. In non-small cell lung cancer (NSCLC), an increased expression of GM3 and GM3 synthase (sialyltransferase-I or SAT-I) mRNA has been detected. However, the cDNA sequences of the cytidine monophospho-N-acetylneuraminic acid hydroxylase (CMAH) suggest an inactivating mutation, similar to that in normal tissues [7]. In this sense, these results suggest the existence of an alternative pathway for NeuGc-containing gangliosides, different from the normal pathway that is mediated by CMAH enzyme activity [30]. In line with this, Yin et al. reported a hypoxic culture induced NeuGc-containing ganglioside expression on human cells as a possible candidate for the alternative pathway because a hypoxic culture markedly induced mRNA for the sialic acid transporter, sialin [31].

In this study, the expression of NeuGcGM3 in NSCLC samples after the routine histopathological procedures was confirmed using both immunohistochemistry after sialidase digestion and TLC-immunostaining with 14F7 Mab. However, GM3 was the major ganglioside detected in this kind of samples, similar to previous report [7]. The tissue expression of NeuGcGM3 was confirmed by mean of mass spectrometry of lipid fraction extracted from FFPE samples. NeuGcGM3 is not completely extracted from NSCLC tissues after formaldehyde fixation and the subsequent histological procedures [8]. In a previous work, our group published the NeuGcGM3 ganglioside biochemical measure in breast cancer using frozen tissues and mass spectrometry [32]. However, to our knowledge, this is the first report of the NeuGcGM3 expression in FFPE tissues using mass spectrometry.

Previously, Van Cruijsen et al. [9] and Blanco et al. [10] reported that NeuGcGM3 expression is associated with a favorable survival of NSCLC patients. However, in recent studies Hayashi et al. [7] obtained opposite data, considering the reduced number of cases used by Blanco et al. responsible for these differences ($n = 28$). Nevertheless, Van Cruijsen et al. used 165 patients in their research [9], which is a larger sample size compared with the rest of studies [7, 10]. According to our experience, other factors such as the immunohistochemical analysis (membrane and/or cytoplasmic staining), the IHC score, the specificity of Mabs, and the differences in the histological type proportion could be also responsible for these controversial results.

Here, the reactivity of 14F7 Mab in both cell membrane and cytoplasm of malignant cells was analyzed, as it was previously described [10]. However, in previous reports the expression of NeuGcGM3 was only considered in the cytoplasm [9] or in plasmatic membranes [7] of malignant cells, excluding part of Mabs staining. Moreover, the expression of NeuGcGM3 was scored (F-score) by mean of the integration of both percentage of 14F7-positive cells and the intensity of reaction. It is known that any scoring decision could directly be influenced by bias because the analysis of IHC assays is visually judged [33]. Nevertheless, the introduction of the score systems in the clinical practice had permitted us to reduce variability, particularly for markers that aim to select patients for specific treatments [34].

Interestingly, NSCLC patients displaying higher levels of NeuGcGM3 expression had a significantly poorer overall survival than those with lower levels of this ganglioside.

It is the first report describing the relation between the 14F7 Mab reactivity and a more aggressive biological behavior of NSCLC. Comparable results were recently obtained in colon adenocarcinoma by mean of a similar integrated IHC score [15]. Notably, when only the intensity of reaction or the percentage of 14F7-positive cells was analyzed, in general, no significant associations with clinicopathological features were noted [15], resembling the present research. In this sense, our data permit us to suggest the use of an IHC score integrating both parameters, although further studies are needed to validate these findings.

On the other hand, increasing levels of NeuGcGM3 expression correlated with higher S-Phase fraction and proliferation index measured by flow cytometry. It is known that the upregulation of EGFR expression by EGF is considered a mechanism that promotes the development and progression of lung tumors [35, 36]. Additionally, GM3 diminishes the cancer cell proliferation inhibiting of EGFR tyrosine kinase [37], modulating the expression of cell cycle regulation proteins [38–40]. However, NeuGcGM3 is not able to inhibit the EGFR tyrosine kinase as compared with GM3 [7]. Interestingly, the triple expression of NeuGcGM3 with EGFR and EGF was detected in the 20.0% of studied patients. In line with this, the aberrant expression of NeuGcGM3 in NSCLC probably causes a disruption in the mechanism of EGFR tyrosine kinase inhibition by GM3, permitting an uncontrolled EGFR system activation mediated by the ligand EGF.

In addition, the simultaneous expression of EGFR and its ligands in tumor and adjacent lung tissues was associated with lower overall and relapse-free survival in NSCLC patients [41]. Here, the dual expression of EGFR and EGF was evidenced in 58.7% of NSCLC samples, while the double expression of NeuGcGM3 and EGFR or EGF was detected in 65.0% and 77.5% of these patients, respectively. Outstandingly, patients with $EGFR^+/EGF^+$, $NeuGcGM3^+/EGFR^+$, and $NeuGcGM3^+/EGFR^+/EGF^+$ phenotypes of NSCLC displayed poor overall survival rates as compared with those with $EGFR^+/EGF^-$, $NeuGcGM3^+/EGFR^-$, and $NeuGcGM3^-/EGFR^+/EGF^+$, respectively. The dual expression of NeuGcGM3 and EGFR in a variety of human malignant tumors, including NSCLC, was evidenced [42]. However, to our knowledge, it is the first report regarding the double and the triple expressions of NeuGcGM3 with EGFR and/or EGF and its relationship with the overall survival of NSCLC patients.

Finally, differences in predominant histological type might also lead to differences in results. In the first two studies using the 14F7 Mab [9, 10] the proportion of squamous subtype and adenocarcinoma was major in favor of squamous carcinoma, while in the third report an opposite relation was obtained [7], resembling the present work. Lung adenocarcinoma had been reported to be the highest levels of SAT-I mRNA expression as compared with epidermoid carcinoma and the rest of tumors [29]. Interestingly, in this study, a statistically significant difference was obtained when the reactivity of 14F7 Mab was compared in function of the histological subtype of tumors. But no differences in NeuGcGM3 expression were evidenced between epidermoid carcinoma and adenocarcinoma (data not shown). In this sense, experiments using increasing number of these tumors of the lung should be designed.

5. Conclusions

In summary, in this paper the expression of NeuGcGM3 in NSCLC is reported for the first time using mass spectrometry and TLC-immunostaining with 14F7 Mab. Interestingly, high levels of NeuGcGM3 expression, by means of an IHC integrated score (*F*-score), correlate with the proliferation index and with a poor overall survival of NSCLC patients. These results support the use of a universal scoring system to assess the prognostic value of NeuGcGM3 expression in NSCLC patients. Moreover, some NSCLC phenotypes with poor overall survival rates based on the simultaneous expression of NeuGcGM3 with EGFR and/or EGF were identified. Our data permit us to consider the immunohistochemical detection of these tumor-associated antigens as a useful complement of established prognostic factors in NSCLC. Moreover, our findings support the potential use of combined passive and active immunotherapy in tumors overexpressing NeuGcGM3, EGFR, and/or EGF.

Conflict of Interests

The authors report no competing interests.

Authors' Contribution

Rancés Blanco, Elizabeth Domínguez, Darel Martínez, Enrique Rengifo, and Adriana Carr designed methods and experiments. Rancés Blanco, Elizabeth Domínguez, Damián Blanco, Orlando Morales, and Charles E. Rengifo carried out the laboratory assays. Rancés Blanco, Charles E. Rengifo, Carmen Viada, Mercedes Cedeño, Enrique Rengifo, and Adriana Carr analyzed the data. Rancés Blanco and Adriana Carr interpreted the results. Rancés Blanco wrote the paper.

Acknowledgments

The authors want to express their gratitude to M.S. Vladimir Peña for the helpful recommendations regarding TLC experiments and to M.S. Janoi Chang for kindly providing them with TLC specific reagents. The authors also want to thank Dr. Rolando Dominguez for his editorial assistance. This work was supported by the Center of Molecular Immunology, Havana, Cuba.

References

[1] A. Barzi and N. A. Pennell, "Targeting angiogenesis in non-small cell lung cancer: agents in practice and clinical development," *European Journal of Clinical and Medical Oncology*, vol. 2, no. 1, pp. 31–42, 2010.

[2] K. Kaira, N. Oriuchi, N. Sunaga, T. Ishizuka, K. Shimizu, and N. Yamamoto, "A systemic review of PET and biology in lung cancer," *American Journal of Translational Research*, vol. 3, no. 4, pp. 383–391, 2011.

[3] X. Jin, Z. Wang, L. Qiu et al., "Potential biomarkers involving IKK/RelA signal in early stage non-small cell lung cancer," *Cancer Science*, vol. 99, no. 3, pp. 582–589, 2008.

[4] Y. Qiu, H. Yang, H. Chen et al., "Detection of CEA mRNA, p53 and AE1/AE3 in haematoxylin-eosin-negative lymph nodes of early-stage non-small cell lung cancer may improve veracity of N staging and indicate prognosis," *Japanese Journal of Clinical Oncology*, vol. 40, no. 2, pp. 146–152, 2010.

[5] R. Blanco, C. E. Rengifo, M. Cedeño, M. Frómeta, and E. Rengifo, "Flow cytometric measurement of aneuploid DNA content correlates with high S-phase fraction and poor prognosis in patients with non-small-cell lung cancer," *ISRN Biomarkers*, vol. 2013, Article ID 354123, 8 pages, 2013.

[6] A. M. Vázquez, M. Alfonso, B. Lanne et al., "Generation of a murine monoclonal antibody specific for N-glycolylneuraminic acid-containing gangliosides that also recognizes sulfated glycolipids," *Hybridoma*, vol. 14, no. 6, pp. 551–556, 1995.

[7] N. Hayashi, H. Chiba, K. Kuronuma et al., "Detection of N-glycolyated gangliosides in non-small-cell lung cancer using GMR8 monoclonal antibody," *Cancer Science*, vol. 104, no. 1, pp. 43–47, 2013.

[8] R. Blanco, C. E. Rengifo, M. Cedeño et al., "Immunodetection of N-glycolyl GM3 ganglioside inlung carcinoma by immunohistochemistry: a technical study using frozen and formalin-fixed and paraffin-embedded tissues," *Acta Microscopica*, vol. 23, no. 3, p. 199, 2014.

[9] H. Van Cruijsen, M. Ruiz, P. van der Valk, T. D. de Gruijl, and G. Giaccone, "Tissue micro array analysis of ganglioside N-glycolyl GM3 expression and signal transducer and activator of transcription (STAT)-3 activation in relation to dendritic cell infiltration and microvessel density in non-small cell lung cancer," *BMC Cancer*, vol. 9, article 180, 2009.

[10] R. Blanco, C. E. Rengifo, M. Cedeño, M. Frómeta, E. Rengifo, and A. Carr, "Immunoreactivity of the 14F7 Mab (raised against N-glycolyl GM3 ganglioside) as a positive prognostic factor in non-small-cell lung cancer," *Pathology Research International*, vol. 2012, Article ID 235418, 12 pages, 2012.

[11] A. Carr, A. Mullet, Z. Mazorra et al., "A mouse IgG1 monoclonal antibody specific for N-glycolyl GM3 ganglioside recognized breast and melanoma tumors," *Hybridoma*, vol. 19, no. 3, pp. 241–247, 2000.

[12] H. Ozawa, I. Kawashima, and T. Tai, "Generation of murine monoclonal antibodies specific for N-glycolylneuraminic acid-containing gangliosides," *Archives of Biochemistry and Biophysics*, vol. 294, no. 2, pp. 427–433, 1992.

[13] J. de Leòn, A. Fernández, C. Mesa, M. Clavel, and L. E. Fernández, "Role of tumour-associated N-glycolylated variant of GM3 ganglioside in cancer progression: effect over CD4 expression on T cells," *Cancer Immunology, Immunotherapy*, vol. 55, no. 4, pp. 443–450, 2006.

[14] J. de León, A. Fernández, M. Clavell et al., "Differential influence of the tumour-specific non-human sialic acid containing GM3 ganglioside on $CD4^{+}CD25^{-}$ effector and naturally occurring $CD4^{+}CD25^{+}$ regulatory T cells function," *International Immunology*, vol. 20, no. 4, pp. 591–600, 2008.

[15] T. Lahera, A. Calvo, G. Torres et al., "Prognostic role of 14F7 Mab immunoreactivity against N-glycolyl GM3 ganglioside in colon cancer," *Journal of Oncology*, vol. 2014, Article ID 482301, 8 pages, 2014.

[16] C. Mateo, E. Moreno, K. Amour, J. Lombardero, W. Harris, and R. Pérez, "Humanization of a mouse monoclonal antibody that blocks the epidermal growth factor receptor: recovery of antagonistic activity," *Immunotechnology*, vol. 3, no. 1, pp. 71–81, 1997.

[17] F. M. Freyre, J. Vázquez, C. Duarte, E. Ferrá, I. López, and N. Arteaga, "Anticuerpos monoclonales que reconocen los factores de crecimiento epidérmico humano y murino," *Interferón y Biotecnología*, vol. 6, no. 1, pp. 32–46, 1989.

[18] E. G. Bligh and W. J. Dyer, "A rapid method of total lipid extraction and purification," *Canadian Journal of Biochemistry and Physiology*, vol. 37, no. 8, pp. 911–917, 1959.

[19] C. E. Rengifo, R. Blanco, D. Blanco, M. Cedeño, M. Frómeta, and E. R. Calzado, "Immunohistochemical characterization of three monoclonal antibodies raised against the epidermal growth factor and its receptor in non-small-cell lung cancer: their potential use in the selection of patients for immunotherapy," *Journal of Biomarkers*, vol. 2013, Article ID 627845, 9 pages, 2013.

[20] M. Kotani and T. Tai, "An immunohistochemical technique with a series of monoclonal antibodies to gangliosides: their differential distribution in the rat cerebellum," *Brain Research Protocols*, vol. 1, no. 2, pp. 152–156, 1997.

[21] C. J. L. Murray and A. D. Lopez, "Measuring the global burden of disease," *The New England Journal of Medicine*, vol. 369, no. 5, pp. 448–457, 2013.

[22] T. Berghmans, M. Paesmans, and J.-P. Sculier, "Prognostic factors in stage III non-small cell lung cancer: a review of conventional, metabolic and new biological variables," *Therapeutic Advances in Medical Oncology*, vol. 3, no. 3, pp. 127–138, 2011.

[23] G. Zalcman, E. Bergot, and E. Lechapt, "Update on nonsmall cell lung cancer," *European Respiratory Review*, vol. 19, no. 117, pp. 173–185, 2010.

[24] G. Marulli, E. Verderi, A. Zuin et al., "Outcomes and prognostic factors of non-small-cell lung cancer with lymph node involvement treated with induction treatment and surgical resection," *Interactive CardioVascular and Thoracic Surgery*, vol. 19, no. 2, pp. 256–262, 2014.

[25] K. Okamura, K. Takayama, K. Kawahara et al., "PICT1 expression is a poor prognostic factor in non-small cell lung cancer," *Oncoscience*, vol. 1, no. 5, pp. 375–382, 2014.

[26] D. M. Parkin, F. Bray, J. Ferlay, and P. Pisani, "Global cancer statistics, 2002," *CA: A Cancer Journal for Clinicians*, vol. 55, no. 2, pp. 74–108, 2005.

[27] R.-P. Perng, C.-Y. Chen, G.-C. Chang et al., "Revisit of 1997 TNM staging system—survival analysis of 1112 lung cancer patients in Taiwan," *Japanese Journal of Clinical Oncology*, vol. 37, no. 1, pp. 9–15, 2007.

[28] K. Tabata, T. Tanaka, T. Hayashi et al., "Ki-67 is a strong prognostic marker of non-small cell lung cancer when tissue heterogeneity is considered," *BMC Clinical Pathology*, vol. 14, article 23, 2014.

[29] M. Noguchi, T. Suzuki, K. Kabayama et al., "GM3 synthase gene is a novel biomarker for histological classification and drug sensitivity against epidermal growth factor receptor tyrosine kinase inhibitors in non-small cell lung cancer," *Cancer Science*, vol. 98, no. 10, pp. 1625–1632, 2007.

[30] Y. N. Malykh, R. Schauer, and L. Shaw, "N-glycolylneuraminic acid in human tumours," *Biochimie*, vol. 83, no. 7, pp. 623–634, 2001.

[31] J. Yin, A. Hashimoto, M. Izawa et al., "Hypoxic culture induces expression of sialin, a sialic acid transporter, and cancer-associated gangliosides containing non-human sialic acid on human cancer cells," *Cancer Research*, vol. 66, no. 6, pp. 2937–2945, 2006.

[32] G. Marquina, H. Waki, L. E. Fernández et al., "Gangliosides expressed in human breast cancer," *Cancer Research*, vol. 56, no. 22, pp. 5165–5171, 1996.

[33] F. Varghese, A. B. Bukhari, R. Malhotra, and A. De, "IHC profiler: an open source plugin for the quantitative evaluation and automated scoring of immunohistochemistry images of human tissue samples," *PLoS ONE*, vol. 9, no. 5, Article ID e96801, 2014.

[34] L. L. de Matos, D. C. Trufelli, M. G. L. de Matos, and M. A. da Silva Pinhal, "Immunohistochemistry as an important tool in biomarkers detection and clinical practice," *Biomark Insights*, vol. 5, pp. 9–20, 2010.

[35] X. Zhao, W. Dai, H. Zhu et al., "Epidermal growth factor (EGF) induces apoptosis in a transfected cell line expressing EGF receptor on its membrane," *Cell Biology International*, vol. 30, no. 8, pp. 653–658, 2006.

[36] M. D. Siegelin and A. C. Borczuk, "Epidermal growth factor receptor mutations in lung adenocarcinoma," *Laboratory Investigation*, vol. 94, no. 2, pp. 129–137, 2014.

[37] E. G. Bremer, J. Schlessinger, and S. Hakomori, "Ganglioside-mediated modulation of cell growth. Specific effects of GM3 on tyrosine phosphorylation of the epidermal growth factor receptor," *The Journal of Biological Chemistry*, vol. 261, no. 5, pp. 2434–2440, 1986.

[38] D.-M. Li and H. Sun, "PTEN/MMAC1/TEP1 suppresses the tumorigenicity and induces G1 cell cycle arrest in human glioblastoma cells," *Proceedings of the National Academy of Sciences of the United States of America*, vol. 95, no. 26, pp. 15406–15411, 1998.

[39] H.-J. Choi, T.-W. Chung, S.-K. Kang et al., "Ganglioside GM3 modulates tumor suppressor PTEN-mediated cell cycle progression—transcriptional induction of $p21^{WAF1}$ and $p27^{kip1}$ by inhibition of PI-3K/AKT pathway," *Glycobiology*, vol. 16, no. 7, pp. 573–583, 2006.

[40] Ü. Coskun, M. Grzybek, D. Drechsel, and K. Simons, "Regulation of human EGF receptor by lipids," *Proceedings of the National Academy of Sciences of the United States of America*, vol. 108, no. 22, pp. 9044–9048, 2011.

[41] O. I. Kostyleva, E. S. Gerstein, A. I. Dykhno, A. V. Vasil'ev, B. E. Polotskiĭ, and N. E. Kushlinskiĭ, "EFR-like peptides and their receptors as prognostic factors for the survival of patients with non-small-cell lung cancer," *Voprosy Onkologii*, vol. 45, no. 6, pp. 617–622, 1999.

[42] A. González, A. Carr, K. León et al., "Pharmaceutical compositions for the treatment of tumours that express EGFR and ganglioside N-glycolyl GM3 (NeuGcGM3) (WO 2013097834 A1)," http://www.google.com/patents/WO2013097834A1?cl=es.

12

Clinicopathological Study of 25 Cases of Diverticular Disease of the Appendix: Experience from Farwaniya Hospital

Nabeel Al-Brahim,[1] Ibrahim Al-Kandari,[2] Musaad Munahai,[2] and Prem Sharma[3]

[1] *Department of Pathology, Farwaniya Hospital, P.O. Box 3313, 22034 Salmiya, Kuwait*
[2] *Department of Surgery, Farwaniya Hospital, 81004 Sabah Al-Naser, Kuwait*
[3] *Faculty of Medicine, Kuwait University, P.O. Box 24923, 13110 Safat, Kuwait*

Correspondence should be addressed to Nabeel Al-Brahim; nabeel.albrahim@gmail.com

Academic Editor: Marco Volante

Background. Diverticular disease of the appendix (DDA) is a rare disease and it has been shown to be associated with locoregional neoplasms. This study was conducted to characterize clinicopathological features and to investigate its association with appendiceal neoplasms. *Methods.* We searched the records of the Department of Pathology at Farwaniya Hospital for cases of diverticular disease of the appendix between 2003 and 2011. Histological slides and patient charts were reviewed for relevant information. Consecutive cases of acute appendicitis were selected as a control group. *Results.* We identified 25 cases of DDA, 24 of which occurred in men. Mean age of DDA patients was 35 ± 10.1 years and was significantly greater than that of appendicitis patients ($P = 0.027$). The mean temperature of cases (37.9°) was significantly higher ($P = 0.012$) than that of the controls (37.3°). The cases had lower white blood cell (WBC) counts compared to controls (13.6 versus 16.7, $P = 0.04$). Pathological diagnosis identified 4 cases of diverticulosis, 5 cases of diverticulitis, 6 cases of diverticulosis with acute appendicitis, and 10 cases of diverticulitis and appendicitis. None of the cases was associated with any type of neoplasm. *Conclusions.* DDA is a rare disease, and clinicians and radiologists should be aware of it. Male sex and adult age seem to be risk factors associated with DDA. The disease may not have any direct association with any neoplasm.

1. Introduction

Diverticular disease of the appendix (DDA) is a rare disease characterized by herniation or outpouching of the appendiceal mucosa through the muscular wall. Congenital DDA is rare, with a reported prevalence of 0.014%. It is equally frequent in both sexes and commonly presents as a single diverticulum [1]. Acquired DDA is also rare; it has been reported in 0.2% to 1.7% of all appendectomy specimens [2, 3]. In the medical literature, there are only few studies on DDA because the disease is extremely rare. Moreover, it is commonly overlooked by clinicians, radiologists, and surgeons because its clinical characterizations are limited, as is awareness of its complications. In relatively recent years, researchers have noticed an association between DDA and appendiceal neoplasms. Lamps et al. [4] reported a 25% association between appendiceal mucinous neoplasms and DDA. A study by Dupre et al. [5] revealed that 48% of appendectomy specimens with diverticulosis harbored appendiceal neoplasms including well-differentiated neuroendocrine tumors (carcinoid), mucinous adenoma, tubular adenoma, and adenocarcinoma. Furthermore, a recent study showed that 43.6% of the cases coincided with appendiceal neoplasm and regional colonic carcinoma [6]. Therefore, the authors considered DDA a marker of regional neoplasms.

This study was conducted at Farwaniya Hospital, a major general hospital in Kuwait, with the following objectives: (1) to further characterize the clinicopathological features of DDA in our population and compare them with the published data from different geographic areas; (2) to compare the cases of DDA with those of acute appendicitis; (3) to determine the association of DDA with appendiceal neoplasms.

2. Materials and Methods

We searched computer files (dated between 2003 and 2011) at the Department of Pathology at Farwaniya Hospital for the following terms: appendix, acute appendicitis, diverticular disease, diverticulosis, and diverticulitis. The cases of DDA in appendectomy specimens were included. Appendectomies associated with other procedures, such as right hemicolectomy and gynecological surgical procedures, were excluded because we used a simple computer software that allowed to enter the name of a single organ only. Therefore, appendectomies associated with other procedures were entered under the names of the procedure on other organs like colon and gynecological organs and thus difficult to identify. Moreover, the focus of this study was to select cases of DDA presenting as acute appendicitis so that they could be compared with actual cases of acute appendicitis (serving as controls). Histological slides were reviewed to confirm the diagnosis of DDA. In 14 cases, all appendices were submitted for histological examination. In the remaining cases ($n = 11$), we examined from 1 to 3 blocks of the appendix. Pathological diagnosis was defined as follows: (1) diverticulosis, defined as appendiceal mucosal herniation beyond the muscularis propria; (2) diverticulitis, which is characterized by the presence of acute inflammation around a diverticulum; (3) acute appendicitis, defined as the presence of transmural acute inflammation away from a diverticulum. Based on whether inflammation was present or absent and, if present, whether it affected a diverticulum or away from it, the pathological diagnosis was classified into four categories: (1) acute diverticulitis with normal appendix; (2) acute diverticulitis with acute appendicitis; (3) diverticulosis with acute appendicitis; (4) diverticulosis. Histological slides were also reviewed carefully for the presence of additional pathological findings—particularly neoplasms—and the number and location of the diverticula. Patient records were reviewed for demographic data, including age, sex, and nationality. Furthermore, clinical presentation, laboratory results, radiological imaging findings, and operative findings were recorded. Thirty-three consecutive patients who presented to hospital in 2010 with usual acute appendicitis were included as controls, and their records were reviewed for similar data.

2.1. Statistical Analysis. The data were entered and analyzed using the Statistical Package for the Social Sciences (SPSS) software, version 19.0 (IBM, Armouk, NY, USA). The normal distribution of age, duration of pain, temperature, white blood cell (WBC) count, and hospital stay were tested using Shapiro-Wilk test. Descriptive statistics were presented as means and standard deviations (SD) as well as medians and ranges, because these variables did not meet the assumptions of normal distribution. The chi-square or Fisher's exact test and Mann-Whitney U or Student's t-tests were used to compare cases and controls. A two-tailed P value of less than 0.05 was considered statistically significant.

The study was approved by a joint committee (Ministry of Health and Faculty of Medicine).

3. Results

We identified 25 cases of DDA in the pathology files of Farwaniya Hospital. Twenty-four (96%) were men. Their ages ranged from 20 to 59 years, with a mean age of 35.0 ± 10.2 years. The mean age of DDA patients was significantly greater ($P = 0.027$) than that of the controls, 29.3 ± 8.69 years. The percentage of men was much higher among DDA group than that in the controls (96% versus 78%). Abdominal pain was found to be common among cases and controls, although the mean duration of pain was longer in patients with DDA. Nausea was slightly more frequent in patient with DDA cases, while vomiting and anorexia were more common among controls. The mean temperature was significantly higher in cases (37.9°) compared to controls (37.3°) ($P = 0.012$). The average duration of symptoms was 3 days with no significant associated diseases. The WBC count among cases was 13.6 ± 3.7, which was significantly lower ($P = 0.041$) than that of the control group, 16.7 ± 5.7. The mean duration of hospital stay was longer for patients with DDA than that for controls (4.7 days versus 4.1 days), although this was not a statistically significant difference ($P = 0.077$) (Table 1).

An ultrasound examination was performed for 10 patients. The findings were diagnostic of acute appendicitis in 4 patients, and no abnormalities were revealed in 3 patients. Fluid collection in the right iliac fossa and dilated bowel loops were observed in 2 patients, and the record for 1 showed fatty liver and no comment about the appendix. None of the cases were diagnosed with DDA based on imaging studies. We reviewed intraoperative findings with particular attention to the presence of perforation, diverticular disease, and pseudomyxoma peritonei. The records were available for 24 patients, 5 of whom had obvious evidence of perforation according to the surgeons. Pseudomyxoma peritonei was reported in 1 patient. DDA was not diagnosed intraoperatively in any of the patients. The remaining patients had an inflamed appendix. Three patients were reported to have an appendiceal mass.

3.1. Pathological Findings. Based on a histological examination of the appendectomy specimen, we differentiated 4 categories of disease in our patients: (1) diverticulosis, which indicates presence of a diverticulum without evidence of inflammation ($n = 4$); (2) diverticulitis, which indicates inflammation around the diverticulum ($n = 5$); (3) diverticular disease with acute appendicitis, which indicates inflammation in the appendix away from the diverticulum ($n = 6$); (4) diverticulitis and acute appendicitis, which indicates acute inflammation around the diverticulum and in the appendix away from the diverticulum ($n = 10$). The number of diverticula varied and ranged from 1 to 6. The tip of the appendix was the most common site of diverticula. There was no associated neoplasm in any of the cases (Figures 1, 2, 3, and 4).

4. Discussion

DDA is rare in appendectomy specimens. The mechanism of DDA was explained long ago by Stout [7]. The appendiceal mucosa herniates through penetrating vessels or the site of a previous perforation. Muscular contraction is also another contributing factor; muscular hypertrophy was seen in numerous patients with DDA. Furthermore, obstruction may play a role in the pathogenesis of DDA, as many cases with inspissated secretions and appendiceal neoplasms led to increased intraluminal pressure resulting from obstruction.

TABLE 1: Summary of clinical presentation of the cases and control.

Demographic and clinical presentation	Diverticular disease of appendix (n = 25)	Acute appendicitis (n = 33)	P
Sex			
Male	24 (96%)	26 (78.2%)	0.121
Female	1 (4%)	7 (21.2%)	
Age, years			
Mean ± SD	35.0 ± 8.33	29.3 ± 8.69	0.027
Median (range)	34 (20–56)	27 (12–51)	
Ethnic group			
Arabs	14 (56%)	16 (48.5%)	0.571
Asian	11 (44%)	17 (51.5%)	
Pain			
Present	25 (100%)	33 (100%)	—
Absent	0	0	
Duration of pain, days			
Mean ± SD	2.89 ± 2.4	2.06 ± 2.05	0.108
Median (range)	2 (0.25–10)	2 (0–12)	
Nausea			
Present	12 (48.0%)	13 (39.4%)	0.512
Absent	13 (62.0%)	20 (60.6%)	
Vomiting			
Present	9 (36.0%)	20 (60.6%)	0.063
Absent	16 (64.0%)	13 (39.4%)	
Temperature			
Mean ± SD	37.9 ± 0.72	32.8 ± 0.73	0.012
Median (range)	37.9 (36.6–39.6)	37.2 (36.3–39.4)	
Anorexia			
Present	7 (28.0%)	21 (63.6%)	0.007
Absent	18 (72.0%)	12 (36.4%)	
WBC			
Mean ± SD	13.6 ± 3.7	16.7 ± 5.75	0.041
Median (range)	14.2 (4.5–20.8)	16.2 (6.8–36.5)	
Hospital stay			
Mean ± SD	4.72 ± 1.67	4.09 ± 2.04	0.077
Median	4 (3–10)	4.0 (1–10)	

DDA is commonly overlooked by clinicians and radiologists because it is so rare and clinicians are unfamiliar with its clinical presentations. Recently, this disease has attracted more attention because of studies reporting an association with appendiceal neoplasms and locoregional tumors [4–6].

In searching patient records at Farwaniya Hospital, which serves 1 million people, we identified only 25 cases of DDA occurring during a period of 9 years (2003–2011). This indicates just how rare the disease is. We found that the mean age of DDA patients (33.6 ± 8.33 years) was significantly older than that of the acute appendicitis group (29 ± 8.6 years). Lee et al. [8] obtained a similar result: the mean age of their study

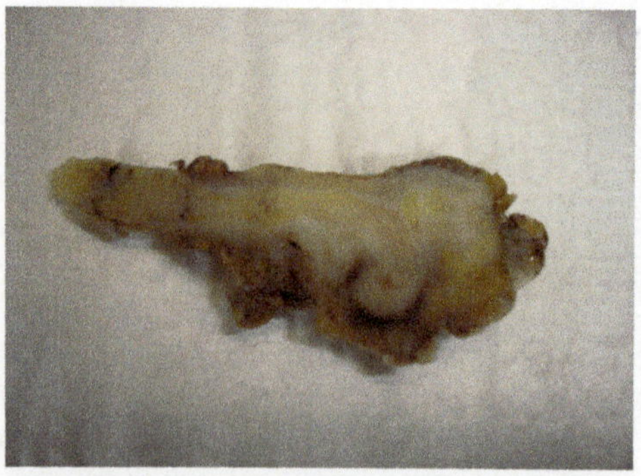

FIGURE 1: Gross picture of appendix with outpouching of the mucosa forming a diverticulum.

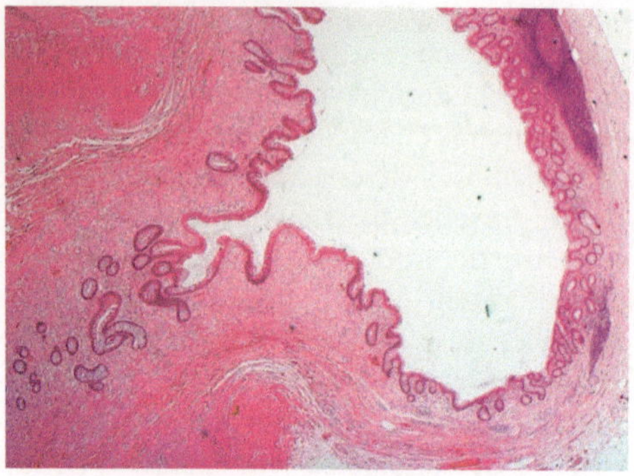

FIGURE 2: Histological picture of diverticulosis at the tip of the appendix (no inflammation around the diverticulum).

group (47.3 ± 3.0 years) was significantly (P = 0.001) greater than the mean age of their control group (31.8 ± 2.9 years). Another recent study also found that patients presenting with acute diverticulitis of the appendix were significantly older than those with acute appendicitis [9]. Various studies have found that DDA is more common in men. A study conducted by Lee and colleagues [8] found that 52% of patients were men, while two other studies [9, 10] reported that 66.6% and 83.3% of their respective series of cases were men. This can be explained by the fact that the majority of single expatriates in Kuwait are located in Farwaniya Governorate, the area served by the hospital. The clinical presentation of DDA in our series was characterized by higher temperature at presentation and lower WBC count, compared with acute appendicitis. Our series of cases in this study included 4 cases (16%) of DDA without inflammation (i.e., diverticulosis), and this explains the lower WBC count. However, there is no obvious explanation for the higher temperature in DDA patients than that in controls.

Imaging studies are important tools that help clinicians to diagnose patients and provide appropriate treatment. In this study, 10 patients (40%) underwent an ultrasound examination prior to surgical intervention, and none of them were diagnosed with DDA. This is likely because DDA is a rare disease and ultrasonographers are unfamiliar with radiologic findings. One study described the appearance of DDA on ultrasonography [11]. The morphology was characterized by an enlarged, swollen appendix and a small finger-like lateral

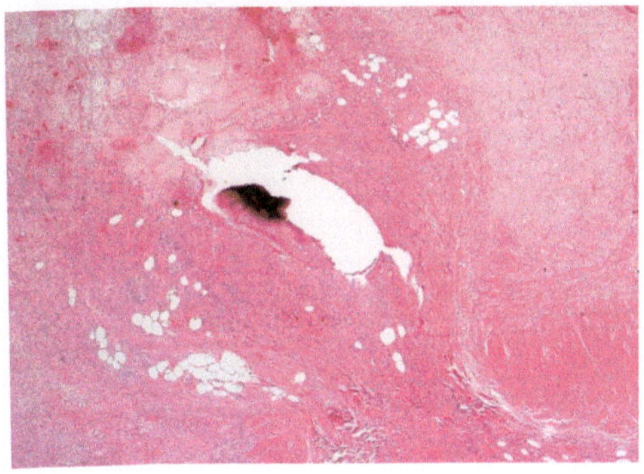

Figure 3: Histological picture of diverticulitis. Note the inflammatory cells around ruptured diverticulum.

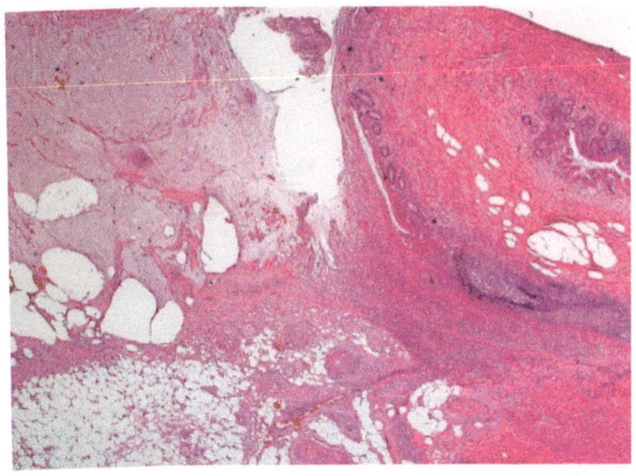

Figure 4: Histological picture of ruptured diverticulum. Note that localized mucinous spillage with epithelium on the serosa may resemble mucinous neoplasm.

projection. However, the literature shows that computed tomography (CT) is a more useful tool for detecting DDA if the practitioner is familiar with the disease. In a study by Lee et al. [8], appendiceal diverticulitis was included in preoperative diagnoses of 15% of the patients. However, with a greater awareness of DDA, the radiologist was able to recognize the disease in 80% of the cases. The CT finding that helped identify appendiceal diverticulitis was the presence of a small round cystic outpouching at the distal appendix with contrast enhancement of the cyst wall.

Pathological classification of DDA, as stated earlier, includes 4 categories: (1) acute diverticulitis with a normal appendix, (2) acute diverticulitis with acute appendicitis, (3) diverticulosis with acute appendicitis, and (4) diverticulosis. The literature shows that the first category is the most common while in our study it was the second category. These findings can be attributed to late presentation of the patients, who live in an area associated with low socioeconomic status and are usually late in seeking medical advice.

Recently, DDA has attracted more attention from clinicians and researchers because an association with locoregional neoplasm has been found. Lamps and colleagues [4] reviewed cases of low-grade mucinous neoplasm, diverticulosis, and adenoma in appendectomy specimens. They identified 32 cases of mucinous neoplasm, of which 8 (25%) were associated with a diverticulum. Therefore, the authors calculated the probability of observed rate of occurrence of mucinous neoplasm and diverticulosis which was 42%. This is higher than the observed rates of each separate condition reported in the literature, which ranged from 1% to 2%. They explained this finding by the fact that the dysplastic epithelium produced mucin, which increased the intraluminal pressure, resulting in mucosal herniation. Another study, by Dupre et al. [5], found that diverticulosis was present in 23 patients (1.7%) of a series of 1361 cases, of which 11 harbored appendiceal neoplasm, including 5 well-differentiated neuroendocrine tumors (carcinoid), 3 mucinous adenomas, 2 mucinous adenocarcinomas, and 1 tubular adenoma. Therefore, they calculated that 45% of the cases of mucinous lesions, either invasive or noninvasive, were associated with diverticular disease. Interestingly, DDA was associated with 5 cases of well-differentiated neuroendocrine tumor. This type of tumor commonly occurs at the tip of the appendix. However, the authors of the previously mentioned study reviewed all cases of carcinoid tumor of the appendix and observed that tumors associated with diverticular disease were located in the mid or proximal appendix rather than the tip. This indicates that DDA resulted from obstruction and increased intraluminal pressure.

There is a difference between the data published in the literature and the data showed herein regarding the association of DDA with appendiceal tumors, particularly mucinous neoplasm. Different explanations for this discrepancy can be extrapolated. For example, sampling of the appendix may play a role in this difference as the more sections from the appendix are taken for histological examination, the more chance of identifying these neoplasms. In addition, understanding the histological morphology of mucinous neoplasm may help in understanding this contradictory finding. These tumors commonly have a flat or villous epithelium with a flat lymphoid follicle. The cells are filled with mucin and the nuclei are columnar with low-grade dysplasia [12]. With such subtle diagnostic features, the interobserver variability of pathologists is high. The distinction of these tumors from retention cysts or reactive atypia that is seen in the presence of inflammation may be difficult. Therefore, these low-grade features may be misinterpreted as low-grade mucinous neoplasm. Another explanation is that ruptured appendiceal diverticula with periappendiceal mucin spillage, particularly in some cases with localized pseudomyxoma peritonei, can mimic low-grade appendiceal neoplasm (as shown in Figure 4). Hsu et al. [13] published a series of consultation cases of ruptured appendiceal diverticula that were misdiagnosed as low-grade mucinous neoplasm or flagged as suspicious by the original pathologist. We conclude that reactive nuclear atypia seen in diverticulitis, ruptured diverticulum, and localized mucin spillage may be overinterpreted as low-grade mucinous neoplasm.

In conclusion, diverticular disease of the appendix is a rare disease; male sex and adult age are risk factors. Clinicians and radiologists are still widely unaware of its clinical features. The literature shows that CT is the best imaging modality for diagnosis. Our study did not show any association of DDA with appendiceal neoplasm. Therefore, pathologists should be alert not to overdiagnose any reactive atypia or ruptured diverticulum as low-grade mucinous neoplasm.

References

[1] D. C. Collins, "A study of 50,000 specimens of the human vermiform appendix," *Surgery, Gynecology & Obstetrics*, vol. 101, no. 4, pp. 437–445, 1955.

[2] N. P. Blair, S. P. Bugis, L. J. Turner, and M. M. MacLeod, "Review of the pathologic diagnoses of 2,216 appendectomy specimens," *American Journal of Surgery*, vol. 165, no. 5, pp. 618–620, 1993.

[3] P. Delikaris, P. S. Teglbjaerg, P. Fisker Sorensen, and I. Balslev, "Diverticula of the vermiform appendix. Alternatives of clinical presentation and significance," *Diseases of the Colon and Rectum*, vol. 26, no. 6, pp. 374–376, 1983.

[4] L. W. Lamps, G. F. Gray Jr., B. R. Dilday, and M. K. Washington, "The coexistence of low-grade mucinous neoplasms of the appendix and appendiceal diverticula: a possible role in the pathogenesis of pseudomyxoma peritonei," *Modern Pathology*, vol. 13, no. 5, pp. 495–501, 2000.

[5] M. P. Dupre, I. Jadavji, E. Matshes, and S. J. Urbanski, "Diverticular disease of the vermiform appendix: a diagnostic clue to underlying appendiceal neoplasm," *Human Pathology*, vol. 39, no. 12, pp. 1823–1826, 2008.

[6] K. Kallenbach, S. V. Hjorth, U. Engel, N. H. Schlesinger, and S. Holck, "Significance of acquired diverticular disease of the vermiform appendix: a marker of regional neoplasms?" *Journal of Clinical Pathology*, vol. 65, pp. 638–642, 2012.

[7] A. P. Stout, "A study of diverticulum formation in the appendix," *Archives of Surgery*, vol. 6, pp. 793–829, 1923.

[8] K. H. Lee, H. S. Lee, S. H. Park et al., "Appendiceal diverticulitis: diagnosis and differentiation from usual acute appendicitis using computed tomography," *Journal of Computer Assisted Tomography*, vol. 31, no. 5, pp. 763–769, 2007.

[9] I. Yamana, S. Kawamoto, K. Inada, S. Nagao, T. Yoshida, and Y. Yamashita, "Clinical characteristics of 12 cases of appendiceal diverticulitis: a comparison with 378 cases of acute appendicitis," *Surgery Today*, vol. 42, pp. 363–367, 2012.

[10] J. Majeski, "Diverticulum of the vermiform appendix is associated with chronic abdominal pain," *American Journal of Surgery*, vol. 186, no. 2, pp. 129–131, 2003.

[11] O. Konen, E. Edelstein, A. Osadchi, M. Shapiro, and V. Rathaus, "Sonographic appearance of an appendiceal diverticulum," *Journal of Clinical Ultrasound*, vol. 30, no. 1, pp. 45–47, 2002.

[12] A. H. Qizilbash, "Mucoceles of the appendix. Their relationship to hyperplastic polyps, mucinous cystadenomas, and cystadenocarcinomas," *Archives of Pathology*, vol. 99, no. 10, pp. 548–555, 1975.

[13] M. Hsu, R. H. Young, and J. Misdraji, "Ruptured appendiceal diverticula mimicking low-grade appendiceal mucinous neoplasms," *American Journal of Surgical Pathology*, vol. 33, no. 10, pp. 1515–1521, 2009.

13

What We Have Learned about Autism Spectrum Disorder from Valproic Acid

Taylor Chomiak, Nathanael Turner, and Bin Hu

Department of Clinical Neurosciences, Hotchkiss Brain Institute, Faculty of Medicine, University of Calgary, 3280 Hospital Drive NW, Calgary, AB, Canada T2N 4N1

Correspondence should be addressed to Taylor Chomiak; tgchomia@ucalgary.ca

Academic Editor: Piero Tosi

Two recent epidemiological investigations in children exposed to valproic acid (VPA) treatment *in utero* have reported a significant risk associated with neurodevelopmental disorders and autism spectrum disorder (ASD) in particular. Parallel to this work, there is a growing body of animal research literature using VPA as an animal model of ASD. In this focused review we first summarize the epidemiological evidence linking VPA to ASD and then comment on two important neurobiological findings linking VPA to ASD clinicopathology, namely, accelerated or early brain overgrowth and hyperexcitable networks. Improving our understanding of how the drug VPA can alter early development of neurological systems will ultimately improve our understanding of ASD.

1. Introduction

The core clinicopathology of autism spectrum disorder (ASD) is currently thought to be characterized by accelerated or early brain tissue overgrowth in regions involved in emotional, social, and communication functions [1–6]. Although much of the earlier evidence regarding accelerated or early brain overgrowth was based on head circumference measurements which may not be as robust as previously thought [7] (but see [8]), more recent longitudinal brain imaging studies have provided further evidence of this abnormal pattern of brain growth in ASD [3, 6]. In fact, abnormal pathological overgrowth in ASD may even persist into adulthood in certain brain regions [9].

Exposure to exogenous chemicals during pregnancy can interfere with cortical development and the maturation of offspring. One such exogenous chemical is the short chain fatty acid valproic acid (VPA). VPA is a drug used in humans primarily for epilepsy and seizure control, although it has been used in many nonepileptic conditions as well [10]. Based on several case studies and small-scale population-based studies in humans [11–16], in addition to mounting experimental evidence in animals [17–32], VPA has known teratogenicity and has long been suspected as a risk factor for ASD. This year, however, both a prospective study and a large-scale population-based study were published providing the most substantial evidence to date linking prenatal VPA exposure to an increased risk of ASD [33, 34]. Thus, in this paper we will review epidemiological evidence linking VPA to ASD and will discuss two promising leads in the study of ASD in light of human clinical findings and the valproic acid animal model of ASD.

2. Valproic Acid and ASD: Epidemiological Evidence

Previous links between the antiepileptic drug VPA and ASD have been found and explored in several case studies and retrospective studies. VPA has long been known to cause physical malformations and developmental disabilities, features of the clinical entity termed fetal valproate syndrome (FVS). Laegreid and colleagues in a 1993 study examined seven children with FVS, two of which were also exposed to benzodiazepines. Two of the seven cases showed autistic traits, with 2 more showing marked developmental delays [16]. The next year Christianson et al. published a case study describing two sibling pairs, all having FVS to various degrees, with one having been diagnosed with infantile autism [11]. A second case of a boy with FVS and ASD was reported by Williams et al. in 1997, followed up with 5 more cases described by the same authors in 2001 [12, 13]. Several larger retrospective studies have also been published providing further support that *in utero* VPA exposure and fetal valproate syndrome may be linked to an increased risk of ASD, where, for example, it has been reported that the rate of ASD in the children of VPA-treated mothers may be roughly eight times larger than that of the general population [14, 15, 35]. Nevertheless, many of these studies had mentioned the need for future study to confirm the association between VPA and ASD.

A recently published prospective cohort study by Bromley et al. [33] explored the relationship between prenatal exposure to anti-epileptic drugs (including VPA) and the risk of neurodevelopmental disorders such as ASD, ADHD, and Dyspraxia. They performed an 11-year study, observing the physical and cognitive development of 415 children born to mothers with epilepsy and nonepileptic controls, with a final outcome of neurodevelopmental diagnosis by 6 years of age. Their results showed a significant increase in the risk of neurodevelopmental disorders in those women taking VPA during pregnancy, with autism being the most frequent diagnosis. The researchers also suspected a dose-dependent mechanism of VPA action but were not able to show it with significance in the study due to low numbers of mothers taking VPA. Although this study had a fairly small cohort and a relatively early endpoint (the average age of diagnosis of ASD in the UK is 5–11 years of age), it was the first prospective study to explore the relationship of VPA to ASD [33].

A much larger and detailed population-based study by Christensen et al. [34] that focused more on ASD than other neurodevelopmental disorders was also published this year. The large sample (655,615 children) and thorough control of the study provide the strongest evidence to date on the relationship between VPA and ASD. Data were from children born in Denmark from 1996 through 2006 over 14 years until the end of 2010. In their analysis they controlled for other known risk factors of ASD and potential confounders such as parental psychiatric disease, parental age at conception, congenital malformations, and maternal epilepsy. They divided the outcomes as Autism Spectrum Disorder (ASD) or childhood autism (the most severe diagnosis, simply referred to as "autism") and reported absolute risks over the 14 years and hazard ratios (HR) for each. The absolute risks for all children studied for ASD and autism were 1.53% and 0.48%, respectively, whereas for those exposed to VPA *in utero*, the risks were 4.42% (HR 2.9) and 2.5% (HR 5.2). In fact, even when looking at all stratifications and controls, it was concluded that there was a significantly increased risk of children developing either ASD or autism in women taking VPA during pregnancy [34].

Accumulating epidemiological studies have shown an increased risk of children developing a neurodevelopmental disorder, and ASD in particular, if their mothers take VPA during pregnancy. These findings should encourage a discussion on the risks and benefits of the treatment during pregnancy and provide an opportunity to explore how this chemical can alter early developing biological systems that may relate to ASD in animal models. This may facilitate the discovery of other VPA-like substances that may subsequently prove to be environmental or nutritional risk factors for the development of ASD, and these could further elucidate the role of exogenous chemicals on ASD pathology. The authors of the two recent papers discussed above also noted a need to define the mechanism behind the increased risk of ASD with VPA exposure. Several questions arise as to the relationship between environmental exposure to chemicals such as VPA in the manifestation of ASD [33, 34]. Christensen et al. suggested several mechanisms by which VPA may increase the risk of ASD that need further study, including interference in neurotransmitter function, neuronal apoptosis or plasticity, histone deacetylase inhibition, and disruption of folic acid metabolism [34]. Studying the effects of VPA on biological tissue will provide many avenues to explore the possible mechanism(s) of ASD.

3. Valproic Acid Rodent Model of ASD

The model of VPA exposure proposed by Rodier et al. in 1996 is one of the most frequently studied animal models of ASD [36, 37] (also see [38] for review). As reviewed by Dufour-Rainfray et al., this model exhibits many of the structural and behavioural features that can be observed in ASD patients [39]. For example, rats exposed to VPA *in utero* can exhibit physical malformations (e.g., ear malformations) which have been compared to similar abnormalities that have been observed in some autistic patients (e.g., posterior rotation of the outer ear) [39]. Furthermore, several independent laboratories have also shown that prenatal VPA exposure can lead to behavioral abnormalities that are strikingly similar to those observed in autistic patients; including decreased social interactions and sensitivity to pain, increased sensitivity to nonpainful stimuli, repetitive/stereotypic-like activity, increased anxiety, abnormally high and longer lasting fear memories which are over-generalized and harder to extinguish, and changes in specific types of pup ultrasonic vocalizations [17–28, 30, 31, 39]. At the cellular level, recent morphological data has also suggested that a decrease in spine density in forebrain structures may be a substrate for distal hypo-connectivity, while the increase in dendritic length might support the enhancement of local hyperconnectivity [40]. As pointed out by the authors, this notion is consistent with the "intense world" theory of ASD which postulates a main neuropathology characterized by hyperfunctioning of local neural microcircuits [40–42].

An animal model, to be considered as a relevant model of a psychiatric condition described in humans, should fit several criteria usually described as construct, face, and predictive validity [43]. Although the effects of VPA have been tested in rodents for many years, only relatively recently it has been used to model ASD in rodents for studying ASD-like behavioural features and potential treatment interventions [1, 26]. Roullet et al. have noted that the VPA model exhibits both construct and face validity [38], and recent work has now provided evidence that it may also exhibit predictive validity [26, 44]. For example, Schneider et al. previously reported that environmental enrichment including multisensory stimulation reversed almost all behavioral alterations observed in pups exposed to VPA *in utero* [26], while Woo and Leon have recently shown in a randomized controlled trial that environmental enrichment in the form of multiple sensorimotor stimuli was also effective in ameliorating some of the symptoms in autistic children [44].

It has been suggested that methodological issues may have limited the effectiveness of utilizing the prenatal VPA rodent model to study ASD [45]. Interestingly, similar to the prenatal model, many ASD-like behavioural and pathological features have also been observed with VPA exposure during the early postnatal period (equivalent to the third trimester and perinatal period in humans) as previously shown by Yochum et al. [46–49]. This suggests a mechanism that is effective over different developmental time points and may offer an additional approach for studying ASD in rodents. Indeed, the postnatal VPA model may partly be explained by the clinical observation that the maternal serum VPA free-fraction increases in the third trimester and is highest at birth [50]. This is consistent with the idea that bioavailability may play an important role in VPA teratogenicity and that pre- and early postnatal VPA exposure may be quite useful in studying the effects of VPA to help elucidate neuropathological mechanisms of ASD [47]. For instance, VPA exposure during prenatal and early postnatal periods in rodents can lead to accelerated or early brain overgrowth that is reminiscent of that observed in humans. Prenatal VPA exposure on the one hand has been shown to induce a more generalized pathology and can induce macrocephaly in rat brain [51], while early postnatal VPA exposure, on the other hand, has been suggested to induce a more regionally selective pattern of aberrant overgrowth that may be particularly prominent in the temporal association cortex [49]. Thus, while it has been reported that the period of exposure to VPA that is likely to result in ASD is the first trimester of pregnancy, the possibility that ASD can also result from later effects should not be excluded [39].

4. Valproic Acid and Epigenetic Regulation

Dysregulated biochemical pathways can have a profound impact on key cellular processes that may ultimately alter neuronal and network developmental trajectories. We know that the coordinated execution of gene programs involved in neural network maturation is highly regulated by epigenetic processes and that many biochemical pathways can converge to influence these processes [52–55] (Figure 1). Some of the mechanisms that may be involved include histone acetylation, histone methylation, and possibly DNA methylation.

Valproic acid is a commonly used antiepileptic drug [39]. Classically, the mechanism of action of VPA has focused on increases in brain concentrations of gamma-aminobutyric acid (GABA), the major inhibitory neurotransmitter [39], but has also included modulation of voltage-gated sodium channels and glutamatergic signaling [59]. However, it was previously shown in an animal model of seizure that VPA treatment did not significantly affect seizure strength or frequency for the first several days following induction but did, interestingly, protect the animals from seizure-induced cognitive impairment [60]. The authors concluded that their results could be explained, at least partially, by histone deacetylase (HDAC) inhibition [60]. In fact, several studies have since been published supporting the notion that VPA may block HDAC activity in neurons [52, 58, 61].

Histone deacetylases (HDACs) play an important role in regulating gene transcription and phenotype differentiation [53–55]. For example, MacDonald and Roskams reported specific expression patterns of HDAC1 and HDAC2 (both class I HDACs) in the murine brain at multiple developmental ages. HDAC1 is expressed in neural stem cells/progenitors and glia, while HDAC2 is upregulated in postmitotic neuroblasts and neurons but not in fully differentiated glia [62]. HDAC modulation in different cell types and at different maturational time points may therefore lead to dramatically different outcomes and may help to explain why HDAC inhibition in adulthood can improve ASD-like symptoms in rodents exposed to VPA *in utero* [63].

VPA is a nonselective HDAC inhibitor. Class I HDACs, which include HDAC1 and HDAC2, are expressed in the CNS, and VPA has the net effect of inhibiting their activity via different mechanisms. VPA inhibits HDAC1 through interaction with the enzyme's catalytic site, while VPA induces proteasomal degradation of HDAC2 [64, 65]. This is important as inhibition of class I HDACs can lead to increases in synapse numbers and a robust facilitation of excitatory synapse maturation [52]. Furthermore, VPA can also lead to increased neurite growth and promote neural proliferation [51, 66], both of which are thought to contribute to the accelerated or early overgrowth observed in ASD [1].

ASD structural pathology is regionally selective, exhibiting changes that are prominent in the prefrontal and temporal association cortices [1–3] that can even persist into adulthood [9]. These areas have been found to exhibit a slow and protracted endogenous pattern of development under normal conditions, remaining relatively immature well into postnatal life [67–72]. This pattern of maturation appears to be needed for appropriate cognitive development and allowing for the maturation and stabilization of lower-order networks with which to build upon [73–75]. However, the protracted maturation pattern of these prefrontal and temporal areas may confer an enhanced vulnerability to HDAC inhibition compared to networks that have already attained full maturity [1]. This vulnerability may lead to prominent increases in the structural assembly of synapses and growth of neural networks, both of which are thought to contribute to the underlying clinicopathology of ASD [1, 76].

Histone methylation is another important epigenetic mechanism related to histone acetylation that can regulate gene transcription, developmental gene programs, and cellular phenotype [55, 77, 78]. Much like that of histone acetylation, it has been proposed that histone methylation may be reversible, dynamic, and also important in the teratogenicity of VPA [78]. For example, Tung and Winn reported that not

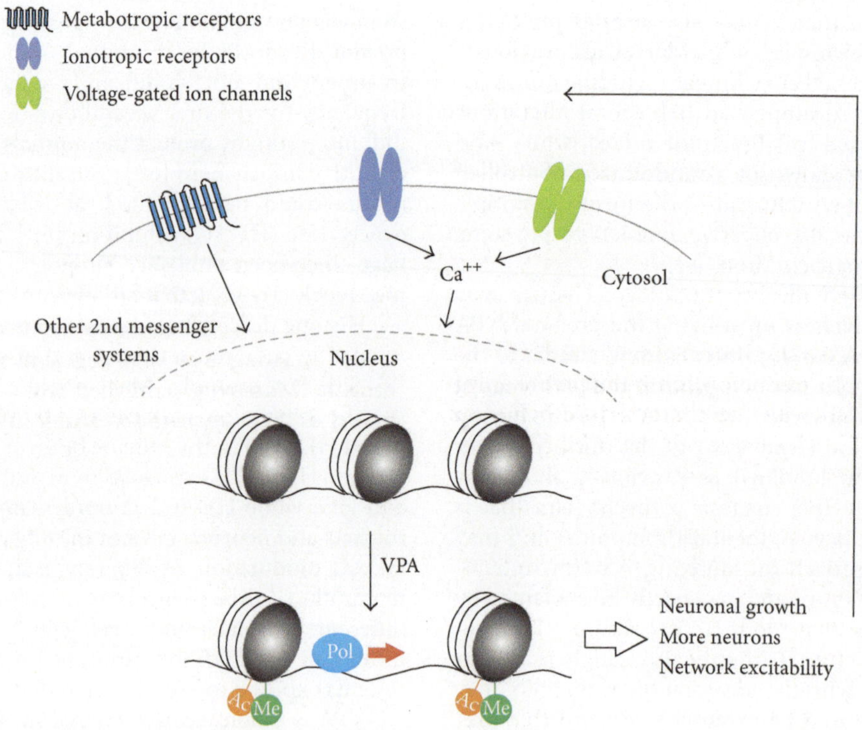

FIGURE 1: A schematic of some key molecular and cellular changes associated with VPA related to ASD neuropathology. Common clinicopathology associated with ASD is accelerated or early brain overgrowth and increased network excitability. Early or accelerated overgrowth may result from more synapses, increased denritic growth, and/or increased number of cells, while increased network excitability may result from hyperconnectivity and/or hyperplasticity of microcircuits, presumably driven by synaptic mechanisms (i.e., enhanced paired-pulse facilitation and long-term potentiation) that have been shown in rat brain both *in vitro* and *in vivo* following prenatal VPA exposure [56, 57]. All of these aspects are also likely regulated by histone acetylation (orange circles "Ac") and/or histone methylation (green circles "Me") and possibly DNA methylation (DNA methylation not shown). VPA has been shown to increase histone acetylation and histone methylation that can promote gene activation (symbolized by blue circle "Pol"; RNA polymerase). While VPA may disrupt the balance between excitatory and inhibitory neuronal activities through histone acetylation modulation [58], the role of histone methylation on VPA-related ASD neuropathology is much less clear. Increased connectivity and network excitability may further influence this process by activating metabotropic, ionotropic, and voltage-gated ion channels and subsequent intracellular signaling cascades.

only did *in utero* exposure to VPA lead to HDAC inhibition and increased histone acetylation of mouse fetal tissue, but it was also associated with changes in histone methylation [78]. In fact, this study found significant increases in di- and trimethylated histone 3-K4 and significant decreases in monomethylated histone 3-K9, which may represent sites involved in gene activation and repression, respectively [77]. Indeed, these epigenetic changes are likely involved in the multiple genes that can be influenced by early VPA exposure [58].

Adding another layer of complexity to the epigenetic control of gene regulation is DNA methylation, where methyl groups covalently bound to the 5′ position of cytosine project into the major groove of DNA, thus inhibiting the binding of transcription factors [78]. While there is interplay between DNA methylation and histone acetylation [79], somewhat surprisingly, the significance of DNA methylation as a mechanism of VPA-induced teratogenesis remains debatable [78]. Thus, the role VPA plays on DNA methylation and the interplay between DNA methylation and histone acetylation will be an important area for future research.

5. Valproic Acid, Overconnectivity, and Hyperexcitable Networks

Clinically apparent seizures are not uncommon in ASD [80]. While there has been a long standing association between ASD and seizure, even children that do not present with clinical seizure can exhibit subclinical seizure and epileptiform electroencephalographic (EEG) abnormalities [80, 81]. Thus, it is postulated that accelerated or early brain overgrowth is accompanied by pathological changes in network excitability.

The rodent VPA model of ASD allows for intrusive electrophysiological study of living tissue unavailable in humans to uncover the nature and potential causes of these suspected electrophysiological abnormalities. One prevailing theory of ASD, the "intense world" theory [41, 42], has been refined through the study of the VPA rat model and postulates that several areas of the brain including the prefrontal cortex and amygdala display hyperreactivity of the microcircuitry of pyramidal cells compared to controls [22, 23, 41, 42, 56, 57]. The amygdala bares particular relevance, for example, as it has been functionally related to ASD due to its role in socioemotional behaviour and can also exhibit enlargement and hyperactivation in autistic children [82, 83]. Markram's group has shown enhanced fear memories, enhanced fear generalization, and impaired fear extinction in prenatally exposed VPA treated rats, along with the other ASD-like behavioural phenotypes [23]. As well, electrophysiological data from lateral amygdaloid nucleus slices showed increased reactivity to stimulation, increased long-term potentiation, and impaired inhibition [23]. A similar result was found by Lin et al. as they also reported hyperexcitability and enhanced LTP in amygdala lateral nucleus pyramidal neurons following prenatal exposure to VPA [17]. These authors stated that the increased ratio of synaptic excitation/inhibition in the amygdala might be associated with the characteristic behaviour in this ASD model [17], which was reiterated by Kim et al. based on their own work showing increased expression of glutamatergic proteins in prefrontal networks of postnatal brains of rat offspring exposed to VPA *in utero* [84]. Finally, as impairments in the GABAergic system may critically contribute to an increased synaptic excitation/inhibition ratio, an additional mechanism may also involve reduced GABAergic inhibition as recently shown in the temporal cortex of rat pups following prenatal VPA exposure [85].

Although functional imaging studies of the autistic brain have long suggested decreased activity, these recent findings from the VPA model propose an alternate explanation wherein electrophysiological abnormalities may cause network hyperactivity within hyperconnected microcircuits [22, 42, 57]. Indeed, a recent imaging study has shown hyperconnectivity in several large-scale brain networks of children with ASD [86]. While previous functional magnetic resonance imaging (fMRI) studies have been somewhat contradictory, these recent findings suggest that further research into brain network connectivity may lead to a better understanding of the pathology of ASD in the brain [86].

Furthermore, prenatal VPA exposure has been shown to increase NMDA receptor NR2A and NR2B subunits [22], with NR2A being important in epileptogenesis [87]. Consequently, this enhanced activity may subsequently lead to greater activity-dependent processes involved in controlling structural aspects neuronal and synaptic network maturation and growth (Figure 1). For example, it has been shown that activity-induced NR2A activation can lead to increased brain-derived neurotrophic factor (BDNF) expression [87]. Thus, given that BDNF is important in neuronal development [88–90] and epileptogenesis [91], this may be one of several signaling pathways involved in the clinicopathology of ASD.

While activity modulates not only structural aspects of neuronal connectivity such as dendritic branching and spine formation, it can also influence the neurochemical landscape of the neural network. For example, an emerging body of the literature is now providing mechanistic insight into neurotransmitter specification and the role of electrical activity in the developing nervous system [92–94]. Consequently, alterations in the proportions of excitatory and inhibitory neural transmitter phenotypes may play a very important role in the pathophysiology associated with ASD [95]. A number of neurodevelopmental processes ranging from early events of cell proliferation and differentiation, to late events involving maturation of the dendritic arbors and synapses, can all be influenced by activity [92, 94]. Thus, further study on the electrophysiological changes associated with rodent brains exposed to VPA is likely to uncover convergent molecular pathway(s) that drive these changes.

6. Conclusion

Based on accumulating clinical data, it is becoming increasingly clear that VPA is an important risk factor associated with ASD. In addition, a growing body of animal literature is also showing that VPA can lead to ASD-like features in rodents. Moreover, published work suggests that the VPA model of ASD appears to exhibit all elements of a relevant model, namely, construct, face, and predictive validity, and therefore is likely to prove useful in elucidating mechanisms of ASD clinicopathology. It is also important to note that the significance of the two recent epidemiological studies discussed in this paper may also lie in the potential of revealing VPA-like environmental or nutritional substances that could increase the risk of ASD. For example, it was recently shown that in certain cell types global histone acetylation and HDAC activity could be regulated by metabolites of intermediate metabolism [96]. Based on studies primarily in nonneuronal cells, it is also now evident that other agents, including those in the human diet, can be converted by metabolism to intermediates that can influence HDAC activity [96, 97]. Thus, improving our understanding of how VPA and VPA-like compounds can alter early nervous system development will ultimately improve our understanding of ASD.

Acknowledgments

The authors would like to thank Johanna Hung for helpful comments on an earlier version of the paper and Dr. Jeffrey Buchhalter for insightful discussion. This study was supported by Canadian Institutes of Health Research and CIHR Regenerative Medicine Initiative. Nathanael Turner is supported by a PURE studentship. Taylor Chomiak and Nathanael Turner are cofirst authors.

References

[1] T. Chomiak and B. Hu, "Alterations of neocortical development and maturation in autism: insight from valproic acid exposure and animal models of autism," *Neurotoxicology and Teratology*, vol. 36, pp. 57–66, 2013.

[2] E. Courchesne, K. Pierce, C. M. Schumann et al., "Mapping early brain development in autism," *Neuron*, vol. 56, no. 2, pp. 399–413, 2007.

[3] C. M. Schumann, C. S. Bloss, C. C. Barnes et al., "Longitudinal magnetic resonance imaging study of cortical development through early childhood in autism," *Journal of Neuroscience*, vol. 30, no. 12, pp. 4419–4427, 2010.

[4] D. G. Amaral, C. M. Schumann, and C. W. Nordahl, "Neuroanatomy of autism," *Trends in Neurosciences*, vol. 31, no. 3, pp. 137–145, 2008.

[5] R. Adolphs, "The neurobiology of social cognition," *Current Opinion in Neurobiology*, vol. 11, no. 2, pp. 231–239, 2001.

[6] H. C. Hazlett, M. D. Poe, G. Gerig et al., "Early brain overgrowth in autism associated with an increase in cortical surface area before age 2 years," *Archives of General Psychiatry*, vol. 68, no. 5, pp. 467–476, 2011.

[7] A. Raznahan, G. L. Wallace, L. Antezana et al., "Compared to what? Early brain overgrowth in autism and the perils of population norms," *Biol Psychiatry*, vol. 74, no. 8, pp. 563–575, 2013.

[8] D. R. Morhardt, W. Barrow, M. Jaworski, and P. J. Accardo, "Head circumference in young children with autism: the impact of different head circumference charts," *Journal of Child Neurology*, 2013.

[9] C. Ecker, J. Suckling, S. C. Deoni et al., "Brain anatomy and its relationship to behavior in adults with autism spectrum disorder: a multicenter magnetic resonance imaging study," *Archives of General Psychiatry*, vol. 69, no. 2, pp. 195–209, 2012.

[10] J. A. Balfour and H. M. Bryson, "Valproic acid," *CNS Drugs*, vol. 2, no. 2, pp. 144–173, 1994.

[11] A. L. Christianson, N. Chesler, and J. G. R. Kromberg, "Fetal valproate syndrome: clinical and neuro-developmental features in two sibling pairs," *Developmental Medicine and Child Neurology*, vol. 36, no. 4, pp. 361–369, 1994.

[12] G. Williams, J. King, M. Cunningham, M. Stephan, B. Kerr, and J. H. Hersh, "Fetal valproate syndrome and autism: additional evidence of an association," *Developmental Medicine and Child Neurology*, vol. 43, no. 3, pp. 202–206, 2001.

[13] P. G. Williams and J. H. Hersh, "A male with fetal valproate syndrome and autism," *Developmental Medicine and Child Neurology*, vol. 39, no. 9, pp. 632–634, 1997.

[14] S. J. Moore, P. Turnpenny, A. Quinn et al., "A clinical study of 57 children with fetal anticonvulsant syndromes," *Journal of Medical Genetics*, vol. 37, no. 7, pp. 489–497, 2000.

[15] A. D. Rasalam, H. Hailey, J. H. G. Williams et al., "Characteristics of fetal anticonvulsant syndrome associated autistic disorder," *Developmental Medicine and Child Neurology*, vol. 47, no. 8, pp. 551–555, 2005.

[16] L. Laegreid, M. Kyllerman, T. Hedner, B. Hagberg, and G. Viggedahl, "Benzodiazepine amplification of valproate teratogenic effects in children of mothers with absence epilepsy," *Neuropediatrics*, vol. 24, no. 2, pp. 88–92, 1993.

[17] H. C. Lin, P. W. Gean, C.-C. Wang, Y. H. Chan, and P. Chen, "The amygdala excitatory/inhibitory balance in a valproate-induced rat autism model," *PLoS ONE*, vol. 8, no. 1, Article ID e55248, 2013.

[18] V. Bambini-Junior, L. Rodrigues, G. A. Behr, J. C. F. Moreira, R. Riesgo, and C. Gottfried, "Animal model of autism induced by prenatal exposure to valproate: behavioral changes and liver parameters," *Brain Research*, vol. 1408, pp. 8–16, 2011.

[19] P. E. Binkerd, J. M. Rowland, H. Nau, and A. G. Hendrickx, "Evaluation of valproic acid (VPA) developmental toxicity and pharmacokinetics in Sprague-Dawley rats," *Fundamental and Applied Toxicology*, vol. 11, no. 3, pp. 485–493, 1988.

[20] D. Dufour-Rainfray, P. Vourc'h, A. Le Guisquet et al., "Behavior and serotonergic disorders in rats exposed prenatally to valproate: a model for autism," *Neuroscience Letters*, vol. 470, no. 1, pp. 55–59, 2010.

[21] K. C. Kim, P. Kim, H. S. Go et al., "The critical period of valproate exposure to induce autistic symptoms in Sprague-Dawley rats," *Toxicology Letters*, vol. 201, no. 2, pp. 137–142, 2011.

[22] T. Rinaldi, K. Kulangara, K. Antoniello, and H. Markram, "Elevated NMDA receptor levels and enhanced postsynaptic long-term potentiation induced by prenatal exposure to valproic acid," *Proceedings of the National Academy of Sciences of the United States of America*, vol. 104, no. 33, pp. 13501–13506, 2007.

[23] K. Markram, T. Rinaldi, D. L. Mendola, C. Sandi, and H. Markram, "Abnormal fear conditioning and amygdala processing in an animal model of autism," *Neuropsychopharmacology*, vol. 33, no. 4, pp. 901–912, 2008.

[24] F. I. Roullet, L. Wollaston, D. deCatanzaro, and J. A. Foster, "Behavioral and molecular changes in the mouse in response to prenatal exposure to the anti-epileptic drug valproic acid," *Neuroscience*, vol. 170, no. 2, pp. 514–522, 2010.

[25] T. Schneider and R. Przewłocki, "Behavioral alterations in rats prenatally to valproic acid: animal model of autism," *Neuropsychopharmacology*, vol. 30, no. 1, pp. 80–89, 2005.

[26] T. Schneider, J. Turczak, and R. Przewłocki, "Environmental enrichment reverses behavioral alterations in rats prenatally exposed to valproic acid: issues for a therapeutic approach in autism," *Neuropsychopharmacology*, vol. 31, no. 1, pp. 36–46, 2006.

[27] T. Schneider, A. Roman, A. Basta-Kaim et al., "Gender-specific behavioral and immunological alterations in an animal model of autism induced by prenatal exposure to valproic acid," *Psychoneuroendocrinology*, vol. 33, no. 6, pp. 728–740, 2008.

[28] C. V. Vorhees, "Behavioral teratogenicity of valproic acid: selective effects on behavior after prenatal exposure to rats," *Psychopharmacology*, vol. 92, no. 2, pp. 173–179, 1987.

[29] C. V. Vorhees, "Teratogenicity and developmental toxicity of valproic acid in rats," *Teratology*, vol. 35, no. 2, pp. 195–202, 1987.

[30] G. C. Wagner, K. R. Reuhl, M. Cheh, P. McRae, and A. K. Halladay, "A new neurobehavioral model of autism in mice: pre- and postnatal exposure to sodium valproate," *Journal of Autism and Developmental Disorders*, vol. 36, no. 6, pp. 779–793, 2006.

[31] A. C. Felix-Ortiz and M. Febo, "Gestational valproate alters BOLD activation in response to complex social and primary sensory stimuli," *PLoS ONE*, vol. 7, no. 5, Article ID e37313, 2012.

[32] R. Mychasiuk, S. Richards, A. Nakahashi, B. Kolb, and R. Gibb, "Effects of rat prenatal exposure to valproic acid on behaviour and neuro-anatomy," *Developmental Neuroscience*, vol. 34, pp. 268–276, 2012.

[33] R. L. Bromley, G. E. Mawer, M. Briggs et al., "The prevalence of neurodevelopmental disorders in children prenatally exposed to antiepileptic drugs," *Journal of Neurology, Neurosurgery & Psychiatry*, vol. 84, no. 6, pp. 637–643, 2013.

[34] J. Christensen, T. K. Grønborg, M. J. Sørensen et al., "Prenatal valproate exposure and risk of autism spectrum disorders and childhood autism," *Journal of the American Medical Association*, vol. 309, no. 16, pp. 1696–1703, 2013.

[35] J. C. Dean, H. Hailey, S. J. Moore, D. J. Lloyd, P. D. Turnpenny, and J. Little, "Long term health and neurodevelopment in children exposed to antiepileptic drugs before birth," *Journal of Medical Genetics*, vol. 39, no. 4, pp. 251–259, 2002.

[36] P. M. Rodier, J. L. Ingram, B. Tisdale, S. Nelson, and J. Romano, "Embryological origin for autism: developmental anomalies of the cranial nerve motor nuclei," *Journal of Comparative Neurology*, vol. 370, no. 2, pp. 247–261, 1996.

[37] P. M. Rodier, J. L. Ingram, B. Tisdale, and V. J. Croog, "Linking etiologies in humans and animal models: studies of autism," *Reproductive Toxicology*, vol. 11, no. 2-3, pp. 417–422, 1997.

[38] F. I. Roullet, J. K. Lai, and J. A. Foster, "*In Utero* exposure to valproic acid and autism—a current review of clinical and animal studies," *Neurotoxicology and Teratology*, vol. 36, pp. 47–56, 2013.

[39] D. Dufour-Rainfray, P. Vourc'h, S. Tourlet, D. Guilloteau, S. Chalon, and C. R. Andres, "Fetal exposure to teratogens: evidence of genes involved in autism," *Neuroscience and Biobehavioral Reviews*, vol. 35, no. 5, pp. 1254–1265, 2011.

[40] M. E. Bringas, F. N. Carvajal-Floresa, T. A. López-Ramírez, M. Atzori, and G. Flores, "Rearrangement of the dendritic morphology in limbic regions and altered exploratory behavior in a rat model of autism spectrum disorder," *Neuroscience*, vol. 241, pp. 170–187, 2013.

[41] K. Markram and H. Markram, "The intense world theory-a unifying theory of the neurobiology of autism," *Frontiers in Human Neuroscience*, vol. 4, p. 224, 2010.

[42] H. Markram, T. Rinaldi, and K. Markram, "The intense world syndrome-an alternative hypothesis for autism," *Frontiers in Neuroscience*, vol. 1, no. 1, pp. 77–96, 2007.

[43] C. Belzung, S. Leman, P. Vourc'h, and C. Andres, "Rodent models for autism: a critical review," *Drug Discovery Today*, vol. 2, no. 2, pp. 93–101, 2005.

[44] C. C. Woo and M. Leon, "Environmental enrichment as an effective treatment for autism: a randomized controlled trial," *Behavioral Neuroscience*, vol. 127, no. 4, pp. 487–497, 2013.

[45] S. E. Lazic and L. Essioux, "Improving basic and translational science by accounting for litter-to-litter variation in animal models," *BMC Neuroscience*, vol. 14, p. 37, 2013.

[46] A. Oguchi-Katayama, A. Monma, Y. Sekino, T. Moriguchi, and K. Sato, "Comparative gene expression analysis of the amygdala in autistic rat models produced by pre- and post-natal exposures to valproic acid," *Journal of Toxicological Sciences*, vol. 38, no. 3, pp. 391–402, 2013.

[47] S. Reynolds, A. Millette, and D. P. Devine, "Sensory and motor characterization in the postnatal valproate rat model of autism," *Developmental Neuroscience*, vol. 34, no. 2-3, pp. 258–267, 2012.

[48] C. L. Yochum, P. Dowling, K. R. Reuhl, G. C. Wagner, and X. Ming, "VPA-induced apoptosis and behavioral deficits in neonatal mice," *Brain Research*, vol. 1203, pp. 126–132, 2008.

[49] T. Chomiak, V. Karnik, E. Block, and B. Hu, "Altering the trajectory of early postnatal cortical development can lead to structural and behavioural features of autism," *BMC Neuroscience*, vol. 11, p. 102, 2010.

[50] E. Jager-Roman, A. Deichl, and S. Jakob, "Fetal growth, major malformations, and minor anomalies in infants born to women receiving valproic acid," *Journal of Pediatrics*, vol. 108, no. 6, pp. 997–1004, 1986.

[51] H. S. Go, K. C. Kim, C. S. Choi et al., "Prenatal exposure to valproic acid increases the neural progenitor cell pool and induces macrocephaly in rat brain via a mechanism involving the GSK-3beta/beta-catenin pathway," *Neuropharmacology*, vol. 63, no. 6, pp. 1028–1041, 2012.

[52] M. W. Akhtar, J. Raingo, E. D. Nelson et al., "Histone deacetylases 1 and 2 form a developmental switch that controls excitatory synapse maturation and function," *Journal of Neuroscience*, vol. 29, no. 25, pp. 8288–8297, 2009.

[53] V. Balasubramaniyan, E. Boddeke, R. Bakels et al., "Effects of histone deacetylation inhibition on neuronal differentiation of embryonic mouse neural stem cells," *Neuroscience*, vol. 143, no. 4, pp. 939–951, 2006.

[54] J. Hsieh and F. H. Gage, "Epigenetic control of neural stem cell fate," *Current Opinion in Genetics and Development*, vol. 14, no. 5, pp. 461–469, 2004.

[55] J. Hsieh and F. H. Gage, "Chromatin remodeling in neural development and plasticity," *Current Opinion in Cell Biology*, vol. 17, no. 6, pp. 664–671, 2005.

[56] L. Sui and M. Chen, "Prenatal exposure to valproic acid enhances synaptic plasticity in the medial prefrontal cortex and fear memories," *Brain Research Bulletin*, vol. 87, no. 6, pp. 556–563, 2012.

[57] T. Rinaldi, C. Perrodin, and H. Markram, "Hyper-connectivity and hyper-plasticity in the medial prefrontal cortex in the valproic Acid animal model of autism," *Frontiers in Neural Circuits*, vol. 2, p. 4, 2008.

[58] M. Fukuchi, T. Nii, N. Ishimaru et al., "Valproic acid induces up- or down-regulation of gene expression responsible for the neuronal excitation and inhibition in rat cortical neurons through its epigenetic actions," *Neuroscience Research*, vol. 65, no. 1, pp. 35–43, 2009.

[59] B. Monti, E. Polazzi, and A. Contestabile, "Biochemical, molecular and epigenetic mechanisms of valproic acid neuroprotection," *Current Molecular Pharmacology*, vol. 2, no. 1, pp. 95–109, 2009.

[60] S. Jessberger, K. Nakashima, G. D. Clemenson Jr. et al., "Epigenetic modulation of seizure-induced neurogenesis and cognitive decline," *Journal of Neuroscience*, vol. 27, no. 22, pp. 5967–5975, 2007.

[61] S. Yasuda, M.-H. Liang, Z. Marinova, A. Yahyavi, and D.-M. Chuang, "The mood stabilizers lithium and valproate selectively activate the promoter IV of brain-derived neurotrophic factor in neurons," *Molecular Psychiatry*, vol. 14, no. 1, pp. 51–59, 2009.

[62] J. L. MacDonald and A. J. Roskams, "Histone deacetylases 1 and 2 are expressed at distinct stages of neuro-glial development," *Developmental Dynamics*, vol. 237, no. 8, pp. 2256–2267, 2008.

[63] A. G. Foley, S. Gannon, N. Rombach-Mullan et al., "Class I histone deacetylase inhibition ameliorates social cognition and cell adhesion molecule plasticity deficits in a rodent model of autism spectrum disorder," *Neuropharmacology*, vol. 63, no. 4, pp. 750–760, 2012.

[64] C. J. Phiel, F. Zhang, E. Y. Huang, M. G. Guenther, M. A. Lazar, and P. S. Klein, "Histone deacetylase is a direct target of valproic acid, a potent anticonvulsant, mood stabilizer, and teratogen," *Journal of Biological Chemistry*, vol. 276, no. 39, pp. 36734–36741, 2001.

[65] O. H. Krämer, P. Zhu, H. P. Ostendorff et al., "The histone deacetylase inhibitor valproic acid selectively induces proteasomal degradation of HDAC2," *EMBO Journal*, vol. 22, no. 13, pp. 3411–3420, 2003.

[66] Y. Hao, T. Creson, L. Zhang et al., "Mood stabilizer valproate promotes ERK pathway-dependent cortical neuronal growth and neurogenesis," *Journal of Neuroscience*, vol. 24, no. 29, pp. 6590–6599, 2004.

[67] C. F. Geier, K. Garver, R. Terwilliger, and B. Luna, "Development of working memory maintenance," *Journal of Neurophysiology*, vol. 101, no. 1, pp. 84–99, 2009.

[68] G. Golarai, D. G. Ghahremani, S. Whitfield-Gabrieli et al., "Differential development of high-level visual cortex correlates with category-specific recognition memory," *Nature Neuroscience*, vol. 10, no. 4, pp. 512–522, 2007.

[69] B. Luna, K. E. Garver, T. A. Urban, N. A. Lazar, and J. A. Sweeney, "Maturation of cognitive processes from late childhood to adulthood," *Child Development*, vol. 75, no. 5, pp. 1357–1372, 2004.

[70] K. S. Scherf, M. Behrmann, K. Humphreys, and B. Luna, "Visual category-selectivity for faces, places and objects emerges along different developmental trajectories," *Developmental Science*, vol. 10, no. 4, pp. F15–F30, 2007.

[71] P. Shaw, K. Eckstrand, W. Sharp et al., "Attention-deficit/hyperactivity disorder is characterized by a delay in cortical maturation," *Proceedings of the National Academy of Sciences of the United States of America*, vol. 104, no. 49, pp. 19649–19654, 2007.

[72] N. Gogtay, J. N. Giedd, L. Lusk et al., "Dynamic mapping of human cortical development during childhood through early adulthood," *Proceedings of the National Academy of Sciences of the United States of America*, vol. 101, no. 21, pp. 8174–8179, 2004.

[73] E. I. Knudsen, J. J. Heckman, J. L. Cameron, and J. P. Shonkoff, "Economic, neurobiological, and behavioral perspectives on building America's future workforce," *Proceedings of the National Academy of Sciences of the United States of America*, vol. 103, no. 27, pp. 10155–10162, 2006.

[74] J. L. Elman, "Learning and development in neural networks: the importance of starting small," *Cognition*, vol. 48, no. 1, pp. 71–99, 1993.

[75] S. R. Quartz, "The constructivist brain," *Trends in Cognitive Sciences*, vol. 3, no. 2, pp. 48–57, 1999.

[76] P. Penzes, M. E. Cahill, K. A. Jones, J. Vanleeuwen, and K. M. Woolfrey, "Dendritic spine pathology in neuropsychiatric disorders," *Nature Neuroscience*, vol. 14, no. 3, pp. 285–293, 2011.

[77] N. Mosammaparast and Y. Shi, "Reversal of histone methylation: biochemical and molecular mechanisms of histone demethylases," *Annual Review of Biochemistry*, vol. 79, pp. 155–179, 2010.

[78] E. W. Tung and L. M. Winn, "Epigenetic modifications in valproic acid-induced teratogenesis," *Toxicology and Applied Pharmacology*, vol. 248, no. 3, pp. 201–209, 2010.

[79] A. E. Handel, G. C. Ebers, and S. V. Ramagopalan, "Epigenetics: molecular mechanisms and implications for disease," *Trends in Molecular Medicine*, vol. 16, no. 1, pp. 7–16, 2010.

[80] R. Tuchman and I. Rapin, "Epilepsy in autism," *Lancet Neurology*, vol. 1, no. 6, pp. 352–358, 2002.

[81] M. G. Chez, M. Chang, V. Krasne, C. Coughlan, M. Kominsky, and A. Schwartz, "Frequency of epileptiform EEG abnormalities in a sequential screening of autistic patients with no known clinical epilepsy from 1996 to 2005," *Epilepsy and Behavior*, vol. 8, no. 1, pp. 267–271, 2006.

[82] K. M. Dalton, B. M. Nacewicz, T. Johnstone et al., "Gaze fixation and the neural circuitry of face processing in autism," *Nature Neuroscience*, vol. 8, no. 4, pp. 519–526, 2005.

[83] C. W. Nordahl, R. Scholz, X. Yang et al., "Increased rate of amygdala growth in children aged 2 to 4 years with autism spectrum disorders: a longitudinal study," *Archives of General Psychiatry*, vol. 69, no. 1, pp. 53–61, 2012.

[84] K. C. Kim, D. K. Lee, H. S. Go et al., "Pax6-dependent cortical glutamatergic neuronal differentiation regulates autism-like behavior in prenatally valproic acid-exposed rat offspring," *Molecular Neurobiology*, 2013.

[85] A. Banerjee, F. García-Oscos, S. Roychowdhury et al., "Impairment of cortical GABAergic synaptic transmission in an environmental rat model of autism," *International Journal of Neuropsychopharmacology*, vol. 16, no. 6, pp. 1309–1318, 2013.

[86] L. Q. Uddin, K. Supekar, C. J. Lynch et al., "Salience network-based classification and prediction of symptom severity in children with autism," *JAMA Psychiatry*, vol. 70, no. 8, pp. 869–879, 2013.

[87] Q. Chen, S. He, X. Hu et al., "Differential roles of NR2A- and NR2B-containing NMDA receptors in activity-dependent brain-derived neurotrophic factor gene regulation and limbic epileptogenesis," *Journal of Neuroscience*, vol. 27, no. 3, pp. 542–552, 2007.

[88] H. W. Horch and L. C. Katz, "BDNF release from single cells elicits local dendritic growth in nearby neurons," *Nature Neuroscience*, vol. 5, no. 11, pp. 1177–1184, 2002.

[89] A. K. McAllister, D. C. Lo, and L. C. Katz, "Neurotrophins regulate dendritic growth in developing visual cortex," *Neuron*, vol. 15, no. 4, pp. 791–803, 1995.

[90] A. K. McAllister, L. C. Katz, and D. C. Lo, "Neurotrophin regulation of cortical dendritic growth requires activity," *Neuron*, vol. 17, no. 6, pp. 1057–1064, 1996.

[91] D. K. Binder, S. D. Croll, C. M. Gall, and H. E. Scharfman, "BDNF and epilepsy: too much of a good thing?" *Trends in Neurosciences*, vol. 24, no. 1, pp. 47–53, 2001.

[92] M. Stamou, K. M. Streifel, P. E. Goines, and P. J. Lein, "Neuronal connectivity as a convergent target of gene x environment interactions that confer risk for autism spectrum disorders," *Neurotoxicology and Teratology*, vol. 36, pp. 3–16, 2013.

[93] N. C. Spitzer, "Activity-dependent neurotransmitter respecification," *Nature Reviews Neuroscience*, vol. 13, no. 2, pp. 94–106, 2012.

[94] N. C. Spitzer, "Electrical activity in early neuronal development," *Nature*, vol. 444, no. 7120, pp. 707–712, 2006.

[95] J. L. Rubenstein and M. M. Merzenich, "Model of autism: increased ratio of excitation/inhibition in key neural systems," *Genes, Brain and Behavior*, vol. 2, no. 5, pp. 255–267, 2003.

[96] M. Vogelauer, A. S. Krall, M . A. McBrian, J.-Y. Li, and S. A. Kurdistani, "Stimulation of histone deacetylase activity by metabolites of intermediary metabolism," *Journal of Biological Chemistry*, vol. 287, no. 38, pp. 32006–32016, 2012.

[97] P. Rajendran, D. E. Williams, E. Ho, and R. H. Dashwood, "Metabolism as a key to histone deacetylase inhibition," *Critical Reviews in Biochemistry and Molecular Biology*, vol. 46, no. 3, pp. 181–199, 2011.

Matrix Metalloproteinases 2 and 9 Immunoexpression in Prostate Carcinoma at the Positive Margin of Radical Prostatectomy Specimens

Romano Oguić,[1] Vladimir Mozetič,[2] Eleonora Cini Tešar,[3] Dora Fučkar Čupić,[4] Elvira Mustać,[4] and Gordana Đorđević[4]

[1] *Department of Urology, Clinical Hospital Centre Rijeka, Krešimirova 42, 51000 Rijeka, Croatia*
[2] *Medico Polyclinic, Agatićeva 8, 51000 Rijeka, Croatia*
[3] *Department of Oncology, Clinical Hospital Centre Rijeka, Krešimirova 42, 51000 Rijeka, Croatia*
[4] *Department of Pathology, School of Medicine, University of Rijeka, Braće Branchetta 20, 51000 Rijeka, Croatia*

Correspondence should be addressed to Gordana Đorđević; gordana.dordevic@medri.uniri.hr

Academic Editor: Shahid Pervez

The aim of this study was to evaluate the expression of matrix metalloproteinase 2 (MMP-2) and matrix metalloproteinase 9 (MMP-9) in prostate cancer in the main tumor mass and tumor cells at the positive margin as well as the influence of these biomarkers on the biochemical recurrence of the disease in prostatectomy patients. Tissue microarrays of 120 archival prostate carcinoma samples were immunohistochemically evaluated for MMP-2 and MMP-9 expression and compared with clinicopathological parameters. Tumors with positive surgical margins showed significantly higher overall expression of MMP-9 versus tumors with negative resection margins ($P = 0.0121$). MMP-9 expression was significantly elevated in tumors from patients who had biochemical recurrence ($P = 0.0207$). In the group of patients with negative margins, MMP-9 expression above the cut-off value was significantly associated with recurrence ($P = 0.0065$). Multivariate analysis indicated that MMP-9 is a good predictor of biochemical recurrence (odds ratio = 10.29; $P = 0.0052$). Expression of MMP-2 in tumor cells was significantly higher at the positive margins than in the main tumor mass ($P = 0.0301$). The present results highlight the potential value of MMP-2 and MMP-9 expression for predicting the behavior of prostate tumors after prostatectomy with both positive and negative surgical margins.

1. Introduction

Extensive studies of the matrix metalloproteinases (MMPs) indicate that a large number of MMP family factors play active roles in carcinogenesis and metastasis [1–3]. Many studies have focused on the role of MMPs and their inhibitors in the prognoses of various types of malignancies. Most published data on MMP-2 and MMP-9 address the role of these proteins in encouraging the aggressiveness of cancers. Increased expression of MMP-2 correlates with low survival in patients with breast cancer [4–8], is associated with a 4.5-fold higher relative risk of mortality from skin melanoma, and predicts the risk of metastasis in uveal melanoma [9, 10]. Increased expression of MMP-2 is a sign of poor prognosis in cancer of the stomach and pancreas [11–13] as well as the prostate [14].

Kuvaja et al. concluded that low levels of serum pro-MMP-2 correlate with aggressive cancer behavior [15]. High MMP-2 expression in hematological malignancies suggests good prognosis; in contrast, high MMP-9 expression is a sign of poor disease outcome [16]. The function of MMP-9 is still controversial in solid tumors. Scorilas et al. proposed that MMP-9 immunoreactive protein can be a favorable sign for node-negative breast cancer [17]. On the other hand, investigations of high MMP-9 levels in plasma or serum samples showed that MMP-9 expression may be associated with increased risk of recurrence and poor prognosis [18, 19]. In prostate carcinoma, MMP-2 and MMP-9 are novel molecular biomarkers that reflect the invasive and metastatic potential of this type of carcinoma [20]. The standard biomarkers that significantly predict the clinical and biochemical recurrence of prostate cancer are preoperative serum prostate-specific antigen (PSA), pathological grade according to Gleason score, positive surgical margins (with and without extraprostatic extension), and capsular incision adding up the following factors as of prognostic significance: presence of perineural, angiolymphatic, seminal vesicle invasion and extraprostatic tissue invasion. However, the real prognostic importance of positive margins remains to be defined. Few studies have emphasized the behavior of the previously mentioned biomarkers on the positive edge of the resection in comparison to their behavior in the bulk tumor mass. Recently, Cao et al. addressed the issue of positive resection margins in radical prostatectomy and found that the Gleason score at the edge of the tumor resection is predictive of biochemical recurrence [21]. There are currently no studies on the predictive value of MMP expression on the edge of the resection in radical prostatectomy.

The aim of this study was to measure the expression levels of MMP-2 and MMP-9 in the main tumor mass and in tumor cells on the positive margin and to compare these expression levels with Gleason score and tumor size in patients treated by radical prostatectomy. We also examined the influence of these biomarkers on biochemical recurrence of the disease in prostatectomy patients.

2. Methods

2.1. Patients. During the period from 2001 to 2006, acinar adenocarcinoma was discovered by ultrasound-guided biopsy of the prostate in 793 patients at the Clinic of Urology, Clinical Hospital Center Rijeka, Croatia. In accordance with the criteria from the European Urological Association, candidates for radical prostatectomy had a Gleason score of 7 or less, PSA levels below 10 ng/mL, and clinically confirmed prostate cancer in stage T1c/T2c (normal preoperative computed tomography findings and pelvic bone scintigraphy) [22]. From 2001 to 2006, 120 patients who had undergone radical prostatectomy were chosen from medical documentation files and adequate clinical data were collected. Two groups of patients were formed: a group of 71 patients having tumors with negative surgical margins and a second group of 49 patients with tumors showing positive surgical margins. Tumor material, obtained from radical prostatectomy, was selected for the construction of tissue microarrays. Representative areas on the hematoxylin and eosin-stained sections were carefully selected and marked on the corresponding paraffin blocks. From each carcinoma, two tissue cores (1 mm in diameter) were obtained from the main tumor mass and two cores were taken from the tumor at the positive surgical margin; these samples were arrayed in a recipient paraffin block using MTA Booster OI Manual Tissue Arrayer (Alphalyse, Plaisir, France).

2.2. Immunohistochemistry. Immunohistochemical staining for MMP-2 (17B11 mouse monoclonal antibody, Vision Biosystems Novocastra, Newcastle, UK) and MMP-9 (17W2 mouse monoclonal antibody NCL-MMP-9-493, Vision Biosystems Novocastra) was carried out with an automated immunostainer (OptiMax Plus, BioGenex) employing a standard biotin-streptavidin method. Heat-induced pretreatment for antigen retrieval (slides were immersed in a 10 mM citrated buffer, pH 6.0, at 95°C for 5 min) was carried out prior to incubation with primary antibody; the Dako En/Vision+/HRP Kit was used to visualize MMP expression. Intestinal tissue of patients with inflammatory bowel disease (as recommended by the manufacturer) and the positive control for MMP-9 were normal liver tissues (as recommended by the manufacturer).

The expression level of each protein was determined with image analysis system ISSA 3.1 software (Zagreb, Croatia). Staining was evaluated as the percentage of cytoplasmic-positive tumor cells multiplied by the staining intensity; this value was expressed as a histoscore. Clinicopathological data obtained from patient medical records included age, tumor size, TNM stage, Gleason score, and margin status of the prostatectomy specimens (Table 1). We separately examined the immunoexpression of the MMPs relative to localization within the tumor mass (MMP expression on the positive surgical margins and in the bulk of the tumor mass).

TABLE 1: Clinical and pathological features of patients with prostate cancer treated with prostatectomy.

Feature	
Age of patients (years, median)	64.12
Preoperative serum PSA (ng/mL, median)	8.50
Tumor size (cm, median)	2.25
Pathologic stage (%)	
pT2	74.00
pT3	26.00
Gleason score (%)	
≤6	65.40
≥7	34.60
Margin status (%)	
Positive	58.82
Negative	41.17
Disease-free survival (months)	
Negative margin group	31.2
Positive margin group	22.6

3. Results

We found a mean Gleason score significantly higher in the group with positive surgical margins than in the group with negative surgical margins ($P = 0.0032$; Figure 1).

Immunohistochemical staining against MMP-2 and MMP-9 in glands with hyperplastic epithelium indicated weak or negative expression of these proteins, except for glands with high-grade PIN, where the expression was stronger (Figures 1). MMP-2 and MMP-9 immunoexpression in tumor cells was cytoplasmic, finely granular, and varied in intensity and percentage. We did not find tumors that were negative for the expression of these proteins (Figures 1).

Table 2: Expression of MMP-2 and MMP-9 in the main tumor mass and on the resection margin.

	N	Average	*P*
MMP-2			
Tumor	95	98.9160	0.0301
Margin	43	109.0237	
Tumor mass, positive surgical margin	43	91.3581	0.1833
Tumor mass, negative surgical margin	52	105.1658	
MMP-9			
Tumor	106	142.1780	0.1214
Margin	45	171.0924	
Tumor mass, positive surgical margin	45	157.2962	0.0121
Tumor mass, negative surgical margin	61	131.0252	

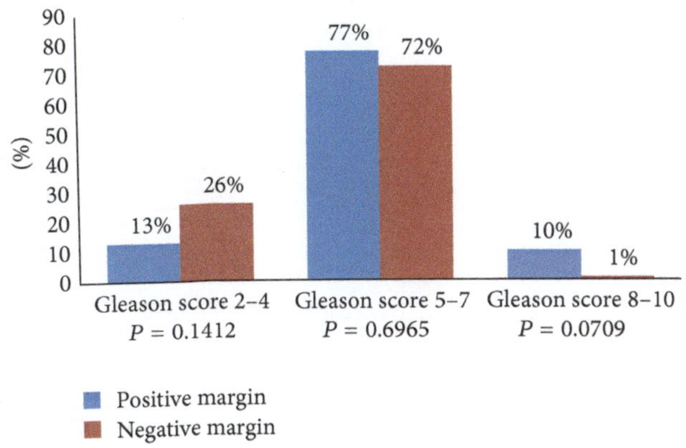

Figure 1: Analysis of Gleason score in patients with positive or negative surgical margins.

Table 3: MMP-2 and MMP-9 expression in terms of total Gleason score and tumor stage and size.

	Average histoscore	*P*
MMP-2 expression in margin		
Gleason <7	98.103	0.7417
Gleason ≥7	127.453	
Stage 2	113.390	0.5867
Stage 3	102.089	
MMP-2 expression in tumor		
Gleason <7	99.121	0.9389
Gleason ≥7	98.146	
Stage 2	94.942	0.1712
Stage 3	110.771	
Size ≤1 cm	114.165	0.5207
Size >1 cm	97.342	
MMP-9 expression in margin		
Gleason <7	173.391	0.7417
Gleason ≥7	166.927	
Stage 2	173.116	0.9093
Stage 3	170.875	
MMP-9 expression in tumor		
Gleason <7	139.472	0.2597
Gleason ≥7	153.812	
Stage 2	137.432	0.1044
Stage 3	155.930	
Size ≤1 cm	95.000	0.0378
Size >1 cm	143.067	

MMP-2 was expressed not only in the cytoplasm of tumor cells but also in the cytoplasm of prostatic stromal cells, endothelium, fibroblasts, smooth muscle cells, macrophages, and lymphocytes. The average histoscore of MMP-2 expression per tumor was 98.9160 (standard deviation (SD) 50.1750). MMP-2 was significantly more strongly expressed in tumor cells on the positive margins than in the main tumor mass, with an average of 109.0237 (SD 64.0751; $P = 0.0301$). In the stroma, the strongest MMP-2 expression occurred in the cytoplasm of inflammatory cells, especially macrophages (Figure 3).

MMP-9 expression was detected in the cytoplasm of tumor cells, while stromal cells were weakly positive for this marker; staining could be categorized as cytoplasmic or nuclear plus cytoplasmic. The cytoplasm of some tumors contained more pronounced luminal expression of MMP-9, while, in other tumors, this staining was diffuse or mostly peripheral. The average amount of MMP-9 immunostaining was higher than that of MMP-2 in both examined locations. The mean MMP-9 expression was 142.1780 (SD 51.0358) in the main tumor mass and 171.0924 (SD 61.9203) at the positive margin of resection. Although there was no significant difference in MMP-9 immunoexpression between the main tumor mass and the edge, a group of tumors with positive surgical margins showed significantly stronger overall expression of MMP-9 compared to a group of tumors with negative resection margins ($P = 0.0121$; Table 2).

Increased expression of MMP-2 and MMP-9 was found in tumors of better differentiation and higher Gleason score but with no significant differences between tumors with Gleason score <7 and high-grade cancers with Gleason score ≥7. Regarding disease stage, MMP-2 staining was slightly stronger in higher-stage tumors but without statistical significance. Tumor size was significantly associated with MMP-9

TABLE 4: ROC analysis.

		AUC	95% confidence interval	P
MMP-2, margin	All	0.589	0.413 to 0.749	0.3596
MMP-2, tumor mass	All	0.524	0.408 to 0.638	0.7610
	Negative margin	0.525	0.352 to 0.694	0.8108
	Positive margin	0.693	0.532 to 0.826	0.0988
MMP-9, margin	All	0.551	0.379 to 0.715	0.6352
MMP-9, tumor mass	All	0.626	0.515 to 0.728	0.0582
	Negative margin	0.513	0.343 to 0.680	0.8970
	Positive margin	0.714	0.567 to 0.834	0.0274

TABLE 5: MMP-2 and MMP-9 expression and recurrence regarding cut-off values determined by the Youden index.

		Youden index	95% CI	Associated criterion	Sensitivity	95% CI	Specificity	95% CI
MMP-2	all margins	0.2609	0.1405 to 0.3344	>52.5	100.00	75.3 to 100.0	26.09	10.2 to 48.4
MMP-2 TM	all	0.1679	0.1203 to 0.1839	>158.33	23.81	8.2 to 47.2	92.98	83.0 to 98.1
	neg. margin	0.2475	0.1605 to 0.2910	≤90	76.92	46.2 to 95.0	47.83	26.8 to 69.4
	pos. margin	0.3456	0.1471 to 0.4632	>90	87.50	47.3 to 99.7	47.06	29.8 to 64.9
MMP-9	all margins	0.1827	0.1314 to 0.189	≤115	30.77	9.1 to 61.4	87.50	67.6 to 97.3
MMP-9 TM	all	0.2553	0.1242 to 0.3941	>141.67	65.22	42.7 to 83.6	60.32	47.2 to 72.4
	neg. margin	0.1731	0.1314 to 0.1795	>195	7.69	0.2 to 36.0	75.00	53.3 to 90.2
	pos. margin	0.3974	0.1729 to 0.5718	>175	50.00	18.7 to 81.3	89.74	75.8 to 97.1

CI: confidence interval; TM: tumor mass.

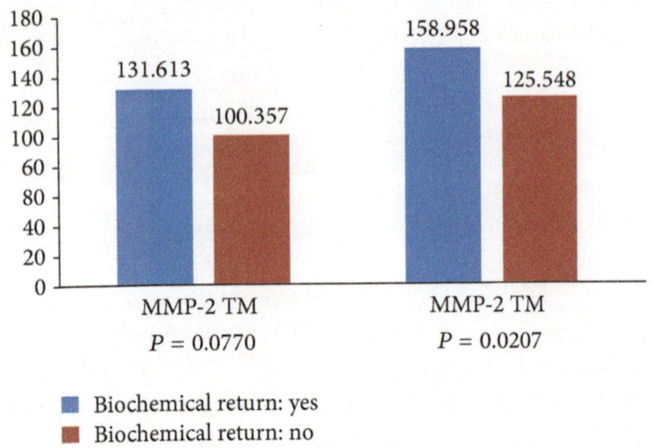

FIGURE 2: Biochemical recurrence with respect to molecular biomarkers in patients with tumors with negative surgical margins.

expression, which was high in tumors larger than 1 cm (P = 0.038; Table 3).

We analyzed the biochemical recurrence of the disease in relation to MMP expression in the group of patients with negative surgical margins that did not receive any therapy after prostatectomy that could have affected the outcome. MMP-9 expression was significantly elevated in tumors from patients who experienced biochemical recurrence (P = 0.0207). MMP-2 expression in tumors tended to be increased in patients with biochemical recurrence (P = 0.0770; Figure 2).

We used a receiver operating characteristic (ROC) analysis, which is widely recognized as a measure of a diagnostic test's discriminatory power. The maximum value for the area under the curve (AUC) is 1.0, indicating a (theoretically) perfect test (100% sensitive and 100% specific). An AUC value of 0.5 indicates no discriminative value. We evaluated MMP-2 and MMP-9 expression as predictors of recurrence in patients with tumors with negative surgical margins. MMP-9 expression was detected in all patients (Table 4). Furthermore, cut-off values for these parameters and groups were determined based on the Youden index (Table 5).

Analysis of the proportions of patients with and without recurrence in terms of increased MMP-9 expression revealed significant differences between the two groups at a significance level of 0.1 (P = 0.0635).

In the group of patients with negative margins, increased MMP-9 expression above the cut-off value of 175 was significantly associated with recurrence (P = 0.0065), while MMP-2 expression was not (Table 6).

Univariate and multivariate analysis showed that MMP-9 expression is a good predictor of biochemical recurrence (Table 7).

Recurrence-free survival was not significantly shorter in the group of patients with tumors with negative margins and high MMP-9 expression (Kaplan-Meier analysis, P = 0.5555).

4. Discussion

Prostate diseases are often present in the older population. Benign enlargement or inflammation of the prostate affect quality of life, while prostate cancer can be life threatening. Unfortunately, the routine diagnostic triad of a combination

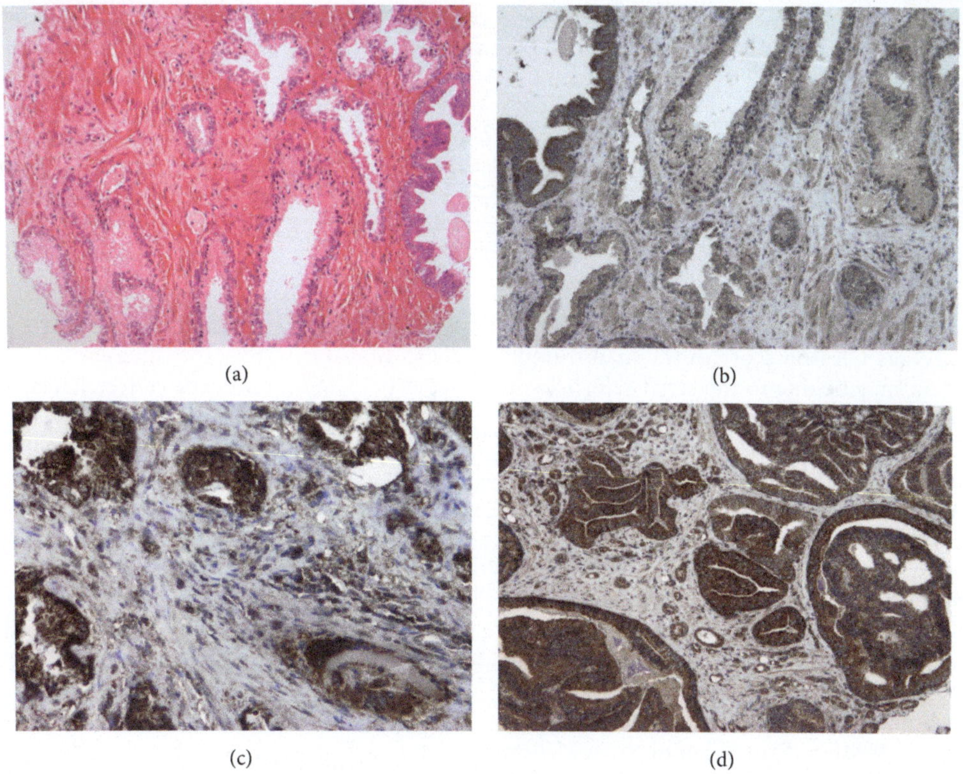

FIGURE 3: (a) Glands lined with hyperplastic epithelium and PIN (hematoxylin and eosin staining, 100x). (b) MMP-2 and MMP-9 immunohistochemistry indicates weak or negative expression in hyperplastic epithelium, except for the PIN, where the expression is strong (100x). (c) MMP-9 immunoexpression in moderately differentiated prostate cancer. Note the intense staining in the cytoplasm of tumor cells and the strongly positive reaction in the cytoplasm of stromal cells (200x). (d) MMP-2 immunoexpression in poorly differentiated prostate cancer. Note the strong cytoplasmic staining intensity (200x).

TABLE 6: MMP-2 and MMP-9 expression in terms of cut-off value in tumors with negative margins.

Tumors with negative margins		Recurrence		
		N	Yes	No
MMP-9, tumor margin	0 (≤175)	35 (90%)	5 (10%)	39
	1 (>175)	4 (44%)	5 (56%)	9
P		0.0065		
MMP-2, tumor margin	0 (≤90)	16 (94%)	1 (6%)	17
	1 (>90)	18 (72%)	7 (28%)	25
P		0.1674		

of an abnormal PSA level, digital rectal examination, and transrectal sonography-guided biopsy of the prostate does not always result in detection of the tumor (sensitivity 75%, specificity 68%). If one or more tests are abnormal, prostate biopsy must be performed to confirm or exclude malignant disease. For now, the best information about limitations, disease stage, and the malignant potential of the prostate cancer are obtained by histopathological examination.

Pathological classification of prostate cancer after radical prostatectomy provides important prognostic information, and an accurate histopathological report is thought to be fundamental for treating and monitoring patients. Preoperative serum PSA levels, pathological grade according to Gleason score, invasion into the seminal vesicle, positive surgical margins with and without extraprostatic extension, and capsular incision are significant predictors of clinical and biochemical recurrence. The real prognostic significance of positive margins and capsule incision remains to be defined [23, 24].

Approximately 5–43% of patients with radical prostatectomy have positive surgical margins, and only 25–47% of them develop biochemical recurrence [25]. These observations suggest the utility of further subclassification of positive margins in order to identify patients with higher risks of recurrence. In our study, the overall rate of positive surgical margins was 29.8% in pT3 tumors and up to 90% in other tumors, which is similar to other studies [26–28].

The time to recurrence, regardless of treatment, was significantly shorter in patients with locally confined tumors with positive surgical margins. This observation is consistent with the results of Bostwick et al., who reported a positive impact of positive prostatectomy margins on biochemical recurrence of the disease [29]. Few studies have emphasized the potential utilities of biomarker expression on positive surgical margins relative to the main tumor mass. In our study, which used tissue microarrays, the average Gleason score was significantly higher in the group of patients with tumors with positive margins, partially confirming the results of Cao et al. [30]. There was no significant difference between

TABLE 7: Analysis of the significance of MMP-9 expression for predicting biochemical recurrence.

	Univariate analysis			Multivariate analysis		
	OR	95% CI	*P*	OR	95% CI	*P*
MMP-2, TM	6.2222	0.6888 to 56.2057	0.1035	5.1721	0.4924 to 54.3318	0.1708
MMP-9, TM	8.7500	1.7411 to 43.9746	0.0078	10.2909	1.6284 to 65.0367	0.0132
					$P = 0.0052$	

OR: odds ratio; CI: confidence interval; and TM: tumor mass.

the average Gleason score on the margins of the tumor resection and the average Gleason score in the main tumor mass; this observation may be due to the strict selection of patients for prostatectomy, which usually requires Gleason scores ≤7.

The human family of MMPs consists of at least 24 proteinases involved in degradation of the extracellular matrix and components of the basement membrane. The MMPs are directly involved in the essential cellular processes of proliferation, differentiation, angiogenesis, and apoptosis through their ability to catalyze the hydrolysis of various substrates, including the precursors of cytokines, growth factors, and hormone receptors. A number of studies revealed positive correlations between tumor invasion and the activities of the gelatinases MMP-2 and MMP-9. Expression of these MMPs is most frequently associated with tumor aggressiveness and overall survival, and they are used as markers of malignant phenotypes [31–33].

In prostate cancer, MMP-2 and MMP-9 expression indicate the tumor's invasive and metastatic potential [34]. Given the development of specific MMP inhibitors, we assumed that the immunohistochemical determination of the expression of these two MMPs would be of particular importance for therapy, especially if it indicated whether the tumor was at high risk of recurrence. In our study, we sought to determine whether MMP-2 and/or MMP-9 expression differed between aggressive cancers on the positive margin of the resection that progress and cancers that remain localized. We detected a significant difference in MMP-2 expression on the positive margin versus that in the main tumor mass ($P = 0.0301$). MMP-9 expression at the margin of the resection did not significantly differ from the expression in the main tumor mass, but, in the group of tumors with positive margins, MMP-9 was significantly more strongly expressed overall versus the group of tumors with negative resection margins ($P = 0.0121$).

In the group of tumors with negative surgical margins, MMP-9 expression was significantly higher in samples from patients with biochemical recurrence of the disease. Therefore, this study yielded additional insight into the potential value of the biomarkers investigated here, particularly, the utility of MMP-2 and MMP-9 expression for predicting the invasive behavior of the tumor and justification for therapy. This utility has been highlighted by numerous works that have explored the expression of MMP-2 and MMP-9 in serum, urine, and tissues from prostate cancers. Sauer and colleagues linked higher expression of MMP-2 and MMP-9 in serum and tissues with higher Gleason scores [34]. In our study, MMP-2 and MMP-9 were expressed in tumors with poor differentiation and higher Gleason scores, but there were no significant differences between low Gleason score (<7) and high-grade cancer (Gleason score >7). These enzymes also displayed significantly higher values in the serum of metastatic carcinoma. In patients with pT3 tumors, increased expression of MMP-2 and MMP-9 was associated with shorter disease-free survival periods; the expression levels of these markers exhibited statistical significance in predicting recurrence. Significant decreases in the levels of these two markers in the sera of patients with metastatic disease after therapy are useful as independent predictors of disease stage in combination with the expression of adhesion molecules [35].

5. Conclusion

The results of this study underscore the potential value of the expression levels of MMP-2 and MMP-9 for predicting the invasive behavior of tumors with positive surgical margins; further investigation of this observation and its utility is warranted. In our patients with tumors with negative surgical margins, increased MMP-9 expression above the cut-off value was a good predictor of biochemical recurrence, whereas MMP-2 expression was associated with an increased risk of relapse.

Conflict of Interests

The authors declare that they have no competing interests.

Acknowledgments

The authors thank their technicians Ozren Štanfel and Ankica Brajenić for technical assistance and Professor of Mathematics Ivan Dražić for statistical analysis. This work was supported by the Ministry of Science, Education, and Sports of the Republic of Croatia, Grant no. 062-0620095-0077.

References

[1] S. Valastyan and R. A. Weinberg, "Tumor metastasis: molecular insights and evolving paradigms," *Cell*, vol. 147, no. 2, pp. 275–292, 2011.

[2] J. Westermarck and V. Kähäri, "Regulation of matrix metalloproteinase expression in tumor invasion," *FASEB Journal*, vol. 13, no. 8, pp. 781–792, 1999.

[3] A. H. Said, J. P. Raufman, and G. Xie, "The role of matrix metalloproteinases in colorectal cancer," *Cancers*, vol. 6, no. 1, pp. 366–375, 2014.

[4] A. Talvensaari-Mattila, P. Pääkkö, M. Höyhtyä, G. Blanco-Sequeiros, and T. Turpeenniemi-Hujanen, "Matrix metalloproteinase-2 immunoreactive protein: a marker of aggressiveness in breast carcinoma," *Cancer*, vol. 83, no. 6, pp. 1153–1162, 1998.

[5] A. Talvensaari-Mattila, P. Pääkkö, and T. Turpeenniemi-Hujanen, "MMP-2 positivity and age less than 40 years increases the risk for recurrence in premenopausal patients with node-positive breast carcinoma," *Breast Cancer Research and Treatment*, vol. 58, no. 3, pp. 287–293, 1999.

[6] A. Talvensaari-Mattila, P. Pääkkö, G. Blanco-Sequeiros, and T. Turpeenniemi-Hujanen, "Matrix metalloproteinase-2 (MMP-2) is associated with the risk for a relapse in postmenopausal patients with node-positive breast carcinoma treated with antiestrogen adjuvant therapy," *Breast Cancer Research and Treatment*, vol. 65, no. 1, pp. 55–61, 2001.

[7] A. Talvensaari-Mattila, P. Pääkkö, and T. Turpeenniemi-Hujanen, "Matrix metalloproteinase-2 (MMP-2) is associated with survival in breast carcinoma," *British Journal of Cancer*, vol. 89, no. 7, pp. 1270–1275, 2003.

[8] A. Sivula, A. Talvensaari-Mattila, J. Lundin et al., "Association of cyclooxygenase-2 and matrix metalloproteinase-2 expression in human breast cancer," *Breast Cancer Research and Treatment*, vol. 89, no. 3, pp. 215–220, 2005.

[9] A. Väisänen, M. Kallioinen, P. J. Taskinen, and T. Turpeenniemi-Hujanen, "Prognostic value of MMP-2 immunoreactive protein (72 kD type IV collagenase) in primary skin melanoma," *The Journal of Pathology*, vol. 186, no. 1, pp. 51–58, 1998.

[10] A. Väisänen, M. Kallioinen, K. von Dickhoff, L. Laatikainen, M. Höyhtyä, and T. Turpeenniemi-Hujanen, "Matrix metalloproteinase-2 (MMP-2) immunoreactive protein—a new prognostic marker in uveal melanoma?" *The Journal of Pathology*, vol. 188, no. 1, pp. 56–62, 1999.

[11] W. F. Grigioni, A. D'Errico, C. Fortunato et al., "Prognosis of gastric carcinoma revealed by interactions between tumor cells and basement membrane," *Modern Pathology*, vol. 7, no. 2, pp. 220–225, 1994.

[12] P. Ring, K. Johansson, M. Höyhtyä, K. Rubin, and G. Lindmark, "Expression of tissue inhibitor of metalloproteinases TIMP-2 in human colorectal cancer—a predictor of tumour stage," *British Journal of Cancer*, vol. 76, no. 6, pp. 805–811, 1997.

[13] A. Juuti, J. Lundin, S. Nordling, J. Louhimo, and C. Haglund, "Epithelial MMP-2 expression correlates with worse prognosis in pancreatic cancer," *Oncology*, vol. 71, no. 1-2, pp. 61–68, 2007.

[14] D. Trudel, Y. Fradet, F. Meyer, F. Harel, and B. Têtu, "Significance of MMP-2 expression in prostate cancer: an immunohistochemical study," *Cancer Research*, vol. 63, no. 23, pp. 8511–8515, 2003.

[15] P. Kuvaja, A. Talvensaari-Mattila, P. Pääkkö, and T. Turpeenniemi-Hujanen, "Low serum level of pro-matrix metalloproteinase 2 correlates with aggressive behavior in breast carcinoma," *Human Pathology*, vol. 37, no. 10, pp. 1316–1323, 2006.

[16] O. Kuittinen, Y. Soini, and T. Turpeenniemi-Hujanen, "Diverse role of MMP-2 and MMP-9 in the clinicopathological behavior of Hodgkin's lymphoma," *European Journal of Haematology*, vol. 69, no. 4, pp. 205–212, 2002.

[17] A. Scorilas, A. Karameris, N. Arnogiannaki et al., "Overexpression of matrix-metalloproteinase-9 in human breast cancer: a potential favourable indicator in node-negative patients," *British Journal of Cancer*, vol. 84, no. 11, pp. 1488–1496, 2001.

[18] S. M. Ranuncolo, E. Armanasco, C. Cresta, E. B. De Kier Joffe, and L. Puricelli, "Plasma MMP-9 (92 kDa-MMP) activity is useful in the follow-up and in the assessment of prognosis in breast cancer patients," *International Journal of Cancer*, vol. 106, no. 5, pp. 745–751, 2003.

[19] A. Talvensaari-Mattila, M. Santala, Y. Soini, and T. Turpeenniemi-Hujanen, "Prognostic value of matrix metalloproteinase-2 (MMP-2) expression in endometrial endometrioid adenocarcinoma," *Anticancer Research B*, vol. 25, no. 6, pp. 4101–4105, 2005.

[20] K. W. Kwak, H. M. Lee, and H. Y. Choi, "Impact of capsular incision on biochemical recurrence after radical perineal prostatectomy," *Prostate Cancer and Prostatic Diseases*, vol. 13, no. 1, pp. 28–33, 2010.

[21] D. Cao, A. S. Kibel, F. Gao, Y. Tao, and P. A. Humphrey, "The gleason score of tumor at the margin in radical prostatectomy is predictive of biochemical recurrence," *American Journal of Surgical Pathology*, vol. 34, no. 7, pp. 994–1001, 2010.

[22] A. Heidenreich, J. Bellmunt, M. Bolla et al., "Guidelines on prostate cancer," *European Urology*, vol. 59, no. 1, pp. 572–583, 2011.

[23] K. W. Kwak, H. M. Lee, and H. Y. Choi, "Impact of capsular incision on biochemical recurrence after radical perineal prostatectomy," *Prostate Cancer and Prostatic Diseases*, vol. 13, no. 1, pp. 28–33, 2010.

[24] W. E. Grizzle, D. G. Bostwick, H. Burke et al., "Biomarkers in prostate cancer," in *AACR Education Book*, pp. 196–204, Intenational Union Against Cancer, Washington, DC, USA, 2005.

[25] D. M. Somford, I. M. van Oort, J. Cosyns, J. A. Witjes, L. A. L. M. Kiemeney, and B. Tombal, "Prognostic relevance of number and bilaterality of positive surgical margins after radical prostatectomy," *World Journal of Urology*, vol. 30, no. 1, pp. 105–110, 2012.

[26] R. Thurairaja, J. Osborn, J. Mcfarlane, A. Bahl, and R. Persad, "Radical prostatectomy with positive surgical margins: how are patients managed?" *BJU International*, vol. 97, no. 3, pp. 445–450, 2006.

[27] S. S. Chang and M. S. Cookson, "Impact of positive surgical margins after radical prostatectomy," *Urology*, vol. 68, no. 2, pp. 249–252, 2006.

[28] Y. Yang, "Treatment of the positive surgical margin following radical prostatectomy," *Chinese Medical Journal*, vol. 121, no. 4, pp. 375–379, 2008.

[29] D. G. Bostwick, D. J. Grignon, M. E. H. Hammond et al., "Prognostic factors in prostate cancer: college of American pathologists consensus statement 1999," *Archives of Pathology and Laboratory Medicine*, vol. 124, no. 7, pp. 995–1000, 2000.

[30] D. Cao, A. S. Kibel, F. Gao, Y. Tao, and P. A. Humphrey, "The gleason score of tumor at the margin in radical prostatectomy is predictive of biochemical recurrence," *American Journal of Surgical Pathology*, vol. 34, no. 7, pp. 994–1001, 2010.

[31] E. Llano, A. M. Pendas, P. Aza-Blanc, T. B. Kornberg, and C. Lopez-Otin, "*Dm1*-MMP, a matrix metalloproteinase from Drosophila with a potential role in extracellular matrix remodeling during neural development," *Journal of Biological Chemistry*, vol. 275, no. 46, pp. 35978–35985, 2000.

[32] G. Klein, E. Vellenga, M. W. Fraaije, W. A. Kamps, and E. S. J. M. De Bont, "The possible role of matrix metalloproteinase (MMP)-2 and MMP-9 in cancer, e.g. acute leukemia," *Critical Reviews in Oncology/Hematology*, vol. 50, no. 2, pp. 87–100, 2004.

[33] A. Di Carlo, A. Mariano, D. Terracciano et al., "Matrix metalloproteinase-2 and -9 in the urine of prostate cancer patients," *Oncology Reports*, vol. 24, no. 1, pp. 3–8, 2010.

[34] C. G. Sauer, A. Kappeler, M. Späth et al., "Expression and activity of matrix metalloproteinases-2 and -9 in serum, core needle biopsies and tissue specimens of prostate cancer patients," *Virchows Archiv*, vol. 444, no. 6, pp. 518–526, 2004.

[35] R. Roy, J. Yang, and M. A. Moses, "Matrix metalloproteinases as novel biomarkers and potential therapeutic targets in human cancer," *Journal of Clinical Oncology*, vol. 27, no. 31, pp. 5287–5297, 2009.

15

A Histomorphological Pattern Analysis of Pulmonary Tuberculosis in Lung Autopsy and Surgically Resected Specimens

Mamta Gupta,[1] Flora D. Lobo,[2] Deepa Sowkur Anandarama Adiga,[2] and Abhishek Gupta[3]

[1]*Department of Pathology, Subharti Medical College, Swami Vivekananda Subharti University, Meerut, Uttar Pradesh 250002, India*
[2]*Department of Pathology, Kasturba Medical College, Mangalore, Manipal University, Karnataka 575001, India*
[3]*Department of Medicine, Subharti Medical College, Swami Vivekananda Subharti University, Meerut, Uttar Pradesh 250002, India*

Correspondence should be addressed to Mamta Gupta; drmamta04@gmail.com

Academic Editor: Piero Tosi

Background. Tuberculosis (TB) is a major cause of morbidity and mortality globally. Many cases are diagnosed on autopsy and a subset of patients may require surgical intervention either due to the complication or sequelae of TB. *Materials and Methods.* 40 cases of resected lung specimens following surgery or autopsy in which a diagnosis of pulmonary tuberculosis was made were included. Histopathological pattern analysis of pulmonary tuberculosis along with associated nonneoplastic changes and identification of *Mycobacterium tuberculosis* bacilli was done. *Results.* The mean age of diagnosis was 41 years with male predominance (92.5%). Tuberculosis was suspected in only 12.1% of cases before death. Seven cases were operated upon due to associated complications or suspicion of malignancy. Tubercular consolidation was the most frequent pattern followed by miliary tuberculosis. The presence of necrotizing granulomas was seen in 33 cases (82.5%). Acid fast bacilli were seen in 57.5% cases on Ziehl-Neelsen stain. *Conclusion.* Histopathology remains one of the most important methods for diagnosing tuberculosis, especially in TB prevalent areas. It should be considered in the differential diagnosis of all respiratory diseases because of its varied clinical presentations and manifestations.

1. Introduction

Tuberculosis (TB) continues to remain one of the most pressing health problems in India. India is the highest TB burden country in the world, accounting for one-fifth of the global incidence with an estimated 1.96 million cases annually [1].

Tuberculosis is endemic in many parts of the world and causes many deaths. The most common form is pulmonary tuberculosis, characterized pathologically by necrotizing granulomas, associated pneumonia, and a great propensity for fibrosis and dystrophic calcification [2].

Due to the stigma associated with this disease, in many cases of active TB, either there is a delay in diagnosis and treatment leading to unrestricted exposure of bacilli to environment or the patient fails to take adequate treatment causing multidrug resistance. A subset of patients may require surgical intervention due to the associated complications. The prevalence of tuberculosis is high in the Indian subcontinent, and cases may not be diagnosed until after an autopsy is performed [3–6].

Various complications of pulmonary tuberculosis significantly contributing to morbidity and mortality of patients include hemoptysis, posttubercular bronchiectasis, aspergilloma, tubercular endobronchitis and tracheitis, spontaneous pneumothorax, scar carcinoma, disseminated calcification in lung, pulmonary function changes, obstructive airway disease, and secondary pyogenic infections. Systemic manifestations in the form of secondary amyloidosis and chronic corpulmonale may also occur [7].

The hallmark of *Mycobacterium tuberculosis* infected tissue is necrotizing granulomatous inflammation, composed of epithelioid histiocytes surrounding a central necrotic zone, and can be accompanied by a variable number of multinucleated giant cells and lymphocytes. Nonnecrotizing granulomas can be present as well. The major function of epithelioid histiocytes is to contain the infection to a localized area, thus avoiding bacterial spread to surrounding healthy tissues and to other organs, and to concentrate the immune response to a limited infectious area [8].

TB is a major cause of morbidity and mortality globally. Many cases may go undetected and are diagnosed only after an autopsy is performed. Another subset of cases present with various complications or sequelae of the disease process. The present study was undertaken to evaluate the histopathological spectrum of pulmonary tuberculosis in surgically resected and autopsy lung specimens.

2. Materials and Methods

A descriptive retrospective and prospective histomorphological study of pulmonary tuberculosis was undertaken in the Department of Pathology, Kasturba Medical College, Mangalore, India, over a period of 4 years from 2008 to 2011. The specimens comprised of 33 autopsy cases in which sections from both lungs were submitted and 7 surgically resected cases including 4 lobectomy, 2 pneumonectomy, and 1 lung tissue for frozen section. Lung biopsies were excluded. Information regarding each patient was obtained from medical records or autopsy files. The specimens were received in 10% formalin. Gross examination was performed and representative sections were submitted. Slides were stained with Haematoxylin and Eosin (H&E) along with Ziehl-Neelsen (ZN) stain for identification of tuberculous bacilli.

The criteria for acceptance of a case as tuberculosis included the following:

(i) Demonstration of acid fast bacilli on ZN stain.

(ii) Presence of necrotizing granulomatous inflammation.

(iii) In absence of caseous necrosis or failure to demonstrate acid fast bacilli, past history of tuberculosis with response to treatment with antituberculous therapy.

(iv) Exclusion of other causes of granulomatous inflammation.

Fungal infections and other noninfectious causes of granulomatous diseases were excluded by careful microscopic examination and application of special stains wherever required.

The histomorphological pattern noted the distribution of the lesions and the morphologic features of the tissue reaction. Other nonneoplastic findings in adjacent lung parenchyma were noted as well.

3. Results

The material for the study comprised 40 cases diagnosed as pulmonary tuberculosis on autopsy and resected lung specimens. Their age ranged from 20 to 75 years with a mean age of 41 years; the majority of the cases were in the 3rd decade (40%). There was a male predominance (92.5%).

The total number of autopsies performed during this period was 3034. Thus, frequency of tuberculosis in local autopsy service was 1.08%.

Prior to autopsy, a clinical diagnosis of pulmonary tuberculosis was known in only 4 of 33 (12.1%) cases. The majority of cases had presented with sudden death (19; 57.6%); 10 cases brought dead to mortuary were destitute; in these cases it was presumed that the death was sudden since they did not seek medical advice for their illness leading to death. These were subsequently diagnosed on histopathology as disseminated tuberculosis (4 cases), fibrocavitary tuberculosis (2 cases), and fibrocaseous tuberculosis (4 cases). Associated pneumonic changes were observed in 4 cases. The remaining 9 admitted patients with sudden death had disseminated TB (6 cases), fibrocaseous tuberculosis (2 cases), and tubercular bronchopneumonia (1 case). These cases had rapid deterioration of symptoms upon admission. Additional finding of left ventricular subendocardial ischemia with block of left coronary artery in a case of disseminated tuberculosis and healed myocardial infarction was observed in a case of fibrocaseous tuberculosis. Death in other cases was attributed to acute respiratory distress syndrome (ARDS) (4; 12.1%), lung abscess (2; 6.0%), and one case each with poisoning, drowning, complicated malaria, and a known diabetic with alcoholic cirrhosis. One patient with ARDS was coinfected with HIV.

Seven cases were operated upon; 2 cases were operated upon due to suspicion of malignancy. The remaining 5 cases were known cases of pulmonary tuberculosis with history of antitubercular treatment (ATT) and associated complications, namely, hemoptysis, empyema, bronchiectasis, and aspergilloma. Resistance to ATT was noted in one case which revealed positive acid fast bacilli in spite of regular treatment and presented with empyema.

On gross examination, pleural thickening was observed in 30 cases. The cut surface revealed caseation, consolidation, and miliary nodules in 10 cases each, cavity in 5 cases, and dilated bronchi, purulent exudates, and calcification in two cases each. Additionally, congestion and hemorrhage were observed in 8 cases and frothing was observed in 2 cases.

The histological evaluation of lung sections (Figure 1) revealed necrotizing granulomas in 32 cases (80%), nonnecrotizing granulomas in 2 cases (5%), caseous necrosis with few Langhans giant cells in 2 cases (5%), and only caseous necrosis in 4 cases (10%).

ZN stain for acid fast bacilli (AFB) was positive in 57.5% of cases including 21 of 33 (63.6%) autopsy cases and 2/7 (28.5%) surgically resected specimens. All these cases showed presence of caseous necrosis on H&E stain.

Treatment history was not available in 12 cases that were brought dead to mortuary; 8 cases including 6 destitute and one case each of poisoning and drowning showed AFB positivity. The remaining were hospital based autopsies, with deaths due to ARDS in 4 cases (all were positive for AFB), lung abscess in 2 cases (AFB positivity in both cases), and unexplained sudden death in 9 cases (AFB positivity in 5 cases). Four were diagnosed cases of pulmonary tuberculosis with history of ATT treatment (one of these patients was positive for AFB). One case was admitted with complicated

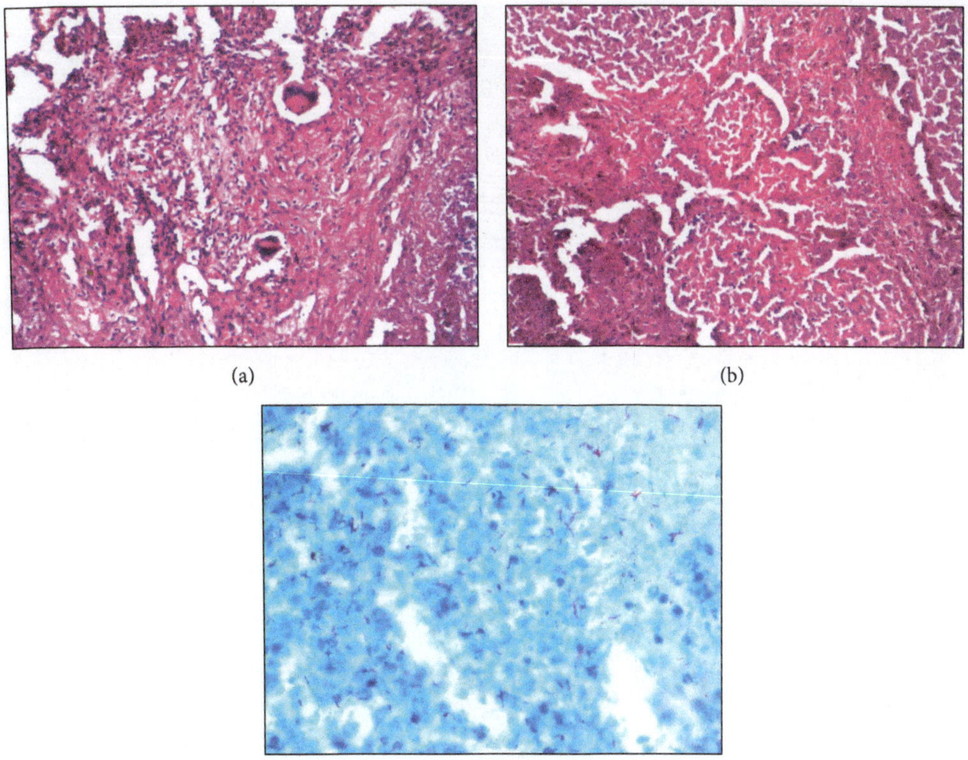

(a) (b) (c)

FIGURE 1: Microscopy examination. (a) Epithelioid granuloma with multinucleated giant cells (H&E, ×400). (b) Necrotic acute inflammatory exudate in alveolar spaces (H&E, ×400). (c) Numerous acid fast bacilli (ZN stain, ×1000).

malaria (AFB negative) and one case was diabetes mellitus with alcoholic cirrhosis (positive for AFB). Among the 7 cases which were operated upon, acid fast bacilli was observed in two cases, including a case with clinical suspicion of malignancy revealing necrotizing granulomatous inflammation with consolidation and another case of empyema associated with fibrocaseous tuberculosis.

16 cases (37.5%) of pulmonary tuberculosis were also associated with other nonneoplastic findings in adjacent lung parenchyma or pleura, with acute bronchopneumonia constituting the most common finding followed by empyema, bronchiectasis, and aspergilloma (Table 1). In 10 cases dissemination to other organs was observed including liver in 9 cases, spleen in 8 cases, and kidney and brain in one case each. Hilar lymph nodes were involved in three cases.

Histopathological pattern analysis revealed primary caseating tuberculosis with involvement of hilar lymph nodes in 3 cases. Postprimary tuberculosis was seen in form of fibrocavitary, fibrocaseating, and tubercular bronchiectasis in 14 cases. Tubercular consolidation, miliary tuberculosis, and empyema were reported in 23 cases; these findings can be a manifestation of both of the above patterns. Tubercular bronchopneumonia was seen associated with fibrocavitary, fibrocaseous, or disseminated tuberculosis reflecting the fact that these finding were associated with postprimary tuberculosis. Miliary tuberculosis was observed especially in patients presenting with dissemination to other organs (Table 2) (Figure 2).

TABLE 1: Various pulmonary diseases associated with tuberculosis.

TB with other diseases	Cases	Percentage
Acute bronchopneumonia	11	68.7
Empyema	02	12.5
Bronchiectasis	02	12.5
Aspergilloma	01	06.3
Total	16	100

TABLE 2: Histopathological pattern of tubercular lesions in lungs.

Final diagnosis	Cases	Percentage
Tubercular consolidation	11	27.5
Miliary tuberculosis	10	25.0
Fibrocaseous tuberculosis	07	17.5
Fibrocavitary tuberculosis	05	12.5
Caseating tuberculosis	03	7.5
Tubercular empyema	02	5.0
Tubercular bronchiectasis	02	5.0
Total	40	100

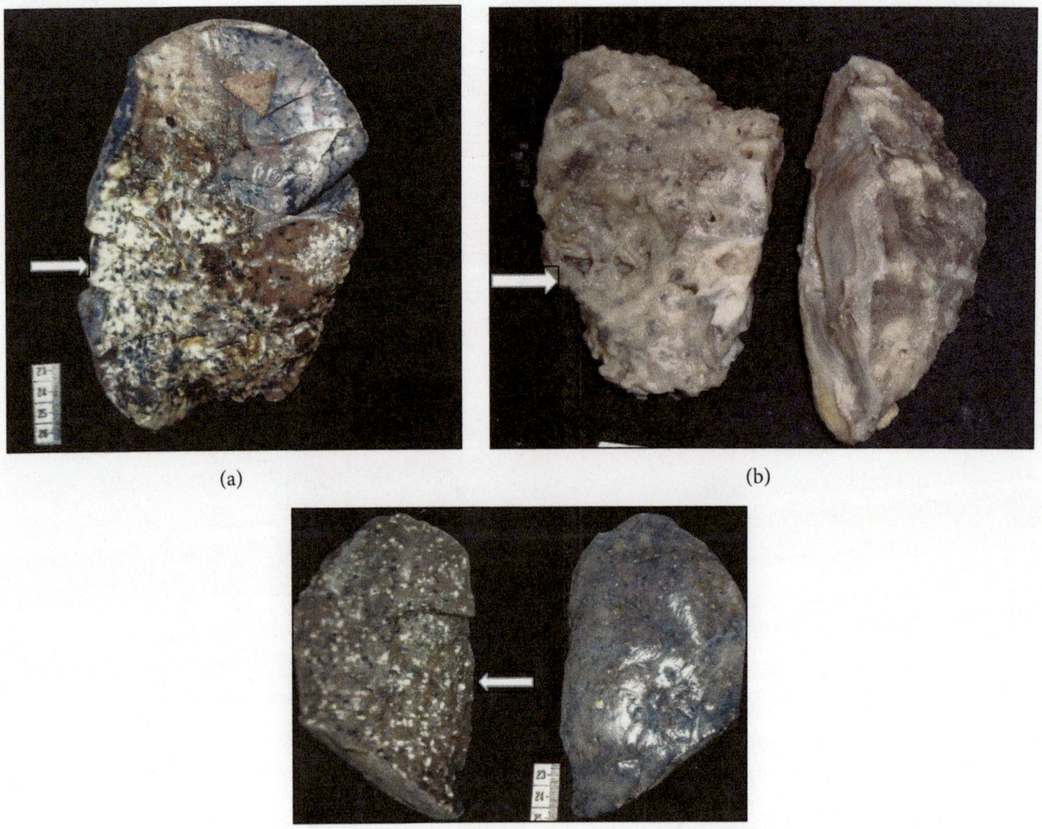

(a) (b)

(c)

Figure 2: Histomorphological patterns on gross examination of lung (a), fibrocaseous tuberculosis (b), fibrocavitary tuberculosis with bronchiectasis, and (c) multiple millet sized tubercles in miliary tuberculosis.

4. Discussion

TB is an infectious disease caused by the bacillus *Mycobacterium tuberculosis*. It typically affects the lungs (pulmonary TB) but can affect other sites as well (extrapulmonary TB). It is more common among men and affects mostly adults in economically productive age groups. The latest estimates included in global tuberculosis report in 2013 were 8.6 million new TB cases in 2012 and 1.3 million deaths due to tuberculosis. The number is unacceptably large especially that deaths can be prevented with access to health care and proper treatment [9]. The present study highlights the magnitude of undetected pulmonary tuberculosis diagnosed at autopsy and of patients presenting with complications/sequelae of the disease.

Aziz et al. [10] in a study on 46 cases of tuberculosis of lung observed a bimodal distribution with a younger age group of less than 30 years and an older age group of more than 50 years. In our study most of the patients were young, in the third decade of life with male predominance.

In India, the Revised National Tuberculosis Programme detects nearly three times more male than female TB patients [11]. In a study conducted in similar region Ganapathy et al. [12] observed a male predilection. The reasons for this are unclear. It could be due to epidemiological differences, exposure to risk of infection, and progression from infection to disease. Due to various stigmata and sociocultural factors associated with this disease, women in developing countries confront more barriers than men in accessing health care services.

Combination drug therapy is the first-line of treatment for pulmonary tuberculosis. Surgery for tuberculosis has been of major concern because of its associated morbidity and mortality [4]. The common complications leading to surgery fall into three main categories: persistent or drug-resistant disease, bronchiectasis, and hemoptysis [13]. Similar findings were observed in the present study.

Tuberculous empyema represents a chronic, active infection of the pleural space that contains a large number of tubercle bacilli. Treatment consists of pleural space drainage and antituberculous chemotherapy. Problematic treatment issues include the inability to reexpand the trapped lung and difficulty in achieving therapeutic drug levels in pleural fluid, which lead to drug resistance. Surgery too is often challenging [14]. Bhattacharya et al. [15] observed tuberculosis to be the cause of bilateral empyema in 58.8% cases.

Bronchiectasis is one of the commonest abnormalities seen in pulmonary tuberculosis. It is rarely gross and is found in the presence of secondary advanced parenchymatous disease [16]. The exact incidence of bronchiectasis as sequela to tuberculosis is difficult to determine as studies are done on selected groups and varies in developed and developing countries [17]. In an Indian study, Sahoo et al. [18] observed 62% cases with posttubercular bronchiectasis.

Fibrocavitary tuberculosis with aspergillosis in right upper lobe was diagnosed in a case. Aspergilloma represents the most common infectious complication of pulmonary tuberculous cavities. A combination of antitubercular drug treatment with surgical resection is the treatment of choice [19].

Two cases were operated upon with suspicion of malignancy. Frozen section was done in one case; while in the other case lobectomy was performed. Both showed necrotizing granulomas with associated pneumonic consolidation. Pulmonary tuberculosis can present with a variety of radiological findings. Tuberculoma and focal organizing pneumonia can mimic neoplasm because of similar radiological findings on plain chest radiographs and CT scans. Also, diffuse form of bronchoalveolar carcinoma can appear radiologically as air space consolidation resembling pneumonia, multiple nodules mimicking disseminated tuberculosis, fungal infection, metastasis or as ill-defined masses, cavitating nodules, or pleural effusions [20–22]. In such cases final diagnosis is made on histopathology.

Clinically undiagnosed TB constitutes a substantial proportion of active TB cases diagnosed at autopsy. In the present study 87.8% of cases were diagnosed on autopsy. These undetected cases at autopsy range from 44% to 70% in various studies [6, 23–25].

In the present study 57.6% had presented with sudden death. Rastogi et al. [5] observed tuberculosis as the most important cause of sudden unexpected death involving respiratory system in 61.64% and it contributed to 16.42% of total sudden deaths. This increase in the frequency of sudden death due to TB despite better facilities is a cause of concern.

Reddy et al. [26] in a study on patterns of tuberculosis in autopsy cases observed that the commonest type of lesion in the lung was fibrocaseous variety (66.56%). Miliary lesions were seen in 22.7% whereas the pneumonic type was seen in 10.74%. In the present study most of the cases were of tuberculous consolidation (27.5%) followed by miliary tuberculosis and fibrocaseous TB (25% and 17.5%, resp.).

Rarely pulmonary tuberculosis may present as an acute pneumonia with respiratory failure. TB misdiagnosed as community acquired pneumonia (CAP) accounts for approximately 35% of microbiologically confirmed pneumonias. Tuberculous consolidation was present in 27.5% of cases in the present study. The incidence of acute respiratory failure is 1.5% among patients hospitalized with pulmonary TB. In the present study 12.1% of deaths were due to ARDS. This acute presentation may result from primary infection, progressive primary disease, reactivation of latent TB, or atelectasis [27].

Miliary TB is a potentially fatal form of TB that results from massive lymphohematogenous dissemination. Diagnosis can perplex even the experienced because of nonspecific symptoms and chest radiographs do not always reveal classical miliary changes. Atypical presentations like cryptic miliary TB and ARDS further lead to delay in diagnosis. It is characterized by high mortality rate, despite the availability of effective treatment [28].

The usual histologic reaction in TB is a granulomatous inflammation with varying numbers of accompanying nonnecrotizing granulomas [29]. Necrotizing granulomas were observed in 80% cases in present study. Similar findings were observed by Das et al. [30]. They observed necrotizing granulomas in 44.7%, nonnecrotizing granuloma in 10.5%, and only caseous necrosis in 44.7% cases.

Granulomatous diseases of lung often present a diagnostic challenge. The diagnosis requires familiarity with the tissue reaction as well as with the morphologic features of the organisms, including appropriate interpretation of special stains. Nonneoplastic granulomatous diseases like Wegener's granulomatosis and Churg-Strauss syndrome microscopically show necrotizing granulomas with features of vasculitis. Granulomas of tuberculosis may also involve blood vessels resembling true primary vasculitic disorder posing a diagnostic difficulty. However, in the present study, involvement of blood vessels was not seen. Many infectious granulomatous lesions may also mimic tuberculosis. Fungal infections especially histoplasma show necrosis similar to tuberculosis. Clue to diagnosis is careful interpretation of surrounding tissue reaction and special stains [31].

Acid fast bacilli (AFB) positivity in smears and histological specimens depends on the bacillary load of the specimen and the type of the material [32]. Acid fast bacilli positivity was seen in 57.5% in the present study. Similarly, Park et al. [33] observed microbiologically confirmed pulmonary tuberculosis in 50% of patients. The bacilli are normally scanty in tuberculous tissue and their identification with ZN stain requires careful examination. Tissue containing necrotizing granulomas is more likely to give positive results than specimens showing only nonnecrotizing granulomas, poorly formed granulomas, or acute inflammation. Failure to demonstrate them does not exclude a diagnosis of tuberculosis. Making a definitive diagnosis in the future may incorporate application of immunohistochemistry or molecular techniques such as polymerase chain reaction to paraffin sections [34].

As the present study included mostly autopsy cases it was subject to various limitations. The complete details of underlying risk factors such as coinfection with HIV, steroid therapy, and BCG exposure were not available. Only one case was known to be infected with HIV. Tuberculosis associated with HIV infection is aggressive and is characterized by widespread dissemination. These patients are susceptible to rapidly progressive tuberculosis. Recurrence of tuberculosis may occur after successful treatment due to exogenous reinfection. The risk of developing tuberculosis disease in HIV-infected patients in India is estimated to be 7 cases per 100 person-years at risk [34, 35].

Also, clinical data or test for confirmation of multidrug-resistant (MDR) tuberculosis was not available in these cases. AFB was positive in a patient on ATT who developed empyema for which he was operated upon and in one patient who died during the course of disease for which autopsy was done. These cases may reflect probable resistance, reactivation, or reinfection.

In conclusion, pulmonary tuberculosis is one of the oldest known diseases with rapidly increasing newer diagnostic modalities and treatment strategies. But still the incidence of disease has not decreased. Histopathology remains one of the important methods for diagnosis. Tuberculosis if diagnosed in time is treatable and patient may get cured without any complications. However, if the patient is immunocompromised or elderly or presents in late stages of the disease or unusual presentations leading to delayed diagnosis, they may have a fulminant course with bilateral involvement and respiratory distress. The morbidity and mortality are high in this population of cases. Undiagnosed tuberculosis may be a health hazard to the public and healthcare providers. These cases form a substantial number in autopsy studies, probably representing the tip of the iceberg and indicating seriousness of the problem of tuberculosis.

Protective strategies like risk assessment, early diagnosis, recognition of lesions, use of methods to reduce infection transmission, and effective regular treatment are advocated to curtail the spread of tuberculosis [5, 19].

Competing Interests

The authors declare that they have no competing interests.

References

[1] V. M. Vashishtha, "Current status of tuberculosis and acute respiratory infections in India: much more needs to be done!," *Indian Pediatrics*, vol. 47, no. 1, pp. 88–89, 2010.

[2] J.-G. Im, H. Itoh, K. S. Lee, and M. C. Han, "CT-pathology correlation of pulmonary tuberculosis," *Critical Reviews in Diagnostic Imaging*, vol. 36, no. 3, pp. 227–285, 1995.

[3] T. Anand, D. Arun Kumar, N. Sharma et al., "Perception of stigma towards TB among patients on DOTS & patients attending general opd in Delhi," *Indian Journal of Tuberculosis*, vol. 61, no. 1, pp. 35–42, 2014.

[4] T. Mohsen, A. Abou Zeid, and S. Haj-Yahia, "Lobectomy or pneumonectomy for multidrug-resistant pulmonary tuberculosis can be performed with acceptable morbidity and mortality: a seven-year review of a single institution's experience," *Journal of Thoracic and Cardiovascular Surgery*, vol. 134, no. 1, pp. 194–198, 2007.

[5] P. Rastogi, T. Kanchan, and R. G. Menezes, "Sudden unexpected deaths due to tuberculosis: an autopsy based study," *Journal of Forensic Medicine and Toxicology*, vol. 28, no. 2, pp. 77–81, 2011.

[6] M. Garg, A. D. Aggarwal, S. Singh, and S. P. Kataria, "Tuberculous lesions at autopsy," *Journal of Indian Academy of Forensic Medicine*, vol. 33, no. 2, pp. 116–119, 2011.

[7] D. Behera, "Complications of pulmonary tuberculosis," in *Tuberculosis*, S. K. Sharma and A. Mohan, Eds., pp. 519–531, Jaypee, New Delhi, India, 2nd edition, 2009.

[8] B. M. Saunders and A. M. Cooper, "Restraining mycobacteria: role of granulomas in mycobacterial infections," *Immunology and Cell Biology*, vol. 78, no. 4, pp. 334–341, 2000.

[9] World Health Organization, *Global Tuberculosis Report 2013*, WHO Press Minimum Graphics, 2013.

[10] R. Aziz, A. R. Khan, I. Qayum, M. ul Mannan, M. T. Khan, and N. Khan, "Presentation of pulmonary tuberculosis at Ayub Teaching Hospital Abbottabad," *Journal of Ayub Medical College, Abbottabad*, vol. 14, no. 1, pp. 6–9, 2002.

[11] G. R. Khatri and T. R. Frieden, "The status and prospects of tuberculosis control in India," *International Journal of Tuberculosis and Lung Disease*, vol. 4, no. 3, pp. 193–200, 2000.

[12] S. Ganapathy, B. E. Thomas, M. S. Jawahar, K. J. A. Selvi, Sivasubramaniam, and M. Weiss, "Perceptions of gender and tuberculosis in a south Indian urban community," *The Indian Journal of Tuberculosis*, vol. 55, no. 1, pp. 9–14, 2008.

[13] C. E. Reed, E. F. Parker, and F. A. Crawford Jr., "Surgical resection for complications of pulmonary tuberculosis," *The Annals of Thoracic Surgery*, vol. 48, no. 2, pp. 165–167, 1989.

[14] S. A. Sahn and M. D. Iseman, "Tuberculous empyema," *Seminars in Respiratory Infections*, vol. 14, no. 1, pp. 82–87, 1999.

[15] S. Bhattacharya, K. N. Sinha, Ramakant, and P. C. Dubey, "Bilateral empyema," *Indian Journal of Tuberculosis*, vol. 34, no. 4, pp. 192–193, 1987.

[16] J. Clark and J. Golding, "Tuberculous bronchiectasis," *Postgraduate Medical Journal*, vol. 35, no. 399, pp. 24–25, 1959.

[17] B. Chakrabarti, P. M. A. Calverley, and P. D. O. Davies, "Tuberculosis and its incidence, special nature, and relationship with chronic obstructive pulmonary disease," *International Journal of COPD*, vol. 2, no. 3, pp. 263–272, 2007.

[18] K. Sahoo, B. N. Panda, V. P. Singh, K. G. Kiran, B. Raha, and J. S. Bhalla, "Bronchographic evaluation of radiologic sequelae of pulmonary tuberculosis after short term chemotherapy," *Indian Journal of Tuberculosis*, vol. 35, no. 3, pp. 128–132, 1988.

[19] A. O. Adeyemo, E. O. Odelowo, and D. I. Makanjuola, "Management of pulmonary aspergilloma in the presence of active tuberculosis," *Thorax*, vol. 39, no. 11, pp. 862–867, 1984.

[20] M. L. B. Bhatt, S. Kant, and R. Bhaskar, "Pulmonary tuberculosis as differential diagnosis of lung cancer," *South Asian Journal of Cancer*, vol. 1, no. 1, pp. 36–42, 2012.

[21] S. W. Chen and J. Price, "Focal organizing pneumonia mimicking small peripheral lung adenocarcinoma on CT scans," *Australasian Radiology*, vol. 42, no. 4, pp. 360–363, 1998.

[22] A. Tandon, R. Tandon, S. K. Bhargava, and N. Kishore, "Bronchoalveolar carcinoma-the great masquerader: a case report," *Journal International Medical Sciences Academy*, vol. 23, no. 4, pp. 239–240, 2010.

[23] R. J. Flavin, N. Gibbons, and D. S. O'Briain, "Mycobacterium tuberculosis at autopsy—exposure and protection: an old adversary revisited," *Journal of Clinical Pathology*, vol. 60, no. 5, pp. 487–491, 2007.

[24] P. Chastonay and D. Gardiol, "Severe active tuberculosis at autopsy: retrospective study of an adult autopsy material 1961–1985," *Schweizerische Medizinische Wochenschrift*, vol. 117, no. 24, pp. 925–927, 1987.

[25] A. Andrion, R. Bona, and F. Mollo, "Active tuberculosis unsuspected until autopsy," *Minerva Medica*, vol. 72, no. 2, pp. 73–80, 1981.

[26] D. B. Reddy, G. C. Raju, and G. S. Kumari, "Pattern of tuberculosis—a review based on an autopsy study," *The Indian Journal of Tuberculosis*, vol. 22, no. 3, pp. 115–118, 1975.

[27] L. M. Pinto, A. C. Shah, K. D. Shah, and Z. F. Udwadia, "Pulmonary tuberculosis masquerading as community acquired pneumonia," *Respiratory Medicine CME*, vol. 4, no. 3, pp. 138–140, 2011.

[28] S. Ray, A. Talukdar, S. Kundu, D. Khanra, and N. Sonthalia, "Diagnosis and management of miliary tuberculosis: current state and future perspectives," *Therapeutics and Clinical Risk Management*, vol. 9, no. 1, pp. 9–26, 2013.

[29] O. A. El-Zammar and A.-L. A. Katzenstein, "Pathological diagnosis of granulomatous lung disease: a review," *Histopathology*, vol. 50, no. 3, pp. 289–310, 2007.

[30] D. K. Das, C. S. Pant, J. N. Pant, and P. Sodhani, "Transthoracic (percutaneous) fine needle aspiration cytology diagnosis of pulmonary tuberculosis," *Tubercle and Lung Disease*, vol. 76, no. 1, pp. 84–89, 1995.

[31] S. Mukhopadhyay and A. A. Gal, "Granulomatous lung disease an approach to the differential diagnosis," *Archives of Pathology and Laboratory Medicine*, vol. 134, no. 5, pp. 667–690, 2010.

[32] H. G. Ahmed, A. S. Nassar, and I. Ginawi, "Screening for tuberculosis and its histological pattern in patients with enlarged lymph node," *Pathology Research International*, vol. 2011, Article ID 417635, 4 pages, 2011.

[33] J. S. Park, Y. A. Kang, S. Y. Kwon et al., "Nested PCR in lung tissue for diagnosis of pulmonary tuberculosis," *European Respiratory Journal*, vol. 35, no. 4, pp. 851–857, 2010.

[34] B. Corrin and A. G. Nicholson, "Infectious diseases—chronic bacterial infections," in *Pathology of the Lungs*, pp. 197–221, Churchill Livingstone, 3rd edition, 2011.

[35] S. Narayanan, S. Swaminathan, P. Supply et al., "Impact of HIV infection on the recurrence of tuberculosis in south India," *Journal of Infectious Diseases*, vol. 201, no. 5, pp. 691–703, 2010.

16

Utility of Tissue Transglutaminase Immunohistochemistry in Pediatric Duodenal Biopsies: Patterns of Expression and Role in Celiac Disease—A Clinicopathologic Review

Saeeda Almarzooqi,[1] Ronald H. Houston,[2] and Vinay Prasad[3]

[1] *Nationwide Children's Hospital, 700 Children's Drive, Columbus, OH 43205, USA*
[2] *Anatomic Pathology ChildLab, Nationwide Children's Hospital, 700 Children's Drive, Columbus, OH 43205, USA*
[3] *Nationwide Children's Hospital, Clinical Ohio State University, 700 Children's Drive, Columbus, OH 43205, USA*

Correspondence should be addressed to Vinay Prasad; vinay.prasad@nationwidechildrens.org

Academic Editor: Hanlin L. Wang

Tissue transglutaminase (tTG) is a ubiquitous multifunctional protein. It has roles in various cellular processes. tTG is a major target of autoantibodies in celiac disease, and its expression by immunohistochemistry in pediatric celiac disease has not been fully examined. We studied tTG expression in 78 pediatric duodenal biopsies by utilizing an antibody to transglutaminase 2. Serum tTG was positive in all celiac cases evaluated. Serum antiserum endomysial antibody (EMA) and tTG were negative in all control subjects and in inflammatory bowel disease and eosinophilic gastroenteritis. There was a statistically significant difference between cases of celiac disease and normal controls in terms of tTG immunohistochemical staining in duodenal biopsies surface epithelium (P value = 0.0012). There was no significant statistical difference in terms of staining of the villous surface or crypt between the cases of celiac disease and cases with IBD (P value = 0.5970 and 0.5227, resp.). There was no detected correlation between serum tTG values and immunohistochemical positivity on duodenal biopsy in cases of celiac disease (P value = 1). There was no relationship between Marsh classification and positivity of villous surface for tTG (P value = 0.4955). We conclude that tTG has limited utility in diagnosis of celiac disease in pediatric duodenal biopsies.

1. Introduction

The diagnosis of celiac disease is based on demonstrating characteristic villous abnormality on duodenal biopsy in a patient with positive celiac serology. Among the serological tests used are antiserum endomysial antibody (EMA) and antitissue transglutaminase antibodies (tTG).

EMA antibodies have a sensitivity of 92.1% and a specificity of 99.8% [1]. EMA antibodies are of the IgA subtype, and thus, false negative cases may be encountered in patients with IgA deficiency [2]. Serum tTG has a sensitivity of 94.8% and specificity of 99.2% [1].

Tissue transglutaminase is an intracellular enzyme present in many tissues. It has roles in various cellular processes including cellular differentiation, matrix production, and tissue repair [3, 4]. Serum tTG has been found to be increased in patients with celiac disease [3]. It has been confirmed that this enzyme is a target in the autoimmune process of celiac disease that is targeted by EMA [1, 5]. tTG deamidates glutamine residues of the glutamine-rich gliadins exposing them and facilitating their presentation by antigen presenting cells to T cells [6].

The validity of utility of tTG immunohistochemistry in duodenal biopsy of celiac disease has conflicting results in the literature, some authors finding it to be a useful test in differentiating celiac disease cases from normal control, while others have failed to demonstrate such usefulness [2, 4, 6]. In addition, its expression by immunohistochemistry in pediatric celiac disease has not been fully examined. The aim of our study was to investigate the pattern of expression of tTG in pediatric patients with celiac disease and compare it with normal duodenal biopsy and patients with other

TABLE 1: Clinical characteristics of subjects.

Group (n)	Age range (median)	Gender		Other diseases (n)	Clinical symptoms
		F	M		
Celiac disease (36)	1–16 (8)	23	13	DM (7) Down syndrome (2) Juvenile RA (1) Hypothyroidism (1)	(i) Abdominal pain (ii) Diarrhea (iii) Failure to thrive/weight loss (iv) Constipation
IBD (7)	5–17 (15)	2	5		(i) Rectal bleeding (ii) Diarrhea (iii) Abdominal pain (iv) Weight loss
*Normal control (33)	0.6–17 (8)	16 17		Asthma (5) Juvenile RA (1)	(i) GERD (ii) Abdominal pain
Eosinophilic GE (2)	1–11 (6)	2			(i) Dysphagia (ii) Vomiting

n: number; IBD: inflammatory bowel disease; GE: gastroenteritis; F: female; M: male; DM: diabetes mellitus; RA: rheumatoid arthritis; GERD: gastroesophageal reflux disease; *diagnoses of control cases were 17 cases with no pathologic diagnosis, 7 chronic gastritis, 6 active esophagitis, 2 reactive gastritis, and 1 candida esophagitis.

duodenal pathology, for example, inflammatory bowel disease (IBD).

2. Materials and Methods

We obtained approval from the Institutional Review Board (IRB) of Nationwide Children's Hospital to undertake this study. 78 cases of duodenal biopsy from the files of the Department of Anatomic Pathology were retrieved; 36 celiac disease, 33 pathologically normal controls, 7 inflammatory bowel disease, and 2 eosinophilic gastroenteritis.

Three micron-thick sections of formalin-fixed, paraffin-embedded duodenal biopsies were cut and mounted on charged slides. An antibody to tissue transglutaminase, clone CUB 7402 (Abcam Inc., Cambridge MA), was used at a dilution factor of 1 : 1280, after antigen retrieval in a citrate buffer, pH 6 (ER1; Leica Microsystems, Buffalo Grove, IL). A negative control was obtained by substituting the primary antibody with Universal Negative Control Serum (cat no. NC49BL, Biocare Medical, Concord CA). All stages of the immunohistochemistry procedure were automated on the BondMax IHC system (Leica Microsystems) using the Refine polymer detection system (Leica Microsystems), with DAB visualization and counterstained with hematoxylin.

Laboratory serological studies for Serum IgA endomysial antibodies (EMA) or tissue tansglutaminase IgA antibodies (tTG) were obtained by review of medical charts.

Results were evaluated by using Fisher's exact test with SAS software (SAS 9.1.3 SAS 9.1.3 by SAS Institute Inc., Cary, NC, USA).

3. Results

A total of 78 cases were evaluated. The diagnosis of celiac disease (36 patients) had been confirmed based on clinical, serological, and histological evaluation. All the cases were biopsied because of clinical symptoms of pain. None of the cases of celiac disease that were biopsied were on a Gluten-free diet. 7 cases of IBD (5 Crohn's disease, 2 ulcerative colitis) were also retrieved. The cases of inflammatory bowel disease did not have small bowel involvement at the time the biopsies were taken. Two patients had eosinophilic gastroenteritis. In addition, 33 cases of histologically normal duodenal biopsies that underwent upper gastrointestinal (GI) endoscopy for evaluation of upper GI symptoms were included. The clinical characteristics of our patients are summarized in Table 1. Among the group with celiac disease there were 23 females and 13 males. The age range was 1–16 years (median 8 years). Comorbidity was noted in a number of the cases and included diabetes mellitus (7), Down syndrome (2), juvenile rheumatoid arthritis (1), and hypothyroidism (1).

In patients with celiac disease, serum tTG was positive in all cases where it was evaluated (26/26). There were 10 cases in which serum tTG was not evaluated before or at the time of biopsy, and these cases were lost to follow up. Therefore, the results of serum tTG testing were available only in 26 cases. Serum EMA was elevated in 26/30 and was not elevated in 4/30, Table 2(b). In the remaining 6 cases, serum EMA was not evaluated. Serum EMA and tTG were negative in all control subjects and in cases with inflammatory bowel disease and eosinophilic gastroenteritis.

Among the cases with celiac disease, the pattern of mucosal staining with tTG was characterized by one of three staining patterns, Table 2(a) and Figure 1. The majority of celiac cases (27/36) demonstrated both surface epithelial staining with localization to enterocyte cytoplasm, superficial lamina propria, and basement membrane. This pattern was accompanied by an absence of staining in mucosal crypts. Three of the cases showed both surface epithelial positivity as well as crypt staining. Absence of staining was noted in six of the celiac cases.

Figure 2 demonstrates the predominant patterns of expression of tTG among cases of celiac disease, normal control, and cases with inflammatory bowel disease. When comparing all groups for the pattern of tTG staining, there was

TABLE 2: (a) Breakdown of cases of celiac disease by pattern of tTG expression. (b) Breakdown of cases of celiac disease by serum tTG and serum EMA results.

(a)

Pattern of expression	tTG surface positive/crypt negative	tTG surface positive/crypt positive	tTG surface/crypt negative
No. of cases (total 36)	27	3	6

(b)

	Serum tTG elevated	Serum EMA elevated	Serum not tested
No. of cases (total cases 36)	26 of 26 tested	26 of 30 tested (4/30 not elevated)	6 not tested for EMA 10 not tested for serum tTG

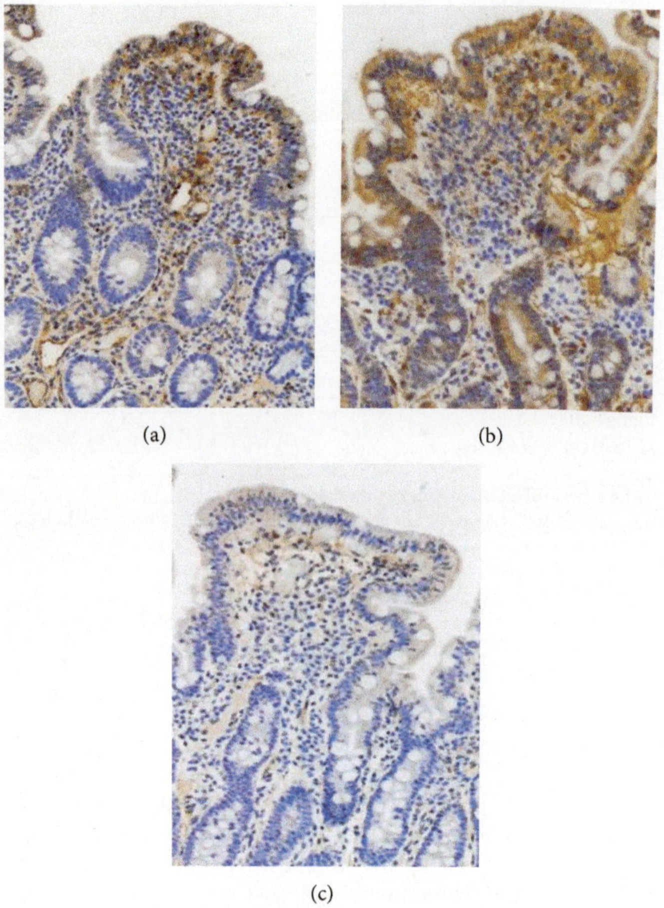

FIGURE 1: Patterns of expression of tissue transglutaminase in duodenal biopsies of celiac disease. (a) Positive surface mucosa labelling with absent staining in crypts. (b) Positive staining in both surface mucosa and in crypts. (c) Absence of staining in both surface epithelium and crypts. (immunoperoxidase 20x).

a statistically significant association between the different groups and tTG villous surface staining (P value = 0.0045). There was no significant association between different groups and tTG staining in duodenal crypts (P value = 0.7272). There was a statistically significant difference between celiac cases and normal control in terms of tTG immunohistochemical staining in duodenal biopsies surface epithelium (P value = 0.0012). No difference was present between immunohistochemical staining of crypt epithelium (P value = 1) (Table 3).

There was no significant difference in terms of villous surface staining between celiac disease cases and cases with IBD (P value = 0.5970). Similarly, there was no significant difference between crypt staining with tTG between the two groups (P value = 0.5227) (Table 4). Combining the cases of eosinophilic gastroenteritis with cases of IBD failed to detect any significant difference between them and patients with celiac disease by evaluation staining in surface villi and crypt (P value = 0.3536 and 1, resp.).

There was no detected correlation between serum tTG values and immunohistochemical positivity on duodenal biopsy in cases of celiac disease (P value = 1). Categorizing cases of celiac disease using the Marsh classification yielded one case of class 0, 5 cases of class 2, 10 cases of class 3a, 19 cases of 3b, and 1 case of class 3c. There was no relationship between Marsh type and positivity of villous surface for tTG (P value = 0.4955) (Table 5).

The results of this small study are significant because we did not observe a specific single pattern of staining. We observed immunohistochemical staining with tTG in different areas within the biopsies, such as crypt epithelium, lamina propria, and basement membrane. The results also showed that there is no significant difference in the pattern of tTG staining among cases of celiac disease versus chronic duodenitis due to inflammatory bowel disease. Additionally, a few cases of celiac disease had no staining with immunohistochemical stain for tTG. In this study, the Marsh grades noted and the tTG staining patterns also did not follow a pattern.

4. Discussion

Tissue transglutaminase is an intracellular enzyme present in many tissues. It has roles in various cellular processes including cellular differentiation, matrix production, and tissue repair [3, 4]. Serum tTG has been found to be increased in patients with celiac disease [3]. It has been confirmed that this enzyme is a target in the autoimmune process of celiac disease that is mediated by endomysial antibodies [1, 5].

The utility of tTG immunohistochemistry in the evaluation of duodenal biopsy for the diagnosis of celiac disease has been reported recently [2–4]. However, results of the different studies had conflicting results in terms of the specificity of the immunohistochemical test in differentiating celiac disease from nonceliac cases [2–4].

Serological screening for celiac disease is based on identification of serum antiendomysial IgA antibodies. The test has a sensitivity and specificity >95% [2]. Limitations encountered with the utility of this paper include lower sensitivity (<90%) in patients below the age of 2 years and the false negativity seen in patients with IgA deficiency [2, 7]. This has been overcome by the measurement of serum IgA in all

TABLE 3: Immunohistochemical staining pattern in celiac disease and control cases.

	Surface tTG		Crypt tTG	
	Positive *n* (%)	Negative *n* (%)	Positive *n* (%)	Negative *n* (%)
Celiac disease	30 (83.33)	6 (16.67)	3 (8.33)	33 (91.67)
Normal control	15 (45.45)	18 (54.55)	2 (6.06)	31 (93.94)
P value	0.0012		1.0	

n: number; %: percentage.

TABLE 4: Immunostaining pattern in celiac and inflammatory bowel disease.

	Surface tTG		Crypt tTG	
	Positive *n* (%)	Negative *n* (%)	Positive *n* (%)	Negative *n* (%)
Celiac disease	30 (83.33)	6 (16.67)	3 (8.33)	33 (91.67)
IBD	5 (71.43)	2 (28.57)	1 (14.29)	6 (85.71)
P value	0.5970		0.5227	

n: number; %: percentage; IBD: inflammatory bowel disease.

TABLE 5: Cases of celiac disease subclassified by Marsh classification.

Marsh classification	No. of cases
0	1
2	5
3a	10
3b	19
3c	1

patients undergoing serological evaluation for celiac disease. Serum tTG levels have a sensitivity and specificity up to 98% [2].

In our series of celiac disease, the findings are in accordance with those reported in the literature. All of our patients who have been tested for serum tTG had a positive result. Of those patients evaluated for serum EMA, 26 out of 30 patients had an elevated serum level. Thus, according to our data, serum EMA has a sensitivity of 86% and a specificity of 100%.

The patterns of localization of tTG in celiac duodenal biopsies were characterized by a predominant surface epithelial staining with absent staining in mucosal crypts. The staining was located in the cytoplasm of enterocytes as well as in superficial lamina propria and subepithelial basement membrane. This pattern was noted in 75% of our celiac disease cases. Three of our cases (3/36) showed both surface epithelial staining as well as staining of crypts. In six cases (6/36), no staining was detected. Among these cases with a negative staining pattern, a positive serologically elevated serum tTG was seen in the four cases where it was measured. Previous studies have shown the patterns of tTG localization in celiac disease duodenal biopsy. Salky et al. have demonstrated that localization of tTG in duodenal mucosa was related to degree of mucosal atrophy. In their series, cases of celiac disease showed an increased expression of the tTG in the basement membrane and lamina propria when compared to control cases. They suggest that this pattern of localization can be explained on the basis that tTG forms complexes with gliadin in the basement membrane and lamina propria in celiac

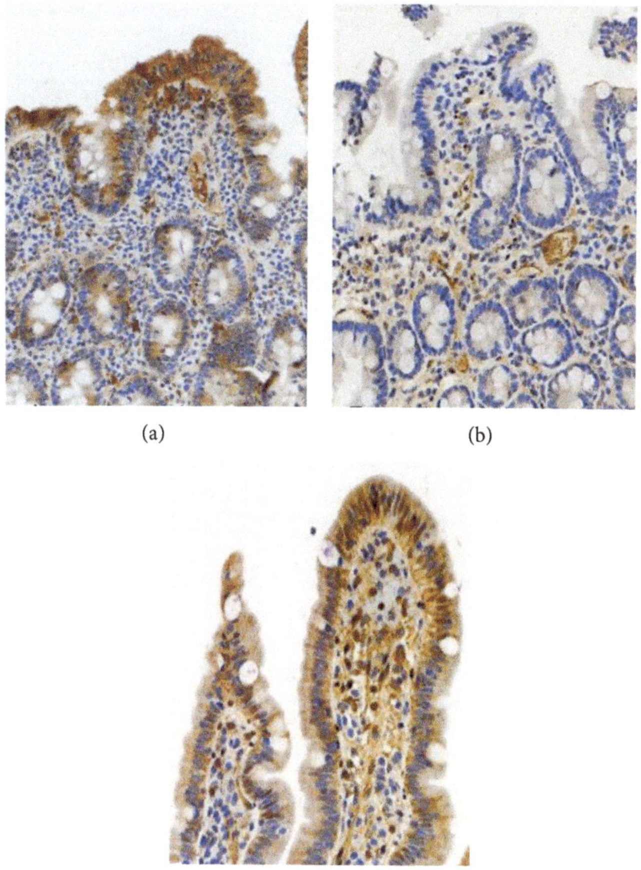

(a) (b) (c)

FIGURE 2: Expression of tissue transglutaminase in duodenal biopsies. (a) Celiac disease. (b) Normal control. (c) Crohn's disease. (immunoperoxidase 20x).

patients [8]. Similar results have been shown by other authors as well [4, 6].

Our data demonstrate that the utility of immunohistochemical tTG in evaluation of duodenal biopsy for suspected celiac disease has a significant value when comparing it to normal controls. Esposito et al. evaluated the expression of tTG in 26 patients (0.9–18 years) and showed an increased expression in duodenal biopsies of their cases. They showed increased staining in subepithelial connective tissue as well as in enterocytes in cases of celiac compared with control subjects. They suggest that the staining is either disease specific or secondary to inflammation [4]. Similar studies were also in support of the utility of this immunohistochemical stain in differentiating celiac disease from normal control [6, 8]. However, Tuncer and colleagues in a review of 12 cases of celiac disease failed to demonstrate a significant difference in comparison to normal controls [2].

A limitation of this study is the possibility of low detectability, perhaps due to technical constraints, leading to the minimal staining within the lamina propria in some cases. We also noted a subset of patients with celiac disease who had no immunohistochemical tTG staining, a confounding factor. Another limitation of this immunohistochemical stain is the demonstration of mucosal positivity in cases of duodenitis due to other etiologies. In our series, seven cases of inflammatory bowel disease and two cases of eosinophilic gastroenteritis were evaluated. We failed to demonstrate any significant statistical difference. This observation has been noted by other investigators [4, 6, 9]. In the series by Gorgun and colleagues, cases of duodenitis other than celiac disease were evaluated. Their cases included one case of Crohn's disease, 5 cases of acid related duodenitis, one case of Campylobacter duodenitis, one case of abetalipoproteinemia, and one case of Waldenström macroglobinemia. Their data failed to show any difference when comparing these cases to cases of celiac disease [6]. Similarly, Esposito et al. demonstrated the expression of tTG in one patient of Crohn's disease. They suggested that the positivity might not be disease specific but rather a marker of an abnormal immune response [4].

Immunohistochemical staining in cases of celiac disease does not correlate with the Marsh type. 80% of the cases were Marsh types 3a or 3b.

In conclusion, the immunohistochemical utility of tTG in celiac duodenal biopsies seems to be of limited value. This is due to expression in inflamed duodenal mucosa in nonceliac cases such as cases of inflammatory bowel disease. This immunohistochemical stain has to be studied in more detail, in a larger number of children. It would also be beneficial to examine the tTG staining of patients who are on gluten-free diets and compare the findings. Therefore, one should not rely on immunohistochemical expression of tTG to make a diagnosis of celiac disease.

Disclosure

This work was presented at the plenary session of the Society for Pediatric Pathology annual spring meeting, 2010, Washington, DC.

References

[1] E. Tonutti, D. Visentini, N. Bizzaro et al., "The role of antitissue transglutaminase assay for the diagnosis and monitoring of coeliac disease: a French-Italian multicentre study," *Journal of Clinical Pathology*, vol. 56, no. 5, pp. 389–393, 2003.

[2] I. Tuncer, I. Bayram, I. Kaba, R. Mercan, and S. Uğraş, "Tissue transglutaminase expression in duodenal mucosa of patients with celiac disease and of normal subjects," *Turkish Journal of Gastroenterology*, vol. 14, no. 3, pp. 185–188, 2003.

[3] G. D'Argenio, I. Sorrentini, C. Ciacci et al., "Human serum transglutaminase and coeliac disease: correlation between serum and mucosal activity in an experimental model of rat small bowel enteropathy," *Gut*, vol. 30, no. 7, pp. 950–954, 1989.

[4] C. Esposito, F. Paparo, I. Caputo et al., "Expression and enzymatic activity of small intestinal tissue transglutaminase in celiac disease," *American Journal of Gastroenterology*, vol. 98, no. 8, pp. 1813–1820, 2003.

[5] W. Dieterich, T. Ehnis, M. Bauer et al., "Identification of tissue transglutaminase as the autoantigen of celiac disease," *Nature Medicine*, vol. 3, no. 7, pp. 797–801, 1997.

[6] J. Gorgun, A. Portyanko, Y. Marakhouski, and E. Cherstvoy, "Tissue transglutaminase expression in celiac mucosa: an immunohistochemical study," *Virchows Archiv*, vol. 455, no. 4, pp. 363–373, 2009.

[7] H. Vogelsang, D. Genser, J. Wyatt et al., "Screening for celiac disease: a prospective study on the value of noninvasive tests," *American Journal of Gastroenterology*, vol. 90, no. 3, pp. 394–398, 1995.

[8] W. Sakly, B. Sriha, I. Ghedira et al., "Localization of tissue transglutaminase and N (epsilon)-(gamma) -glutamyl lysine in duodenal cucosa during the development of mucosal atrophy in coeliac disease," *Virchows Archiv*, vol. 446, no. 6, pp. 613–618, 2005.

[9] V. Villanacci, T. Not, D. Sblattero et al., "Mucosal tissue transglutaminase expression in celiac disease," *Journal of Cellular and Molecular Medicine*, vol. 13, no. 2, pp. 334–340, 2009.

17

Upregulation of Serum Vascular Endothelial Growth Factor in Patients with Salivary Gland Tumor

Azadeh Andisheh Tadbir,[1] Bijan Khademi,[2] Mahyar Malekzadeh,[3] Maryam Mardani,[4] and Bahar Khademi[5]

[1] *Department of Oral and Maxillofacial Pathology, School of Dentistry, Shiraz University of Medical Sciences, Ghom Abad, Ghasrodasht Avenue, Shiraz 71956-15878, Iran*

[2] *Department of Otolaryngology, Khalili Hospital, Shiraz Institute for Cancer Research, Shiraz University of Medical Sciences, Shiraz 71348-45794, Iran*

[3] *Shiraz Institute for Cancer Research, Shiraz University of Medical Sciences, Shiraz 71348-45794, Iran*

[4] *Department of Oral Medicine, School of Dentistry, Shiraz University of Medical Sciences, Ghom Abad, Ghasrodasht Avenue, Shiraz 71956-15878, Iran*

[5] *School of Dentistry, Shiraz University of Medical Sciences (International Branch), Azadi Square, Jahad Sazandegi Street, Shiraz 71447-16699, Iran*

Correspondence should be addressed to Azadeh Andisheh Tadbir; andisheh@sums.ac.ir

Academic Editor: Piero Tosi

Neoangiogenesis is essential for tumor development, invasion, and dissemination. The most potent of the cytokines associated with angiogenesis is vascular endothelial growth factor (VEGF). The aim of the present study was to determine VEGF serum level in patients with salivary gland tumor. Using an ELISA kit, the circulating levels of VEGF in sera from 58 patients with salivary gland tumor and 30 healthy controls were assessed. Mean VEGF levels in sera of patients with salivary gland tumors (574.9 ± 414.3) were significantly higher than those in controls (263.9 ± 310.0) ($P = 0.009$). Within the salivary gland tumor group, mean serum VEGF concentration in malignant tumors ($n = 27$) was 727.3 ± 441.8 pg/mL, and that in benign tumors ($n = 31$) was 442.2 ± 343.3 pg/mL. Mean serum VEGF concentration was significantly higher in malignant tumors than in benign tumors ($P = 0.008$) and was higher in benign tumors than in controls ($P = 0.03$). The data in the present study clearly show that VEGF level was consistently upregulated in benign and malignant tumors in comparison to healthy controls. However, the role of VEGF as a prognostic factor in salivary gland tumor and its application in antiangiogenic therapy require further clinical research.

1. Introduction

Neoangiogenesis, the development of new vessels from preexisting ones, is necessary for tumor development, invasion, and dissemination. Angiogenic process not only delivers nutrients for tumor growth but also increases the chance for tumor cells to enter the circulation and metastasis [1].

A variety of signals such as diminished nutrition or oxygen in tissue or genetic changes in oncogenes or tumor suppressor genes can start angiogenic process. Different factors produced from stromal and tumor cells such as growth factors, cytokines, enzymes, and adhesion molecules are involved in this process, and the most potent of them is vascular endothelial growth factor (VEGF) [2].

Among the VEGF family, which consists of VEGF-A, VEGF-B, VEGF-C, VEGF-D, and VEGF-F, VEGF-A is a key angiogenic factor and is mostly used to promote angiogenic phenotype by a tumor [3].

VEGF-A is a dimeric glycoprotein with a molecular weight of 34–45 KDa, consisting of two subunits. Increased VEGF expression was seen in different physiologic and pathologic conditions which was associated with hypoxia [4].

VEGF is expressed in several malignant tumors which indicates its importance in angiogenesis process.

Table 1: Serum VEGF level in benign, malignant salivary gland tumors and normal controls as measured by Sandwich ELISA.

Groups	Mean serum VEGF (pg/mL)	P value
Controls	263.9 ± 310 ± 0.0	Controls versus benign tumors $P = 0.03$
Benign salivary gland tumor	442.2 ± 343.3	Controls versus malignant tumors $P = 0.001$
Malignant salivary gland tumor	727.3 ± 441.8	Benign tumors versus malignant tumors $P = 0.008$

Overexpression of VEGF was found in body fluids and solid tumors such as brain, colon, breast, kidney, bladder, lung, and oral cancer [5].

However, no investigations have been conducted regarding serum VEGF levels in patients with salivary gland tumor, so the aim of the present study was to determine VEGF serum level in patients with salivary gland tumor.

2. Materials & Methods

2.1. Subjects. For the purpose of this case-control study, 58 serum samples from the patients diagnosed with salivary gland tumor (24 males, 34 females, age: 44.8 ± 16.6 years) consisting of 31 pleomorphic adenoma, 17 adenoid cystic carcinoma, and 10 mucoepidermoid carcinoma and 30 serum samples from healthy control subjects (12 males, 18 females, age: 44.6 ± 16.6 years) were collected.

Study subjects were the patients admitted to the Department of Otolaryngology, Khalili Hospital, Shiraz University of Medical Sciences, and diagnosed with salivary gland tumor histopathologically.

Control cases were healthy blood donors, who were matched for age and gender. Exclusion criteria for both groups were based on the presence of any systemic disease, use of corticosteroid or nonsteroid anti-inflammatory medication, or a history of malignancy of any type.

All the participants were informed about the research study and agreed to participate by signing an informed consent form.

2.2. Serum Analysis. Serum samples were obtained from clotted blood following the centrifugation at 4°C and storing at −80°C until analysis. VEGF concentrations were measured by Sandwich ELISA, in accordance with the manufacturer's instructions (BMS, GmbH, Germany).

2.3. Statistical Analysis. Statistical analysis was performed using Mann-Whitney test. A P value less than 0.05 was considered significant.

3. Results

Mean serum VEGF levels in malignant tumors, benign tumors, and controls are shown in Table 1. Mean VEGF levels in sera of patients with salivary gland tumors (574.9 ± 414.3) were significantly higher than those in controls (263.9 ± 310.0) ($P = 0.009$). Within the salivary gland tumor group, mean serum VEGF concentration in malignant tumors ($n = 27$) was 727.3 ± 441.8 pg/mL, and that in benign tumors ($n = 31$) was 442.2 ± 343.3 pg/mL. Mean serum VEGF concentration was significantly higher in malignant tumors than in benign tumors ($P = 0.008$) and was higher in benign tumors than in controls ($P = 0.03$).

No relation was found between mean VEGF levels and sex and age of the patients and controls.

4. Discussion

Angiogenesis is necessary for tumor growth. It is a multifaceted process which is regulated by a variety of inducers and inhibitors, which are produced by different cell types like stromal cells, endothelial cells, and tumor cells [6]. Different angiogenic factors have been described. VEGF plays an important role in both pathologic and physiologic conditions [7].

VEGF is one of the most important angiogenic factors involved in tumor angiogenesis. It has been suggested that VEGF is a potent mitogen for endothelial cells and can directly induce new blood vessels formation. Concurrently, increased VEGF will enhance microvascular permeability and will lead to plasma protein extravasation (e.g., fibrinogen) into the extravascular area. Then, extra vascular fibrinogen causes clot formation and other proteins like fibronectin are added to fibrin clot and formed a suitable matrix for growth of endothelial cells [8].

Numerous studies have shown that VEGF is involved in tumor progression. VEGF can increase tumor cell extravasation and metastasis through inducing angiogenesis, enhancing vascular permeability, and stimulating immunosuppression [8–10].

Clearly, identification of different biologic markers and understanding of underlying mechanisms may provide useful markers for determining prognosis and effective treatment.

Recently, different functions such as lymphangiogenesis, enhanced vascular permeability, and antiapoptosis activity have been recognized for VEGF which all have a role in tumor progression [10, 11].

VEGF overexpression has been reported in different tumors. Kulapaditharom et al. (2012) found that the most aggressive head and neck squamous cell carcinoma showed the highest VEGF expression. These findings suggest that VEGF has a role in the progression of head and neck squamous cell carcinoma toward an aggressive and invasive phenotype [12].

Lequerica-Fernández et al. (2007) showed that VEGF can contribute to the progression of salivary gland carcinomas and seems to be associated with lymph node metastasis and worse survival [13].

Recently, Ke-Xiong et al. (2011) suggested that inducible nitric oxide synthase can motivate the expression of VEGF, and its expression status may help evaluate tumor malignancy and prognosis of the patient [14].

A study conducted by Hao et al. (2010) showed that overexpression of VEGF was seen in adenoid cystic carcinoma and its expression was higher in solid form and in advanced-stage group. Also VEGF expression was related to invasion and metastasis and proposed as a prognostic factor [15].

Swelam et al. (2005) suggest that tumor cells of pleomorphic adenoma secrete functional VEGF in different forms that induce their proliferation and differentiation, and VEGF expression is regulated by hypoxic conditions [16].

Recently, circulating VEGF levels have been reported to be a reliable and noninvasive marker of angiogenic activity and were shown to be independent prognostic factors which are correlated with survival in various malignant neoplasms [17], but fewer studies were carried out to evaluate its circulating level.

Shang et al. showed serum VEGF levels to be significantly elevated in oral cancers compared to control group [18].

Dirix et al. (1996) showed that high serum VEGF was associated with the large size of the primary tumor in advanced colorectal cancer [19].

Khademi et al. (2013) reported that increased preoperative or postoperative serum levels of VEGF can predict disease recurrence and are associated with poor disease-free and overall survival of patients with HNSCC [20].

In the present study, ELISA kit was used to measure serum VEGF concentrations in patients with salivary gland tumor. By reviewing the articles, this study was the first report to do so.

Results of this study indicate a significant increase in VEGF level from healthy controls to benign and malignant tumors.

So VEGF levels can significantly discriminate patients from controls and malignant from benign tumors. Also our results suggest that VEGF levels play a role in the progression of salivary gland tumors which was similar to those of Doi et al. (1999) and de Faria et al. (2011) [21, 22].

5. Conclusion

The data in the present study clearly show that VEGF level was consistently upregulated in benign and malignant tumors in comparison to healthy controls. However, the role of VEGF as a prognostic factor in salivary gland tumor and its application in antiangiogenic therapy require further clinical research.

Acknowledgments

This paper has been extracted from Mrs. Bahar Khademi's DDS thesis which was conducted under supervision of Dr. Azadeh Andisheh Tadbir and Dr. Bijan Khademi. This study was approved, registered with ID Grant no. 8591019, and supported by the Vice-Chancellery of International Branch of Shiraz University of Medical Sciences.

References

[1] S. Pourshahidi, A. A. Tadbir, H. Ebrahimi et al., "Serum level of vascular endothelial growth factor-c in patients with head and neck squamous cell carcinoma," *Australian Journal of Basic and Applied Sciences*, vol. 5, no. 9, pp. 426–429, 2011.

[2] D. Hodorowicz-Zaniewska, W. Kibil, A. Małek, J. Szpor, J. Kulig, and K. Sztefko, "Evaluation of serum concentrations of vascular endothelial growth factor (VEGF) in breast cancer patients," *Polish Journal of Pathology*, vol. 63, no. 4, pp. 255–260, 2012.

[3] S. Nayak, M. M. Goel, S. Chandra et al., "VEGF-A immunohistochemical and mRNA expression in tissues and its serum levels in potentially malignant oral lesions and oral squamous cell carcinomas," *Oral Oncology*, vol. 48, no. 3, pp. 233–239, 2012.

[4] M. Farzin, M. Mardani, J. Ghabanchi et al., "Serum level of matrix metalloproteinase-3 in patients with oral Lichen planus," *Iranian Red Crescent Medical Journal*, vol. 14, no. 1, 2012.

[5] C.-J. Liu, K.-W. Chang, S.-C. Lin, and H.-W. Cheng, "Presurgical serum levels of matrix metalloproteinase-9 and vascular endothelial growth factor in oral squamous cell carcinoma," *Oral Oncology*, vol. 45, no. 10, pp. 920–925, 2009.

[6] D. Hanahan and J. Folkman, "Patterns and emerging mechanisms of the angiogenic switch during tumorigenesis," *Cell*, vol. 86, no. 3, pp. 353–364, 1996.

[7] M. Sawatsubashi, T. Yamada, N. Fukushima, H. Mizokami, O. Tokunaga, and T. Shin, "Association of vascular endothelial growth factor and mast cells with angiogenesis in laryngeal squamous cell carcinoma," *Virchows Archiv*, vol. 436, no. 3, pp. 243–248, 2000.

[8] Z.-J. Shang, J.-R. Li, and Z.-B. Li, "Upregulation of serum and tissue vascular endothelial growth factor correlates with angiogenesis and prognosis of oral squamous cell carcinoma," *Journal of Oral and Maxillofacial Surgery*, vol. 65, no. 1, pp. 17–21, 2007.

[9] M. E. Baldwin, S. A. Stacker, and M. G. Achen, "Molecular control of lymphangiogenesis," *BioEssays*, vol. 24, no. 11, pp. 1030–1040, 2002.

[10] J. A. Nagy, E. Vasile, D. Feng et al., "Vascular permeability factor/vascular endothelial growth factor induces lymphangiogenesis as well as angiogenesis," *Journal of Experimental Medicine*, vol. 196, no. 11, pp. 1497–1506, 2002.

[11] J. E. Ohm, D. I. Gabrilovich, G. D. Sempowski et al., "VEGF inhibits T-cell development and may contribute to tumor-induced immune suppression," *Blood*, vol. 101, no. 12, pp. 4878–4886, 2003.

[12] B. Kulapaditharom, V. Boonkitticharoen, and C. Sritara, "Plasma vascular endothelial growth factor dysregulation in defining aggressiveness of head and neck squamous cell carcinoma," *Journal of Oncology*, vol. 2012, Article ID 687934, 7 pages, 2012.

[13] P. Lequerica-Fernández, A. Astudillo, and J. C. De Vicente, "Expression of vascular endothelial growth factor in salivary gland carcinomas correlates with lymph node metastasis," *Anticancer Research*, vol. 27, no. 5 B, pp. 3661–3666, 2007.

[14] O. Y. Ke-Xiong, L. Jun, and H. Zhi-Quan, "Association of clinicopathologic parameters with the expression of inducible nitric oxide synthase and vascular endothelial growth factor in mucoepidermoid carcinoma," *Oral Diseases*, vol. 17, no. 6, pp. 590–596, 2011.

[15] L. Hao, N. Xiao-lin, C. Qi, Y. Yi-ping, L. Jia-quan, and L. Yanning, "Nerve growth factor and vascular endothelial growth factor: retrospective analysis of 63 patients with salivary adenoid cystic carcinoma," *International journal of oral science*, vol. 2, no. 1, pp. 35–44, 2010.

[16] W. Swelam, H. Ida-Yonemochi, S. Maruyama, K. Ohshiro, J. Cheng, and T. Saku, "Vascular endothelial growth factor in

salivary pleomorphic adenomas: one of the reasons for their poorly vascularized stroma," *Virchows Archiv*, vol. 446, no. 6, pp. 653–662, 2005.

[17] R. T.-P. Poon, S.-T. Fan, and J. Wong, "Clinical implications of circulating angiogenic factors in cancer patients," *Journal of Clinical Oncology*, vol. 19, no. 4, pp. 1207–1225, 2001.

[18] Z.-J. Shang, J.-R. Li, and Z.-B. Li, "Circulating levels of vascular endothelial growth factor in patients with oral squamous cell carcinoma," *International Journal of Oral and Maxillofacial Surgery*, vol. 31, no. 5, pp. 495–498, 2002.

[19] L. Y. Dirix, P. B. Vermeulen, G. Hubens et al., "Serum basic fibroblst growth factor and vascular endothelial growth factor and tumour growth kinetics in advanced colorectal cancer," *Annals of Oncology*, vol. 7, no. 8, pp. 843–848, 1996.

[20] B. Khademi, M. Soleimanpour, A. Ghaderi, and M. Mohammadianpanah, "Prognostic and predictive value of serum vascular endothelial growth factor (VEGF) in squamous cell carcinoma of the head and neck," *Oral and Maxillofacial Surgery*, 2013.

[21] R. Doi, I. Kuratate, E. Okamoto, K. Ryoke, and H. Ito, "Expression of p53 oncoprotein increases intratumoral microvessel formation in human salivary gland carcinomas," *Journal of Oral Pathology and Medicine*, vol. 28, no. 6, pp. 259–263, 1999.

[22] P. R. de Faria, R. A. Lima, F. L. Dias et al., "Vascular endothelial growth factor and thymidine phosphorylase expression in salivary gland tumors with distinct metastatic behavior," *Journal of Oral Pathology and Medicine*, vol. 40, no. 6, pp. 456–459, 2011.

18

Pathology of Experimental *Encephalitozoon cuniculi* Infection in Immunocompetent and Immunosuppressed Mice in Iraq

Hafidh I. Al-Sadi[1] and Saevan S. Al-Mahmood[2]

[1] *Department of Oral and Maxillofacial Surgery, College of Dentistry, University of Mosul, Mosul, Iraq*
[2] *Department of Pathology and Poultry Diseases, College of Veterinary Medicine, University of Mosul, Mosul, Iraq*

Correspondence should be addressed to Saevan S. Al-Mahmood; saevan981@yahoo.com

Academic Editor: Maria M. Picken

This study was performed to evaluate pathology of experimental *Encephalitozoon cuniculi* (Iraqi isolate) infection in normal and immunosuppressed mice. Pathological changes were not seen in negative control mice while secondary bacterial infections were noted in the lungs, kidneys, and heart of mice given dexamethasone. Typical *E. cuniculi* infection lesions were found in brain, livers, lungs, and kidneys of mice given 10^7 *E. cuniculi* spores/mouse orally. These lesions were in the form of nonsuppurative meningoencephalitis with vasculitis in brain, interstitial inflammation with infiltration of both lymphocytes and plasma cells in lung tissue, and nonsuppurative interstitial (focal and diffuse) nephritis, presence of vacuole containing mature and immature spores in enterocytes within the tips of villi, and lymphoiod hyperplasia of the white pulp and vasculitis of the intratrabecular vessels. Mice that were given 10^7 *E. cuniculi* spores/mouse orally showed lesions similar to those observed in the previous group (vasculitis and granulomas) but the lesions were more severe and widespread. In conclusion, this is the first report of experimental *E. cuniculi* infection induced by *E. cuniculi* isolated from a naturally infected rabbit in Iraq and that infection became more severe and widespread upon the administration of dexaethasone.

1. Introduction

Microsporidia are obligate intracellular microorganisms that infect a wide range of invertebrate and vertebrate species [1]. Traditionally, they were considered protozoa but recently have been reclassified phylogenetically as fungi [2]. These microorganisms have been reported as causing economic losses in honeybee, fish, mink, and other fur-bearing animals [3].

The phylum Microsporidia is subdivided into a variety of families and genera, which includes the genus *Encephalitozoon* which in turn includes the important species *Encephalitozoon cuniculi, E. hellem, E. intestinalis,* and *E. lacerate* [4]. Microsporidian spores have been reported in foods and water sources [3]. The natural route of entry of microsporidia into the host was found to be through ingestion or inhalation of infective spores or via wounds and transplacentally [3].

E. cuniculi has been considered the most common and most important pathogen in animals; most of the knowledge available now on microsporidia is based on *E. cuniculi* [5]. Additionally, *E. cuniculi* was also the first mammalian microsporidium that was isolated and cultured in vitro [6].

In immunocompetent host, microsporidial infection is characterized by a short acute diarrheal phase followed by asymptomatic infection, while chronic malabsorptive diarrhea and systemic disease can develop in immunocompromised individuals [7].

Although microsporidia have been known as pathogenic agents in a wide range of wild, laboratory, and domestic animals for several decades, further studies are required to completely understand the epidemiology and pathobiology of microsporidiosis; also these parasites have not been isolated or identified before in Iraq; furthermore, their pathology in different species was not studied. The present study was designed to determine the pathology of experimental *E. cuniculi* (using *E. cuniculi* isolated from rabbit infected in Iraq) in immunocompetent and immunosuppressed mice.

2. Materials and Methods

2.1. Ethics Statement. All of the experimental procedures were conducted in accordance with the regulations of the College of Veterinary Medicine, University of Mosul, concerning protection of animals against cruelty.

2.2. Experimental Animals. A total of 240 inbred Balb/c, 35- to 42-day-old male mice were housed in the Animal House of the College of Veterinary Medicine, University of Mosul, given food and water ad libitum, and maintained on a 12-hour light/dark cycle. Mice were allowed to acclimate for one week prior to their use in the experiments. To prevent reinfection, microisolator cages, feed, water, and bedding were sterilized and changed daily. All animals were tested daily (fecal examination) for the presence of microsporidia. Only mice without microsporidial infection were used. Additionally, mice were treated orally with albendazol (25 mg/kg b.w.) and five days later with 0.5 mg/kg b.w. of fumagillin to get rid of any possible microsporidial or other parasitic infections [8].

2.3. Preparation of Inoculum. Spores of microsporidia (*Encephalitozoon cuniculi*) were obtained from fecal samples of a naturally infected rabbit isolated by Al-Sadi and Al-Mahmood [9]. Infected spores of *E. cuniculi* were prepared as described by [10].

2.4. Experimental Design. Mice ($n = 240$) were divided into 4 equal groups randomly: first group (control group, nontreated), second group (microsporidia group) which was given 10^7 spores of *E. cuniculi*/mouse orally, third group (*E. cuniculi* and dexamethasone) which was given 10^7 *E. cuniculi* spores/mouse orally and given dexamethasone 125 μg/mouse intraperitoneally during the first day of the experimentation and repeated once a week for the rest of the experimental period, and fourth group (control group, dexamethasone treated) which was given dexamethasone 125 μg/mouse intraperitoneally during the first day of the experimentation and repeated once a week for the rest of the experimental period [11]. Fecal samples were collected from mice at 3, 7, 10, 15, 30, and 60 postinoculation days (PID). Smears were prepared from the samples and the slides were stained with Giemsa, quick-hot Gram-chromotrope, Weber-green modified trichrome, Ryan-blue modified trichrome, and Calcofluor-white stains [12–15]. Slides were examined under a light microscope to determine the presence of *E. cuniculi* spores and to determine the mean shedding of microsporidia.

2.5. Histopathological Examination. Ten mice from each group were euthanized at each of the 3rd, 7th, 10th, 15th, 30th, and 60th postinoculation days using chloroform [16]. Following gross pathological examination, tissue specimens were collected from the brain, kidneys, liver, lungs, intestines, pancreas, heart, and spleen; these tissue specimens were fixed as described by [15]. Following fixation these tissues were processed and stained by routine stain as described by [10, 12, 15].

3. Results

There were no significant clinical signs or gross lesions in immunocompetent mice inoculated with *E. cuniculi*, at the third PID. Microscopically, renal tissues exhibited focal infiltration of mononuclear cells in the interstitium. Fatty change of hepatocytes and mild vasculitis were found within the portal areas (Figure 1(a)). Pulmonary tissue showed heavy infiltration of mononuclear cells. In the lumen of intestines, large numbers of spores were detected (Figure 1(b)). Similar changes were found at the 7th PID. However, at the 10th PID, focal granulomatous inflammation and vasculitis were seen in the hepatic parenchyma and lymphocytic cholangitis was found in the portal areas (Figure 1(c)). The lungs exhibited vasculitis in the interstitium and lymphoid hyperplasia of the peribronchial lymph nodes. Other lesions included lymphocytic enteritis and granulomatous splenitis. At the 15th PID, the brain showed vasculitis in the meninges, gliosis in cerebral cortex, and granulomas in the cerebrum (Figure 1(d)). The lungs showed vasculitis and granulomatous pneumonia (Figure 2(a)). In the intestines, the parasites were seen in parasitophorous vacuoles in enterocytes within the villi (Figure 2(b)). At the 30th PID, grossly, there were congestions of meninges, brain, liver, and spleen. The lungs, stomach, and intestines were pale with presence of hemorrhagic area in the lungs. Microscopically, the nervous tissue showed vasculitis and granulomas in the cerebrum and vasculitis in the cerebellum (Figure 2(c)). At the 60th PID, the mice were anorexic and depressed. Grossly, there were congestions of meninges, brain, and liver and paleness of intestines and lungs. The latter also exhibited scattered nodular lesions. Histologically, granulomas were seen in the liver as well as thickening of blood vessels and bile ducts in portal areas (Figure 2(d)).

In immunosuppressed mice, at the 7th PID, microscopically, there was infiltration of mononuclear cells in cerebral cortex and cerebellum (Figure 3(a)). Hyperplasia of the lymphoid follicles was seen in the submucosa of the intestines (Figure 3(b)). At the 10th PID, anorexia, sneezing, coughing, and staggering of mice were seen. Vasculitis, cholangitis, and granulomas were seen in the liver (Figure 3(c)). The intestines showed lymphocytic enteritis and the presence of the parasites in parasitophorous vacuoles in enterocytes (Figure 3(d)). At the 15th PID, the parasite was seen in parasitophorous vacuoles in enterocytes (Figure 4(a)). At the 30th PID, microscopically, vasculitis and heavy infiltration of mononuclear cells were found in meninges, cerebrum, and cerebellum (Figure 4(b)), and vasculitis and focal interstitial nephritis were noted. At the 60th PID, microscopically, diffuse mononuclear cell infiltrations were seen in brain and meninges (Figure 4(c)). In the intestines, there were lymphocytic enteritis, thickening of the serosa due to proliferation

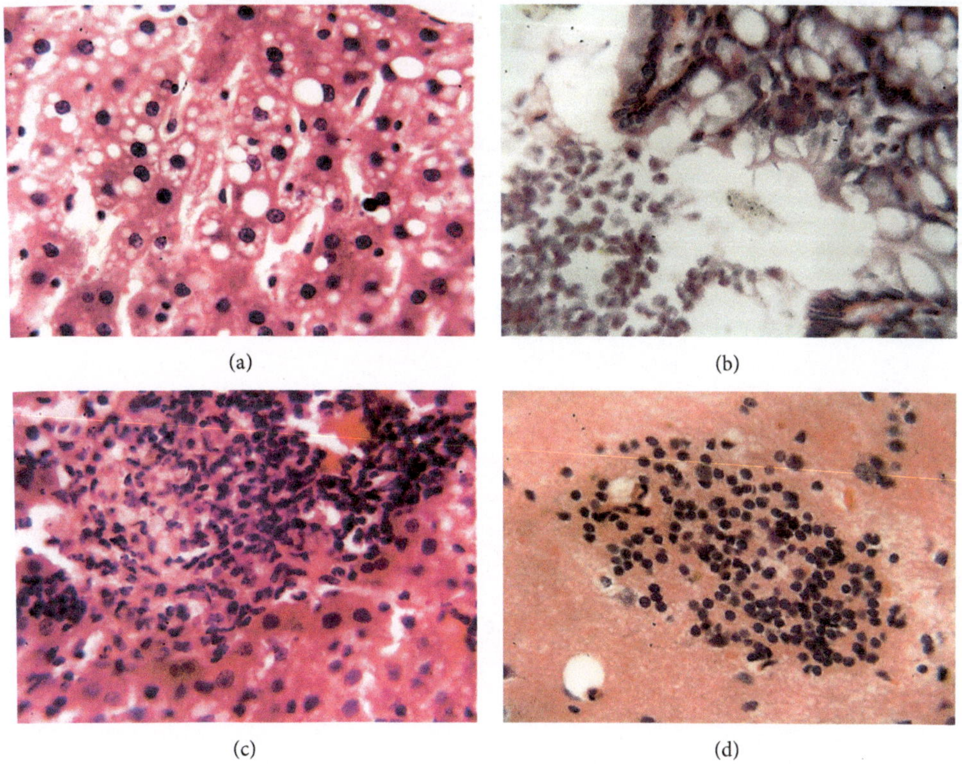

FIGURE 1: (a) Vacuolar degeneration of hepatocytes; (b) *E. cuniculi* spores in intestinal lumen; (c) hepatic granuloma; (d) glial nodule in the cerebral cortex. All HE; 400x.

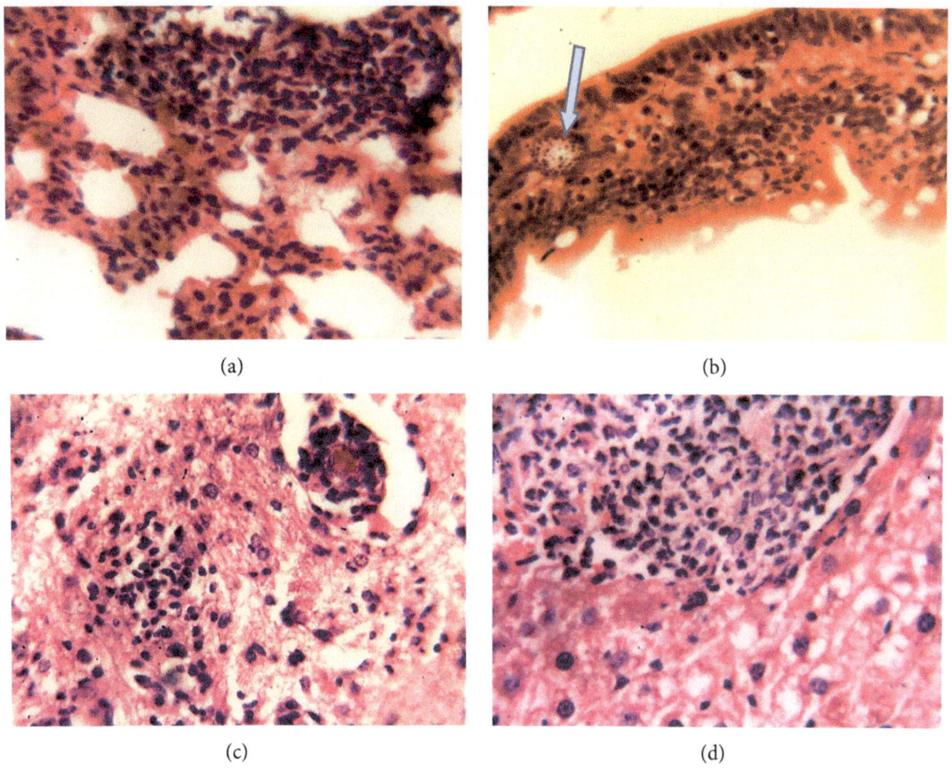

FIGURE 2: (a) Granulomatous lesion in the lung; (b) parasitophorous vacuole containing spores of *E. cuniculi* in enterocyte (arrow); (c) cerebral granuloma; (d) hepatic granuloma. All HE; 400x.

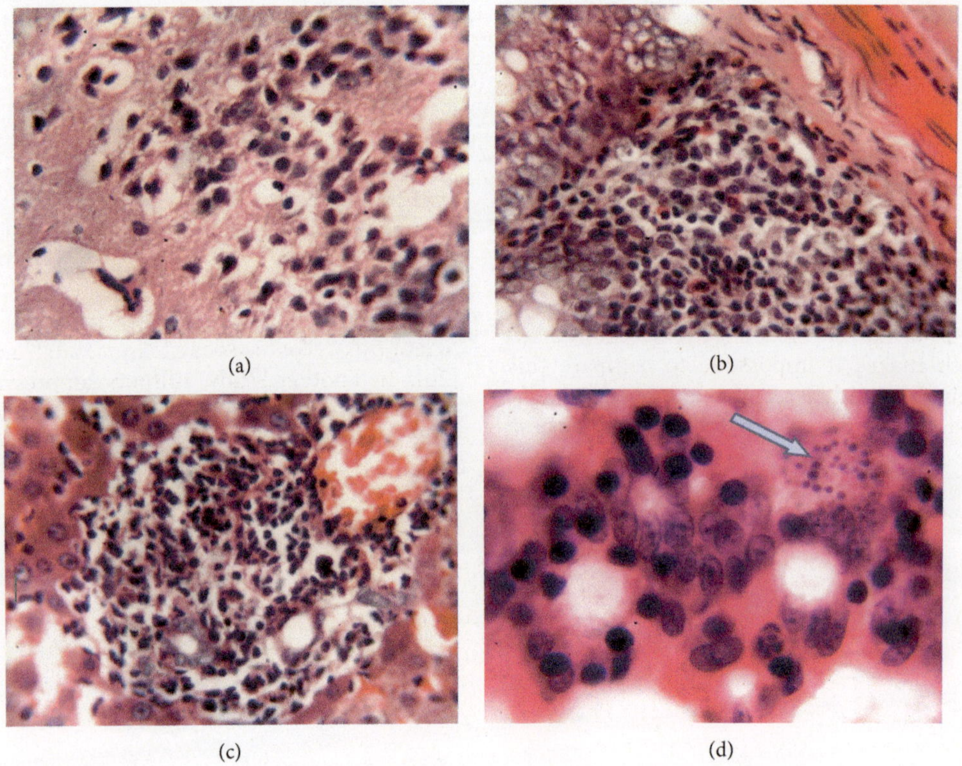

FIGURE 3: (a) Focal infiltration of inflammatory mononuclear cells in the cerebrum; (b) lymphoid hyperplasia in intestinal submucosa; (c) hepatic granuloma; (d) *E. cuniculi* spores in enterocytes (arrow). All HE; 400x.

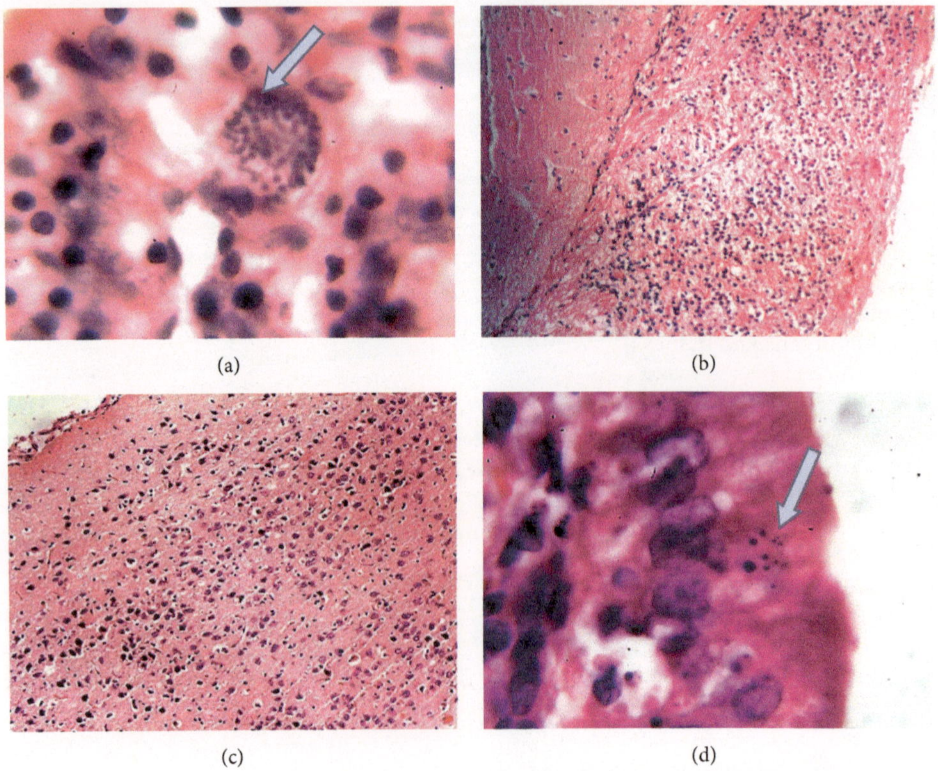

FIGURE 4: (a) *E. cuniculi* spores in parasitophorous vacuole in enterocytes (arrow) (1000x); (b) heavy infiltration of inflammatory mononuclear cells in the meninges and cerebral cortex (100x); (c) diffuse infiltration of inflammatory mononuclear cells in the cerebral cortex (100x); (d) *E. cuniculi* spores in enterocytes (arrow) (1000x). All HE.

of smooth muscle, and mesothelial cells and presence of the parasites in enterocytes (Figure 4(d)).

4. Discussion

In the present study, *E. cuniculi* spores of rabbit origin isolated in Iraq were used to induce the infection in mice, and a special emphasis was made on pathology of the infection in immunocompetent and immunosuppressed mice. Previously, there are no studies on the presence or occurrence and pathology of microsporidial species in Iraq, in both human and animals, which makes it impossible to compare this study with others in Iraq and also makes the current study the first one that identified and diagnosed presence of these microorganisms in Iraq.

Two basic patterns of encephalitozoonosis are known to occur, an acute and clinically detectable disease, frequently resulting in death. This form has been induced in neonates as well as immunocompromised animals [17, 18]. The second form is recognized as a chronic and silent infection, which is mostly seen in healthy animals [17–19].

In second group, histological lesions seen at seven days after infection were in the form of mononuclear inflammatory foci in the brain, liver, lungs, kidneys, and intestines. After that and up to the sixty days after infection, the lesions included vasculitis, gliosis and granulomas of the cerebral cortex, focal interstitial nephritis, vasculitis cholangitis and granulomas in the liver, granulomas in the lungs, enteritis, and depletion of lymphocytes from the germinative centers of the spleen. These lesions have been attributed to subclinical *E. cuniculi* infection; they are similar to what have been found by [20, 21]. Infection with the *E. cuniculi* has been shown to originate in either the intestinal or respiratory epithelia; dissemination of *E. cuniculi* can cause nephritis as well as infections of the sinuses, urinary bladder, and skin; *E. cuniculi* has been also shown to cause keratoconjunctivitis and is capable of infecting the heart, brain, kidneys, and even the tongue; this is due to its ability to disseminate to other parts of the body for the ability of these species to infect macrophages and be transported to other organs and tissues.

Immunosuppressed mice infected with *E. cuniculi* showed similar clinical signs and gross lesions to those exhibited by immunocompetent mice. However, at the ten days after infection necrotic areas were seen in the lungs, and at the sixty days after infection nodular lesions raised over the surface of the lung and hearts were found. Histological lesions included vasculitis and granulomas in meninges and brain, vasculitis and hyperplasia of the peribronchial lymphoid follicles, purulent bronchopneumonia and pleuritis, focal interstitial nephritis, vasculitis, cholangitis and granulomas in the liver, enteritis, and presence of numerous macrophages and cellular debris in the spleen. These changes were similar to those described in experimental infection in athymic nude or severely combined immunodeficient mice [22–24]. Many studies concluded that resistance to infection was mediated by one or more cytokines but not antibody responses; many studies reported that the infection with *E. cuniculi* is dependent on the secretion of IL-12 and INF-γ and then the role of T_1 helper lymphocytes in clearing the pathogens from these organs, this is manifested from infection of *E. cuniculi* to INF-γ null mice and IL-12 deficient mice could not eliminate the infection without presence of T_1 helper lymphocytes [25], so the following sentence is clearly right: resistance or susceptibility to *E. cuniculi* infection is interdependent upon interactions of T_1 helper lymphocytes with the innate arm of immunity.

It has been shown previously that immunosuppression in mice with 100 mg/kg of cyclophosphamide, twice a week by intraperitoneal route, produced an acute form of encephalitozoonosis, recognized as a disseminated and lethal infection [26]. In another study, immunosuppression was induced using intraperitoneal injection of 50 mg/kg of cyclophosphamide twice a week and the infection was chronic [17]. In the present study, the dose schedule of dexamethasone 125 μg/mouse intraperitoneally once a week for 9 weeks leads to the occurrence of chronic infection, and this effect of immunosuppression of dexamethasone is studied widely by other researchers in which they recommended the dose of 125 μg/mouse intraperitoneally once a week to overcome the immune system of mice [11], so it does not need any evaluation of the immunosuppression achieved with the use of dexamethasone [11, 27].

The present study provided evidence that mice and rabbit isolates of *E. cuniculi* are identical and that any difference in the nature and distribution of lesions in the two species may be due to dissimilarities in the hosts. These findings were in accordance with those reported by others [28].

5. Conclusions

In this study, the microsporidial species generally and *Encephalitozoon cuniculi* especially are present in Iraq. This study is considered the first one to report its presence and pathology in Iraq. Also the pathological lesions in both immunocompetent and immunosuppressed mice were typical of *Encephalitozoon cuniculi* infection; however, the lesions were more severe, extensive, and widespread in immunosuppressed mice.

Conflict of Interests

The authors declare that there is no conflict of interests regarding the publication of this paper.

Acknowledgment

This research was supported by the College of Veterinary Medicine, University of Mosul, Mosul, Iraq.

References

[1] P. J. Keeling and C. H. Slamovits, "Simplicity and complexity of microsporidian genomes," *Eukaryotic Cell*, vol. 3, no. 6, pp. 1363–1369, 2004.

[2] E. E. Gill and N. M. Fast, "Assessing the microsporidia-fungi relationship: combined phylogenetic analysis of eight genes," *Gene*, vol. 375, no. 1-2, pp. 103–109, 2006.

[3] A. Mathis, R. Weber, and P. Deplazes, "Zoonotic potential of the microsporidia," *Clinical Microbiology Reviews*, vol. 18, no. 3, pp. 423–445, 2005.

[4] E. S. Didier and L. M. Weiss, "Microsporidiosis: current status," *Current Opinion in Infectious Diseases*, vol. 19, no. 5, pp. 485–492, 2006.

[5] M. Kotkova, B. Sak, D. Kvetonova, and M. Kvac, "Latent microsporidiosis caused by *Encephalitozoon cuniculi* in immunocompetent hosts: a murine model demonstrating the ineffectiveness of the immune system and treatment with albendazole," *Plos One*, vol. 8, no. 4, Article ID e60941, 2013.

[6] J. A. Shadduck, "*Nosema cuniculi*: in vitro isolation," *Science*, vol. 166, no. 3904, pp. 516–517, 1969.

[7] D. Waywa, S. Kongkriengdaj, S. Chaidatch et al., "Protozoan enteric infection in aids related diarrhea in Thailand," *Southeast Asian Journal of Tropical Medicine and Public Health*, vol. 32, no. 2, pp. 151–155, 2001.

[8] P. J. Didier, J. N. Phillips, D. J. Kuebler et al., "Antimicrosporidial activities of fumagillin, TNP-470, ovalicin, and ovalicin derivatives in vitro and in vivo," *Antimicrobial Agents and Chemotherapy*, vol. 50, no. 6, pp. 2146–2155, 2006.

[9] H. I. Al-Sadi and S. S. Al-Mahmood, "Microsporidial infection in some domestic and laboratory animals in Iraq," *International Journal of Basic and Applied Medical Sciences*, vol. 3, no. 3, pp. 78–91, 2013.

[10] L. S. Garcia, *Clinical Microbiology Procedures Handbook*, LSG & Associates, Santa Monica, Calif, USA, 2nd edition, 2007.

[11] L. F. Da Costa De Avila, J. S. V. Da Fonseca, G. F. Dutra et al., "Evaluation of the immunosuppressive effect of cyclophosphamide and dexamethasone in mice with visceral toxocariasis," *Parasitology Research*, vol. 110, no. 1, pp. 443–447, 2012.

[12] L. S. Garcia, "Laboratory identification of the microsporidia," *Journal of Clinical Microbiology*, vol. 40, no. 6, pp. 1892–1901, 2002.

[13] R. Weber, R. T. Bryan, R. L. Owen, C. M. Wilcox, L. Gorelkin, and G. S. Visvesvara, "Improved light-microscopical detection of microsporidia spores in stool and duodenal aspirates," *The New England Journal of Medicine*, vol. 326, no. 3, pp. 161–166, 1991.

[14] N. J. Ryan, G. Sutherland, K. Coughlan et al., "A new trichrome-blue stain for detection of microsporidial species in urine, stool, and nasopharyngeal specimens," *Journal of Clinical Microbiology*, vol. 31, no. 12, pp. 3264–3269, 1993.

[15] S. K. Suvarna, C. Layuton, and J. D. Bancroft, *Bancroft's Theory and Practice of Histological Techniques*, Churchill Livingstone Press, New York, NY, USA, 7th edition, 2013.

[16] K. A. Cooney, J. R. Chappell, R. J. Calle, and B. A. Connally, *Veterinary Euthanasia Techniques: A Practical Guide*, John Wiley & Sons, San Francisco, Calif, USA, 1st edition, 2013.

[17] M. A. Lallo and E. F. Bondan, "Experimental meningoencephalomyelitis by *Encephalitozoon cuniculi* in cyclophosphamide-immunosuppressed mice," *Arquivos de Neuro-Psiquiatria*, vol. 63, no. 2, pp. 246–251, 2005.

[18] J. Gannon, "The course of infection of *Encephalitozoon cuniculi* in immunodeficient and immunocompetent mice," *Laboratory Animals*, vol. 14, no. 3, pp. 189–192, 1980.

[19] E. C. Schmidt and J. A. Shadduck, "Murine encephalitozoonosis model for studying the host-parasite relationship of a chronic infection," *Infection and Immunity*, vol. 40, no. 3, pp. 936–942, 1983.

[20] K. Wasson and R. L. Peper, "Mammalian microsporidiosis," *Veterinary Pathology*, vol. 37, no. 2, pp. 113–128, 2000.

[21] J. R. M. Innes, W. Zeman, J. K. Frenkel, and G. Borner, "Occult endemic encephalitozoonosis of the central nervous system of mice (Swiss-Bagg-O'Grady strain)," *Journal of neuropathology and experimental neurology*, vol. 21, pp. 519–533, 1962.

[22] B. Koudela, J. Vítovec, Z. Kucerová, O. Ditrich, and J. Trávnícek, "The severe combined immunodeficient mouse as a model for *Encephalitozoon cuniculi* microsporidiosis," *Folia Parasitologica*, vol. 40, no. 4, pp. 279–286, 1993.

[23] E. S. Didier, P. W. Varner, P. J. Didier et al., "Experimental microsporidiosis in immunocompetent and immunodeficient mice and monkeys," *Folia Parasitologica*, vol. 41, no. 1, pp. 1–11, 1994.

[24] J. Hermánek, B. Koudela, Z. Kucerová, O. Ditrich, and J. Trávnícek, "Prophylactic and therapeutic immune reconstitution of SCID mice infected with *Encephalitozoon cuniculi*," *Folia Parasitologica*, vol. 40, no. 4, pp. 287–291, 1993.

[25] I. A. Khan and E. S. Didier, *Insights Into the Immune Microsporidia*, Kluwer Academic, Boston, Mass, USA, 2004.

[26] J. M. Castro, M. A. Lallo, D. D. Spadacci-Morena, E. F. Bondan, and M. M. P. Hirschfeld, "Behavior of Encephalitozoon cuniculi with in macrophages from immunosuppressed mice," *Acta Microscopica*, vol. 8, pp. 445–446, 1999.

[27] S. Yang and M. C. Healey, "The immunosuppressive effects of dexamethasone administered in drinking water to C57BL/6N mice infected with *Cryptosporidium parvum*," *Journal of Parasitology*, vol. 79, no. 4, pp. 626–630, 1993.

[28] J. A. Shadduck, W. T. Watson, S. P. Pakes, and A. Cali, "Animal infectivity of *Encephalitozoon cuniculi*," *Journal of Parasitology*, vol. 65, no. 1, pp. 123–129, 1979.

19

Correlation of Various Techniques in Diagnosis of Tuberculous Lymphadenitis on Fine Needle Aspiration Cytology

Brijesh Thakur,[1] Ravi Mehrotra,[2] and Jitendra Singh Nigam[3]

[1] *Department of Pathology, SGRRIM & HS, Patel Nagar Industrial Area, Niranjanpur, Dehradun, Uttarakhand 248001, India*
[2] *Institute of Cytology and Preventive Oncology (ICPO), I-7 Sector 39, Noida, Uttar Pradesh 201303, India*
[3] *Department of Pathology, Deen Dayal Upadhyay Hospital, Harinagar, New Delhi 110066, India*

Correspondence should be addressed to Jitendra Singh Nigam; nigamjs@gmail.com

Academic Editor: Luigi M. Terracciano

Objective. To study the correlation of cytomorphological features in fine needle aspiration smears from patients suspected of having tuberculous lymphadenitis with Ziehl-Neelsen staining (ZN), auramine-rhodamine staining (ARS), and autofluorescence (AF). *Methods.* A total of 145 lymph nodes were aspirated, 3 air-dried smears were stained with Giemsa, Ziehl-Neelsen, and auramine-rhodamine stains, and 1 smear was wet fixed for Papanicolaou staining. Needle washes were incubated in Lowenstein-Jensen medium for culture. Papanicolaou and auramine-rhodamine stained smears were examined under fluorescent microscope using a blue excitation filter (450–480 nm). *Results.* Ninety aspirates were reported on cytomorphology as suggestive of tuberculous lymphadenitis. Smear positivity for *Mycobacteria* by Ziehl-Neelsen method was 26.67% (24/90), while positivity increased to 34.44% (31/90) by auramine-rhodamine and 42.22% (38/90) on autofluorescence. Culture was positive in 27.78% (25/90) aspirates. Using culture as the reference method, the statistical values of ZN, ARS, and AF were as follows: sensitivity 80.0%, 88.0%, 96.0%; specificity 93.85%, 86.15%, 78.46%; positive predictive values 83.33%, 70.97%, 63.16%; and negative predictive values 92.42%, 94.92%, 98.08%, respectively. *Conclusion.* There is a definite advantage of autofluorescence over Ziehl-Neelsen and auramine-rhodamine which is to detect *Mycobacteria*, being more sensitive as well as an inexpensive technique. Autofluorescence can be a useful addition to routine cytology for early diagnosis and effective treatment.

1. Introduction

Tuberculosis (TB) is a major health problem in developing countries. Lymphadenopathy is the most common presentation of extrapulmonary tuberculosis [1, 2]. The precise cause of these enlarged lymph nodes is often difficult to establish by history, physical examination, and radiographic studies alone. Fine needle aspiration cytology (FNAC) has assumed an important role in the evaluation of peripheral adenopathy as a possible noninvasive alternative to excisional biopsy [3].

The cytological criteria for the diagnosis of possible tubercular lymphadenitis have been clearly defined as epithelioid cell granulomas with or without multinucleated giant cells and caseation necrosis [4]. Culture is essential for a definitive diagnosis; however, it takes weeks for identification, and its sensitivity is also relatively low in paucibacillary conditions [5, 6]. Conventional Ziehl-Neelsen (ZN) method for acid-fast bacilli (AFB) plays a key role in the diagnosis and the monitoring of treatment in tuberculosis [7]. Its major disadvantages are low sensitivity, time consuming, and oil immersion use.

Fluorescent microscopy plays an important role for detection of *Mycobacteria* because lower magnifications are used as well as less time is required to examine smears. Fluorescence microscopy using auramine-rhodamine (AR) or Papanicolaou (PAP) staining has been considered to be superior to ZN staining [8, 9]. The method is quick and inexpensive, and it can be focused on those specimens felt to harbour the above infections on morphologic grounds. This suggests that it can provide a rapid, safe, and inexpensive

Table 1: Comparative chart of the results of detection of *Mycobacteria* by Ziehl-Neelsen, auramine-rhodamine stain, and autofluorescence in various types of needle aspirates and cytomorphological patterns in the present study.

Appearance of aspirate	ZN	AR	AF
Blood mixed material	08	15	20
Pus-like material	06	07	09
Cheesy white material	10	08	08
Clear fluid	00	01	01
Cytomorphological patterns			
Granulomatous	10	16	26
Caseating necrotising	12	11	08
Acute inflammation with granuloma	02	04	04

technique for early provisional diagnosis of mycobacterial infection in cytological specimens, but it shows proclivity towards observer bias and problems associated with artifacts.

Basically, the study was an attempt to find out cost-effective, rapid, and sensitive technique which can be used routinely in developing countries for early diagnosis and effective treatment of tuberculous lymphadenitis. The study demonstrated the correlation of the cytomorphological features with various techniques in FNA smears from patients who are suspected of having tuberculous lymphadenitis. We tried to use fluorescent microscopy (auramine-rhodamine staining (ARS) and autofluorescence (AF)) to detect *Mycobacterium* and to compare it with conventional ZN method on lymph node aspirates in cytology.

2. Material and Methods

A total of 145 patients suspected clinically of having tuberculosis with peripheral lymphadenopathy were referred for FNAC to the cytology unit of the Department of Pathology, from August, 2010 to July, 2011. A pretested proforma was used for collection of demographic information, relevant clinical history, and physical examination findings of each patient. Routine investigations including hemogram, mantoux test, and chest radiogram were performed.

Both males and females (>1 yr) with well palpable and enlarged peripheral lymph node were included. Patients with multiple enlarged lymph nodes were enrolled, but a separate study form was not used for each lymph node. Exclusion criteria were age <1 year, very small or nonpalpable lymph nodes, or known cases of malignant, allergic, or skin disorders.

Four smears were made from each aspirate: three air-dried smears were stained with Giemsa, ZN, and AR stains and one was wet fixed for PAP stain for autofluorescence. Needle washes were incubated for culture over Lowenstein-Jensen medium at the same time. If aspirate was found to be inadequate, FNA was repeated at the same time for better retrieval of aspirate. Culture over Lowenstein-Jensen medium was taken as a reference method. PAP and AR stained slides were examined under fluorescent microscope using the blue excitation filter (450–480 nm). *Mycobacteria* appear as greenish yellow, slender, and slightly curved rod-shaped (400X). ZN stained smears were examined for AFB under oil immersion (1000X) using light microscopy which appeared as pinkish, thin curved rod-shaped bacterium measuring 0.5 to 3 micrometer and sometimes as beaded.

3. Results

Out of the 145 cases, 90 (62.1%) aspirates were reported as cytomorphology suggestive of tuberculous lymphadenitis. Rest of the aspirates showed either blood or a reactive population of lymphoid cells only. Culture was also negative for these aspirates. Mantoux test was positive in 64.4% (58/90) cases, but significantly positivity (more than 10 mm.) was in 38.8% of the cases. Chest radiograms showed features of pulmonary tuberculosis in 32.2% (29/90) cases. Depending upon cytomorphological features, three patterns were found in tuberculous lymphadenitis: (1) granulomatous lymphadenitis, (2) caseating necrotising lymphadenitis, and (3) acute inflammation with granulomas. The cytomorphological features observed were granulomatous lymphadenitis in 57.8% (52/90), caseating necrotising lymphadenitis in (left lower inset Figure 1(a)) 31.1% (28/90), and acute inflammation with granuloma (right upper inset Figure 1(a)) in 11.1% (10/90) cases. (Figure 1(a)).

The age ranged from 2–60 years. Sixty% (54/90) of the cases with suggestive cytomorphology of tubercular lymphadenitis were in the range of 10–30 years of age. Male preponderance was noted accounting for 61.1% (55/90) of cases. In this study, the most common site of involved lymph nodes was of the cervical region in 83.3% (75/90) of the cases. On the basis of appearance of aspirate, blood mixed aspirates were found more commonly in 51.1% cases (46/90), followed by pus in 31.1% (28/90), cheesy white material in 15.6% (14/90), and clear fluid in 2.2% (2/90). Smear positivity for *Mycobacteria* by conventional ZN method was 26.7% (24/90), while positivity increased to 34.4% (31/90) by ARS and to 42.2% (38/90) on AF (Figures 1(b), 1(c), and 1(d)). Comparative results of positivity for *Mycobacteria* in various appearances of aspirates and cytomorphological patterns are shown in Table 1. Culture was positive in 27.8% (25/90) cases with suggestive cytomorphology of tubercular lymphadenitis. Using culture as reference method, a comparative chart of ZN, AR, and AF in cases that were reported as cytomorphology suggestive of tuberculous lymphadenitis was shown in Table 2, and the statistical values of ZN, AR, and AF were compared in Table 3.

4. Discussion

FNAC is an easy, reliable outpatient procedure for the diagnosis of tubercular lymphadenitis in palpable superficial lymph nodes, and it is ideally suited for use in resource limited settings, especially in developing countries where tuberculosis is a major cause of morbidity and mortality [10]. Several conditions, including mycosis, bacterial, and viral adenitis, can present the same cytology as does *Mycobacterium* Tubercular adenitis does. Laboratory tests may be essential to establish the cause of such adenopathy correctly, because treatment

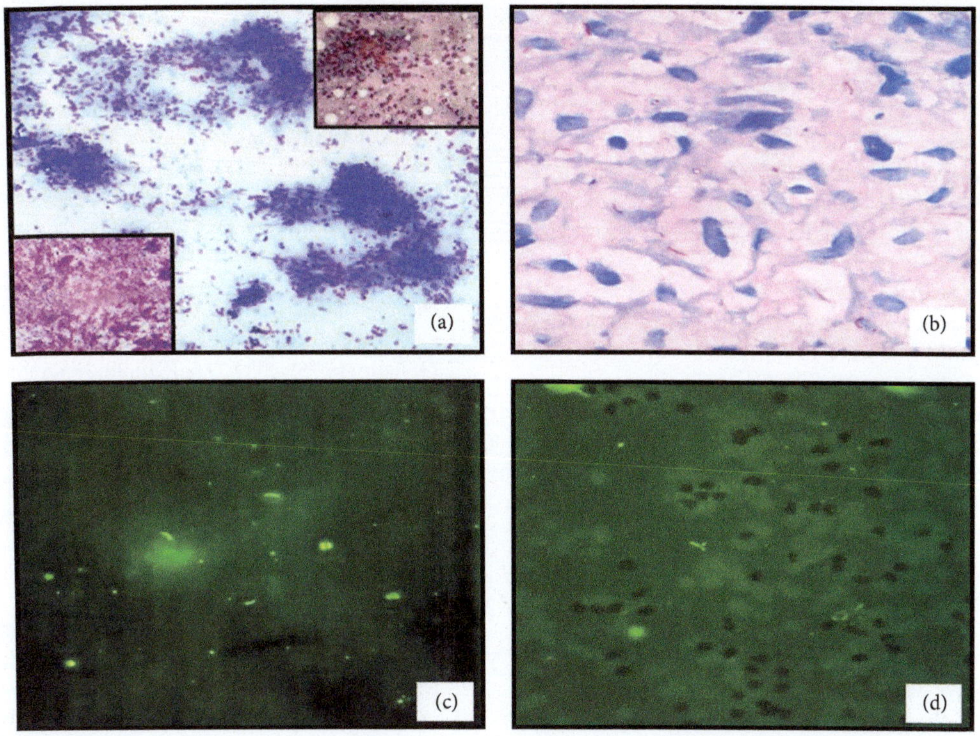

Figure 1: (a) Tuberculous lymphadenitis showing many well-formed epithelioid cell granulomas (Giemas ×100) with Caseating tuberculous lymphadenitis (left lower inset, Giemas ×400) and granuloma along with numerous neutrophils (right upper inset PAP, ×400). (b) Acid fast bacilli (arrows) in a case of tuberculous lymphadenitis (ZN ×1000). (c) Demonstration of bacilli through autofluorescence technique on Papanicolaou stained smears (Pap ×400). (d) Demonstration of bacilli on Auramine-rhodamine stained smear under fluorescent microscopy using blue excitation filter (Auramine-rhodamine ×400).

Table 2: Comparative chart of results of the detection of *Mycobacteria* by Ziehl-Neelsen, auramine-rhodamine stain, and autofluorescence.

	ZN	AR	AF
TP (true positive)	20	22	24
FN (false negative)	05	03	01
FP (false positive)	04	09	14
TN (true negative)	61	56	51

Table 3: Taking culture as a reference method, analysis of statistical values of Ziehl-Neelsen, auramine-rhodamine stain, and autofluorescence.

	ZN	AR	AF
Sensitivity	80.0%	88.0%	96.0%
Specificity	93.85%	86.15%	78.46%
Positive predictive value	83.33%	70.97%	63.16%
Negative predictive value	92.42%	94.42%	98.08%

and prognosis may differ. Demonstration of *Mycobacterium* tuberculosis in fine needle aspirates becomes necessary for an early and accurate treatment. Directed treatment may decrease morbidity and prolong life expectancy.

Auramine-rhodamine involves the use of toxic and carcinogenic substances, but it requires less time, low power examination and shows superiority to ZN staining as auramine combined more readily with mycolic acid than the conventional carbol-fuchsin acid-fast stain. In comparison to both, AF on PAP stained smears provides a safe, inexpensive, and exposure-free diagnostic procedure along with more positive results. Even this technique does not require any addition to the standard PAP stain. Single PAP stained smear can be used for routine light microscopy to determine cytological diagnosis and for demonstrating *Mycobacteria* using fluorescent microscope. *Mycobacteria* AF, also known as primary fluorescence, is seen as brilliant yellowish green bacilli, thin, and slightly curved with polar enhancement and sometimes even beaded appearance.

Previous studies for detection of AFB from various clinical specimens, comprising sputum, CSF, fine needle aspirate, pus, and miscellaneous body fluids which were examined by ZN and AR staining techniques, showed that AR was 86.6% sensitive as compared to ZN 67.3% sensitive with more marked difference in extrapulmonary samples [8]. In other studies on FNA smears of lymph nodes, autofluorescence was found to be more sensitive than ZN staining [11, 12], but as compared to cytodiagnosis, it was less sensitive [9].

The present study was an attempt to use fluorescent microscopy (ARS and AF) to detect *Mycobacterium* and to compare it with conventional ZN method on lymph node aspirates in cytology. During the present study by using culture as the reference method, true statistical values of these techniques were given in Table 3. By these results, AF was noted to be more sensitive in identifying the acid fast bacilli than ZN stain; however, ZN was found to be more specific than AF.

A comparison between AF and ARS was also done in the present study. It was found that autofluorescence was more sensitive for identifying the bacilli. There was only one case (1.1%) which showed ARS positivity on smear but was negative by AF. However, 8 cases (8.89%) were AF positive, but they were found to be ARS negative. No comparative study between autofluorescence and auramine-rhodamine staining on FNAC smears could be found in literature searched.

However, some organisms exhibiting spontaneous emission spectra following excitation at specific wavelengths may pose problem in the detection of *Mycobacteria*. These organisms such as spore-forminglike *Bacillus subtilis*, nonspore-forming bacteria like *Staphylococcus aureus*, *Nocardia*, budding yeast may produce fluorescence [13]. Even air-drying artifacts in Papanicolaou stained smears may produce problems in identifying *Mycobacteria* by fluorescent microscopy. There is also increased frequency of false positivity of AF due to subjective biased errors and interobserver's variability.

5. Conclusion

FNAC as a primary diagnostic procedure in tubercular lymphadenitis has demonstrated the adaptability of autofluorescence on Papanicolaou stain which is the most frequently utilized stain for cytologic specimens and autofluorescence on the Pap smear is a rapid and relatively simple method. This study explores the utility of autofluorescence as an adjunct to routine cytology as it is simple, rapid, and cost-effective screening technique especially in developing countries where tuberculosis is widely prevalent and shows continued presence of infection in the community. However, limited and cautious use of AF is necessary because of its increased false-positivity rate and subjective-biased errors. AF should be used in addition to other ancillary techniques.

References

[1] M. C. Dandapat, B. M. Mishra, S. P. Dash, and P. K. Kar, "Peripheral lymph node tuberculosis: a review of 80 cases," *British Journal of Surgery*, vol. 77, no. 8, pp. 911–912, 1990.

[2] S. K. Lau, S. Kwan, J. Lee, and W. I. Wei, "Source of tubercle bacilli in cervical lymph nodes: a prospective study," *Journal of Laryngology and Otology*, vol. 105, no. 7, pp. 558–561, 1991.

[3] R. Pahwa, S. Hedau, S. Jain et al., "Assessment of possible tuberculous lymphadenopathy by PCR compared to non-molecular methods," *Journal of Medical Microbiology*, vol. 54, no. 9, pp. 873–878, 2005.

[4] K. K. Singh, M. Muralidhar, A. Kumar et al., "Comparison of in house polymerase chain reaction with conventional techniques for the detection of Mycobacterium tuberculosis DNA in granulomatous lymphadenopathy," *Journal of Clinical Pathology*, vol. 53, no. 5, pp. 355–361, 2000.

[5] V. S. Rajan and Y. S. Goh, "Intermittent chemotherapy in the treatment of tuberculosis cutis. A preliminary report," *British Journal of Dermatology*, vol. 87, no. 3, pp. 270–273, 1972.

[6] T. M. Daniel, "The rapid diagnosis of tuberculosis: a selective review," *Journal of Laboratory and Clinical Medicine*, vol. 116, no. 3, pp. 277–282, 1990.

[7] V. Annam, M. H. Kulkarni, and R. B. Puranik, "Comparison of the modified fluorescent method and conventional Ziehl-Neelsen method in the detection of acidfast bacilli in lymphnode aspirates," *CytoJournal*, vol. 6, article 13, 2009.

[8] A. Jain, A. Bhargava, and S. K. Agarwal, "A comparative study of two commonly used staining techniques for acid fast bacilli in clinical specimens," *Indian Journal of Tuberculosis*, vol. 49, pp. 161–162, 2002.

[9] C. A. Wright, Y. van Zyl, S. M. Burgess, L. Blumberg, and G. Leiman, "Mycobacterial autofluorescence in papanicolaou-stained lymph node aspirates: a glimmer in the dark?" *Diagnostic Cytopathology*, vol. 30, no. 4, pp. 257–260, 2004.

[10] C. A. Wright, A. C. Hesseling, C. Bamford, S. M. Burgess, R. Warren, and B. J. Marais, "Fine-needle aspiration biopsy: a fi rst-line diagnostic procedure in paediatric tuberculosis suspects with peripheral lymphadenopathy?" *International Journal of Tuberculosis and Lung Disease*, vol. 13, no. 11, pp. 1373–1379, 2009.

[11] C. A. Wright, M. van der Burg, D. Geiger, J. G. Noordzij, S. M. Burgess, and B. J. Marais, "Diagnosing mycobacterial lymphadenitis in children using fine needle aspiration biopsy: cytomorphology, ZN staining and autofluorescence-making more of less," *Diagnostic Cytopathology*, vol. 36, no. 4, pp. 245–251, 2008.

[12] P. Joshi, M. Singh, A. Bhargava, M. Singh, and R. Mehrotra, "Autofluorescence—an important ancillary technique for the detection of Mycobacterium tuberculosis: revisited," *Diagnostic Cytopathology*, vol. 41, no. 4, pp. 330–334, 2012.

[13] S. Patiño, L. Alamo, M. Cimino et al., "Autofluorescence of mycobacteria as a tool for detection of Mycobacterium tuberculosis," *Journal of Clinical Microbiology*, vol. 46, no. 10, pp. 3296–3302, 2008.

Specimens from Biopsies of Colorectal Polyps Often Harbor Additional Diagnoses

Shefali Chopra and Mark Li-cheng Wu

Department of Pathology and Laboratory Medicine, University of California Irvine School of Medicine, Irvine, CA 92868, USA

Correspondence should be addressed to Mark Li-cheng Wu; mlwu@uci.edu

Academic Editor: Oscar Cummings

Objectives. The utility of examining specimens from colorectal biopsies of polyps for nonneoplastic diseases is currently unknown. Our objectives were to characterize such additional diagnoses that could be rendered. *Methods.* We retrospectively and prospectively reviewed specimens from endoscopic biopsies of colorectal polyps obtained during routine screening or surveillance. *Results.* 17 of 168 specimens (10.1%) contained additional diagnoses, including schistosomiasis, eosinophilic colitis, intestinal spirochetosis, melanosis coli, and other entities. These findings were easily overlooked because they often affected mucosa that was spared by the polyps or were often evident only at high magnification. Schistosomiasis, eosinophilic colitis, and intestinal spirochetosis were clinically occult. *Conclusions.* Specimens from biopsies of colorectal polyps often harbor other diagnoses, in addition to polyps, and can be simultaneously screened for polyps and examined for nonneoplastic diseases. Detection of other diagnoses in addition to polyps requires awareness, examination at high magnification, and examination of areas spared by the polyps.

1. Introduction

Specimens from endoscopic biopsies of putative colorectal lesions usually show traditional nonserrated adenomas, serrated polyps, or variants of normal mucosa. These entities generally are easily and rapidly diagnosed at low magnification. Consequently, pathologists are tempted to examine these specimens quickly and only at low magnification, to assume that these specimens will harbor only polyps or variants of normal mucosa, and to refrain from examining these specimens further at high magnification once polyps are diagnosed. Directed review of these specimens might reveal other diagnoses, in addition to polyps. Pathologists might overlook such second diagnoses for various reasons. However, such second diagnoses might be significant. We reviewed specimens from biopsies of colorectal polyps to characterize second diagnoses that could be rendered in this setting and to demonstrate that these specimens could be examined for nonneoplastic diseases.

2. Materials and Methods

The study was approved by the Institutional Review Board of the University of California, Irvine, USA, on November 7, 2005 as protocol HS number: 2005-4646. The study was carried out in 2 phases. The first phase was designed to determine prevalence, and the second phase was designed to determine incidence.

During the first phase, consecutive specimens from endoscopic colorectal biopsies of polyps accessioned at our institution during a 1-month interval, from July 1, 2003 to August 1, 2003, were retrospectively reviewed by both of us, who are gastrointestinal pathologists, with special effort to render second diagnoses in addition to polyps. Only specimens that had polyps, broadly defined as protruding pathologic mucosal lesions [1], confirmed histologically were eligible for review. All original diagnoses were made by 5 other pathologists, who were general surgical pathologists. These pathologists were unaware of our study. During the second phase, specimens from 100 consecutive histologically confirmed polyps obtained from endoscopic colorectal biopsies accessioned to 1 of us (M. L.-c. Wu) at our institution during the course of normal signout were prospectively accrued during the interval July 1, 2007–September 11, 2007. These specimens were examined with knowledge of our study and with special effort to render second diagnoses in addition to polyps. For both phases, this special effort consisted of examining all sections on each slide, at low magnification and high magnification, and examining the entire surface area of each section including mucosa affected by polyps and mucosa spared by polyps. Specimens from both phases with additional diagnoses were reviewed by both of us for confirmation.

Pathology reports and requisitions for all specimens were reviewed. Corresponding reports from endoscopy were reviewed for each specimen, in either phase, for which additional diagnoses were rendered. Diagnoses were considered clinically occult if the requisitions or corresponding reports from endoscopy lacked the mention of the diagnoses or lacked the mention of findings that could be reasonably attributed to the diagnoses. Excluded from the entire study were specimens from biopsies of putative lesions that lacked polyps histologically. All specimens were processed routinely, formalin-fixed, and paraffin-embedded. All histologic sections were cut 4 microns thick and stained with hematoxylin and eosin. Microscopy was performed with a conventional multiheaded optical microscope (BX45, Olympus, Melville, NY, USA). All diagnoses were rendered according to standard criteria [1–4].

3. Results

For the first phase, 78 specimens were diagnosed as polyps by original pathologists in the 1-month interval. We reclassified 3 hyperplastic polyps and 1 tubular adenoma as normal mucosa and excluded these specimens from further study. We reclassified 1 mucosal prolapse, 1 hyperplastic polyp, and 1 inflammatory polyp, as leiomyoma, sessile serrated adenoma, and tubular adenoma, respectively. We confirmed all other original diagnoses. A few specimens had multiple polyps. The first phase therefore eventually consisted of 74 specimens, with 78 histologically confirmed polyps. These polyps were from 52 patients, ages 43 to 74, including 31 men and 21 women. The 78 polyps included 48 polyps in men and 30 polyps in women.

Of the 74 specimens, additional diagnoses were retrospectively detected by us in 7 specimens (9.5%). These diagnoses included the following: mucosal prolapse (Figure 1) (in 2 specimens with hyperplastic polyps and 1 specimen with tubular adenoma), melanosis coli (Figures 2(a) and 2(b)) (in 2 specimens with tubular adenomas), hyperplastic polyp (in 1 specimen with tubular adenoma), and eosinophilic colitis (Figure 3) (in 1 specimen with tubular adenoma).

The patient for whom we diagnosed eosinophilic colitis was asymptomatic. With this caveat, we rendered the diagnosis of eosinophilic colitis based on compelling morphology that satisfied recently proposed criteria [3]. Microscopy showed the entire specimen, including areas remote from the polyp, to have an extremely high density of eosinophils with greater than 120 eosinophils per 600x field, frequent eosinophilic cryptitis and crypt abscesses, degranulated eosinophils, submucosal eosinophils, and absence of neutrophils in nonpolypoid mucosa.

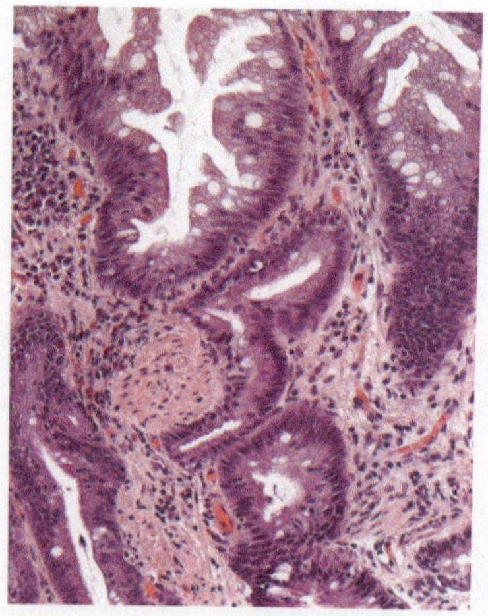

FIGURE 1: Mucosal prolapse in specimen with hyperplastic polyp. Only small focus of smooth muscle present (left of center) (H&E, ×200).

Mention of all of these additional diagnoses, except for eosinophilic colitis, was absent from the original pathology reports. Therefore, 6 of 7 additional diagnoses were potentially overlooked by original pathologists.

For the second phase, the 100 polyps were accrued after examining 94 specimens. A few specimens had multiple polyps. The 94 specimens were from 55 patients, including 27 men and 28 women, ages 45 to 82. The 100 polyps included 57 polyps in men and 43 polyps in women.

Of the 94 specimens, additional diagnoses were prospectively detected in 10 specimens (10.6%) by 1 of us (M. L.-c. Wu). These diagnoses included the following: melanosis coli (in 4 specimens with tubular adenomas and 1 specimen with hyperplastic polyp), mucosal prolapse (in 2 specimens with hyperplastic polyps), schistosomiasis (Figures 4(a), 4(b), and 4(c)) (in 1 specimen with adenocarcinoma and 1 specimen with hyperplastic polyp), and intestinal spirochetosis (Figure 5) (in 1 specimen with sessile serrated adenoma), and they were confirmed retrospectively by both of us.

For the entire study, a final total of 168 specimens were included, and 17 additional diagnoses were rendered, for a rate of 10.1%. Clinical information obtained from pathology requisitions and corresponding notes from endoscopy indicated that all endoscopies were performed for screening or surveillance for polyps and that all patients were asymptomatic.

Several factors potentially contributed to difficulty in rendering additional diagnoses. The additional diagnostic findings were easily overlooked in many scenarios (Figures 1, 2(a), 2(b), 3, 4(a), 4(b), 4(c), and 5), including when the findings were small, focal, in nonpolypoid mucosa, in otherwise normal mucosa, or clinically occult.

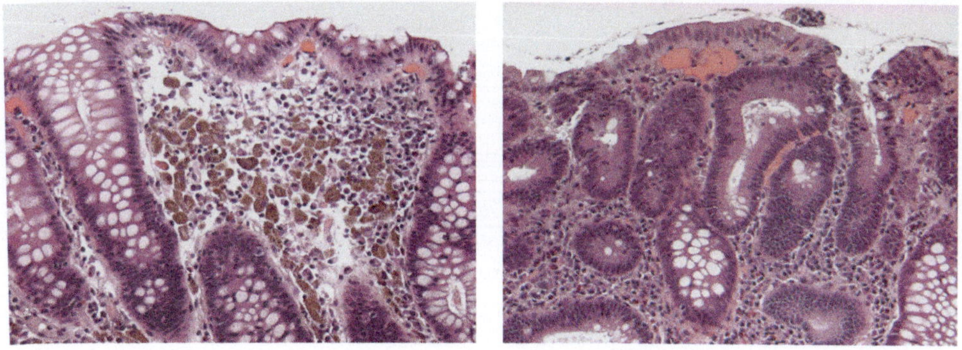

(a) (b)

FIGURE 2: Melanosis coli in specimen with tubular adenoma. (a) Melanosis affects nonpolypoid mucosa (H&E, ×200) and (b) spares adenoma (H&E, ×200).

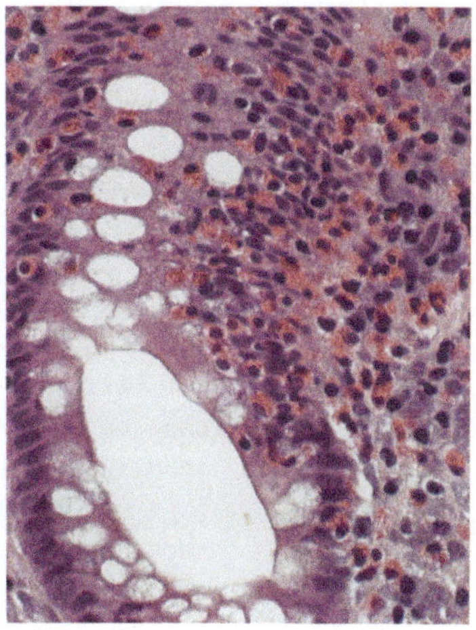

FIGURE 3: Eosinophilic colitis in specimen with tubular adenoma. Nonpolypoid mucosa contains abundant eosinophils in lamina propria, eosinophilic cryptitis, and absence of neutrophils (H&E, ×600).

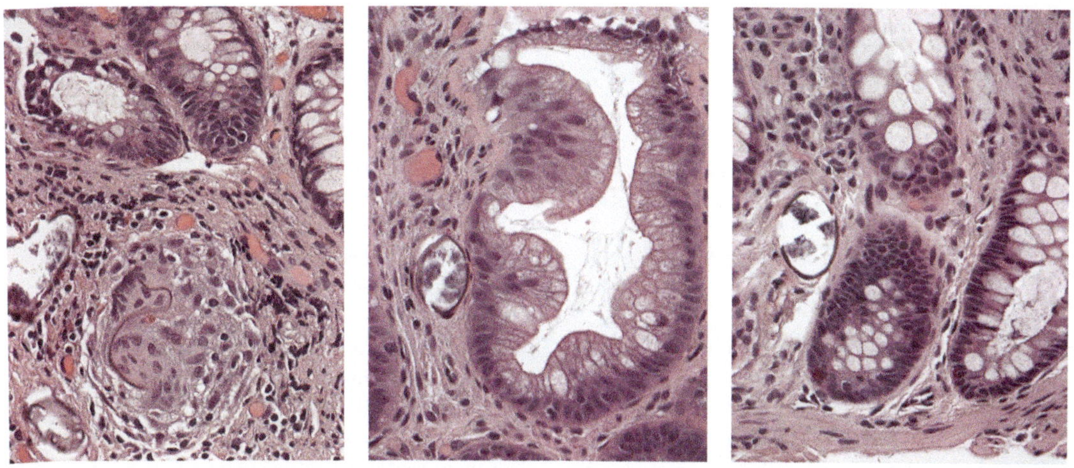

(a) (b) (c)

FIGURE 4: Schistosomiasis in specimens with adenocarcinoma and hyperplastic polyp. (a) Nonpolypoid mucosa beside adenocarcinoma (not shown) shows schistosomiasis and granuloma (H&E, ×400). (b) Schistosomiasis affects hyperplastic polyp (H&E, ×400) and (c) adjacent, otherwise normal nonpolypoid mucosa (H&E, ×400).

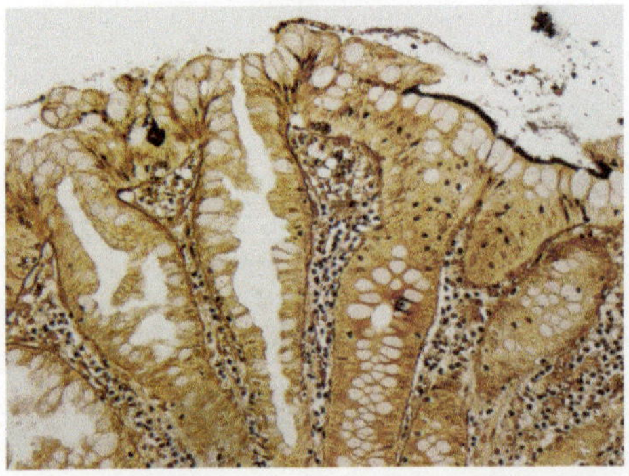

Figure 5: Intestinal spirochetosis in specimen with sessile serrated adenoma. Spirochetes colonize surface of otherwise normal mucosa present beside polyp (top right) and present focally between serrated crypts (top left) (Warthin-Starry, ×200).

Table 1: Histology of polyps.

Histology	Phase 1	Phase 2
Tubular adenomas	49	34
Tubulovillous adenomas	2	10
Adenocarcinomas	2	2
Hyperplastic polyps	22	46
Sessile serrated adenomas	2	7
Leiomyomas	1	0
Neuroendocrine tumors	0	1

Table 2: Distribution of polyps.

Site	Phase 1	Phase 2
Cecum	9	11
Ascending colon	15	11
Hepatic flexure	1	3
Transverse colon	1	11
Splenic flexure	2	1
Descending colon	9	9
Sigmoid colon	12	28
Rectum	15	24
Unspecified	14	2

Tables 1, 2, and 3 summarize the histology and distribution of the polyps and the additional diagnoses.

4. Discussion

Specimens taken for the purpose of evaluating 1 disease may contain additional, incidental diagnostic findings, which may be related or unrelated to the primary disease. These additional diagnoses are easily overlooked, because of many reasons: (1) additional diagnoses may be associated with morphologic changes that are considerably smaller than those of the primary disease and might only be appreciated at high magnification or by purposefully examining the slide for incidental findings; (2) attention of pathologists is usually directed toward the primary disease due to habit and due to bias from the clinical request, and hence attention is diverted away from incidental findings; (3) incidental findings may occupy seemingly extraneous tissue, from the same organ or unrelated organs, that usually is histologically normal [5]; (4) even if incidental findings are detected, pathologists that lack expertise in a particular specialty may fail to recognize incidental findings as significant. It is important for pathologists to report such additional diagnoses because these additional diagnoses may have pathologic, endoscopic, or clinical significance or may be clinically occult. This process transforms these specimens into invaluable, cost-effective tools to detect unexpected diagnoses. Examining for additional diagnoses detects disease early, guides therapy, and eliminates morbidity and financial burden associated with repeat biopsies and advanced disease. Colonoscopy carries a 0.07% incidence of iatrogenic perforation [6] and costs approximately $3081 by itself but costs significantly more with biopsy, anesthesia, or immunohistochemistry or if performed on an inpatient [7].

Table 3: Additional diagnoses detected at colorectal biopsy for polyps.

Additional diagnoses	Factors potentially contributing to diagnostic difficulty
Mucosal prolapse	Only small focus affected
Melanosis coli	Nonpolypoid mucosa preferentially affected Polyps relatively or completely spared
Eosinophilic colitis	Confusion with reaction to adenoma Clinically occult
Schistosomiasis	Minute ova Affected nonpolypoid mucosa otherwise normal or focally normal Clinically occult
Intestinal spirochetosis	Minute bacteria Confined to nonpolypoid mucosa Affected nonpolypoid mucosa otherwise normal Clinically occult

The concept of purposefully examining specimens to detect other, secondary diagnoses has been studied in the setting of genitourinary pathology and hepatic pathology. Specimens from nephrectomies performed to stage primary renal neoplasia were recently shown to occasionally contain incidental nonneoplastic disease [8]. Specimens from prostatic core biopsies often contain incidental pieces of rectal mucosa that occasionally harbors clinically significant rectal pathology or causes diagnostic difficulty [5]. Specimens from hepatic core biopsies obtained for the purpose of grading and staging chronic viral hepatitis often contain other diagnoses [9]. To our knowledge, our study is the first to apply this concept to colorectal biopsies.

Our results show that the rate of additional diagnoses in specimens from biopsies of colorectal polyps in asymptomatic patients at time of screening or surveillance is approximately 10%. This rate is predictably similar to that found in a recent study, which detected abnormal histology in 11% of specimens from colorectal biopsies of patients with normal endoscopy and without diarrhea [10]. Furthermore, this rate is predictably much less than that found in a previous study, which detected abnormal histology in 32.1% of patients with normal colonoscopy and with chronic diarrhea [11].

Although some additional diagnoses had minor clinical impact, all had pathologic or endoscopic significance. For reasons yet to be elucidated, melanosis coli generally avoids adenomas, as our study demonstrated. Adenomas spared by melanosis coli appear endoscopically as pale patches, which help endoscopists locate adenomas [12]. Our study also demonstrated that intestinal spirochetosis and schistosomiasis may be asymptomatic, involve normal or abnormal mucosa, and involve polyps [13–19]. To our knowledge, our study is the first to report schistosomiasis coincidentally affecting a hyperplastic polyp. Although our case of eosinophilic colitis was easily diagnosed, caution must be exercised to avoid overdiagnosing colitis, because polyps commonly attract eosinophils and lymphocytes [20–22]. Mucosal prolapse may mimic hyperplastic polyps, sessile serrated adenomas, traditional nonserrated adenomas, inflammatory bowel disease, and other entities [4, 23].

Specimens from colorectal biopsies of polyps can and should be simultaneously screened for polyps and examined for additional diagnoses. Awareness of the possibility of second diagnoses, examination of nonpolypoid areas, and examination at high magnification are necessary to avoid overlooking these diagnoses.

Conflict of Interests

The authors declare that there is no conflict of interests regarding the publication of this paper.

Acknowledgment

This research was performed without specific financial support and was presented in part in abstract form at the College of American Pathologists '08 annual meeting, poster exhibits session, San Diego, CA, USA, September 25, 2008.

References

[1] K. J. Lewin, R. H. Riddell, and W. M. Weinstein, Eds., *Gastrointestinal Pathology and Its Clinical Implications*, Igaku-Shoin, New York, NY, USA, 1992.

[2] D. C. Snover, J. R. Jass, C. Fenoglio-Preiser, and K. P. Batts, "Serrated polyps of the large intestine: a morphologic and molecular review of an evolving concept," *The American Journal of Clinical Pathology*, vol. 124, no. 3, pp. 380–391, 2005.

[3] J. M. Hurrell, R. M. Genta, and S. D. Melton, "Histopathologic diagnosis of eosinophilic conditions in the gastrointestinal tract," *Advances in Anatomic Pathology*, vol. 18, no. 5, pp. 335–348, 2011.

[4] B. Singh, N. J. M. Mortensen, and B. F. Warren, "Histopathological mimicry in mucosal prolapse," *Histopathology*, vol. 50, no. 1, pp. 97–102, 2007.

[5] A. Ashton-Sager and M. L. Wu, "Incidental rectal mucosa obtained via transrectal ultrasound-guided prostatic core biopsies," *International Journal of Surgical Pathology*, vol. 15, no. 1, pp. 26–30, 2007.

[6] N. E. Samalavicius, D. Kazanavicius, R. Lunevicius et al., "Incidence, risk, management, and outcomes of iatrogenic full-thickness large bowel injury associated with 56, 882 colonoscopies in 14 Lithuanian hospitals," *Surgical Endoscopy*, vol. 27, pp. 1628–1635, 2013.

[7] "Cost of a Colonoscopy: Consumer information and prices paid," 2008, http://health.costhelper.com/colonoscopy.html.

[8] B. Sarsık, A. Simşir, M. Yılmaz, K. Yörükoğlu, and S. Sen, "Spectrum of nontumoral renal pathologies in tumor nephrectomies: nontumoral renal parenchyma changes," *Annals of Diagnostic Pathology*, vol. 17, pp. 176–182, 2013.

[9] V. Nair, S. E. Fischer, and O. A. Adeyi, "Non-viral-related pathologic findings in liver needle biopsy specimens from patients with chronic viral hepatitis," *The American Journal of Clinical Pathology*, vol. 133, no. 1, pp. 127–132, 2010.

[10] O. H. O'Mahony, M. Burgoyne, and J. J. Going, "Specific histological abnormalities are more likely in biopsies of endoscopically normal large bowel after the age of 60 years," *Histopathology*, vol. 61, pp. 1209–1213, 2012.

[11] J. G. N. Da Silva, T. De Brito, A. O. M. Cintra Damião, A. A. Laudanna, and A. M. Sipahi, "Histologic study of colonic mucosa in patients with chronic diarrhea and normal colonoscopic findings," *Journal of Clinical Gastroenterology*, vol. 40, no. 1, pp. 44–48, 2006.

[12] S. J. van Weyenberg, F. Hoentjen, F. Thunnissen, and C. J. Mulder, "Pseudomelanosis coli and adenomatous polyps," *Journal of Gastrointestinal and Liver Diseases*, vol. 20, no. 3, p. 233, 2011.

[13] J. J. Godyn, R. Siderits, and A. Hazra, "Schistosoma mansoni in colon and liver," *Archives of Pathology and Laboratory Medicine*, vol. 129, no. 4, pp. 544–545, 2005.

[14] X. Yu, P. Chen, J. Xu, X. S. Xiao Sen, and Z. Shan, "Histological classification of schistosomal egg induced polyps of colon and their clinical significance: An analysis of 272 cases," *Chinese Medical Journal*, vol. 104, no. 1, pp. 64–70, 1991.

[15] M. Körner and J.-O. Gebbers, "Clinical significance of human intestinal spirochetosis: a morphologic approach," *Infection*, vol. 31, no. 5, pp. 341–349, 2003.

[16] A. Kansagra, N. Nagaria, and S. Ahlawat, "Asymptomatic colon adenoma associated with Schistosoma mansoni," *Digestive and Liver Disease*, vol. 42, no. 7, pp. 526–527, 2010.

[17] A. R. E.-S. Mohamed, M. A. Al Karawi, and M. I. Yasawy, "Schistosomal colonic disease," *Gut*, vol. 31, no. 4, pp. 439–442, 1990.

[18] A. Calderaro, C. Gorrini, S. Montecchini et al., "Intestinal spirochaetosis associated with hyperplastic and adenomatous colonic polyps," *Pathology Research and Practice*, vol. 208, no. 3, pp. 177–180, 2012.

[19] W.-C. Li, Z.-G. Pan, and Y.-H. Sun, "Sigmoid colonic carcinoma associated with deposited ova of Schistosoma japonicum: a case report," *World Journal of Gastroenterology*, vol. 12, no. 37, pp. 6077–6079, 2006.

[20] J. Moezzi, N. Gopalswamy, R. J. Haas Jr., R. J. Markert, S. Suryaprasad, and M. S. Bhutani, "Stromal eosinophilia in colonic epithelial neoplasms," *The American Journal of Gastroenterology*, vol. 95, no. 2, pp. 520–523, 2000.

[21] S. Kiziltaş, S. Sezgin Ramadan, A. Topuzoğlu, and S. Küllü, "Does the severity of tissue eosinophilia of colonic neoplasms reflect their malignancy potential?" *Turkish Journal of Gastroenterology*, vol. 19, pp. 239–244, 2008.

[22] A. D. Polydorides, B. Mukherjee, S. B. Gruber, B. J. McKenna, H. D. Appelman, and J. K. Greenson, "Adenoma-infiltrating Lymphocytes (AILs) are a potential marker of hereditary non-polyposis colorectal cancer," *The American Journal of Surgical Pathology*, vol. 32, no. 11, pp. 1661–1666, 2008.

[23] C. C. Huang, W. L. Frankel, T. Doukides, X. P. Zhou, W. Zhao, and M. M. Yearsley, "Prolapse-related changes are a confounding factor in misdiagnosis of sessile serrated adenomas in the rectum," *Human Pathology*, vol. 44, pp. 480–486, 2013.

Comparison of Immunohistochemical Expression of Antiapoptotic Protein Survivin in Normal Oral Mucosa, Oral Leukoplakia, and Oral Squamous Cell Carcinoma

Amita Negi,[1] Abhiney Puri,[2] Rakhi Gupta,[2] Rajat Nangia,[2] Alisha Sachdeva,[2] and Megha Mittal[2]

[1] *Department of Oral Pathology & Microbiology, Himachal Dental College, Sunder Nagar, District Mandi, Himachal Pradesh 175002, India*
[2] *Department of Oral Pathology & Microbiology, Himachal Institute of Dental Sciences, Paonta Sahib, District Sirmour, Himachal Pradesh 173025, India*

Correspondence should be addressed to Amita Negi; dramitanegi@gmail.com

Academic Editor: Runjan Chetty

Background. Oral squamous cell carcinoma is the sixth most frequent malignant tumor worldwide and the third most common cancers in developing countries. Oral leukoplakia is the best-known precursor lesion of oral squamous cell carcinoma. The aim of the present study was to compare immunohistochemical expression of antiapoptotic protein survivin in normal oral mucosa, oral leukoplakia, and oral squamous cell carcinoma. *Method.* Total 45 specimens of formalin fixed paraffin embedded tissue blocks, 15 in each of the following: normal oral mucosa, leukoplakia, and oral squamous cell carcinoma were used for the study. Immunohistochemical reaction for survivin protein was performed for the 4 μm thick histological sections taken on positively charged slides. *Results.* 20% normal mucosa cases, 53.33% cases of leukoplakia, and 80% of oral squamous cell carcinoma were found out to be survivin positive. One way ANOVA test indicated statistically significant difference of survivin expression between the three different groups ($p < 0.001$). *Conclusion.* A high incidence of survivin protein expression in oral epithelial dysplasia and squamous cell carcinoma samples indicate that survivin protein expression may be an early event in initiation and progression of oral squamous cell carcinoma.

1. Introduction

Carcinoma in the oral region is the sixth most frequent malignant tumor throughout the world and the third commonly occurring cancer in developing countries, with especially high incidence in South-East Asian countries and India [1, 2]. Oral cavity is amongst one of the five major locations of cancer in India, representing 19% of the total count of cancer in males and 7% cases of cancer in females. Approximately 90% of oral malignancies are squamous cell carcinomas (SCC), arising in the mucosal lining. The predominance of oral carcinoma is because of extensive consumption of tobacco and its products in India [3].

In the oral mucosa, almost all carcinomas are preceded by occurrence of a precancerous lesion, progressing into cancer at a later stage. Oral leukoplakia is the most well recognized forerunner of oral cancer. Risk of malignant transformation is variable but many studies have reported that the progression of precursor lesions into cancer is between <1 and 18% [4].

Oral cancer develops as a result of increased lack of genetic stability that involves stimulation of oncogenes and switching off the tumor suppressor genes. In their early stages, most of the human cancers are characterized by loss of cellular systems that regulate cell cycle progress, cell death versus growth balance, and apoptosis [5].

It is now well established that, in a tumor cell, active inhibition of apoptosis occurs due to unchecked division along with numerous genetic modifications. The molecular mechanisms in the progression of apoptosis as well as its regulating factors are extremely conserved in evolution. In recent years, a unique gene known as survivin that encodes for a structurally distinctive suppressor of apoptosis has been recognized [5].

Survivin is a 16.5 kDa intracellular protein from the inhibitor of apoptosis (IAP) gene family. All metazoans genomes contain IAP molecules that characteristically consist of 1–3 copies of ~70-amino-acid zinc-finger fold, known as the baculovirus IAP repeat (BIR). These proteins get physically associated with initiator and effector caspases, intercepting their proteolytic maturation and enzyme activity and hence inhibiting apoptosis [6].

The survivin gene, locus 17q25, is expressed in the G2/M phase of the cell cycle and inhibits apoptosis following physical association with the mitotic spindle. It is now evident that survivin occurs in two immunohistochemically different pools. The nuclear pool is circumscribed to kinetochores of metaphase chromosomes and to the central spindle midzone at anaphase, and the cytosolic pool integrated with interphase microtubules, centrosomes, spindle poles, and mitotic spindle microtubules at metaphase and anaphase [7–9].

Therefore, in the present study, we intended to evaluate the immunohistochemical expression of IAP protein survivin in formalin fixed paraffin embedded (FFPE) sections of normal oral mucosa, oral leukoplakia, and oral squamous cell carcinoma (OSCC) and to find out the correlation between the expressions of survivin within the three groups.

2. Material and Methods

The sample for the study consisted of total 45 specimens of FFPE tissue blocks, 15 in each of the following: normal oral mucosa, leukoplakia, and OSCC. The leukoplakia cases were histopathologically categorized as mild dysplasia (5 cases), moderate dysplasia (9 cases), and severe dysplasia (1 case). The cases of the OSCC group were histopathologically categorized as histopathologically categorized as well differentiated SCC (4 cases), moderately differentiated SCC (9 cases), and poorly differentiated SCC (2 cases). Immunohistochemical reaction for survivin protein was performed for the 4 μm thick histological sections taken on *positively charged slides.* Antigen retrieval was performed by heat induced epitope retrieval (HIER) technique using microwave (EZ retriever system, BioGenex). For this, sections were immersed in 10 mM sodium citrate buffer (pH6.0) in the containers supplied with the retrieval system and two cycles were run: first cycle at 85°C for 10 minutes and second cycle at 100°C for 15 minutes. Anti-survivin rabbit monoclonal antibody (BioGenex, Fremont CA, USA) and Super Sensitive Polymer Detection System (BioGenex, Fremont CA, USA) were used for detection of survivin. The high grade human breast carcinoma specimen showing strong expression for survivin was used as a positive control. For negative control, primary antibody was replaced with PBS.

Survivin positivity was detected in each section. 1000 cells per section were counted under 400x magnification and percentage of survivin positive cells was calculated. The percentage of positive cells was scored according to the method of Nakagawa et al. [10] as follows:

3+ = strong staining (more than 50% stained).

2+ = moderate staining (between 25 and 50% stained).

1+ = weak staining (between 5 and 25% stained).

0 = negative (less than 5% stained).

One way ANOVA (analysis of variance) test was done to test the statistical significance of the difference in the number of survivin positive cells between the three groups.

3. Results

Three out of fifteen normal mucosa cases (20%) showed survivin positivity and the rest were all negative (Figures 1(a) and 1(b)). All the positive cases were having number of positive cells less than 5% and hence all were given a score of 0. Eight out of fifteen (53.33%) cases of leukoplakia were found to be survivin positive (Figures 2(a), 2(b), and 4(b)). Total 13 (86.67%) cases were having a score of 0 (total survivin positive cells count less than 5%) and two cases (13.33%) were given a score of 1+ (total survivin positive cells count between 5 and 25%). Twelve out of fifteen cases (80%) of OSCC were found out to be survivin positive (Figures 3(a), 3(b), and 4(a)). Total four cases (26.67%) were given a score of 0, six cases (40%) were given a score of 1+, and five cases (33.33%) were given a score of 2+.

The statistical analysis (one way ANOVA, Table 1) indicated that the difference of survivin positive cells/1000 cells observed between the three different groups, that is, normal oral mucosa, leukoplakia, and OSCC, was statistically significant ($p < 0.001$).

Furthermore, *Bonferroni test* (Table 2) was applied to evaluate each comparison (i.e., normal oral mucosa with leukoplakia and OSCC, leukoplakia with normal oral mucosa and OSCC, and OSCC with normal oral mucosa and leukoplakia) of the significance test. This analysis showed that the difference in number of survivin positive cells was statistically insignificant between normal oral mucosa and leukoplakia, whereas it was found to be statistically significant between leukoplakia and OSCC ($p < 0.001$). Also, the difference between normal oral mucosa and OSCC was found to be significant ($p < 0.001$).

4. Discussion

Oral carcinoma is the most prevalent cancer in the head and neck region with unfavourable outcome. In spite of the advancements in the treatment protocols like radiation therapy, advanced surgical procedures, and the emergence of aggressive chemotherapy regimens, the 5-year survival rate of OSCC is only 35–50% [11]. One of the major causes for the unfavourable prognosis in oral cancer is the inability to detect the disease at an early stage and its progression. Therefore, a strong need arises for distinct and specific molecular tumor markers to predict the tumor progression and prognosis. Although plenty of tumor markers and predisposing factors are well recognized for oral carcinoma, their role in determining the prognosis is still not established [12].

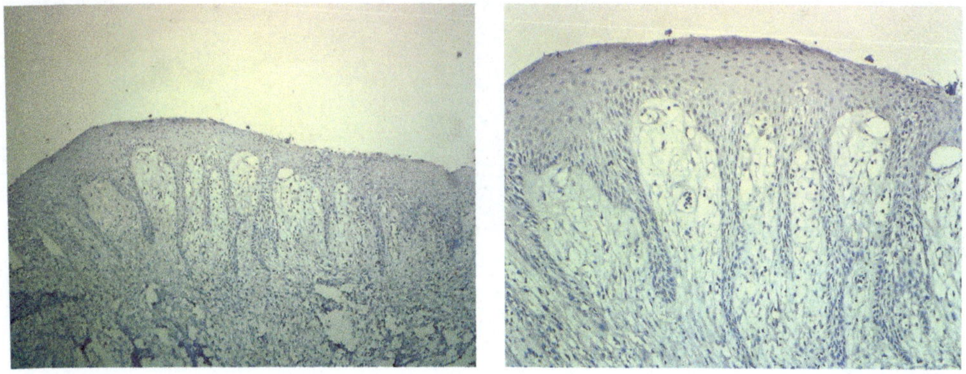

(a) (b)

FIGURE 1: Representative photomicrographs of the immunohistochemical staining for survivin in normal oral mucosa at (a) 40x and (b) 100x magnification showing negative staining.

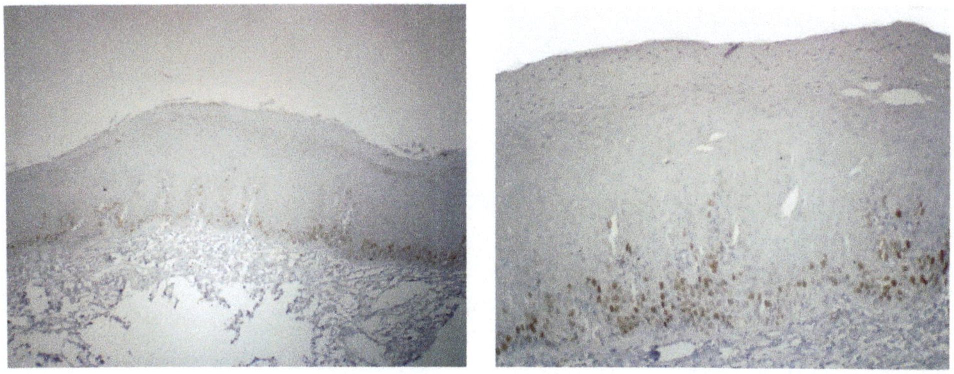

(a) (b)

FIGURE 2: Representative photomicrographs of the immunohistochemical staining for survivin in a case of oral leukoplakia (a) 40x and (b) 100x magnification showing positive nuclear staining.

A tumor establishes itself whenever there are compromises in the regulation of cell proliferation as well as in the control of cell death. In this direction, many gene products are known to be potentially responsible for modifications in tumor cell viability, the resistance to apoptosis, and the magnification of tumor progression. IAP proteins are now known as modulators of downstream events in the progression of apoptosis directly involving the inhibition of terminal effector caspases 3 and 7 and ultimately hampering apoptosis [13].

Survivin has been initially seen to be expressed in fetal life and not in differentiated adult tissue. However, further studies showed positive expression of survivin in normal endometrium, thymus, and placenta, all of them representing tissues with higher proliferation capacity [14]. Survivin has also been reported to be expressed in several human cancers including cancers of lung, breast, bladder, gastrointestinal tract, and haematological tumors [7, 13, 15].

Survivin is the one representative of the IAP group of proteins which has been recognized to have a role in the nucleus; hence it could be presumed that normal epithelium is dedifferentiated while development and progression of carcinoma result in reexpression of survivin [11]. Therefore survivin expression can be helpful for evaluating the progress of head and neck carcinomas.

In the present study, we calculated 1000 cells per section showing positive survivin expression and the results were compared for the test of significance using one way ANOVA test. We found a statistically significant difference between the three groups ($p < 0.001$).

Further Bonferroni analysis was performed to do the multiple comparisons. This test showed that the difference in number of survivin positive cells and their percentage was statistically insignificant between normal oral mucosa and leukoplakia. These results were in accordance with study done by Lo Muzio et al. [16].

In our study, survivin positivity in normal oral mucosa was observed sporadically in basal layer only and all the positive cases were scored as 0; that is, the number of positive cells/1000 cells was between 0 and 5%. This was in accordance with the studies done by Lo Muzio et al. [17].

Further Bonferroni analysis was performed to do the multiple comparisons. This test showed that the difference in number of survivin positive cells and their percentage was statistically insignificant between normal oral mucosa and

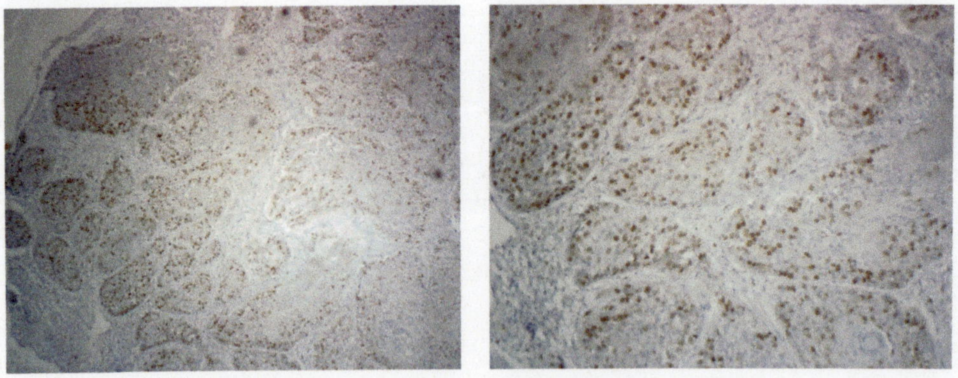

(a) (b)

FIGURE 3: Representative photomicrographs of the immunohistochemical staining for survivin in a case of oral squamous cell carcinoma at (a) 40x and (b) 100x magnification showing positive nuclear staining.

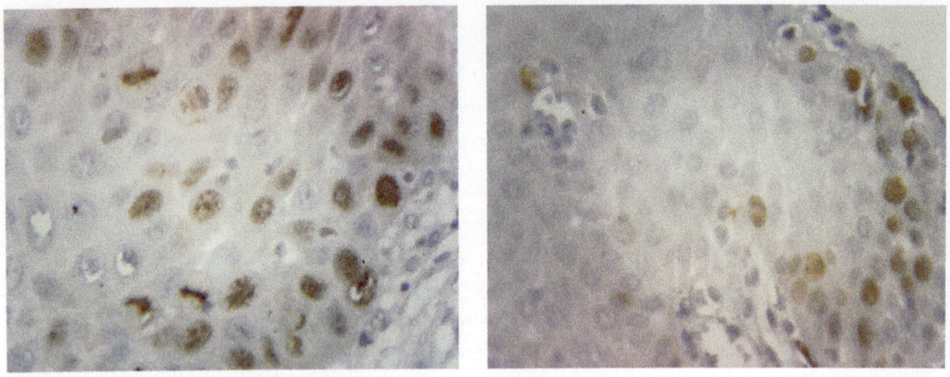

(a) (b)

FIGURE 4: Representative photomicrographs of the immunohistochemical staining for survivin in a case of (a) oral squamous cell carcinoma and (b) oral leukoplakia at 400x magnification showing positive nuclear staining.

TABLE 1: One way ANOVA analysis between the three groups showing statistically significant difference.

	Sum of squares	df	Mean square	F	p value
Number of positive cells/1000 cells					
Between groups	237224.711	2	118612.356	16.547	<0.001*
Within groups	301064.933	42	7168.213		
Total	538289.644	44			

* p value statistically significant.

TABLE 2: Bonferroni analysis showing multiple comparison.

Dependent variable			Std. error	p value
Number of positive cells/1000 cells	Normal mucosa	Leukoplakia	30.91540	1.000
		Squamous cell carcinoma	30.91540	<0.001*
	Leukoplakia	Normal mucosa	30.91540	1.000
		Squamous cell carcinoma	30.91540	<0.001*
	Squamous cell carcinoma	Normal mucosa	30.91540	<0.001*
		Leukoplakia	30.91540	<0.001*

* p value statistically significant.

leukoplakia. These results were similar to the study done by Lo Muzio et al. [17]. In contrast to these results, the difference was significant in studies by Khan et al. [5] and Tanaka et al. [18]. This could be attributed to comparatively small sample size in our study.

The difference in number of survivin positive cells was statistically significant ($p < 0.001$) between normal oral mucosa and OSCC and between leukoplakia and OSCC. These findings are similar to study conducted by Pannone et al. [19].

We observed an upregulation of survivin expression in leukoplakia and OSCC. More than half of the cases of leukoplakia in our study showed positive survivin expression. Thus, we can postulate that, during the development of oral cancer, antiapoptotic protein survivin might accumulate within the involved tissue at an early stage. Numerous types of precancerous lesions or initial stages of cancer have been reported to show positive expression of survivin, including colon polyps and Bowen disease [20] and precancerous colorectal lesion [21].

Upregulation of survivin in OSCC and highly significant difference with leukoplakia were observed in our study. However, we did not observe any significant relation between degree of survivin expression and the histological grade of OSCC. Along with small sample size, the nonuniform proportion of various grades of dysplasia and histological grades of OSCC could be the reason for not significant difference in survivin expression within the groups.

Hence, in conclusion, our study demonstrated a high expression of survivin protein in leukoplakia and SCC cases. This expression may occur as an early phenomenon in the beginning and advancement of OSCC. Also, survivin may act as an important therapeutic target because of its unique expression in tumor cells and its absence in most adult tissues.

Although our study demonstrated the positive immune-expression of survivin as a reliable marker for OSCC, further studies are required with larger number of samples to assess the relation of survivin with different histological grades of squamous cell carcinoma. Also, to confirm the role of survivin as a guide to prognosis of OSCC, studies with clinical follow-up are desired.

Conflict of Interests

The authors declare that there is no conflict of interests regarding the publication of this paper.

References

[1] J. C. De Vicente, L. M. J. Gutiérrez, A. H. Zapatero, M. F. F. Forcelledo, G. Hernández-Vallejo, and J. S. López Arranz, "Prognostic significance of p53 expression in oral squamous cell carcinoma without neck node metastases," *Head and Neck*, vol. 26, no. 1, pp. 22–30, 2004.

[2] A. S. Bodhade and A. M. Dive, "Chemoprevention of premalignant and malignant lesions of oral cavity: recent trends," *European Journal of Dentistry*, vol. 7, no. 2, pp. 246–250, 2013.

[3] C. Jane, A. V. Nerurkar, N. V. Shirsat, R. B. Deshpande, A. D. Amrapurkar, and F. R. Karjodkar, "Increased survivin expression in high-grade oral squamous cell carcinoma: a study in Indian tobacco chewers," *Journal of Oral Pathology and Medicine*, vol. 35, no. 10, pp. 595–601, 2006.

[4] J. Reibel, "Prognosis of oral pre-malignant lesions: significance of clinical, histopathological, and molecular biological characteristics," *Critical Reviews in Oral Biology and Medicine*, vol. 14, no. 1, pp. 47–62, 2003.

[5] Z. Khan, R. P. Tiwari, R. Mulherkar et al., "Detection of survivin and p53 in human oral cancer: correlation with clinicopathologic findings," *Head & Neck*, vol. 31, no. 8, pp. 1039–1048, 2009.

[6] D. C. Altieri, "The molecular basis and potential role of survivin in cancer diagnosis and therapy," *Trends in Molecular Medicine*, vol. 7, no. 12, pp. 542–547, 2001.

[7] G. Ambrosini, C. Adida, and D. C. Altieri, "A novel anti-apoptosis gene, survivin, expressed in cancer and lymphoma," *Nature Medicine*, vol. 3, no. 8, pp. 917–921, 1997.

[8] F. Li, G. Ambrosini, E. Y. Chu et al., "Control of apoptosis and mitotic spindle checkpoint by survivin," *Nature*, vol. 396, no. 6711, pp. 580–584, 1998.

[9] P. Fortugno, N. R. Wall, A. Giodini et al., "Survivin exists in immunochemically distinct subcellular pools and is involved in spindle microtubule function," *Journal of Cell Science*, vol. 115, no. 3, pp. 575–585, 2002.

[10] K. Nakagawa, K. Yamamura, S. Maeda, and M. Ichihashi, "BCL-2 expression in epidermal keratinocytic diseases," *Cancer*, vol. 74, no. 6, pp. 1720–1724, 1994.

[11] Y.-H. Kim, S.-M. Kim, Y.-K. Kim, S.-P. Hong, M.-J. Kim, and H. Myoung, "Evaluation of survivin as a prognostic marker in oral squamous cell carcinoma," *Journal of Oral Pathology and Medicine*, vol. 39, no. 5, pp. 368–375, 2010.

[12] H. Schliephake, "Prognostic relevance of molecular markers of oral cancer—a review," *International Journal of Oral and Maxillofacial Surgery*, vol. 32, no. 3, pp. 233–245, 2003.

[13] C.-D. Lu, D. C. Altieri, and N. Tanigawa, "Expression of a novel antiapoptosis gene, survivin, correlated with tumor cell apoptosis and p53 accumulation in gastric carcinomas," *Cancer Research*, vol. 58, no. 9, pp. 1808–1812, 1998.

[14] G. Lodi, R. Franchini, C. Bez et al., "Detection of survivin mRNA in healthy oral mucosa, oral leucoplakia and oral cancer," *Oral Diseases*, vol. 16, no. 1, pp. 61–67, 2010.

[15] M. Falleni, C. Pellegrini, A. Marchetti et al., "Survivin gene expression in early-stage non-small cell lung cancer," *The Journal of Pathology*, vol. 200, no. 5, pp. 620–626, 2003.

[16] L. Lo Muzio, G. Pannone, R. Leonardi et al., "Survivin, a potential early predictor of tumor progression in the oral mucosa," *Journal of Dental Research*, vol. 82, no. 11, pp. 923–928, 2003.

[17] L. Lo Muzio, G. Pannone, S. Staibano et al., "Survivin expression in oral squamous cell carcinoma," *British Journal of Cancer*, vol. 89, no. 12, pp. 2244–2248, 2003.

[18] C. Tanaka, K. Uzawa, T. Shibahara, H. Yokoe, H. Noma, and H. Tanzawa, "Expression of an inhibitor of apoptosis, survivin, in oral carcinogenesis," *Journal of Dental Research*, vol. 82, no. 8, pp. 607–611, 2003.

[19] G. Pannone, P. Bufo, R. Serpico et al., "Survivin phosphorylation and M-phase promoting factor in oral carcinogenesis," *Histology and histopathology*, vol. 22, no. 11, pp. 1241–1249, 2007.

[20] R. Gianani, E. Jarboe, D. Orlicky et al., "Expression of survivin in normal, hyperplastic, and neoplastic colonic mucosa," *Human Pathology*, vol. 32, no. 1, pp. 119–125, 2001.

[21] H.-Y. Tan, J. Liu, S.-M. Wu, and H.-S. Luo, "Expression of a novel apoptosis inhibitor-survivin in colorectal carcinoma," *World Journal of Gastroenterology*, vol. 11, no. 30, pp. 4689–4692, 2005.

Barrett's Esophagus: Emerging Knowledge and Management Strategies

Atul Bhardwaj,[1] Douglas B. Stairs,[2] Haresh Mani,[2] and Thomas J. McGarrity[1]

[1] *Division of Gastroenterology and Hepatology, Penn State Milton S. Hershey Medical Center, 500 University Drive, P.O. Box 850, HU33, Hershey, PA 17033, USA*
[2] *Department of Pathology, Penn State Milton S. Hershey Medical Center, 500 University Drive, P.O. Box 850, HO83, Hershey, PA 17033, USA*

Correspondence should be addressed to Thomas J. McGarrity, tmcgarrity@hmc.psu.edu

Academic Editor: Hala El-Zimaity

The incidence of esophageal adenocarcinoma (EAC) has increased exponentially in the last 3 decades. Barrett's esophagus (BE) is the only known precursor of EAC. Patients with BE have a greater than 40 folds higher risk of EAC compared with the general population. Recent years have witnessed a revolution in the clinical and molecular research related to BE. However, several aspects of this condition remain controversial. Data regarding the true prevalence of BE have varied widely. Recent studies have suggested a lower incidence of EAC in nondysplastic BE (NDBE) than previously reported. There is paucity of prospective data showing a survival benefit of screening or surveillance for BE. Furthermore, the ever-increasing emphasis on healthcare cost containment has called for reexamination of the screening and surveillance strategies for BE. There is a need for identification of reliable clinical predictors or molecular biomarkers to risk-stratify patients who might benefit the most from screening or surveillance for BE. Finally, new therapies have emerged for the management of dysplastic BE. In this paper, we highlight the key areas of controversy and uncertainty surrounding BE. The paper discusses, in detail, the current literature about the molecular pathogenesis, biomarkers, histopathological diagnosis, and management strategies for BE.

1. Introduction

In the last 3 decades, the incidence of esophageal adenocarcinoma (EAC) has increased at a faster rate than any other cancer in the US and Western Europe [1–4]. Despite advances in therapies, the 5-year survival rate for EAC remains less than 15% [5]. Barrett's esophagus (BE), a condition in which the squamous epithelium of the distal esophagus is replaced by columnar epithelium with intestinal metaplasia (IM), is a well-established precursor of EAC. BE increases the risk of EAC by greater than 40-fold compared with the general population [6, 7]. Our understanding of BE has increased significantly over the past half a century. However, many aspects of the natural history and pathophysiology of BE have not been fully elucidated.

Some of the controversial areas of BE include the following:

(i) There is a lack of consensus regarding the definition of BE and whether IM should be a requirement for the diagnosis of BE [8–10].

(ii) True prevalence of BE in the general population and its risk of progression to EAC remain unclear. Recent studies have suggested a lower risk of malignant transformation of BE than previously reported [11–14].

(iii) A clear survival benefit of screening or surveillance for BE has not been demonstrated in prospective studies [8].

(iv) There is a lack of reliable predictive biomarkers that might enable us to risk-stratify BE patients and identify those who would benefit the most from endoscopic surveillance and therapy [15].

The aim of this paper is to review the current evidence related to the definition of BE, the cancer risk of nondysplastic and dysplastic BE, screening and surveillance for BE, management of dysplasia in BE, and chemo-prevention of BE. The molecular pathogenesis, biomarkers, and histopathological diagnosis of BE will also be discussed in detail.

2. Historical Perspective and Definition of Barrett's Esophagus

In 1950, Norman Barrett, an Australian-born, British surgeon suggested that the finding of gastric-type mucosa in the esophagus was in most cases, due to a congenitally shortened esophagus resulting in extension of the stomach into the mediastinum. He proposed that ulcers occurring in these areas (described as *"peptic ulcers of the oesophagus"* by most pathologists of that era) were a different entity than the ulcers and strictures of the esophagus that occur as a result of acid reflux. He coined the term *"reflux oesophagitis"* for the latter disease process [17]. In 1953, Allison and Johnstone published an article titled *"The oesophagus lined with gastric mucous membrane"* to emphasize that the areas of columnar mucosa described by Barrett were actually part of the esophagus and not stomach. They proposed that ulcers in these areas be called *"Barrett's ulcers"* [18]. Seven years after his original article, Barrett agreed with Allison and Johnstone and suggested that these findings be called the *"lower oesophagus lined by columnar epithelium"* [19]. With time, the replacement of the normal squamous lining of the esophagus by columnar epithelium became known as *"Barrett's oesophagus"* [20].

In North America, BE is defined as a change in the distal esophageal epithelium of any length, recognized as columnar-type epithelium on endoscopy, and confirmed to have IM by biopsy of the tubular esophagus [8, 21]. However, differences of opinion surround this definition. There is a lack of consensus regarding the precise anatomical landmarks defining the distal limit of esophagus (gastroesophageal junction (GEJ)). According to one school of thought, the GEJ is at the proximal aspect of gastric mucosal folds. However, these landmarks can shift during phases of respiration, distension of the stomach and esophagus, and gut peristalsis [22]. Others consider GEJ as the distal end of the palisade vessels in the lamina propria of the esophagus. This landmark can be obscured by pathology in the distal esophagus and lends itself to interobserver variability [23, 24]. Three types of columnar epithelia can be seen on biopsies from Barrett's like mucosa: (a) cardia type metaplasia composed of mucin secreting glands, (b) gastric-fundus-type metaplasia comprising of parietal cells, chief cells, and mucus secreting cells, and (c) specialized IM, containing predominantly goblet cells. The first 2 types can be indistinguishable from the gastric mucosa, unless the biopsy specimen contains esophageal submucosal glands or islands of squamous epithelium [25]. If cardia- or fundic-type mucosa are obtained from the biopsies from the distal esophagus, the possibility of inadvertent sampling from the stomach should be considered. Conversely, IM can be seen in gastric biopsies due to *Helicobacter pylori* infection. To add to the complexity of this issue, studies have shown that 10–15% of normal population can have IM in the gastric cardia or GEJ [26–28]. Therefore, even the presence of IM does not completely rule out sampling error [28].

If predisposition to EAC is an essential tenet of BE, do all of the 3 types of columnar metaplasia described above increase the risk of EAC? There is robust scientific evidence that IM increases the risk of EAC [3, 29]. Some studies have suggested that cardia-type (nongoblet) metaplasia may also predispose to EAC, perhaps to a lesser extent [30, 31]. However, the true population-based risk of progression of nongoblet metaplasia to EAC is not known. There is scant scientific evidence at this time to include nongoblet metaplasia in the definition of BE.

Table 1: Definition of Barrett's esophagus proposed by major professional organizations of various countries [8, 9, 21, 42].

	ACG (USA)	AGA (USA)	BSG (England)	SFED (France)
Endoscopic documentation of columnar lined mucosa in the tubular esophagus required	Yes	Yes	Yes	Yes
IM required on biopsies from the tubular esophagus	Yes	Yes	No	Yes

ACG: American College of Gastroenterology; AGA: American Gastroenterological Association; BSG: British Society of Gastroenterology; SFED: French Society of Digestive Endoscopy.

There is also a lack of consensus among various professional organizations whether goblet metaplasia, that is, IM, should be a requirement for diagnosis of BE (also see related discussion below, in the section on histopathology). The *British Society of Gastroenterology* (*BSG*) no longer considers IM as a diagnostic criterion for BE [9]. Experts in favor of this school of thought contend that the yield of IM drops as the length of columnar lining and number of biopsies taken decrease [32, 33]. Multiple biopsies must be obtained to adequately assess for IM in patients with >1 cm of columnar lined esophagus [34]. Several arguments can be made in favor of requiring IM for a diagnosis of BE. Studies suggest that a diagnosis of BE may have a negative impact on overall quality of life of the patients. Patients with BE tend to overestimate their risk of cancer, and this leads to higher utilization of healthcare resources. A diagnosis of BE can result in higher health insurance premium and difficulty in obtaining health insurance [35–37]. The *American College of Gastroenterology* (*ACG*) and the *American Gastroenterological Association* (*AGA*) recommend documentation of IM for a diagnosis of BE [8, 21]. Table 1 summarizes definition of BE proposed by major professional organizations.

Historically, BE has been classified into short-segment (<3 cm) and long-segment BE (≥3 cm), based on the length of metaplastic epithelium seen on endoscopy [38]. A more recent classification takes into consideration the circumferential (C) and maximum (M) extent of the endoscopically visualized BE, above the GEJ. This system is called the Prague "C" and "M" criteria (Figures 1(a), 1(b) and 1(c)). The original C&M criteria were developed by an international working group using videoendoscopic recordings in 29 patients. To validate these standardized criteria, a separate panel of 29 expert endoscopists scored these recordings. The overall reliability coefficients (RCs) for the assessment of C and M extent were 0.95 and 0.94, respectively. The RCs for

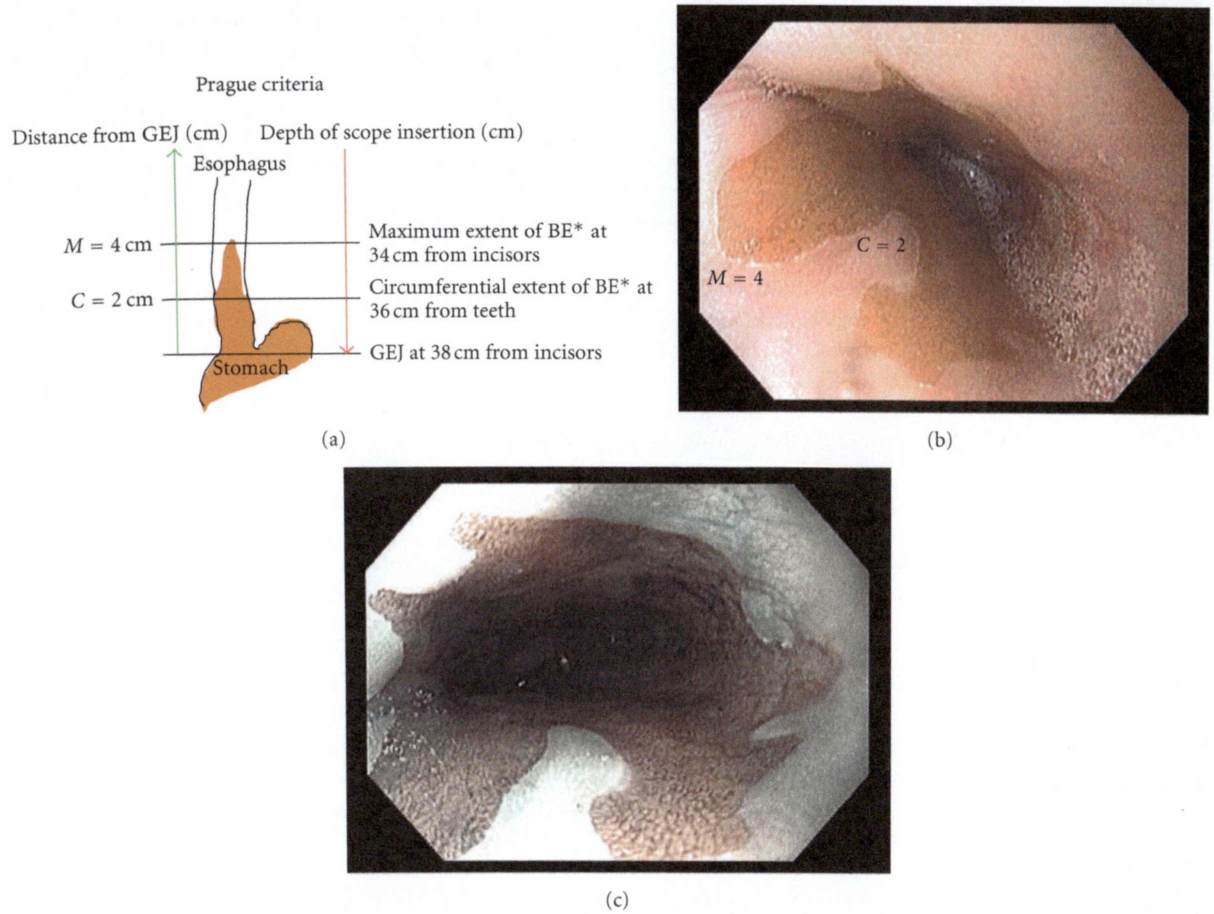

Figure 1: (a) Schematic representation of the Prague criteria for endoscopically suspected esophageal columnar metaplasia/Barrett's esophagus, Step 1: recognize the presence of hiatal hernia; Step 2: identify GEJ and record depth of scope insertion; Step 3: recognize suspected BE mucosa above the GEJ; Step 4: record the depth of scope insertion at the most proximal circumferential extent of BE; Step 5: record the depth of scope insertion at maximum extent of BE; Step 6: subtract the depth of insertion for circumferential and maximum extents from the depth of scope insertion at the GEJ to calculate C and M, respectively. *Endoscopically suspected columnar mucosa. Adapted from [16]. (b) endoscopic image of Barrett's esophagus for circumferential (C) and maximum (M) extent of columnar mucosa, corresponding to the schematic representation shown in Figure 1(a), (c) another endoscopic image of BE using narrow-band imaging (NBI). NBI is a high-resolution endoscopic tool that enhances mucosal surface details without the need for special dyes (electronic chromoendoscopy).

recognizing the location of the GEJ and the diaphragmatic hiatus were 0.88 and 0.85, respectively [16]. A recent multicenter study of gastroenterology trainees demonstrated correlation coefficients of 0.94 and 0.96, respectively, for assessment of the C and M extent of the endoscopically visualized BE. The correlation coefficients for recognition of GEJ and diaphragmatic hiatus were 0.92 and 0.90, respectively [39]. Kinjo et al. prospectively compared endoscopic BE diagnoses using the Japanese criteria (GEJ defined as the distal limit of the longitudinal or palisade vessels in the lamina propria of the esophagus) and Prague C&M criteria in 110 Japanese patients. A higher proportion of patients were diagnosed with endoscopic BE using the Japanese criteria (39%) compared with C&M criteria (26%) ($P = 0.044$). The GEJ identification rates were also higher using the Japanese criteria than with C&M criteria (95% versus 86% ($P = 0.039$)). The authors concluded that, in the Japanese population, the Japanese criteria may be more suitable for the diagnosis of endoscopic BE and for recognition of GEJ than the C&M criteria. The important limitations of this study are that only 2 endoscopists interpreted the findings, and the study was not designed to assess interobserver correlation for the 2 criteria [40]. No formal studies have evaluated the "clinical benefit" of using any standardized classification for the assessment of the endoscopic extent of BE segment. However, data suggest a direct relationship between the endoscopic extent of BE and the probability of finding IM on histology. Greater BE surface area may translate into greater cancer risk [29, 41]. Major professional societies recommend that information about the extent of metaplasia should be recorded using standardized methods [8, 21].

3. Epidemiology and Clinical Features

BE is usually detected on upper endoscopy for various indications, during the 6th decade of life or later [51, 52]. The male-to-female ratio for BE is approximately 2 : 1 [53].

White subjects have a 4–6 times higher incidence of BE compared to black subjects [2, 12, 51, 54]. Patients with chronic heart burn are 6–10 times more likely to have BE than those without heartburn [55–57]. A high body mass index and a centripetal distribution of body fat also increased the risk of BE in multiple studies [58–61]. Data suggest that *Helicobacter pylori* infection, red wine, and diet rich in fruits and vegetables may have protective effect against BE [62–67].

The reported prevalence of BE in different studies has varied widely, depending on the population studied and the definition used. A study of 733 unselected autopsies from Olmsted county, MN, USA, estimated the prevalence of BE to be 376 per 100,000 population [68]. A retrospective analysis of a US rural white population in the Marshfield Epidemiologic Study Area (MESA), estimated the prevalence of endoscopically and histologically confirmed BE to be 261.8 per 100,000 persons [69]. BE was diagnosed in 6.8% patients in a study of 961 US patients who were scheduled for a colonoscopy and had no prior history of an upper endoscopy. However, the study population comprised of predominantly white males [12]. There is a lack of large population-based studies on the prevalence of BE in the United States. A Swedish study reported the prevalence of BE to be 1.6%, when both endoscopic and histological criteria were used to define BE [70].

The presence of columnar mucosa in the distal esophagus does not cause symptoms per se. The symptoms in these patients are mostly related to sequelae of long-standing gastroesophageal reflux disease (GERD) (e.g., esophagitis, peptic stricture, etc.). Absence of chronic reflux symptoms does not exclude the possibility of BE. Indeed, in the Swedish study, about 44% of the patients found to have BE did not report significant symptoms of heart burn and dyspepsia [70]. BE is seen in about 10–15% of the patients undergoing upper endoscopy for chronic GERD, and in 5.6% of those without chronic reflux symptoms [71]. The frequency of long-segment BE is 3–5% and short-segment BE is 10–15% among patients with chronic GERD [72].

4. The Pathogenesis of Barrett's Metaplasia

4.1. Cell of Origin. A very important step in understanding the development of BE and its progression to EAC is identifying the cell of its origin. Unfortunately, the cell of origin in BE is not known. There exist currently 2 conflicting hypotheses. The first possibility is that BE arises from a stem cell. To complicate this question further, the origin of this putative stem cell is also up for debate. It is possible that the BE stem cell originates from the stratified squamous epithelium compartment, the submucosal glands of the distal esophagus, bone-marrow-derived stem cells (BMDCs), or stem cells located in the proximal stomach [73–77]. Search for a putative BE stem cell is hindered by the lack of knowledge regarding stem cells of the esophagus. To date, only one group has identified a population of squamous epithelial-derived cells enriched for stem cell properties which can be isolated by flow cytometry sorting for CD34, a marker for stem cells in other tissues [78].

A second hypothesis for the cell of origin of BE is that of a differentiated esophageal keratinocyte. One presumption for this hypothesis would be that the squamous epithelium would undergo at least a partial dedifferentiation. Recent work to generate pluripotent-induced progenitor stem cells (iPS) by introduction of c-myc, KLF4, Sox2, and Oct3/4 into adult fibroblasts has lent credence to this possibility [79]. In fact, several of these genes have been demonstrated to play a role in esophageal and BE biology. Sox2 has been determined to be a lineage-specific transcription factor in the esophagus specifying squamous cell differentiation [80]. KLF4 and c-myc expressions are upregulated in Barrett's esophagus and may contribute to a transdifferentiation process [81, 82]. Further work on stem cells and the molecular pathways involved in the transdifferentiation process of BE will be necessary to address the cell of origin question.

4.2. Reflux Exposure and Inflammation. One of the most strongly associated clinical symptoms for the development of BE is the recurrent reflux of acid and bile salts. Epidemiologic data suggests that GERD is important for the development of BE [83]. Approximately 13% of patients that have been diagnosed with GERD develop BE [84]. These data suggest a role for GERD in the development of BE. In fact, surgical anastomosis of the esophagus to the small intestine by either joining to the duodenum (EDA or EGDA models) or jejunum (EJA) in rats has verified this hypothesis [85–87].

The chronic reflux associated with GERD induces a significant amount of epithelial damage and a commensurate inflammatory response. Research over the last several decades has begun to illustrate the role inflammation plays in many disease processes, and this is likely true with the development of BE and esophageal adenocarcinoma. Work has focused on cytokines secretion in BE, signaling events induced in the esophageal epithelium in response to GERD, and the accompanying inflammation that may be responsible for the metaplastic process in BE cells. Acid and bile salt exposure may impair the barrier function as well [88]. This loss of barrier function and damage to the epithelium may be the precipitating events for the initial inflammatory response. This induces a Th2 inflammatory response replete with the expression of IL1β, IL4, IL6, IL8, TNFα, and IFNγ [89]. This type of a response has been associated with tumor formation and progression by recruiting immature myeloid cells, tumor-associated macrophages, and neutrophils [90–94]. This type of immune response may have a similar role in triggering signaling events that result in metaplasia of the epithelium.

Several signaling pathways associated with inflammation have been implicated in BE. Cyclooxygenase (Cox) gene expression appears to be induced by acid reflux. In fact, its expression level is positively correlated with the degree of acid reflux which occurs in a given patient. Interestingly, Cox2 expression increases as BE progresses to EAC, suggesting that Cox2 may functionally contribute to the pathogenesis of EAC [95]. Indeed, epidemiologic data demonstrate that anti-inflammatory treatment decreases cancer risk due to Cox2 inhibition [96, 97].

In addition to Cox genes expression, NFκB expression has also been implicated in the initial stages of the development of BE. Induction of NFκB in esophageal cells subsequent to inflammation-inducing reflux many have effects within the epithelium including the induction of cell survival pathways as well as the transcription of target genes involved in the development and progression of BE. Indeed, NFκB has been demonstrated to be a direct transcriptional regulator of the caudal, homeodomain-containing transcription factors, Cdx1 and Cdx2 [98, 99]. Cdx genes have been implicated in the earliest stages in the transdifferentiation process of BE [81].

5. Biomarkers of Barrett's Esophagus

Genome-wide examination of BE lesions had been performed in order to characterize BE for gene expression changes when compared to normal esophagi, EAC, gastric epithelia, gastric cancers, small intestinal epithelia, and colonic epithelia. The use of microarray expression analyses has generated a large amount of data characterizing the differences between these tissues. Many of the arrays have identified genes that function in cell growth and proliferation, apoptosis, cell metabolism, lipid metabolism, catabolism, cell adhesion, signal transduction, migration, stress response, cell adhesion, signal transduction, and transcription factors [100–106]. While these lists cover a wide array of cellular functions, many of these categorizations seem logical based on what is currently known about BE.

One interesting publication describes the identification of two distinct subcategories of BE dubbed as BE1 and BE2 [102]. BE1 identifies a group similar to that of normal stomach mucosal samples and includes several tumor suppressor genes. BE2 identifies a group that may lie closer to EA than does BE1. BE2 gene expression contains genes that have been either overexpressed in cancers such as carboxylesterase 2, galectin-4, glycoprotein A33, and LI-cadherin. These classifications of different BE samples are intriguing and may be reflected in two other microarray studies. One study from Barrett et al. subclassified BE samples into several categories including their own BE1 group which had a higher correlation coefficient with squamous samples while sample their BE4 group had a higher correlation with their gastric samples [100]. A third study from the University of Pennsylvania suggested that two populations of BE may exist [81]. Principle component analysis placed BE samples into 2 groups spatially that were distinct from each other yet closely related based on global gene analysis. A meta-analysis of all BE samples to determine if classifications extend beyond these data sets would be very informative. Differences between BE groups may identify biomarkers that would predict progression. Several microarray expression analyses have begun to identify genes that may predict the progression of BE to EAC [103, 104, 106]. These genes include MMP7, CXCL3, GATA6, HoxB7, and SPRR3. Pepe et al. have defined five phases of biomarker development to establish a gene as a *bone fide* biomarker of disease [107]. Few biomarkers have been evaluated for risk stratification using this systematic approach in BE. Unfortunately, most of the microarray data published to date have lacked followup work to identify those genes contained within the data sets that contribute to the cause of BE or its progression to EAC or in the alternative to serve as true biomarkers for disease progression.

6. Signaling Pathways

As had been previously discussed, many factors such as acid, bile salts, and inflammation are likely to contribute to the pathogenesis of BE. What remains less well defined are the intracellular signaling events responsible for the transition to BE which is likely due to several signaling pathways altering the differentiation of the epithelium of the esophagus. As a result, an approach whereby several signaling pathways are manipulated at one time is needed. As previously mentioned, Cdx gene expression has been detected in BE and is likely a result of NFκB expression subsequent to the inflammatory response elicited by acid reflux. Indeed, Cdx gene expression is one of the most likely candidates for transcription factors that induce intestinal metaplasia due to its well-established role in embryonic intestine development. Additional signaling events that may induce Cdx expression are retinoic acid (RA) and hedgehog signaling [108–112].

Another transcription factor, c-myc, is important for the development of BE [81, 113]. Interestingly, c-myc expression increases in dysplastic lesions and reaches its highest expression in EAC. Also, c-myc activation has been implicated in BE by microarray analysis [81]. To test whether c-myc was involved in BE, c-myc was coexpressed with Cdx1 in squamous esophageal cell lines and induced several genes expressed in BE, suggesting a partial shift in differentiation.

7. Histopathology Diagnosis and Dysplasia Grading

7.1. Definition: Intestinal Metaplasia or No Intestinal Metaplasia. As discussed above, the definition of BE varies worldwide [114]. Countries such as USA require the presence of goblet cells (IM), whereas England and Japan accept any endoscopically visible columnar metaplasia as sufficient to define BE. The requirement of IM has been supported by studies that have claimed IM to be a prerequisite for the development of adenocarcinoma [115, 116]. More recently, there has been a suggestion to move away from this view [10]. Gatenby et al. evaluated clinical followup for 934 patients, including 322 with intestinal metaplasia and 612 with nongoblet columnar cell metaplasia of the distal esophagus, and found no difference with respect to dysplasia and/or cancer incidence between the two groups (19.8% versus 15.2%, resp.), suggesting that nongoblet glandular epithelium in the distal esophagus may also be at risk for neoplastic transformation [117]. As suggested by DeMeester, a practical approach may be to consider that patients with ≥ 3 cm of columnar-lined esophagus nearly always either have or will develop IM, and these patients should be considered to have BE along with those with shorter lengths of columnar mucosa who show IM on biopsy [118].

Goblet cells may be identified on routine histological stains (hematoxylin and eosin, H&E), although many institutions routinely employ PAS-Alcian blue stains to highlight acidic mucin in goblet cells (blue by Alcian blue at pH 2.5) against a backdrop of gastric neutral mucin (magenta caps by PAS). This stain is helpful in differentiating true IM from so-called columnar blue cells or pseudogoblet cells, which are gastric foveolar cells that have been "injured" by acid reflux disease. The Alcian blue stain also helps in easy identification of IM and saves time in evaluating a biopsy. Another clue to the presence of IM is the presence of so-called "multilayered epithelium" which is characterized by the presence of an overlay of columnar cells over basal layers of squamous cells. In their study of 17 cases, Glickman et al. found that glandular cells of multilayered epithelium express different mucin types with similar frequencies to IM and also frequently express CDX2 and MUC2, similar to goblet cells that occur in the esophagus. They proposed that multilayered epithelium is a precursor to intestinal metaplasia; presence of multilayered epithelium should prompt a more detailed search for goblet cells [119].

The IM of gastric cardia mucosa does not equate to BE, since BE has to involve the tubular esophagus. Also, IM of gastric cardia may be less likely to progress to dysplasia than true BE [120]. Thus a diagnosis of BE cannot be made histologically when the exact site of biopsy of the metaplastic fragment is not known. BE is a clinicopathologic diagnosis and the biopsy must be from an endoscopically visualized abnormality in the tubular esophagus. IM may be either "complete" (when goblet cells are accompanied by absorptive and/or Paneth cells) or "incomplete" (absence of absorptive and/or Paneth cells). Conceptually speaking, incomplete IM is less differentiated and therefore more likely to be a dysplasia precursor. In practice, incomplete and complete IM may exist adjacent to each other, and their identification may purely be a result of sampling. Hence, subtypes of IM are not generally mentioned in pathology reports.

7.2. Dysplasia: Negative and Indefinite. All biopsies for BE diagnosis and surveillance should include a qualifier regarding presence or absence of dysplasia. Dysplasia is assessed in columnar mucosa, preferably away from squamous mucosa, and where the surface lining is intact. Biopsies are categorized as being "negative for dysplasia" if the cells show maturation towards the surface in the form of decreasing nuclear size, decreasing nuclear hyperchromasia, increasing cytoplasmic volume and a mucus cap on surface cells (Figure 2(a)). In some cases, there may be some changes that are deemed insufficient to characterize as dysplasia, and these are categorized as "indefinite for dysplasia". Cases that are classified as being indefinite for dysplasia are either those with minimal to mild cytologic atypia or those that have more than mild cytologic atypia but are accompanied by significant inflammation, raising a possibility of atypia reactive to the inflammatory response. These cases need rebiopsy after control of inflammation. Reactive changes tend to be more diffuse rather than abrupt, the latter being a feature of dysplasia. The category of "indefinite" should not be used to downgrade dysplasia, but rather to identify cases that may need followup biopsies.

7.3. Dysplasia: Intestinal Type. Most dysplasias occurring in a setting of IM are of the "intestinal type." Criteria used to classify dysplasia in this setting are similar to what has been used in colonic adenomas. This pattern of dysplasia is therefore morphologically recognized by the presence of hyperchromatic elongate nuclei, with lack of surface maturation and presence of nuclear crowding, such that the surface epithelium appears generally similar to the glands at the depth. In low-grade dysplasia (LGD), architecture is by and large preserved, true nuclear stratification is absent, and, as a rule, nuclear polarity is maintained (Figure 2(b)). Changes are usually patchy or focal with relatively abrupt transformation between dysplastic and nondysplastic foci, although this transition may not always be evident.

High-grade dysplasia (HGD) is usually identifiable at low-power examination by architectural abnormalities such as glandular crowding, branching, and complexity. Nuclear atypia is also more pronounced, with increasing nuclear stratification and nuclei reaching the surface of the lining cells, without a clear cytoplasmic zone at the apex (Figure 2(c)). There is chromatin smudging, increasing nuclear irregularity, and presence of surface mitoses. Loss of nuclear polarity is the single most helpful feature to identify HGD at the cytologic level. In a setting of HGD, presence of cribriform ("back to back") glands, luminal necrosis, glandular budding, and incomplete glands may indicate intramucosal carcinoma (Figure 2(d)) [121].

7.4. Dysplasia: Basal Crypt Dysplasia and Foveolar Dysplasia. Basal crypt dysplasia was recently described as another variant of dysplasia. This entity is recognized by the presence of dysplasia-like atypia affecting the deep/basal crypts with the presence of surface maturation. Lomo et al. consider this to be true dysplasia in view of the presence of molecular abnormalities (significantly increased rate of 17p (TP53) LOH and aneuploidy), and a high association with conventional dysplasia and/or adenocarcinoma, despite the morphologic appearance of surface maturation. The clinical, pathologic, immunohistochemical, and molecular abnormalities were similar in cases showing low-grade and high-grade histological changes in the basal crypts, except that high-grade cases tended to occur in older patients [122]. Presently, there are no clear guidelines on followup of patients with basal crypt dysplasia. Many pathologists tend to diagnose these cases as indefinite for dysplasia with a comment that dysplasia is restricted to the basal crypts.

Gastric foveolar-type dysplasia is another distinct variant of dysplasia in BE. This dysplasia is similar to the so-called type II dysplasia that is known to occur in the stomach [123, 124]. The diagnosis of gastric foveolar-type dysplasia in BE can be challenging, since there are no standardized diagnostic or grading criteria. Mahajan et al. evaluated the prevalence, morphology, and natural history of gastric foveolar-type dysplasia in a cohort of 200 BE patients. The prevalence of gastric foveolar-type dysplasia was 15% at the

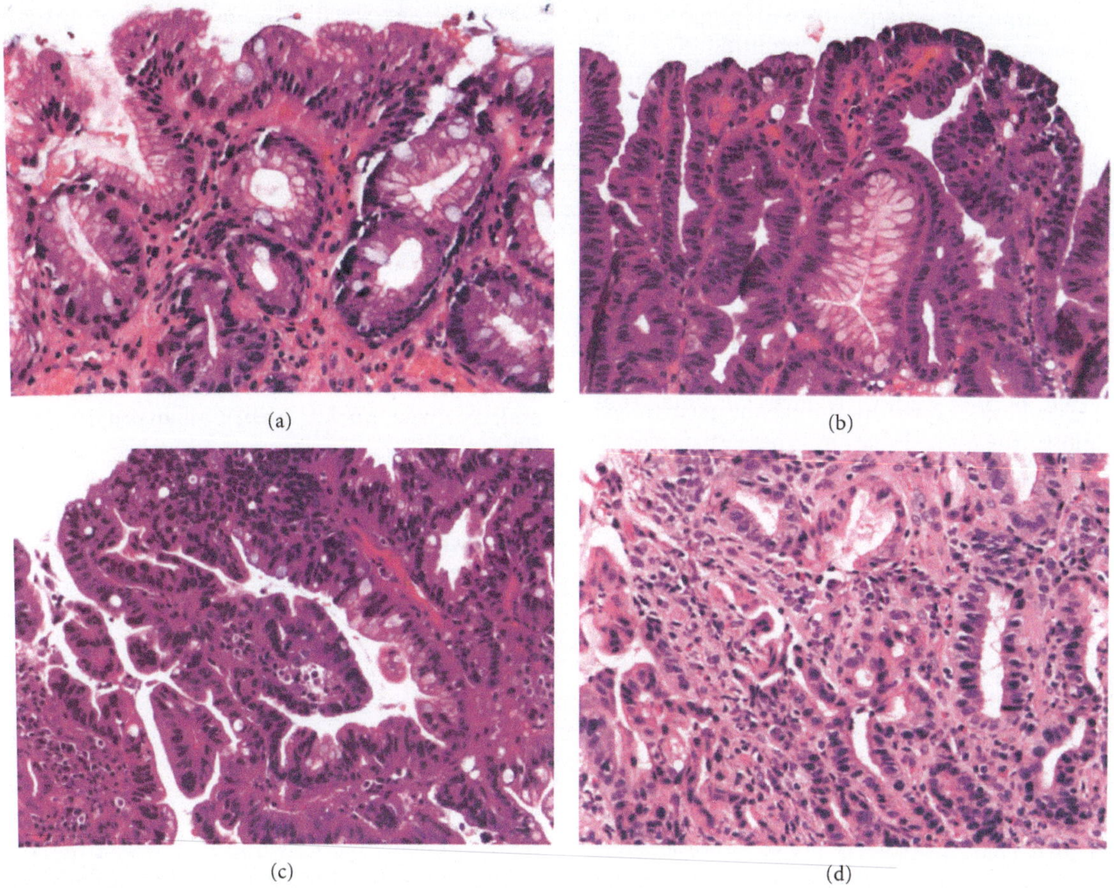

FIGURE 2: (a) Intestinal metaplasia is defined by the presence of goblet cells distended with mucin. In this photomicrograph there is no dysplasia, as evidenced by presence of surface maturation. Surface epithelial cells show uniform mucin caps and well-polarized nuclei. (b) Low-grade dysplasia of the intestinal type is characterized by hyperchromatic elongate nuclei that are seen in both the crypts and the surface epithelium (i.e., loss of surface maturation). (c) Presence of glandular crowding, nuclear stratification, and loss of nuclear polarity signifies high-grade dysplasia. (d) Glandular complexity, budding, and presence of incomplete glandular profiles are evidence of lamina propria invasion (intramucosal carcinoma).

patient level and 20% at the biopsy level. Unlike intestinal-type dysplasia, gastric foveolar-type dysplasia uniformly showed nonstratified, basally oriented nuclei, explaining the difficulty in its recognition. This uniformity therefore precludes the use of loss of nuclear polarity in identifying HGD within this group. Rather, the most important feature permitting a diagnosis of high-grade gastric foveolar-type dysplasia was significantly increased nuclear size (to approximately 3-4 times the size of a mature lymphocyte). Other features in high-grade lesions included villiform architecture, crowded, irregular glandular architecture, eosinophilic and oncocytic cytoplasm, prominent nucleoli, and mild nuclear pleomorphism. During followup, 64% (7 of 11) of patients with pure gastric and 26% (5 of 19) with mixed gastric and intestinal dysplasia underwent neoplastic progression [125].

7.5. Interobserver Variation in Dysplasia Grading. Given the subjectivity in identifying and grading dysplasia, it is not surprising that there is a fair amount of interobserver variability in the pathologic evaluation of BE biopsies. In a study by Kerkhof et al., general pathologists were found to overdiagnose HGD [126]. Nearly 40% of patients who were initially diagnosed with HGD by a general pathologist were downgraded (11% no dysplasia, 12% indefinite for dysplasia, 16% LGD) when the samples were reviewed by three experienced gastrointestinal (GI) pathologists. Downs-Kelly et al., however, reported overall poor interobserver reproducibility even among GI pathologists who see a high volume of Barrett's cases, calling into question treatment regimens based on the assumption that HGD, intramucosal adenocarcinoma, and submucosal adenocarcinoma can reliably be distinguished in biopsy specimens [127]. Montgomery et al. evaluated reproducibility of diagnoses among expert GI pathologists and found that reproducibility improved only after a consensus meeting to decide on criteria to be used. Interobserver variation was better for clinically relevant separation into two groups (BE indefinite and LGD; versus HGD and carcinoma), than into four groups (BE; indefinite and LGD; HGD; carcinoma). Agreement was least for distinction between indefinite and low-grade categories [128]. Followup data collected on 138 cases from the above study were separately analyzed. Dysplasia grade on initial biopsy correlated significantly with progression to invasive carcinoma. Using the initial submitting diagnoses, carcinomas were detected on followup in 18% of indefinite, 15% of LGD, and 61% of HGD cases. When majority diagnoses (among 12 GI pathologists) were used for analysis, carcinomas were detected in 14% indefinite, 20% of LGD, and 60% of HGD cases. There were 39 cases without a majority diagnosis, among which carcinomas were detected in 43% cases with an average score between indefinite and LGD and 70% cases with an average score between LGD and HGD [129]. Interestingly, interobserver reproducibility for basal crypt dysplasia has been reported to be better than conventional LGD but poorer than that for HGD and BE without dysplasia [130]. Notwithstanding the relative lack of reproducibility, it is opined that, in general, pathologists perform extremely well when diagnosing lesions of the highest and lowest risk [131].

7.6. Dysplasia: Role of Immunohistochemistry. Studies have also addressed the utility of immunohistochemical markers in identifying and grading dysplasia. Immunohistochemistry for p53 has been reported to assist in diagnosis in difficult cases [132]. Immunohistochemistry for p53 and Ki67 has also been reported to correlate with the severity of dysplasia in assessing Barrett's biopsies [133, 134]. In another study of 86 biopsies, protein overexpression of β-catenin helped diagnose LGD, whereas overexpression of cyclin D1 and p53 discriminated HGD from LGD [135]. However, most pathologists rely on routine stains and morphology to diagnose and grade dysplasia and immunohistochemistry is rarely, if ever, used in routine day-to-day practice in most centers.

8. Risk of Progression of Nondysplastic Barrett's to Esophageal Adenocarcinoma

Initial studies observed that the risk of progression of BE to EAC ranged between 2 and 4% per year [136–138]. Shaheen et al. noted that these studies might have overestimated the risk due to publication bias in favor of smaller studies reporting relatively higher incidence [139]. Data from subsequent studies showed a lower risk. A meta-analysis of 41 studies with a total followup of 36,635 person years showed 0.7% annual risk of progression from BE to EAC. There was no evidence of significant geographic variation between US, UK, and Europe. There was a trend towards decreased risk of EAC in short-segment BE [29]. Another exhaustive review of forty-seven studies reported a pooled annual estimate of 0.61% for cancer incidence in patients with BE. When early-incident cancers were excluded, the risk decreased to 0.53% per year. When both early incident cancers and HGD at baseline were excluded, the risk was noted to be 0.41% per year [3].

More recent studies have suggested a lower risk of progression of BE to EAC. Bhat et al. analyzed data on 8522 patients with BE from the Northern Ireland Barrett's esophagus register (NIBR). The mean followup was 7 years. Incidence of EAC, carcinoma of the gastric cardia, and HGD was reported to be 0.22% per year in the entire study cohort. Of note, this study used the British definition of BE whereby IM was not required for diagnosis of BE. The incidence of EAC, carcinoma of the gastric cardia, and HGD in patients with IM on index biopsies (criteria used in the US) was 0.38% per year versus 0.07% in those without IM (HR = 3.54, 95% CI = 2.09 to 6.00, $P < 0.001$). The risk was significantly higher in males versus females (HR = 2.11) [7]. A recent study from Denmark reported the incidence of EAC to be 0.29% per year when 11,028 patients with BE were followed for 67,105 person-years. When the EAC cases diagnosed within first year of followup were excluded, the overall annual incidence decreased to 0.12%. The incidence of EAC was 0.1% per year among patients with NDBE on index endoscopies [14].

9. Risk of Progression of Nondysplastic Barrett's to Adenocarcinoma of the Gastric Cardia

Data suggest that chronic reflux and BE increase not only the risk of EAC but also that of adenocarcinoma of the gastric cardia. Ruol et al. compared the epidemiological, clinical, and pathological characteristics of 26 patients with EAC in BE and 16 patients with adenocarcinoma of the gastric cardia. They observed that IM was present in the mucosa adjacent to 25/26 (96%) patients with EAC in BE, and 11/16 (69%) patients with adenocarcinoma of the gastric cardia. Authors concluded that IM may be a common precursor of adenocarcinoma in BE and adenocarcinoma of the gastric cardia [116]. In a retrospective study of the pathology specimen of 100 patients who underwent esophagectomy for adenocarcinoma of the esophagus, cardia, or proximal stomach, specialized IM was identified in the resected specimen in 13/31 (42%) of patients with adenocarcinoma of the cardia as opposed to 1/21 (5%) in those with adenocarcinoma of the proximal stomach [140]. In the Northern Ireland Barrett's esophagus registry, 16 incident cases of adenocarcinoma of the gastric cardia were reported during a mean followup of 7 years in 8522 patients [7].

10. Risk of Progression of Dysplastic Barrett's to Esophageal Adenocarcinoma

10.1. Risk of Progression of Low-Grade Dysplasia to Esophageal Adenocarcinoma. Reported incidence of EAC in patients with LGD has ranged between 0.6% and 13.4% per year, with most studies suggesting the risk to be less than 1% per year. Table 2 summarizes the key findings of the studies evaluating the risk of progression of LDG to EAC [7, 14, 43–46].

10.2. Risk of Progression of High-Grade Dysplasia to Esophageal Adenocarcinoma. Patients with HGD are at high risk of progression to EAC [141]. Table 3 summarizes the key findings of the studies that have evaluated the risk of progression of HGD to EAC [47–49]. Based on the current literature, the risk of EAC in HGD may be more than 10% per patient-year [49, 142, 143]. The extent of HGD may also

TABLE 2: Incidence of neoplastic progression of low-grade dysplasia*.

Study (reference)	Number of BE patients followed	Duration of followup	Incidence of EAC/HGD
Bhat et al. [7]	8522 with BE, (no IM required)	7 years (mean)	1.4% per year (EAC)
Hvid-Jensen et al. [14]	11,028 with BE	5.2 years (median)	0.5% per year (EAC)
Sharma et al. [43]	618 with BE; LGD diagnosed in 156 during f/u	2546 patient years (mean 4.12 years)	0.6% per year (EAC)
Lim et al. [44]	357 with BE; LGD diagnosed in 34 during f/u	8 years	9/34 cases of HGD/EAC; 3.3% per year
Schouten et al. [45]	12,0852 with BE	5.7 years (median)	0.41% per year (EAC)
Curvers et al. [46]	147 LGD patients, but only 15% of these had a consensus diagnosis of LGD	51.1 months (mean)	13.4% per year in those with a consensus diagnosis of LGD

*Includes some of the important studies, not intended to include all studies published in the literature; f/u: followup; LGD: low-grade dysplasia; HGD: high-grade dysplasia; EAC: esophageal adenocarcinoma.

TABLE 3: Incidence of esophageal adenocarcinoma in high-grade dysplasia*.

Study (reference)	Number of patients with HGD	Duration of followup	Incidence of EAC
Schnell et al. [47]	75 HGD patients who didn't have EAC after 1 year f/u	7.3 years (mean)	12/75 (16%) during 7 years; 2.19% per year
Weston et al. [48]	15 patients with unifocal HGD	36.8 ± 23.2 months (mean)	4/15 (26.7%) during f/u; ~8.7% per year
Rastogi et al. [49]	236 HGD patients (meta-analysis of 4 studies)	1241 patient years	Crude = 5.57% per year; weighted = 6.58% per year

*Includes some of the important studies, not intended to include all studies published in the literature; f/u: followup; HGD: high-grade dysplasia; EAC: esophageal adenocarcinoma.

be an important determinant of malignant potential. Diffuse HGD was noted to have a 3.7-fold higher risk of progressing to EAC compared with focal HGD in a retrospective cohort study [144].

11. Screening for Barrett's Esophagus

Approximately 40% of adults in the US experience symptoms of heart burn at least once a month and about 20% report these symptoms once a week [145]. Considering, chronic GERDs is the strongest risk factor for BE, theoretically a large proportion of adult US population would be eligible for screening for BE based on this screening criteria. However, about 40% of the patients diagnosed with EAC do not report chronic GERD symptoms [6]. Thus, if chronic GERD were to be used as a screening criterion, close to half of the targeted population will be missed. Despite a rapid increase in the incidence of EAC in the past 3 decades, the absolute number of EAC cases diagnosed annually in the United States is approximately 10,000. This is a small percentage of patients with chronic GERD. Even when diagnosed with BE, a vast majority of these patients will not develop EAC during their lifetime [47]. Multiple studies have shown that a diagnosis of BE does not necessarily translate into an increased all-cause mortality compared with age- and sex-matched controls. A vast majority of patients with BE die due to causes other than esophageal cancer (e.g., cardiovascular disease) [45, 146, 147]. There is a lack of data showing a clear benefit of screening for BE. The current position of the *AGA* is that *"inadequate evidence exists to endorse endoscopic screening for BE based solely on the presence of GERD symptoms."* The decision regarding screening should be individualized after discussion about the benefits and limitations of screening with the patient [8]. The *ACG* guidelines state that *"screening for BE in general population cannot be recommended at this time."* The use of screening in high-risk population remains to be established and should therefore be individualized [21]. The *American Society of Gastrointestinal Endoscopy* (ASGE) guidelines consider an initial screening endoscopy to be appropriate in select patients with frequent (several times per week), chronic, long-standing GERD (>5 years), who are white, males, aged >50 years, and those with nocturnal heart burn. No further screening is needed if the initial esophagogastroduodenoscopy (EGD) is negative for BE [50]. The *BSG* and the *French Society of Digestive Endoscopy* (*FSDE*) do not recommend routine screening for BE [9, 42, 71]. Table 4 summarizes guidelines for screening for BE by major professional organizations.

12. Surveillance of Patients with Barrett's Esophagus

Multiple studies have demonstrated that cases of EAC diagnosed as a result of endoscopic surveillance are associated with an earlier stage of disease and improved survival compared with clinically diagnosed cases [148–152]. These data present a rationale for surveillance of patients with BE. However, several arguments can be made to the contrary.

Table 4: Guidelines for screening for Barrett's esophagus by major professional organization [8, 9, 21, 42, 50].

	ACG (USA)	AGA (USA)	ASGE (USA)	BSG (England)	SFED (France)
Screening of general population	No	No	No	No	No
Screening of certain high-risk groups	Individualized*	Individualized*	Yes†	No	No

ACG: American College of Gastroenterology; AGA: American Gastroenterological Association; BSG: British Society of Gastroenterology; SFED: French Society of Digestive Endoscopy.
* After careful discussion of the potential risks, benefits, and limitations of screening with the patient.
† Initial screening appropriate in select patients, no further screening needed if initial EGD is normal (see text).

There are no prospective data showing survival advantage with surveillance. The observational studies demonstrating benefit of surveillance are limited by design flaws and lead time bias. A vast majority of patients diagnosed with EAC do not carry a prior diagnosis of BE [147, 151, 153, 154]. Current surveillance methods have limitations. Our ability to detect dysplasia is highly dependent on adherence to rigorous biopsy protocols. One such protocol, called the Seattle Protocol, recommends 4 quadrant biopsies every 1-2 cm throughout the length of columnar-lined esophagus and separate biopsies from other areas of mucosal abnormalities such as ulcers or nodules [155, 156]. Studies have shown that overall adherence to validated biopsy protocols among gastroenterologists is suboptimal and decreases even further as the length of columnar lined mucosa increases [156, 157]. Interobserver variability among expert GI pathologists in diagnosing the presence and degree of dysplasia has been demonstrated in multiple studies [128]. As noted above, the overall risk of EAC in patients with BE is low, with recent studies showing annual incidence much lower than 0.5% [14]. Despite limitations of the scientific evidence, most professional societies recommend endoscopic surveillance for patients with BE. As discussed in previous sections, the risk of EAC increases as NDBE progresses in a sequential manner to LGD and HGD. The frequency of surveillance is therefore based on the grade of dysplasia.

The *ACG* recommends that all patients with documented BE should be assessed for surveillance. The decision should take into consideration patient's age, likelihood of survival over the next 5 years, and willingness to adhere to the surveillance program after understanding the risks, benefits, and limitations of surveillance. In order to avoid interference due to inflammation from reflux esophagitis, patients' symptoms of GERD should be controlled with proton pump inhibitors (PPIs). Surveillance EGD should include 4 quadrant biopsies from every 2 cm of Barrett's mucosa. Separate biopsies must be taken from other areas of mucosal abnormalities such as ulcers or nodules. Patients with BE with no evidence of dysplasia on index endoscopy should undergo a repeat endoscopy with protocol biopsies within 1 year. If no dysplasia is found, surveillance should be done every 3 years. Finding of LGD should be confirmed by an expert GI pathologist. If LGD is confirmed, an upper endoscopy should be repeated 6 months later to rule out a higher grade of dysplasia. If this is not found to be the case, endoscopy should be done annually until no dysplasia is seen on 2 consecutive endoscopies. Mucosal abnormalities (e.g., nodules) in a background of HGD should undergo endoscopic mucosal resection (EMR) [21]. Finding of HGD should also be confirmed by an expert GI pathologist, and an upper endoscopy with biopsies should be repeated within 3 months. Most experts agree that finding of HGD should trigger intensive surveillance endoscopies every 3 months and a detailed discussion with the patient about endoscopic therapeutic options (see below). Mucosal abnormalities (e.g., nodules) in a background of HGD should undergo endoscopic mucosal resection (EMR) [21].

Other major gastroenterology organizations in the US endorse most components of ACG guidelines on surveillance for BE. Table 5 summarizes the guidelines for surveillance of BE by major professional organizations in the United States.

13. Management of Barrett's Esophagus

13.1. Management of Nondysplastic Barrett's Esophagus. All patients with BE should be on acid-suppressive therapy to control symptoms related to GERD. However, there is no convincing evidence that acid-suppressive therapy or antireflux surgery reverses the IM or dysplasia [8, 158]. Although endoscopic eradiation therapies (EET) have been tried successfully in NDBE, at this time most professional organizations do not recommend EET for NDBE [8, 21, 159].

13.2. Management of Barrett's with Low-Grade Dysplasia. The conventional approach for management of LGD has been that of careful endoscopic surveillance biopsies and EMR for all mucosal nodules or irregularities [21]. However, data from some studies showing relatively high malignant risk of LGD and growing literature on safety and efficacy of endoscopic ablation therapies has sparked a debate about the appropriate management of LGD. Those in favor of watchful waiting view the data on high malignant risk of LGD with skepticism. These studies are small in size, and most do not distinguish between prevalent LGD and incident LGD. The latter issue is important to recognize because malignant risk may be different between prevalent and incident LGD. Some of the studies have lumped together HGD and EAC as their final outcome of interest which can skew the data towards a higher risk. The important issue of interobserver variability (see above) in LGD has not been addressed in most of these studies [160]. One also needs to be cognizant of the phenomenon of regression reported in LGD [43]. It is not clear whether this occurs due to initial overdiagnosis,

Table 5: Guidelines for Barrett's esophagus surveillance by major professional organizations in the United States.

Grade of dysplasia	ACG	AGA	ASGE[¥]
NDBE	2 EGD within 1st year, then every 3 years if still NDBE	2 EGD within 1st year, then every 3–5 years if still NDBE	2 EGD within 1st year, then every 3 years if still NDBE
LGD[†]	Repeat EGD within 6 months; if no higher-grade dysplasia, then every 1 year	Repeat EGD within 6 months; if no higher-grade dysplasia, then every 6–12 months	Repeat EGD in 6 months; if no higher-grade dysplasia, then every 1 year
HGD[†£]	Repeat EGD within 3 months to rule out EAC, then every 3 months	Repeat EGD within 3 months to rule out EAC, then every 3 months	Repeat EGD within 3 months to rule out EAC, then every 3 months

[†] Should be confirmed by an expert GI pathologist.
[£] Detailed discussion should be initiated regarding therapeutic options.
[¥] Jumbo biopsy forceps should be used to increase yield.
ACG: American College of Gastroenterology; AGA: American Gastroenterological Association; NDBE: nondysplastic Barrett's esophagus; LGD: low-grade dysplasia; HGD: high-grade dysplasia.

sampling errors, or true regression. Finally, the cost and risks of endoscopic therapies need to be weighed against the benefit of treating LGD, a condition whose malignant risk has not been clearly defined at this time [161, 162].

Endoscopic therapies for LGD have been used successfully. Those in favor of endoscopic ablation for LGD view this therapy as safe, effective, and durable. In a trial of RFA in dysplastic BE, among the patients with LGD, complete eradication of dysplasia was seen in 90.5% patients who received RFA compared with 22.7% in controls (sham procedure) ($P < 0.001$) [163]. Complete ablation of LGD and NDBE may also give the patients peace of mind, although data backing this assumption are lacking. However, radiofrequency ablation (RFA) can result in upper GI bleeding and about 6% rate of esophageal strictures [163]. Esophageal strictures and photosensitivity reaction to chemosensitizing agent were reported in 36% and 69% patients, respectively, who underwent photodynamic therapy (PDT) [142]. Some experts recommend an individualized approach based on risk startification and patient preference. Based on the available data, the ACG, AGA, and ASGE guidelines do not recommend routine endoscopic ablation for LGD at this time [8, 21, 50].

13.3. Management of Barrett's with High-Grade Dysplasia. Before the advent of endoscopic therapies, esophagectomy was the primary treatment option for patients with HGD. Data from older series showed up to 40% coexisting cancer in patients who underwent esophagectomy for HGD [164]. However, recent studies suggest that 12.7% prevalence of EAC in these cases may be a more accurate estimate. If patients without any endoscopically visible lesions are analyzed, the rate drops to about 3% [165]. Furthermore, even in expert hands, esophagectomy carries a mortality risk of 1–5% and morbidity risk of 30–50% [164, 166]. There are no prospective, randomized trials comparing EET directly with esophagectomy for management of HGD or intramucosal adenocarcinoma of the esophagus. However, this question has been evaluated in retrospective studies. Prasad et al. retrospectively compared data on 129 patients who received endoscopic therapy (PDT ± adjunctive EMR) and 70 patients who underwent esophagectomy for HGD at their institution. The patients in the PDT group were followed for a mean of 59 ± 2.7 months and those in the esophagectomy group for a mean of 61 ± 5.8 months. The overall mortality was similar in the 2 groups at the end of followup period (9% in the PDT group versus 8.5% in the esophagectomy group, $P = 0.76$) [167]. Another study identified 742 patients with early esophageal cancer, in a review of surveillance epidemiology and end results (SEER) database. About 13% of these patients were treated with endoscopic therapy and rest with surgical resection. The risk of esophageal cancer-related mortality was similar between the endoscopic and surgical groups (HR = 0.89; CI = 0.51 – 1.56; $P = 0.68$) [168].

EMR is an important tool in accurate staging of the disease that can in turn guide appropriate therapy. The specimens obtained from EMR are larger than the mucosal biopsies and provide a better assessment of the depth of tumor invasion into mucosa and submucosa. Larghi and colleagues performed EUS to stage the disease of 48 BE patients with biopsy-proven HGD/intramucosal carcinoma. EUS showed mucosal disease in 40 patients (25 HGD and 15 intramucosal carcinomas). Eight patients found to have submucosal invasion on EUS were excluded. EMR was done in the 40 patients with disease confined to the mucosa. Compared with EUS, the EMR upstaged the disease from HGD to intramucosal carcinoma in 6/25 (24%) patients and from intramucosal carcinoma to submucosal invasion in 6/15 (40%) patients [169]. A systematic review showed that EMR resulted in change of diagnosis in about 25% of cases when compared with mucosal biopsies (upstaging or downstaging) [170]. Role of circumferential EMR in eradication of BE with HGD has been evaluated. In one study, 12 patients with BE and HGD or intramucosal cancer underwent circumferential EMR (median of 2.5 sessions, median of 5 snare resections per session). No recurrence of BE or cancer occurred during a median followup of 9 months. Complications included esophageal strictures in 2 patients treated successfully by bougienage, and minor bleeding during 4/31 EMR sessions [171]. Other studies on circumferential EMR have reported 86–100% complete eradication rate, and recurrence of malignancy in up to 11% cases. A high stricture rate is a limitation of this technique [172, 173].

Although a variety of endoscopic ablation therapies have been studied for eradication of HGD, the best evidence is available for RFA and PDT. In a multicenter, sham-controlled trial, 127 patients with dysplastic BE were randomized to RFA ($N = 84$) or sham procedure ($N = 43$). Among patients with HGD, complete eradication of dysplasia was achieved in 81% in the ablation group compared with 19% in the control group ($P < 0.001$). One patient developed upper GI hemorrhage and 5 (6%) developed esophageal stricture in the ablation group. All complications were successfully managed endoscopically [163]. As a separate study, in the same population, subjects in the sham group were offered crossover to the RFA treatment after the completion of first 12 months. All subjects were followed for 2 years from initial enrollment. Those who had achieved complete eradication of IM at 2 years were followed for 3 additional years with annual surveillance EGD and biopsies. At the end of study period, dysplasia remained eradicated in >85% patients and intestinal metaplasia in >75% without maintenance RFA. The authors concluded that RFA offers safe, effective, and durable therapy for dysplastic BE [174].

Overholt et al. performed porfimer-PDT in 103 patients with BE and used supplemental Nd:YAG laser to ablate small areas of residual Barrett's mucosa. Mean followup for the 82 patients who completed the study was 58.5 months. About 94% (60/65) patients with HGD had eradication of dysplasia. Three (4.6%) patients developed subsquamous adenocarcinoma. Strictures occurred in 30% patients [175]. In a multicenter, randomized trial, 208 patients with HGD were randomized to receive PDT plus omeprazole (PORPDT group, $N = 138$) or omeprazole only (OM group, $N = 70$). Complete ablation of HGD was seen in 106/138 (77%) patients in the PORPDT group versus 27/70 (39%) patients in the OM group. PORPDT group experienced photosensitivity reactions in 69% patients. About 36% patients in this group developed esophageal strictures that were managed successfully with endoscopic dilatation [142].

The current *ACG* guidelines state that treatment for HGD should be individualized. Patient should be presented the options of EET, surgical resection, or intensive surveillance. Careful consideration should be given to patient's preferences, surgical risk, and available expertise. If esophagectomy is planned, patient should be referred to a center of expertise and high volume (at least 20 esophagectomies per year) to reduce operative mortality to less than 5%. The *AGA* concludes that EET is a reasonable therapeutic option for patients with HGD, especially in those with advanced age and comorbidities. If EET is used, any visible mucosal abnormalities should be resected by EMR. With regards to question of esophagectomy, AGA states that this option should be considered in young and otherwise fit patients with HGD. The Society of Thoracic Surgeons also adopts a position very similar to the ACG and AGA for the management of BE with HGD [176].

The patients who undergo EET for dysplastic BE should continue to undergo surveillance after the therapy. The surveillance interval is dependent on the highest degree of dysplasia documented before the ablative therapy. This surveillance protocol should be continued until lack of dysplasia is documented to a reasonable degree of certainty on 3 consecutive endoscopies. However, periodic surveillance should still be continued because of the potential of BE to recur. The precise interval for these surveillance endoscopies has not been clearly defined at this time [21, 50].

14. Chemoprevention of Barrett's Esophagus

14.1. Proton Pump Inhibitors. Studies have evaluated the role of acid and acid suppression in BE. Acid exposure has been shown to induce DNA double-strand break (DSB), increase reactive oxygen species (ROS), andactivate MAP kinase pathway, suggesting its potential role in carcinogenesis [177, 178]. Observational studies have reported decreased incidence of dysplasia with chronic PPI therapy [179, 180]. In one study, 188 BE patients treated with PPI therapy for 1–13 years were prospectively followed (mean follow-up 5.1 years). During the study period, no decrease in the length of BE was noted, but 48% of the patients developed squamous islands in the BE segments. The squamous islands correlated with the duration of PPI therapy (RR: 0.43; 95% CI: 0.35–0.65) but not with the PPI dose. All 7 patients who received PPI for 12-13 years developed squamous islands [181]. Conversely, there are reports suggesting an association between chronic PPI use and increased risk of EAC. However, these findings may have been confounded by the indication for chronic PPI. Thus, the increased incidence of EAC might have been related to the original condition for which PPI was prescribed rather than the PPI itself [182]. In summary, the evidence on the chemo preventive effects of PPI for BE is equivocal and not backed by prospective studies. Nonetheless, PPI use is recommended in BE, to control the symptoms of GERD and prevent related complications like esophagitis and ulcerations. Higher than once daily dosing of PPI cannot be recommended based on available data [8].

14.2. Nonsteroidal Anti-Inflammatory Drugs and Aspirin. Data suggest that COX-2-derived prostaglandin E2 (PGE2) promotes tumor growth by promoting cell proliferation, migration, apoptosis, and angiogenesis. Inhibition of COX-2 attenuates cell growth and proliferation, inhibits angiogenesis, and restores apoptosis [183–185]. The cardiovascular adverse effects associated with the long-term use of selective COX-2 inhibitors have dampened the enthusiasm about their role in cancer chemoprophylaxis. However, studies have shown that chronic use of nonsteroidal anti-inflammatory drugs (NSAIDs) or aspirin can decrease the risk of colorectal cancer, gastric cancer, and several non-GI malignancies [186]. A systematic review of 9 studies including more than 1800 patients evaluated the association between aspirin or NSAIDs use and esophageal cancer. Any use of aspirin or NSAIDs was associated with a 43% reduced risk of esophageal cancer (odds ratio (OR) = 0.57; 95% confidence interval (CI) = 0.47–0.71). Frequent use of aspirin or NSAIDs was associated with 46% risk reduction (OR = 0.54; CI = 0.43–0.67), whereas intermittent use was associated with 18% risk reduction (OR = 0.82; CI = 0.67–0.99). Analyzed separately, both aspirin use (OR = 0.5; CI, 0.38–0.66) and

NSAIDs use (OR = 0.75; CI = 0.54–1.0) were associated with reduced risk of esophageal cancer. The association between any use of aspirin or NSAIDs and decreased cancer risk was seen for both esophageal adenocarcinoma (OR = 0.67; CI = 0.51–0.87) and squamous cell carcinoma (OR = 0.58; CI = 0.43–0.78) [187]. Vaughan et al. prospectively followed a cohort of 350 Barrett's patients for 20,770 person months (median followup 65.5 months). Current use of NSAIDs was associated with 68% risk reduction of EAC (HR = 0.32; 95% CI = 0.14–0.76) and past use with 30% risk reduction (HR = 0.70; 95% CI = 0.31–1.58) [188]. In a recent study from Netherlands, 570 BE patients were prospectively followed for a median of 4.5 years. Use of NSAIDs (median duration 2 months) was associated with 53% lower risk of progression to HGD/EAC ($P = 0.03$) [189]. Despite the above data, there is lack of evidence to suggest that the chemopreventive benefits of NSAIDs outweigh the potential cardiovascular side effects, risk of major GI and non-GI bleeding, and nephrotoxicity associated with their chronic use. Most experts agree that it is appropriate to use low-dose aspirin in patients with BE who have a cardiovascular indication for this medication. The concomitant use of PPI, as is the case in most BE patients, should decrease the risk of serious GI complications [8].

14.3. Statins. Statins exert their cholesterol-lowering effect by inhibiting the enzyme 3-hydroxy-3-methylglutaryl coenzyme A reductase. However, this class of drugs has also been shown to have other pleiotropic properties. Statins promote apoptosis and inhibit proliferation in BE cells by reducing serum-stimulated Ras activity and inhibiting activation of extracellular signal-regulated kinase (ERK) and protein kinase B (Akt) [190, 191]. A case-control study of approximately 12,000 BE patients in the Department of Veterans' Affairs database showed that statin use was associated with a reduction in EAC risk (HR = 0.55; 95% confidence interval, 0.36–0.86), with a significant trend toward greater risk reduction with longer duration of statin use [192]. In the Dutch study mentioned above, long-term use of statins (median duration of 5 years) was associated with a 54% reduction in the risk of malignant progression of BE. A combination of NSAIDs and statins was associated with a risk reduction of 78% ($P = 0.028$) [189]. Although the above studies suggest an association between statin use and decreased cancer risk in BE, a cause-effect relation cannot be established based on the available evidence.

15. Future Directions

BE will continue to be an area of active research in the foreseeable future due to areas of uncertainty and controversy. With recent studies showing a much lower cancer risk in BE, and the growing emphasis on health care cost containment, the rationale of screening and surveillance for BE, is likely to come under greater scrutiny [193]. More research is anticipated on the development of less invasive and more cost-effective modalities for detection of BE. Further studies are needed on non-endoscopic means for BE diagnosis such as cytosponge with immunohistochemistry, spectroscopy and colorimetric techniques [194–196]. A panel of molecular biomarkers that can stratify patients based on risk of progression to cancer might help develop a more tailored approach to BE surveillance [15]. The current limitations of high-resolution white light endoscopy and protocol biopsies in detecting dysplasia call for continued research on better techniques for optical recognition of dysplasia (e.g., confocal laser endomicroscopy, spectroscopy, optical coherence tomography, chromoendoscopy, etc.) to guide targeted biopsies for a higher diagnostic yield [197–200]. Debate is likely to intensify on the appropriate management of LGD and even NDBE as the safety, effectiveness, and durability of endoscopic ablation of BE is better defined [71, 160, 174, 201]. Finally, the chemoprevention of BE is likely to remain an active area of research.

References

[1] J. Steevens, A. A. M. Botterweck, M. J. M. Dirx, P. A. Van Den Brandt, and L. J. Schouten, "Trends in incidence of oesophageal and stomach cancer subtypes in Europe," *European Journal of Gastroenterology and Hepatology*, vol. 22, no. 6, pp. 669–678, 2010.

[2] M. B. Cook, W. H. Chow, and S. S. Devesa, "Oesophageal cancer incidence in the United States by race, sex, and histologic type, 1977–2005," *British Journal of Cancer*, vol. 101, no. 5, pp. 855–859, 2009.

[3] F. Yousef, C. Cardwell, M. M. Cantwell, K. Galway, B. T. Johnston, and L. Murray, "The incidence of esophageal cancer and high-grade dysplasia in Barrett's esophagus: a systematic review and meta-analysis," *American Journal of Epidemiology*, vol. 168, no. 3, pp. 237–249, 2008.

[4] H. Pohl and H. G. Welch, "The role of overdiagnosis and reclassification in the marked increase of esophageal adenocarcinoma incidence," *Journal of the National Cancer Institute*, vol. 97, no. 2, pp. 142–146, 2005.

[5] M. A. Eloubeidi, A. C. Mason, R. A. Desmond, and H. B. El-Serag, "Temporal trends (1973–1997) in survival of patients with esophageal adenocarcinoma in the United States: a glimmer of hope?" *American Journal of Gastroenterology*, vol. 98, no. 7, pp. 1627–1633, 2003.

[6] J. Lagergren, "Adenocarcinoma of oesophagus: what exactly is the size of the problem and who is at risk?" *Gut*, vol. 54, supplement 1, pp. i1–i5, 2005.

[7] S. Bhat, H. G. Coleman, F. Yousef et al., "Risk of malignant progression in Barrett's Esophagus patients: results from a large population-based study," *Journal of the National Cancer Institute*, vol. 103, no. 13, pp. 1049–1057, 2011.

[8] S. J. Spechler, P. Sharma, R. F. Souza, J. M. Inadomi, and N. J. Shaheen, "American gastroenterological association technical review on the management of Barrett's esophagus," *Gastroenterology*, vol. 140, no. 3, pp. e18–e52, 2011.

[9] R. J. Playford, "New British Society of Gastroenterology (BSG) guidelines for the diagnosis and management of Barrett's oesophagus," *Gut*, vol. 55, no. 4, pp. 442–443, 2006.

[10] R. H. Riddell and R. D. Odze, "Definition of barrett's esophagus: time for a rethinkis intestinal metaplasia dead," *American Journal of Gastroenterology*, vol. 104, no. 10, pp. 2588–2594, 2009.

[11] L. B. Gerson, K. Shetler, and G. Triadafilopoulos, "Prevalence of Barrett's esophagus in asymptomatic individuals," *Gastroenterology*, vol. 123, no. 2, pp. 461–467, 2002.

[12] D. K. Rex, O. W. Cummings, M. Shaw et al., "Screening for Barrett's esophagus in colonoscopy patients with and without heartburn," *Gastroenterology*, vol. 125, no. 6, pp. 1670–1677, 2003.

[13] J. Ronkainen, P. Aro, T. Storskrubb et al., "Prevalence of Barrett's esophagus in the general population: an endoscopic study," *Gastroenterology*, vol. 129, no. 6, pp. 1825–1831, 2005.

[14] F. Hvid-Jensen, L. Pedersen, A. M. Drewes, H. T. Sorensen, and P. Funch-Jensen, "Incidence of adenocarcinoma among patients with Barrett's esophagus," *The New England Journal of Medicine*, vol. 365, no. 15, pp. 1375–1383, 2011.

[15] L. H. Moyes and J. J. Going, "Still waiting for predictive biomarkers in Barrett's oesophagus," *Journal of Clinical Pathology*, vol. 64, no. 9, pp. 742–750, 2011.

[16] P. Sharma, J. Dent, D. Armstrong et al., "The development and validation of an endoscopic grading system for Barrett's esophagus: the prague C & M criteria," *Gastroenterology*, vol. 131, no. 5, pp. 1392–1399, 2006.

[17] N. R. Barrett, "Chronic peptic ulcer of the oesophagus and 'oesophagitis'," *The British Journal of Surgery*, vol. 38, no. 150, pp. 175–182, 1950.

[18] P. R. Allison and A. S. Johnstone, "The oesophagus lined with gastric mucous membrane," *Thorax*, vol. 8, no. 2, pp. 87–101, 1953.

[19] N. R. Barrett, "The lower esophagus lined by columnar epithelium," *Surgery*, vol. 41, no. 6, pp. 881–894, 1957.

[20] S. J. Spechler and R. K. Goyal, "The columnar-lined esophagus, intestinal metaplasia, and Norman Barrett," *Gastroenterology*, vol. 110, no. 2, pp. 614–621, 1996.

[21] K. K. Wang and R. E. Sampliner, "Updated guidelines 2008 for the diagnosis, surveillance and therapy of Barrett's esophagus," *American Journal of Gastroenterology*, vol. 103, no. 3, pp. 788–797, 2008.

[22] S. A. McClave, H. W. Boyce, and M. R. Gottfried, "Early diagnosis of columnar-lined esophagus: a new endoscopic diagnostic criterion," *Gastrointestinal Endoscopy*, vol. 33, no. 6, pp. 413–416, 1987.

[23] D. W. Choi, S. N. Oh, S. J. Baek et al., "Endoscopically observed lower esophageal capillary patterns," *The Korean Journal of Internal Medicine*, vol. 17, no. 4, pp. 245–248, 2002.

[24] A. Vianna, P. C. Hayes, G. Moscoso et al., "Normal venous circulation of the gastroesophageal junction: a route to understanding varices," *Gastroenterology*, vol. 93, no. 4, pp. 876–889, 1987.

[25] A. Paull, J. S. Trier, and M. D. Dalton, "The histologic spectrum of Barrett's esophagus," *New England Journal of Medicine*, vol. 295, no. 9, pp. 476–480, 1976.

[26] W. K. Hirota, T. M. Loughney, D. J. Lazas, C. L. Maydonovitch, V. Rholl, and R. K. H. Wong, "Specialized intestinal metaplasia, dysplasia, and cancer of the esophagus and esophagogastric junction: prevalence and clinical data," *Gastroenterology*, vol. 116, no. 2, pp. 277–285, 1999.

[27] M. Peck-Radosavljevic, A. Puspok, R. Potzi, and G. Oberhuber, "Histological findings after routine biopsy at the gastrooesophageal junction," *European Journal of Gastroenterology & Hepatology*, vol. 11, no. 11, pp. 1265–1270, 1999.

[28] S. J. Spechler, "Intestinal metaplasia at the gastroesophageal junction," *Gastroenterology*, vol. 126, no. 2, pp. 567–575, 2004.

[29] T. Thomas, K. R. Abrams, J. S. De Caestecker, and R. J. Robinson, "Meta analysis: cancer risk in Barrett's oesophagus," *Alimentary Pharmacology and Therapeutics*, vol. 26, no. 11-12, pp. 1465–1477, 2007.

[30] W. Liu, H. Hahn, R. D. Odze, and R. K. Goyal, "Metaplastic esophageal columnar epithelium without goblet cells shows DNA content abnormalities similar to goblet cell-containing epithelium," *American Journal of Gastroenterology*, vol. 104, no. 4, pp. 816–824, 2009.

[31] H. P. Hahn, P. L. Blount, K. Ayub et al., "Intestinal differentiation in metaplastic, nongoblet columnar epithelium in the esophagus," *American Journal of Surgical Pathology*, vol. 33, no. 7, pp. 1006–1015, 2009.

[32] S. Öberg, J. Johansson, J. Wenner et al., "Endoscopic surveillance of columnar-lined esophagus: frequency of intestinal metaplasia detection and impact of antireflux surgery," *Annals of Surgery*, vol. 234, no. 5, pp. 619–626, 2001.

[33] T. F. Jones, P. Sharma, B. Daaboul et al., "Yield of intestinal metaplasia in patients with suspected short-segment Barrett's esophagus (SSBE) on repeat endoscopy," *Digestive Diseases and Sciences*, vol. 47, no. 9, pp. 2108–2111, 2002.

[34] R. Harrison, I. Perry, W. Haddadin et al., "Detection of intestinal metaplasia in Barrett's Esophagus: an observational comparator study suggests the need for a minimum of eight biopsies," *American Journal of Gastroenterology*, vol. 102, no. 6, pp. 1154–1161, 2007.

[35] S. D. Crockett, Q. K. Lippmann, E. S. Dellon, and N. J. Shaheen, "Health-related quality of life in patients with Barrett's esophagus: a systematic review," *Clinical Gastroenterology and Hepatology*, vol. 7, no. 6, pp. 613–623, 2009.

[36] N. J. Shaheen, B. Green, R. K. Medapalli et al., "The perception of cancer risk in patients with prevalent Barrett's esophagus enrolled in an endoscopic surveillance program," *Gastroenterology*, vol. 129, no. 2, pp. 429–436, 2005.

[37] N. J. Shaheen, G. S. Dulai, B. Ascher, K. L. Mitchell, and S. M. Schmitz, "Effect of a new diagnosis of Barrett's esophagus on insurance status," *American Journal of Gastroenterology*, vol. 100, no. 3, pp. 577–580, 2005.

[38] P. Sharma, T. G. Morales, and R. E. Sampliner, "Short segment Barrett's esophagus—the need for standardization of the definition and of endoscopic criteria," *American Journal of Gastroenterology*, vol. 93, no. 7, pp. 1033–1036, 1998.

[39] B. Vahabzadeh, A. B. Seetharam, M. B. Cook et al., "Validation of the Prague C & M criteria for the endoscopic grading of Barrett's esophagus by gastroenterology trainees: a multicenter study," *Gastrointestinal Endoscopy*, vol. 75, no. 2, pp. 236–241, 2012.

[40] T. Kinjo, C. Kusano, I. Oda, and T. Gotoda, "Prague C&M and Japanese criteria: shades of Barrett's esophagus endoscopic diagnosis," *Journal of Gastroenterology*, vol. 45, no. 10, pp. 1039–1044, 2010.

[41] J. Alcedo, A. Ferrandez, J. Arenas et al., "Trends in Barrett's esophagus diagnosis in Southern Europe: implications for surveillance," *Diseases of the Esophagus*, vol. 22, no. 3, pp. 239–248, 2009.

[42] J. Boyer, R. Laugier, M. Chemall et al., "French society of digestive endoscopy SFED guideline: monitoring of patients with Barrett's esophagus," *Endoscopy*, vol. 39, no. 9, pp. 840–842, 2007.

[43] P. Sharma, G. W. Falk, A. P. Weston, D. Reker, M. Johnston, and R. E. Sampliner, "Dysplasia and cancer in a large multicenter cohort of patients with Barrett's esophagus," *Clinical Gastroenterology and Hepatology*, vol. 4, no. 5, pp. 566–572, 2006.

[44] C. H. Lim, D. Treanor, M. F. Dixon, and A. T. R. Axon, "Low-grade dysplasia in Barrett's esophagus has a high risk of progression," *Endoscopy*, vol. 39, no. 7, pp. 581–587, 2007.

[45] L. J. Schouten, J. Steevens, and C. J. Huysentruyt, "Total cancer incidence and overall mortality are not increased among patients with Barrett's esophagus," *Clinical Gastroenterology and Hepatology*, vol. 9, no. 9, pp. 754–761, 2011.

[46] W. L. Curvers, F. J. Ten Kate, K. K. Krishnadath et al., "Low-grade dysplasia in barrett's esophagus: overdiagnosed and underestimated," *American Journal of Gastroenterology*, vol. 105, no. 7, pp. 1523–1530, 2010.

[47] T. G. Schnell, S. J. Sontag, G. Chejfec et al., "Long-term non-surgical management of Barrett's esophagus with high-grade dysplasia," *Gastroenterology*, vol. 120, no. 7, pp. 1607–1619, 2001.

[48] A.P. Weston, P. Sharma, M. Topalovski, R. Richards, R. Cherian, and A. Dixon, "Long-term follow-up of Barrett's high-grade dysplasia," *The American Journal of Gastroenterology*, vol. 95, no. 8, pp. 1888–1893, 2000.

[49] A. Rastogi, S. Puli, H. B. El-Serag, A. Bansal, S. Wani, and P. Sharma, "Incidence of esophageal adenocarcinoma in patients with Barrett's esophagus and high-grade dysplasia: a meta-analysis," *Gastrointestinal Endoscopy*, vol. 67, no. 3, pp. 394–398, 2008.

[50] W. K. Hirota, M. J. Zuckerman, D. G. Adler et al., "ASGE guideline: the role of endoscopy in the surveillance of premalignant conditions of the upper GI tract," *Gastrointestinal Endoscopy*, vol. 63, no. 4, pp. 570–580, 2006.

[51] J. A. Abrams, S. Fields, C. J. Lightdale, and A. I. Neugut, "Racial and ethnic disparities in the prevalence of Barrett's esophagus among patients who undergo upper endoscopy," *Clinical Gastroenterology and Hepatology*, vol. 6, no. 1, pp. 30–34, 2008.

[52] Z. R. Edelstein, M. P. Bronner, S. N. Rosen, and T. L. Vaughan, "Risk factors for barrett's esophagus among patients with gastroesophageal reflux disease: a community clinic-based case-control study," *American Journal of Gastroenterology*, vol. 104, no. 4, pp. 834–842, 2009.

[53] P. Yachimski, R. A. Lee, A. Tramontano, N. S. Nishioka, and C. Hur, "Secular trends in patients diagnosed with Barrett's esophagus," *Digestive Diseases and Sciences*, vol. 55, no. 4, pp. 960–966, 2010.

[54] D. A. Corley, A. Kubo, T. R. Levin et al., "Race, ethnicity, sex and temporal differences in Barrett's oesophagus diagnosis: a large community-based study, 1994–2006," *Gut*, vol. 58, no. 2, pp. 182–188, 2009.

[55] M. A. Eloubeidi and D. Provenzale, "Clinical and demographic predictors of Barrett's esophagus among patients with gastroesophageal reflux disease: a multivariable analysis in veterans," *Journal of Clinical Gastroenterology*, vol. 33, no. 4, pp. 306–309, 2001.

[56] G. M. Eisen, R. S. Sandler, S. Murray, and M. Gottfried, "The relationship between gastroesophageal reflux disease and its complications with Barrett's esophagus," *American Journal of Gastroenterology*, vol. 92, no. 1, pp. 27–31, 1997.

[57] B. Avidan, A. Sonnenberg, T. G. Schnell, and S. J. Sontag, "Hiatal hernia and acid reflux frequency predict presence and length of Barrett's esophagus," *Digestive Diseases and Sciences*, vol. 47, no. 2, pp. 256–264, 2002.

[58] Z. R. Edelstein, D. C. Farrow, M. P. Bronner, S. N. Rosen, and T. L. Vaughan, "Central adiposity and risk of Barrett's esophagus," *Gastroenterology*, vol. 133, no. 2, pp. 403–411, 2007.

[59] H. B. El-Serag, P. Kvapil, J. Hacken-Bitar, and J. R. Kramer, "Abdominal obesity and the risk of Barrett's esophagus," *American Journal of Gastroenterology*, vol. 100, no. 10, pp. 2151–2156, 2005.

[60] P. Kamat, S. Wen, J. Morris, and S. Anandasabapathy, "Exploring the association between elevated body mass index and Barrett's esophagus: a systematic review and meta-analysis," *Annals of Thoracic Surgery*, vol. 87, no. 2, pp. 655–662, 2009.

[61] D. A. Corley, A. Kubo, T. R. Levin et al., "Abdominal obesity and body mass index as risk factors for Barrett's esophagus," *Gastroenterology*, vol. 133, no. 1, pp. 34–41, 2007.

[62] L. A. Anderson, M. M. Cantwell, R. G. P. Watson et al., "The association between alcohol and reflux esophagitis, Barrett's esophagus, and esophageal adenocarcinoma," *Gastroenterology*, vol. 136, no. 3, pp. 799–805, 2009.

[63] A. Kubo, T. R. Levin, G. Block et al., "Alcohol types and sociodemographic characteristics as risk factors for Barrett's esophagus," *Gastroenterology*, vol. 136, no. 3, pp. 806–815, 2009.

[64] A. Kubo, T. R. Levin, G. Block et al., "Dietary antioxidants, fruits, and vegetables and the risk of barrett's esophagus," *American Journal of Gastroenterology*, vol. 103, no. 7, pp. 1614–1624, 2008.

[65] A. Kubo, T. R. Levin, G. Block et al., "Dietary patterns and the risk of Barrett's esophagus," *American Journal of Epidemiology*, vol. 167, no. 7, pp. 839–846, 2008.

[66] O. M. Thompson, S. A. A. Beresford, E. A. Kirk, and T. L. Vaughan, "Vegetable and fruit intakes and risk of Barrett's esophagus in men and women," *American Journal of Clinical Nutrition*, vol. 89, no. 3, pp. 890–896, 2009.

[67] T. Rokkas, D. Pistiolas, P. Sechopoulos, I. Robotis, and G. Margantinis, "Relationship between Helicobacter pylori infection and esophageal neoplasia: a meta-analysis," *Clinical Gastroenterology and Hepatology*, vol. 5, no. 12, pp. 1413–1417, 2007.

[68] A. J. Cameron, A. R. Zinsmeister, D. J. Ballard, and J. A. Carney, "Prevalence of columnar-lined (Barrett's) esophagus: comparison of population-based clinical and autopsy findings," *Gastroenterology*, vol. 99, no. 4, pp. 918–922, 1990.

[69] A. K. Musana, J. M. Resnick, C. F. Torbey, B. N. Mukesh, and R. T. Greenlee, "Barrett's esophagus: incidence and prevalence estimates in a rural mid-western population," *American Journal of Gastroenterology*, vol. 103, no. 3, pp. 516–524, 2008.

[70] J. Ronkainen, P. Aro, T. Storskrubb et al., "High prevalence of gastroesophageal reflux symptoms and esophagitis with or without symptoms in the general adult Swedish population: a Kalixanda study report," *Scandinavian Journal of Gastroenterology*, vol. 40, no. 3, pp. 275–285, 2005.

[71] P. Sharma, "Clinical practice. Barrett's esophagus," *The New England Journal of Medicine*, vol. 361, no. 26, pp. 2548–2556, 2009.

[72] S. J. Spechler, "Clinical practice. Barrett's esophagus," *The New England Journal of Medicine*, vol. 346, no. 11, pp. 836–842, 2002.

[73] J. N. Glickman, Y. Y. Chen, H. H. Wang, D. A. Antonioli, and R. D. Odze, "Phenotypic characteristics of a distinctive multilayered epithelium suggests that it is a precursor in the development of Barrett's esophagus," *American Journal of Surgical Pathology*, vol. 25, no. 5, pp. 569–578, 2001.

[74] J. A. Jankowski, N. A. Wright, S. J. Meltzer et al., "Molecular evolution of the metaplasia-dysplasia-adenocarcinoma sequence in the esophagus," *American Journal of Pathology*, vol. 154, no. 4, pp. 965–973, 1999.

[75] M. Pera and M. Pera, "Experimental Barrett's esophagus and the origin of intestinal metaplasia," *Chest Surgery Clinics of North America*, vol. 12, no. 1, pp. 25–37, 2002.

[76] G. Sarosi, G. Brown, K. Jaiswal et al., "Bone marrow progenitor cells contribute to esophageal regeneration and metaplasia in a rat model of Barrett's esophagus," *Diseases of the Esophagus*, vol. 21, no. 1, pp. 43–50, 2008.

[77] J. P. Seery, "Stem cells of the oesophageal epithelium," *Journal of Cell Science*, vol. 115, no. 9, pp. 1783–1789, 2002.

[78] J. Kalabis, K. Oyama, T. Okawa et al., "A subpopulation of mouse esophageal basal cells has properties of stem cells with the capacity for self-renewal and lineage specification," *Journal of Clinical Investigation*, vol. 118, no. 12, pp. 3860–3869, 2008.

[79] K. Takahashi and S. Yamanaka, "Induction of pluripotent stem cells from mouse embryonic and adult fibroblast cultures by defined factors," *Cell*, vol. 126, no. 4, pp. 663–676, 2006.

[80] A. J. Bass, H. Watanabe, C. H. Mermel et al., "*SOX2* is an amplified lineage-survival oncogene in lung and esophageal squamous cell carcinomas," *Nature Genetics*, vol. 41, no. 11, pp. 1238–1242, 2009.

[81] D. B. Stairs, H. Nakagawa, A. Klein-Szanto et al., "Cdx1 and c-Myc foster the initiation of transdifferentiation of the normal esophageal squamous epithelium toward Barrett's esophagus," *PLoS ONE*, vol. 3, no. 10, Article ID e3534, 2008.

[82] H. Kazumori, S. Ishihara, Y. Takahashi, Y. Amano, and Y. Kinoshita, "Roles of Krüppel-like factor 4 in oesophageal epithelial cells in Barrett's epithelium development," *Gut*, vol. 60, no. 5, pp. 608–617, 2011.

[83] M. F. Vaezi and J. E. Richter, "Role of acid and duodenogastroesophageal reflux in gastroesophageal reflux disease," *Gastroenterology*, vol. 111, no. 5, pp. 1192–1199, 1996.

[84] B. Westhoff, S. Brotze, A. Weston et al., "The frequency of Barrett's esophagus in high-risk patients with chronic GERD," *Gastrointestinal Endoscopy*, vol. 61, no. 2, pp. 226–231, 2005.

[85] X. Chen, G. Y. Yang, W. Y. Ding, F. Bondoc, S. K. Curtis, and C. S. Yang, "An esophagogastroduodenal anastomosis model for esophageal adenocarcinogenesis in rats and enhancement by iron overload," *Carcinogenesis*, vol. 20, no. 9, pp. 1801–1808, 1999.

[86] S. R. Goldstein, G. Y. Yang, S. K. Curtis et al., "Development of esophageal metaplasia and adenocarcinoma in a rat surgical model without the use of a carcinogen," *Carcinogenesis*, vol. 18, no. 11, pp. 2265–2270, 1997.

[87] Y. Seto and O. Kobori, "Role of reflux oesophagitis and acid in the development of columnar epithelium in the rat oesophagus," *British Journal of Surgery*, vol. 80, no. 4, pp. 467–470, 1993.

[88] R. C. Orlando, "Pathophysiology of gastroesophageal reflux disease," *Journal of Clinical Gastroenterology*, vol. 42, no. 5, pp. 584–588, 2008.

[89] L. M. G. Moons, J. G. Kusters, E. Bultman et al., "Barrett's oesophagus is characterized by a predominantly humoral inflammatory response," *Journal of Pathology*, vol. 207, no. 3, pp. 269–276, 2005.

[90] C. E. Clark, S. R. Hingorani, R. Mick, C. Combs, D. A. Tuveson, and R. H. Vonderheide, "Dynamics of the immune reaction to pancreatic cancer from inception to invasion," *Cancer Research*, vol. 67, no. 19, pp. 9518–9527, 2007.

[91] K. E. De Visser, L. V. Korets, and L. M. Coussens, "De novo carcinogenesis promoted by chronic inflammation is B lymphocyte dependent," *Cancer Cell*, vol. 7, no. 5, pp. 411–423, 2005.

[92] D. G. DeNardo, J. B. Barreto, P. Andreu et al., "$CD4^+$ T cells regulate pulmonary metastasis of mammary carcinomas by enhancing protumor properties of macrophages," *Cancer Cell*, vol. 16, no. 2, pp. 91–102, 2009.

[93] L. Yang, L. M. DeBusk, K. Fukuda et al., "Expansion of myeloid immune suppressor Gr+CD11b+ cells in tumor-bearing host directly promotes tumor angiogenesis," *Cancer Cell*, vol. 6, no. 4, pp. 409–421, 2004.

[94] L. Yang, J. Huang, X. Ren et al., "Abrogation of TGFβ signaling in mammary carcinomas recruits Gr-1+CD11b+ myeloid cells that promote metastasis," *Cancer Cell*, vol. 13, no. 1, pp. 23–35, 2008.

[95] C. D. Morris, G. R. Armstrong, G. Bigley, H. Green, and S. E. A. Attwood, "Cyclooxygenase-2 expression in the barrett's metaplasia-dysplasia-adenocarcinoma sequence," *American Journal of Gastroenterology*, vol. 96, no. 4, pp. 990–996, 2001.

[96] L. Duan, A. H. Wu, J. Sullivan-Halley, and L. Bernstein, "Nonsteroidal anti-inflammatory drugs and risk of esophageal and gastric adenocarcinomas in Los Angeles County," *Cancer Epidemiology Biomarkers and Prevention*, vol. 17, no. 1, pp. 126–134, 2008.

[97] S. Sadeghi, C. J. Bain, N. Pandeya, P. M. Webb, A. C. Green, and D. C. Whiteman, "Aspirin, nonsteroidal anti-inflammatory drugs, and the risks of cancers of the esophagus," *Cancer Epidemiology Biomarkers and Prevention*, vol. 17, no. 5, pp. 1169–1178, 2008.

[98] H. Kazumori, S. Ishihara, M. A. K. Rumi, Y. Kadowaki, and Y. Kinoshita, "Bile acids directly augment caudal related homeobox gene Cdx2 expression in oesophageal keratinocytes in Barrett's epithelium," *Gut*, vol. 55, no. 1, pp. 16–25, 2006.

[99] N. A. C. S. Wong, J. Wilding, S. Bartlett et al., "CDX1 is an important molecular mediator of Barrett's metaplasia," *Proceedings of the National Academy of Sciences of the United States of America*, vol. 102, no. 21, pp. 7565–7570, 2005.

[100] M. T. Barrett, K. Y. Yeung, W. L. Ruzzo et al., "Transcriptional analyses of Barrett's metaplasia and normal upper GI mucosae," *Neoplasia*, vol. 4, no. 2, pp. 121–128, 2002.

[101] H. B. El-Serag, Z. Nurgalieva, R. F. Souza, C. Shaw, and G. Darlington, "Is genomic evaluation feasible in endoscopic studies of Barrett's esophagus? A pilot study," *Gastrointestinal Endoscopy*, vol. 64, no. 1, pp. 17–26, 2006.

[102] C. A. Fox, L. M. Sapinoso, H. Zhang et al., "Altered expression of TFF-1 and CES-2 in Barrett's esophagus and associated adenocarcinomas," *Neoplasia*, vol. 7, no. 4, pp. 407–416, 2005.

[103] J. Helm, S. A. Enkemann, D. Coppola, J. S. Barthel, S. T. Kelley, and T. J. Yeatman, "Dedifferentiation precedes invasion in the progression from barrett's metaplasia to esophageal adenocarcinoma," *Clinical Cancer Research*, vol. 11, no. 7, pp. 2478–2485, 2005.

[104] E. T. Kimchi, M. C. Posner, J. O. Park et al., "Progression of Barrett's metaplasia to adenocarcinoma is associated with the suppression of the transcriptional programs of epidermal differentiation," *Cancer Research*, vol. 65, no. 8, pp. 3146–3154, 2005.

[105] P. Lao-Sirieix, A. Boussioutas, S. R. Kadri et al., "Non-endoscopic screening biomarkers for Barrett's oesophagus: from

microarray analysis to the clinic," *Gut*, vol. 58, no. 11, pp. 1451–1459, 2009.

[106] S. Wang, M. Zhan, J. Yin et al., "Transcriptional profiling suggests that Barrett's metaplasia is an early intermediate stage in esophageal adenocarcinogenesis," *Oncogene*, vol. 25, no. 23, pp. 3346–3356, 2006.

[107] M. S. Pepe, R. Etzioni, Z. Feng et al., "Phases of biomarker development for early detection of cancer," *Journal of the National Cancer Institute*, vol. 93, no. 14, pp. 1054–1061, 2001.

[108] C. L. Chang, P. Lao-Sirieix, V. Save, G. D. L. C. Mendez, R. Laskey, and R. C. Fitzgerald, "Retinoic acid-induced glandular differentiation of the oesophagus," *Gut*, vol. 56, no. 7, pp. 906–917, 2007.

[109] A. S. Ioannides, D. J. Henderson, L. Spitz, and A. J. Copp, "Role of Sonic hedgehog in the development of the trachea and oesophagus," *Journal of Pediatric Surgery*, vol. 38, no. 1, pp. 29–36, 2003.

[110] Y. Litingtung, L. Lei, H. Westphal, and C. Chiang, "Sonic hedgehog is essential to foregut development," *Nature Genetics*, vol. 20, no. 1, pp. 58–61, 1998.

[111] D. H. Wang, N. J. Clemons, T. Miyashita et al., "Aberrant epithelial-mesenchymal hedgehog signaling characterizes Barrett's metaplasia," *Gastroenterology*, vol. 138, no. 5, pp. 1810–1822, 2010.

[112] J. Que, M. Choi, J. W. Ziel, J. Klingensmith, and B. L. M. Hogan, "Morphogenesis of the trachea and esophagus: current players and new roles for noggin and Bmps," *Differentiation*, vol. 74, no. 7, pp. 422–437, 2006.

[113] C. Tselepis, I. Perry, C. Dawson et al., "Tumour necrosis factor-α in Barrett's oesophagus: a potential novel mechanism of action," *Oncogene*, vol. 21, no. 39, pp. 6071–6081, 2002.

[114] K. Takubo, M. Vieth, J. Aida et al., "Differences in the definitions used for esophageal and gastric diseases in different countries: endoscopic definition of the esophagogastric junction, the precursor of Barrett's adenocarcinoma, the definition of Barrett's esophagus, and histologic criteria for mucosal adenocarcinoma or high-grade dysplasia," *Digestion*, vol. 80, no. 4, pp. 248–257, 2009.

[115] K. P. Batts, "Barrett esophagus—more steps forward," *Human Pathology*, vol. 32, no. 4, pp. 357–359, 2001.

[116] A. Ruol, A. Parenti, and G. Zaninotto, "Intestinal metaplasia is the probable common precursor of adenocarcinoma in barrett esophagus and adenocarcinoma of the gastric cardia," *Cancer*, vol. 88, no. 11, pp. 2520–2528, 2000.

[117] P. A. C. Gatenby, J. R. Ramus, C. P. J. Caygill, N. A. Shepherd, and A. Watson, "Relevance of the detection of intestinal metaplasia in non-dysplastic columnar-lined oesophagus," *Scandinavian Journal of Gastroenterology*, vol. 43, no. 5, pp. 524–530, 2008.

[118] S. R. DeMeester, "Letter to the editor regarding "Definition of Barrett's esophagus: time for a rethink-is intestinal metaplasia dead?"," *The American Journal of Gastroenterology*, vol. 105, no. 5, pp. 1201–1203, 2010.

[119] J. N. Glickman, S. J. Spechler, R. F. Souza, T. Lunsford, E. Lee, and R. D. Odze, "Multilayered epithelium in mucosal biopsy specimens from the gastroesophageal junction region is a histologic marker of gastroesophageal reflux disease," *American Journal of Surgical Pathology*, vol. 33, no. 6, pp. 818–825, 2009.

[120] P. Sharma, A. P. Weston, T. Morales, M. Topalovski, M. S. Mayo, and R. E. Sampliner, "Relative risk of dysplasia for patients with intestinal metaplasia in the distal oesophagus and in the gastric cardia," *Gut*, vol. 46, no. 1, pp. 9–13, 2000.

[121] W. Zhu, H. D. Appelman, J. K. Greenson et al., "A histologically defined subset of high-grade dysplasia in Barrett mucosa is predictive of associated carcinoma," *American Journal of Clinical Pathology*, vol. 132, no. 1, pp. 94–100, 2009.

[122] L. C. Lomo, P. L. Blount, C. A. Sanchez et al., "Crypt dysplasia with surface maturation: a clinical, pathologic, and molecular study of a Barrett's esophagus cohort," *American Journal of Surgical Pathology*, vol. 30, no. 4, pp. 423–435, 2006.

[123] D. Y. Park, A. Srivastava, G. H. Kim et al., "Adenomatous and foveolar gastric dysplasia: distinct patterns of mucin expression and background intestinal metaplasia," *American Journal of Surgical Pathology*, vol. 32, no. 4, pp. 524–533, 2008.

[124] A. Srivastava and G. Y. Lauwers, "Gastric epithelial dysplasia: the Western perspective," *Digestive and Liver Disease*, vol. 40, no. 8, pp. 641–649, 2008.

[125] D. Mahajan, A. E. Bennett, X. Liu, J. Bena, and M. P. Bronner, "Grading of gastric foveolar-type dysplasia in Barrett's esophagus," *Modern Pathology*, vol. 23, no. 1, pp. 1–11, 2010.

[126] M. Kerkhof, H. Van Dekken, E. W. Steyerberg et al., "Grading of dysplasia in Barrett's oesophagus: substantial interobserver variation between general and gastrointestinal pathologists," *Histopathology*, vol. 50, no. 7, pp. 920–927, 2007.

[127] E. Downs-Kelly, J. E. Mendelin, A. E. Bennett et al., "Poor interobserver agreement in the distinction of high-grade dysplasia and adenocarcinoma in pretreatment Barrett's esophagus biopsies," *The American Journal of Gastroenterology*, vol. 103, no. 9, pp. 2333–2341, 2008.

[128] E. Montgomery, M. P. Bronner, J. R. Goldblum et al., "Reproducibility of the diagnosis of dysplasia in Barrett esophagus: a reaffirmation," *Human Pathology*, vol. 32, no. 4, pp. 368–378, 2001.

[129] E. Montgomery, J. R. Goldblum, J. K. Greenson et al., "Dysplasia as a predictive marker for invasive carcinoma in barrett esophagus: a follow-up study based on 138 cases from a diagnostic variability study," *Human Pathology*, vol. 32, no. 4, pp. 379–388, 2001.

[130] D. P. Coco, J. R. Goldblum, J. L. Hornick et al., "Interobserver variability in the diagnosis of crypt dysplasia in barrett esophagus," *American Journal of Surgical Pathology*, vol. 35, no. 1, pp. 45–54, 2011.

[131] J. R. Goldblum, "Controversies in the diagnosis of Barrett esophagus and Barrett-related dysplasia," *Archives of Pathology and Laboratory Medicine*, vol. 134, no. 10, pp. 1479–1484, 2010.

[132] P. V. Kaye, S. A. Haider, M. Ilyas et al., "Barrett's dysplasia and the Vienna classification: reproducibility, prediction of progression and impact of consensus reporting and p53 immunohistochemistry," *Histopathology*, vol. 54, no. 6, pp. 699–712, 2009.

[133] E. Lörinc, B. Jakobsson, G. Landberg, and B. Veress, "Ki67 and p53 immunohistochemistry reduces interobserver variation in assessment of Barrett's oesophagus," *Histopathology*, vol. 46, no. 6, pp. 642–648, 2005.

[134] M. Binato, R. R. Gurski, R. B. Fagundes, L. Meurer, and M. I. Edelweiss, "P53 and Ki-67 overexpression in gastroesophageal reflux disease–Barrett's esophagus and adenocarcinoma sequence," *Diseases of the Esophagus*, vol. 22, no. 7, pp. 588–595, 2009.

[135] H. Van Dekken, W. C. J. Hop, H. W. Tilanus et al., "Immunohistochemical evaluation of a panel of tumor cell markers during malignant progression in Barrett esophagus," *American Journal of Clinical Pathology*, vol. 130, no. 5, pp. 745–753, 2008.

[136] C. S. Robertson, J. F. Mayberry, D. A. Nicholson, P. D. James, and M. Atkinson, "Value of endoscopic surveillance in the detection of neoplastic change in Barrett's oesophagus," *British Journal of Surgery*, vol. 75, no. 8, pp. 760–763, 1988.

[137] B. J. Reid, P. L. Blount, C. E. Rubin, D. S. Levine, R. C. Haggitt, and P. S. Rabinovitch, "Flow-cytometric and histological progression to malignancy in Barrett's esophagus: prospective endoscopic surveillance of a cohort," *Gastroenterology*, vol. 102, no. 4, pp. 1212–1219, 1992.

[138] J. F. Bartlesman, W. Hameeteman, and G. N. Tÿtgat, "Barrett's oesophagus," *European Journal of Cancer Prevention*, vol. 1, no. 4, pp. 323–325, 1992.

[139] N. J. Shaheen, M. A. Crosby, E. M. Bozymski, and R. S. Sandler, "Is there publication bias in the reporting of cancer risk in Barrett's esophagus?" *Gastroenterology*, vol. 119, no. 2, pp. 333–338, 2000.

[140] G. W. B. Clark, T. C. Smyrk, P. Burdiles et al., "Is Barrett's metaplasia the source of adenocarcinomas of the cardia?" *Archives of Surgery*, vol. 129, no. 6, pp. 609–614, 1994.

[141] J. R. Headrick, F. C. Nichols III, D. L. Miller et al., "High-grade esophageal dysplasia: long-term survival and quality of life after esophagectomy," *The Annals of Thoracic Surgery*, vol. 73, no. 6, pp. 1697–1702, 2002.

[142] B. F. Overholt, C. J. Lightdale, K. K. Wang et al., "Photodynamic therapy with porfimer sodium for ablation of high-grade dysplasia in Barrett's esophagus: international, partially blinded, randomized phase III trial," *Gastrointestinal Endoscopy*, vol. 62, no. 4, pp. 488–498, 2005.

[143] B. J. Reid, D. S. Levine, G. Longton, P. L. Blount, and P. S. Rabinovitch, "Predictors of progression to cancer in Barrett's esophagus: baseline histology and flow cytometry identify low- and high-risk patient subsets," *American Journal of Gastroenterology*, vol. 95, no. 7, pp. 1669–1676, 2000.

[144] N. S. Buttar, K. K. Wang, T. J. Sebo et al., "Extent of high-grade dysplasia in Barrett's esophagus correlates with risk of adenocarcinoma," *Gastroenterology*, vol. 120, no. 7, pp. 1630–1639, 2001.

[145] G. R. Locke III, N. J. Talley, S. L. Fett, A. R. Zinsmeister, and L. J. Melton, "Prevalence and clinical spectrum of gastroesophageal reflux: a population-based study in Olmsted County, Minnesota," *Gastroenterology*, vol. 112, no. 5, pp. 1448–1456, 1997.

[146] L. A. Anderson, L. J. Murray, S. J. Murphy et al., "Mortality in Barrett's oesophagus: results from a population based study," *Gut*, vol. 52, no. 8, pp. 1081–1084, 2003.

[147] K. Oude Rengerink, B. C. Opmeer, S. L. M. Logtenberg et al., "IMproving participation of patients in clinical trials—rationale and design of IMPACT," *BMC Medical Research Methodology*, vol. 10, article 85, 2010.

[148] J. M. Streitz Jr., C. W. Andrews, F. H. Ellis, D. B. Skinner, V. F. Trastek, and J. R. Benfield, "Endoscopic surveillance of Barrett's esophagus: does it help?" *Journal of Thoracic and Cardiovascular Surgery*, vol. 105, no. 3, pp. 383–388, 1993.

[149] J. H. Peters, G. W. B. Clark, A. P. Ireland et al., "Outcome of adenocarcinoma arising in Barrett's esophagus in endoscopically surveyed and nonsurveyed patients," *Journal of Thoracic and Cardiovascular Surgery*, vol. 108, no. 5, pp. 813–822, 1994.

[150] A. Fountoulakis, K. D. Zafirellls, K. Dolan, S. P. L. Dexter, I. G. Martin, and H. M. Sue-Ling, "Effect of surveillance of Barrett's oesophagus on the clinical outcome of oesophageal cancer," *British Journal of Surgery*, vol. 91, no. 8, pp. 997–1003, 2004.

[151] D. A. Corley, T. R. Levin, L. A. Habel, N. S. Weiss, and P. A. Buffler, "Surveillance and survival in Barrett's adenocarcinomas: a population-based study," *Gastroenterology*, vol. 122, no. 3, pp. 633–640, 2002.

[152] J. W. Van Sandick, J. J. B. Van Lanschot, B. W. Kuiken, G. N. J. Tytgat, G. J. A. Offerhaus, and H. Obertop, "Impact of endoscopic biopsy surveillance of Barrett's oesophagus on pathological stage and clinical outcome of Barrett's carcinoma," *Gut*, vol. 43, no. 2, pp. 216–222, 1998.

[153] G. S. Dulai, S. Guha, K. L. Kahn, J. Gornbein, and W. M. Weinstein, "Preoperative prevalence of Barrett's esophagus in esophageal adenocarcinoma: a systematic review," *Gastroenterology*, vol. 122, no. 1, pp. 26–33, 2002.

[154] P. Bytzer, P. B. Christensen, P. Damkier, K. Vinding, and N. Seersholm, "Adenocarcinoma of the esophagus and Barrett's esophagus: a population- based study," *American Journal of Gastroenterology*, vol. 94, no. 1, pp. 86–91, 1999.

[155] R. C. Fitzgerald, I. T. Saeed, D. Khoo, M. J. G. Farthing, and W. R. Burnham, "Rigorous surveillance protocol increases detection of curable cancers associated with Barrett's esophagus," *Digestive Diseases and Sciences*, vol. 46, no. 9, pp. 1892–1898, 2001.

[156] J. A. Abrams, R. C. Kapel, G. M. Lindberg et al., "Adherence to biopsy guidelines for Barrett's esophagus surveillance in the community setting in the United States," *Clinical Gastroenterology and Hepatology*, vol. 7, no. 7, pp. 736–742, 2009.

[157] W. L. Curvers, F. P. Peters, B. Elzer et al., "Quality of Barrett's surveillance in The Netherlands: a standardized review of endoscopy and pathology reports," *European Journal of Gastroenterology and Hepatology*, vol. 20, no. 7, pp. 601–607, 2008.

[158] W. A. Williamson, F. H. Ellis Jr., S. P. Gibb, D. M. Shahian, and H. T. Aretz, "Effect of antireflux operation on Barrett's mucosa," *Annals of Thoracic Surgery*, vol. 49, no. 4, pp. 537–542, 1990.

[159] S. Wani, H. Sayana, and P. Sharma, "Endoscopic eradication of Barrett's esophagus," *Gastrointestinal Endoscopy*, vol. 71, no. 1, pp. 147–166, 2010.

[160] S. Wani, S. Mathur, and P. Sharma, "How to manage a Barrett's esophagus patient with low-grade dysplasia," *Clinical Gastroenterology and Hepatology*, vol. 7, no. 1, pp. 27–32, 2009.

[161] N. J. Shaheen and D. J. Frantz, "When to consider endoscopic ablation therapy for Barrett's esophagus," *Current Opinion in Gastroenterology*, vol. 26, no. 4, pp. 361–366, 2010.

[162] A. Das, C. Wells, H. J. Kim, D. E. Fleischer, M. D. Crowell, and V. K. Sharma, "An economic analysis of endoscopic ablative therapy for management of nondysplastic Barrett's esophagus," *Endoscopy*, vol. 41, no. 5, pp. 400–408, 2009.

[163] N. J. Shaheen, P. Sharma, B. F. Overholt et al., "Radiofrequency ablation in Barrett's esophagus with dysplasia," *New England Journal of Medicine*, vol. 360, no. 22, pp. 2277–2288, 2009.

[164] R. F. Heitmiller, M. Redmond, and S. R. Hamilton, "Barrett's esophagus with high-grade dysplasia: an indication for prophylactic esophagectomy," *Annals of Surgery*, vol. 224, no. 1, pp. 66–71, 1996.

[165] V. J. Konda, A. S. Ross, and M. K. Ferguson, "Is the risk of concomitant invasive esophageal cancer in high-grade dysplasia in Barrett's esophagus overestimated?" *Clinical Gastroenterology and Hepatology*, vol. 6, no. 2, pp. 159–164, 2008.

[166] J. B. F. Hulscher, J. W. Van Sandick, A. G. E. M. De Boer et al., "Extended transthoracic resection compared with limited transhiatal resection for adenocarcinoma of the esophagus,"

New England Journal of Medicine, vol. 347, no. 21, pp. 1662–1669, 2002.

[167] G. A. Prasad, K. K. Wang, N. S. Buttar et al., "Long-term survival following endoscopic and surgical treatment of high-grade dysplasia in Barrett's esophagus," *Gastroenterology*, vol. 132, no. 4, pp. 1226–1233, 2007.

[168] A. Das, V. Singh, D. E. Fleischer, and V. K. Sharma, "A comparison of endoscopic treatment and surgery in early esophageal cancer: an analysis of surveillance epidemiology and end results data," *American Journal of Gastroenterology*, vol. 103, no. 6, pp. 1340–1345, 2008.

[169] A. Larghi, C. J. Lightdale, L. Memeo, G. Bhagat, N. Okpara, and H. Rotterdam, "EUS followed by EMR for staging of high-grade dysplasia and early cancer in Barrett's esophagus," *Gastrointestinal Endoscopy*, vol. 62, no. 1, pp. 16–23, 2005.

[170] H. Sayana, S. Wani, J. Keighley et al., "Endoscopic mucosal resection (EMR) as a diagnostic tool in Barrett's esophagus (BE) patients with high-grade dysplasia (HGD) and early esophageal adenocarcinoma (EAC): a systemic review," *Gastroenterology*, vol. 134, p. W1878, 2008.

[171] S. Seewald, T. Akaraviputh, and U. Seitz, "Circumferential EMR and complete removal of Barrett's epithelium: a new approach to management of Barrett's esophagus containing high-grade intraepithelial neoplasia and intramucosal carcinoma," *Gastrointestinal Endoscopy*, vol. 57, no. 7, pp. 854–859, 2003.

[172] F. P. Peters, M. A. Kara, W. D. Rosmolen et al., "Stepwise radical endoscopic resection is effective for complete removal of Barrett's esophagus with early neoplasia: a prospective study," *American Journal of Gastroenterology*, vol. 101, no. 7, pp. 1449–1457, 2006.

[173] N. Soehendra, S. Seewald, S. Groth et al., "Use of modified multiband ligator facilitates circumferential EMR in Barrett's esophagus (with video)," *Gastrointestinal Endoscopy*, vol. 63, no. 6, pp. 847–852, 2006.

[174] N. J. Shaheen, B. F. Overholt, R. E. Sampliner et al., "Durability of radiofrequency ablation in Barrett's esophagus with dysplasia," *Gastroenterology*, vol. 141, no. 2, pp. 460–468, 2011.

[175] B. F. Overholt, M. Panjehpour, and D. L. Halberg, "Photodynamic therapy for Barrett's esophagus with dysplasia and/or early stage carcinoma: long-term results," *Gastrointestinal Endoscopy*, vol. 58, no. 2, pp. 183–188, 2003.

[176] H. C. Fernando, S. C. Murthy, W. Hofstetter et al., "The society of thoracic surgeons practice guideline series: guidelines for the management of Barrett's esophagus with high-grade dysplasia," *Annals of Thoracic Surgery*, vol. 87, no. 6, pp. 1993–2002, 2009.

[177] N. J. Clemons, K. E. L. McColl, and R. C. Fitzgerald, "Nitric oxide and acid induce double-strand DNA breaks in Barrett's esophagus carcinogenesis via distinct mechanisms," *Gastroenterology*, vol. 133, no. 4, pp. 1198–1209, 2007.

[178] R. F. Souza, K. Shewmake, L. S. Terada, and S. J. Spechler, "Acid exposure activates the mitogen-activated protein kinase pathways in Barrett's esophagus," *Gastroenterology*, vol. 122, no. 2, pp. 299–307, 2002.

[179] H. B. El-Serag, T. V. Aguirre, S. Davis, M. Kuebeler, A. Bhattacharyya, and R. E. Sampliner, "Proton pump inhibitors are associated with reduced incidence of dysplasia in Barrett's esophagus," *American Journal of Gastroenterology*, vol. 99, no. 10, pp. 1877–1883, 2004.

[180] L. C. Hillman, L. Chiragakis, B. Shadbolt, G. L. Kaye, and A. C. Clarke, "Proton-pump inhibitor therapy and the development of dysplasia in patients with Barrett's oesophagus," *Medical Journal of Australia*, vol. 180, no. 8, pp. 387–391, 2004.

[181] B. T. Cooper, W. Chapman, C. S. Neumann, and J. C. Gearty, "Continuous treatment of Barrett's oesophagus patients with proton pump inhibitors up to 13 years: observations on regression and cancer incidence," *Alimentary Pharmacology and Therapeutics*, vol. 23, no. 6, pp. 727–733, 2006.

[182] L. A. Garcia Rodriguez, J. Lagergren, and M. Lindblad, "Gastric acid suppression and risk of oesophageal and gastric adenocarcinoma: a nested case control study in the UK," *Gut*, vol. 55, no. 11, pp. 1538–1544, 2006.

[183] L. A. Anderson, B. T. Johnston, R. G. P. Watson et al., "Nonsteroidal anti-inflammatory drugs and the esophageal inflammation-metaplasia-adenocarcinoma sequence," *Cancer Research*, vol. 66, no. 9, pp. 4975–4982, 2006.

[184] R. F. Souza, K. Shewmake, D. G. Beer, B. Cryer, and S. J. Spechler, "Selective inhibition of cyclooxygenase-2 suppresses growth and induces apoptosis in human esophageal adenocarcinoma cells," *Cancer Research*, vol. 60, no. 20, pp. 5767–5772, 2000.

[185] N. S. Buttar, K. K. Wang, M. A. Anderson et al., "The effect of selective cyclooxygenase-2 inhibition in Barrett's esophagus epithelium: an in vitro study," *Journal of the National Cancer Institute*, vol. 94, no. 6, pp. 422–429, 2002.

[186] D. Wang and R. N. Dubois, "Prostaglandins and cancer," *Gut*, vol. 55, no. 1, pp. 115–122, 2006.

[187] D. A. Corley, K. Kerlikowse, R. Verma, and P. Buffler, "Protective association of aspirin/NSAIDs and esophageal cancer: a systematic review and meta-analysis," *Gastroenterology*, vol. 124, no. 1, pp. 47–56, 2003.

[188] T. L. Vaughan, L. M. Dong, P. L. Blount et al., "Non-steroidal anti-inflammatory drugs and risk of neoplastic progression in Barrett's oesophagus: a prospective study," *The Lancet Oncology*, vol. 6, no. 12, pp. 945–952, 2005.

[189] F. Kastelein, M. C. Spaander, K. Biermann, E. W. Steyerberg, E. J. Kuipers, and M. J. Bruno, "Nonsteroidal anti-inflammatory drugs and statins have chemopreventative effects in patients with Barrett's esophagus," *Gastroenterology*, vol. 141, no. 6, pp. 2000–2008, 2011.

[190] O. O. Ogunwobi and I. L. P. Beales, "Statins inhibit proliferation and induce apoptosis in Barrett's esophageal adenocarcinoma cells," *American Journal of Gastroenterology*, vol. 103, no. 4, pp. 825–837, 2008.

[191] P. C. Konturek, G. Burnat, and E. G. Hahn, "Inhibition of Barret's adenocarcinoma cell growth by simvastatin: involvement of COX-2 and apoptosis-related proteins," *Journal of Physiology and Pharmacology*, vol. 58, supplement 3, pp. 141–148, 2007.

[192] D. M. Nguyen, P. Richardson, and H. B. El-Serag, "Medications (NSAIDs, Statins, Proton Pump Inhibitors) and the risk of esophageal adenocarcinoma in patients with Barrett's esophagus," *Gastroenterology*, vol. 138, no. 7, pp. 2260–2266, 2010.

[193] P. J. Kahrilas, "The problems with surveillance of Barrett's esophagus," *The New England Journal of Medicine*, vol. 365, no. 15, pp. 1437–1438, 2011.

[194] S. R. Kadri, P. Lao-Sirieix, M. O'Donovan et al., "Acceptability and accuracy of a non-endoscopic screening test for Barrett's oesophagus in primary care: cohort study," *British Medical Journal*, vol. 341, Article ID c4372, 2010.

[195] L. Quaroni, R. Zhao, and A. G. Casson, "Shining light on Barrett's esophagus," *Expert Review of Gastroenterology and Hepatology*, vol. 3, no. 6, pp. 577–580, 2009.

[196] A. K. Dattamajumdar, P. L. Blount, J. A. Myers et al., "A low-cost fiber-optic instrument to colorimetrically detect patients with Barrett's esophagus for early detection of esophageal adenocarcinoma," *IEEE Transactions on Biomedical Engineering*, vol. 48, no. 6, pp. 695–705, 2001.

[197] H. Pohl, T. Rösch, M. Vieth et al., "Miniprobe confocal laser microscopy for the detection of invisible neoplasia in patients with Barrett's oesophagus," *Gut*, vol. 57, no. 12, pp. 1648–1653, 2008.

[198] I. Georgakoudi, B. C. Jacobson, J. Van Dam et al., "Fluorescence, reflectance, and light-scattering spectroscopy for evaluating dysplasia in patients with Barrett's esophagus," *Gastroenterology*, vol. 120, no. 7, pp. 1620–1629, 2001.

[199] J. A. Evans, J. M. Poneros, B. E. Bouma et al., "Optical coherence tomography to identify intramucosal carcinoma and high-grade dysplasia in Barrett's esophagus," *Clinical Gastroenterology and Hepatology*, vol. 4, no. 1, pp. 38–43, 2006.

[200] H. C. Wolfsen, J. E. Crook, M. Krishna et al., "Prospective, controlled tandem endoscopy study of narrow band imaging for dysplasia detection in Barrett's esophagus," *Gastroenterology*, vol. 135, no. 1, pp. 24–31, 2008.

[201] R. A. Ganz, "Barrett's esophagus," *New England Journal of Medicine*, vol. 362, no. 15, pp. 1448–1449, 2010.

p40 as a Basal Cell Marker in the Diagnosis of Prostate Glandular Proliferations: A Comparative Immunohistochemical Study with 34betaE12

Hermann Brustmann

Department of Pathology, Landesklinikum Baden-Moedling, Wimmergasse 19, 2500 Baden, Austria

Correspondence should be addressed to Hermann Brustmann; ddrbrustmann@hotmail.com

Academic Editor: Shahid Pervez

Immunohistochemistry is important for the accurate diagnosis of basal cells in atypical glandular proliferations of the prostate. p40, an isoform of p63, may be an adjunct to a marker panel in this setting. Biopsies of 68 patients were analyzed by immunohistochemistry using antibodies to 34betaE12 and p40. Basal cell staining was classified as negative, partial (<60%), or diffuse (≥60%); irregular staining was defined as discordant staining patterns. In acinar proliferations ($N = 41$), partial staining for both markers was seen in 42%, and diffuse staining in 46% of reactive cases. An irregular reactivity was noted in one case only (2%). Finally, these lesions were signed out as benign. Acinar proliferations negative for both markers and limited amount of glands (≤4) were termed atypical small acinar proliferations (ASAP). Out of six PIN lesions two cases showed partial, three cases showed diffuse reactivity for both markers, and one case was stained irregular. All cases diagnosed as prostate carcinomas ($N = 20$) had no evidence of basal cell staining for neither of the markers. p40 expression is closely correlated to 34betaE12 with respect to demonstration of basal cells of prostate glands and may provide further information on the dignity of glandular proliferations of the prostate.

1. Introduction

Immunohistochemistry is an important tool in the differential diagnosis of prostate cancer. In particular, this is true in many instances of prostate needle biopsies presenting with limited amounts of atypical glandular proliferations. Small atypical foci may be challenging for the diagnosing pathologist by raising a suspicion for malignancy [1]. The identification of basal cells is considered helpful in excluding a diagnosis of prostate adenocarcinoma [2]. There is a small number of immunohistochemical markers that have been shown valuable in the demonstration of basal cells in prostate glandular tissues. The antikeratin antibody 34betaE12 (also known as keratin 903) is well recognized in this setting [2, 3]. Another standard marker of basal cells of the prostate gland is p63 [4].

p63 is normally expressed in the basal cell layer of stratified epithelia like squamous or urothelial tissues as well as in basal cells of prostatic epithelia, myoepithelial cells of breast and salivary glands, trophoblasts, and thymic epithelial cells [5]. It consists of several isoforms. They fall into two major groups: TAp63 and ΔNp63. The latter was noted as the predominant p63 transcript in squamous lung cancers and carcinomas of other sites. The antibody designated as p40 recognizes exclusively ΔNp63 and not TAp63 [5]. In the prostate gland recent work has shown that p40 stains prostatic basal cells as reliable as p63 in most cases. Aberrant staining of tumor cells was seen more rarely with p40 than with p63 [4]. p63 immunostaining has been compared with 34betaE12 previously [6]. These authors concluded that for diagnosing prostate carcinoma in needle biopsies p63 is as specific and sensitive as 34betaE12 and therefore can be used as a complementary basal cell-specific stain in difficult cases. Others noted that a basal cell cocktail consisting of 34betaE12 and p63 improves the detection of prostate basal cells [7, 8].

Since p40 is just the ΔNp63 isoform of p63, it seems justified evaluating its value as a marker on its own different diagnostic settings. This study compared the performance of a p40 versus a 34betaE12 antibody in a series of prostate needle biopsies to test whether p40 is another diagnostically valuable basal cell marker in prostate glands to differentiate atypical glandular proliferations from prostate cancers and to determine potential limitations of this staining protocol.

2. Material and Methods

All cases of prostate specimens diagnosed at our institution between October 2012 and December 2013 were retrieved from the department's files. Among a total of 338 patients 62 cases with needle biopsies and 6 cases with TURP (transurethral resection of the prostate) investigated by 34betaE12 and p40 immunohistochemistry at the time of histopathologic work-up were identified and retrospectively analysed. Patients' age ranged from 43 to 82 years, with a median of 69 years. All original hematoxylin-and-eosin (H&E) and immunohistochemically stained sections as well as the clinical histories were reviewed. The specimens were fixed in formalin and embedded in paraffin. Formalin fixation did not exceed 24 h. The study was approved by the local ethical committee (# GS4-EK-4/270/2014).

Step sections of the same paraffin-embedded tissues as those used for the H&E -stained sections were used for immunohistochemistry, applying the same staining protocol for all cases. They were cut at 3 μm. Subsequently, the sections were deparaffinized in xylene and rehydrated via graded ethanol. A standard immunohistochemical technique was performed using a Ventana BenchMark XT immunostainer with a ready-to-use monoclonal mouse anti-human 34betaE12 antibody (code IR051, DakoCytomation, Denmark, incubation time 32 minutes), and a prediluted ready-to-use rabbit polyclonal antibody to p40 (catalog no. API 3030 AA, Biocare Medical, Concord, CA, incubation time 40 minutes). Heat epitope retrieval as provided by the immunostainer was done in a TRIS based buffer supplied by the manufacturer (CCl cell conditioning solution, Ventana Medical Systems, Illkirch, Cedex, France) at pH8 for 30 minutes for all antibodies used. The enzymatic reactivity was visualized by 3-3 diaminobenzidine (DAB). Cases of a normal prostatic tissue with periglandular basal cells retrieved from a prostatectomy specimen and a normal epidermis served as external positive control, indicative for strong staining intensity. For negative controls serial sections of the same specimens were used, omitting the primary antibody from the staining protocol and substituting it by commercially available mouse nonimmune IgG serum. The immunohistochemical slides were evaluated and interpreted without knowledge of the clinical data in a blinded manner.

Immunoreactivity was scored by screening the slides at low power for any staining of basal cells; higher magnification (×100) was used to determine staining pattern which was evaluated semiquantitatively as follows: no staining (0%), partial staining (<60%), diffuse staining (≥60%), and compared casewise. This method of quantification is similar to protocols applied for 34betaE12 and p63 previously [4, 8].

The statistical tests were calculated with GraphPad Prism statistical analysis software (GraphPad Software, version 6.0, San Diego, CA), applying chi-square test or Fisher's exact test for different reactivity patterns and groups of patients, and column statistics for patients' ages (median, standard deviation (SD), minimum, maximum, and range). A P value of <0.05 was considered significant.

3. Results

At the time of diagnosis 34betaE12 and p40 immunostaining was employed to study glandular proliferations of the prostatic tissue present in small amounts and felt to be "atypical." In particular this was true for small acinar glands raising some suspicion for acinar carcinoma. The differential diagnosis for these cases encompassed lobular and partial atrophy, postatrophic hyperplasia, adenosis, normal structures like verumontanum glands, and inflammation associated changes. In some lesions suspicious for high grade prostatic intraepithelial neoplasia (PIN) staining was done to differentiate them from cribriform adenocarcinoma. This setting occurred in PINs with somewhat irregular outlines raising the question of cribriform carcinoma or to determine the Gleason grade in acinar carcinomas associated with such glands.

Staining for 34betaE12 was cytoplasmic, p40 staining was nuclear. A fine granular cytoplasmic p40 and 34betaE12 immunoprecipitate was noted in some cases of glandular epithelial cells or stromal cells and considered nonspecific, in occasional association with mild crush artifacts. Benign prostate glands showed strong and diffuse basal cell staining with both markers. Three main categories of prostate tissues were distinguished. Group 1 consisted of acinar proliferations ($N = 42$), group 2 of prostatic intraepithelial neoplasia (high grade, $N = 6$), and group 3 of adenocarcinomas ($N = 20$). The latter displayed Gleason grade 3+3 ($N = 11$), 3+4 ($N = 4$), 4+3 ($N = 2$), and 4+4 ($N = 3$). One case of group one had to be excluded from this study since there was not sufficient glandular tissue left in deeper step sections performed for immunohistochemistry.

In group 1, four cases (10%) of atypical glandular proliferations were completely negative for basal cell staining with both markers; due to the limited amount of glands (≤4) these cases were termed atypical small acinar proliferations (ASAP). 17 cases (42%) showed partial and 19 cases (46%) diffuse staining patterns. An irregular pattern was recorded in one case (2%) with a diffuse staining for 34betaE12 and partial staining for p40. Casewise comparison in partially and diffusely stained cases revealed identical quantities of immunoreactive basal cells for both markers (Figures 1–3). In PINs there were no cases negative for basal cells (Figures 4–6). Partial staining was seen in two cases and diffuse staining in three cases. One case belonged to the category of irregular staining, with diffuse 34betaE12 reactivity. There was no statistical difference between staining patterns for 34betaE12 and p40 ($P = 1.0000$, chi-square test). All cases with evidence of basal cells were signed out as benign.

All cases signed out as carcinomas were completely negative for both markers (Figures 4–6). The biopsy diagnoses were confirmed as carcinomas in subsequent prostatectomy specimens. Staining between benign glandular proliferations

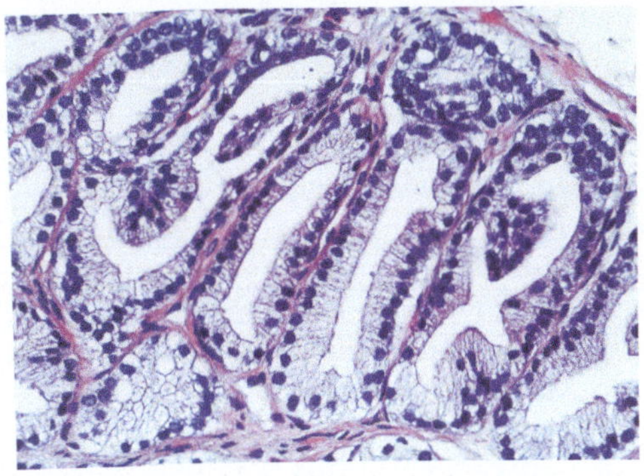

FIGURE 1: A case showing tightly clustered glands, with few intervening stomata. This architecture raised some suspicion, and the cytology advocates for a benign lesion. After basal cell staining a hyperplastic nodule was diagnosed (H&E, ×400).

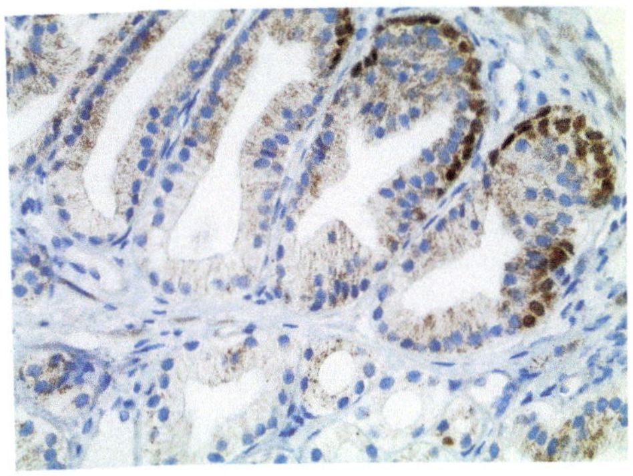

FIGURE 2: Same case as shown in Figure 1. There is evidence of basal cells on p40 immunohistochemistry in a partial pattern. Immunoreactivity is nuclear (×400).

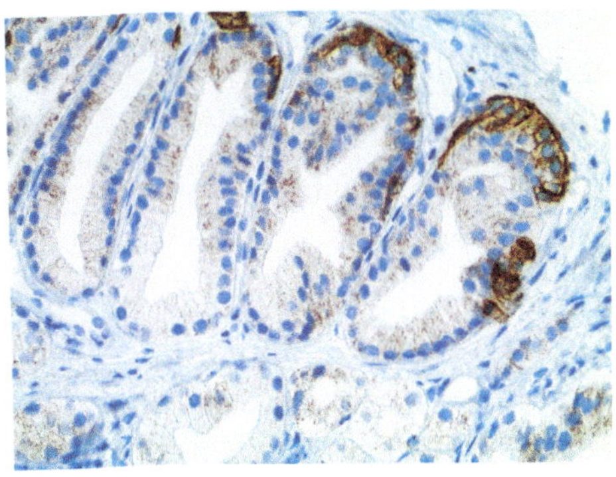

FIGURE 3: Same case as shown in Figure 1. There is evidence of basal cells on 34betaE12 immunohistochemistry in a partial pattern. Immunoreactivity is cytoplasmic (×400).

and prostate cancers differed significantly ($P < 0.0001$, Fisher's exact test).

4. Discussion

In this study a close correlation of prostate gland basal cell staining for antibodies to 34betaE12 and p40 was noted in the vast majority of cases, with concordant staining patterns.

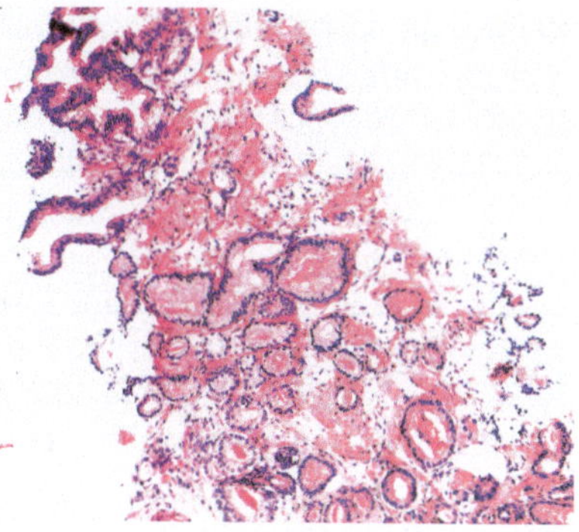

FIGURE 4: Well-differentiated acinar glands in a haphazard pattern are considered suspicious for carcinoma. The cytoplasm is pale and abundant; there is some nuclear atypia, and intraluminal eosinophilic bodies are occasionally seen. After immunohistochemistry for basal cells this focus was signed out as acinar adenocarcinoma: Gleason 3+3 (H&E, ×100).

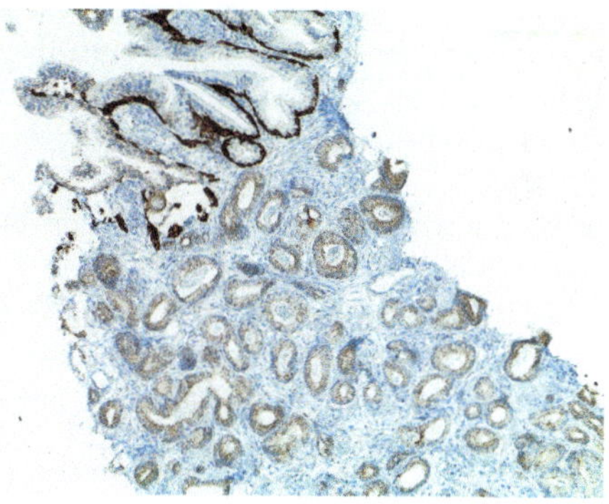

FIGURE 5: Same case as shown in Figure 4. Complete lack of basal cells in the atypical glandular proliferation is noted on 34betaE12 immunohistochemistry. Basal cells are evident in adjacent noninfiltrative glands displaying features of intraepithelial neoplasia/PIN (×100).

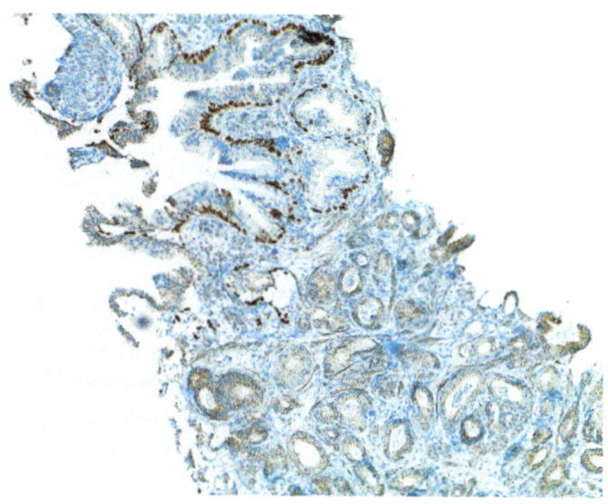

FIGURE 6: Same case as shown in Figure 4. Complete lack of basal cells on p40 immunohistochemistry. There is some weak nonspecific cytoplasmic staining of tumor cells. Basal cells are evident in adjacent noninfiltrative glands displaying features of intraepithelial neoplasia/PIN (×100).

Irregular staining was observed in one case only. The findings presented herein thus indicate that p40 may be used to label basal cells of prostate glands and may be included in a marker panel to demonstrate the latter in diagnostic difficult settings. This situation emanates primarily from needle biopsies with a limited amount of suspicious glands. Looking at such glands on H&E stained sections we use an approach of "favoring benign" or "favoring malignant." This first evaluation is based on previously defined criteria for minimal carcinoma in prostate biopsy specimens [9]. The most important features are nucleomegaly, infiltrative growth pattern, intraluminal secretions, prominent nucleoli, association with high grade PIN, amphophilic cytoplasm, nuclear hyperchromasia, absence of basal cells, and intraluminal crystalloids [10]. An infiltrative growth pattern is an important feature in Gleason 3 acinar minimal carcinomas with a dimension of <1 mm recognized in needle biopsies, displaying a few malignant glands between benign glands. In contrast to PIN lesions, high grade carcinomas of Gleason scores 4 and/or 5 show a ragged pattern of invasion; however, it is challenging to differentiate atypical high grade PINs and carcinomas in some instances on needle biopsies [11]. Evaluation of nuclear atypia may be difficult in a setting of rather well-differentiated Gleason 3 acinar glands [9, 10].

The appreciation of basal cells in prostatic glands may be problematic in some instances on H&E staining; they may seem lacking, or fibroblasts from the periglandular stroma closely adjacent to the epithelial cells may mimic basal cells. Immunostains for basal cell markers like 34betaE12, p63, or p40, respectively, may assist in the diagnosis in such instances. However, such negative stains are not necessarily indicative for malignancy. In an early study, Hedrick and Epstein [2] noted a complete lack of basal cells by keratin 903 (34betaE12) in 8% of atrophic glands, 12% of glands in basal cell hyperplasia, and 39% of glands in atypical adenosis; however, all grades of adenocarcinoma lacked any immunoreactivity. Others found that a fragmented basal cell layer is characteristic of atypical adenomatous hyperplasia (adenosis), with a lack of a basal cell layer in approximately 50% of glands [3]. Thus, evaluating immunostains for the abovementioned basal cell markers should be made with caution, and neglecting basic morphologic features of the glands under suspicion is to be avoided.

The definition of the minimal number of glands to diagnose prostatic adenocarcinoma on needle biopsy is a crucial matter. Diagnostic criteria of malignancy as described above have to be met in these glands. Additionally, these few glands must not show any evidence of basal cells by immunohistochemistry. The cut-off value in such instances considered diagnostic of carcinoma at our institute is five glands. This is in agreement with van der Kwast et al., who felt that foci comprising < 6 glands are equivocal [1]. Others concluded that three glands constituted the lowest numerical cut-off [12].

In agreement with recent literature it is evident that immunohistochemistry is frequently used in prostate biopsy practice to establish or confirm a limited cancer diagnosis [13]. Besides the use of a racemase (AMACR), 34betaE12 and p63 are well-established markers in this setting [2–4, 13]. Since there are many entities entering the differential diagnosis of prostatic adenocarcinoma, sensitivity and specificity of such markers need to be established and, on the other hand, the immunoreactivity patterns of potential mimickers are to be characterized. Normal structures like crowded glands as well as Cowper's glands or seminal vesicles, verumontanum glands, atrophy in its variants, and postatrophic hyperplasia as well as adenosis (atypical adenomatous hyperplasia) are the probably most common conditions to be misinterpreted for adenocarcinoma, as are rarer entities like nephrogenic adenomas or mesonephric hyperplasia [14, 15]. Previously, Kahane et al. have described that the use of high molecular weight cytokeratin decreased the rate of an atypical prostate biopsy from 8.3% to 0.4% [16]. Shah et al. noted the usefulness of a basal cell cocktail consisting of 34betaE12 and p63 in the diagnosis of atypical glandular proliferations of the prostate [8]. These studies also emphasized the cost-effective improvement in analyzing difficult prostatic lesions by these markers. Single cribriform glands may pose a differential diagnosis between cribriform carcinoma and high-grade PIN. Amin et al. analyzed cribriform morphology in prostatic neoplasia using HMWKs [17]. They concluded that HMWK staining to detect basal cells in isolated cribriform glands encountered in biopsy specimens may be a useful diagnostic discriminant between high-grade PIN and prostatic carcinoma. However, they observed focal and isolated HMWK positivity amid prostatic carcinoma and, thus, emphasized that the overall pattern of staining together with morphological features is critical to exclude carcinomas [17]. The study presented herein provides evidence that p40 is a sensitive and specific nuclear marker in the basal cell detection of such atypical glands in prostate biopsies, with a high concordance with the HMWK 34betaE12, therefore offering another complementary basal cell stain.

Atypical small acinar proliferations (ASAP) are represented by a small focus of atypical glands suspicious for carcinoma that cannot be safely diagnosed as benign or malignant on H&E as well as immunostains. Features of ASAP are summarized by Schlesinger et al. [18]. In the study at hand four cases displaying acinar morphology of ≤4 glands accompanied by low grade cytological atypia and lack of evidence of any basal cells were placed into this category. There is no available recent follow-up of these cases. However, in such small lesions the lack of basal cells should not be overinterpreted, since staining may only be evident in partial patterns in many benign instances as discussed above and, thus, may be missed in single glands found on biopsy.

Recently, p40 immunostaining has gained a wide recognition in tumor diagnosis, with special regard to squamous cell and urothelial carcinomas [19, 20]. In the prostate, p40 has been shown to stain basal cells as reliable as p63, with only minor differences [4]. As also noted in the study at hand, some weak granular cytoplasmic reactivity of p40 narrows its eligibility for antibody cocktails containing AMACR [4]. Tacha et al. included three cases of prostatic tissues in their study on p40 in a large number of carcinomas of different origins and observed basal cell staining in benign prostate as well as PIN glands [19]. In the differential diagnostic workup of atypical glandular lesions of the breast it has been suggested that p40 can also be used to label breast myoepithelial cells [21].

In conclusion, this study provides evidence for the usefulness of p40 in the diagnosis of suspicious prostate glands, and for the first time a close correlation with the well-established basal cell marker 34betaE12. Still, morphological assessment of prostate glandular tissues remains the gold standard, and any immunohistochemical ancillary testing should be considered as aid to the final diagnosis only.

Conflict of Interests

The author declares no potential conflict of interests with respect to the research, authorship and/or publication of this paper.

References

[1] T. H. van der Kwast, A. Evans, G. Lockwood et al., "Variability in diagnostic opinion among pathologists for single small atypical foci in prostate biopsies," *The American Journal of Surgical Pathology*, vol. 34, no. 2, pp. 169–177, 2010.

[2] L. Hedrick and J. I. Epstein, "Use of keratin 903 as an adjunct in the diagnosis of prostate carcinoma," *American Journal of Surgical Pathology*, vol. 13, no. 5, pp. 389–396, 1989.

[3] D. G. Bostwick, J. Srigley, D. Grignon et al., "Atypical adenomatous hyperplasia of the prostate: morphologic criteria for its distinction from well-differentiated carcinoma," *Human Pathology*, vol. 24, no. 8, pp. 819–832, 1993.

[4] V. Sailer, C. Stephan, N. Wernert et al., "Comparison of p40 (ΔNp63) and p63 expression in prostate tissues—which one is the superior diagnostic marker for basal cells?" *Histopathology*, vol. 63, no. 1, pp. 50–56, 2013.

[5] J. A. Bishop, J. Teruya-Feldstein, W. H. Westra, G. Pelosi, W. D. Travis, and N. Rekhtman, "P40 (ΔNp63) is superior to p63 for the diagnosis of pulmonary squamous cell carcinoma," *Modern Pathology*, vol. 25, no. 3, pp. 405–415, 2012.

[6] H. H.-J. Wu, O. Lapkus, and M. Corbin, "Comparison of 34βE12 and P63 in 100 consecutive prostate carcinoma diagnosed by needle biopsies," *Applied Immunohistochemistry and Molecular Morphology*, vol. 12, no. 4, pp. 285–289, 2004.

[7] M. Zhou, R. Shah, R. Shen, and M. A. Rubin, "Basal cell cocktail (34βE12 + p63) improves the detection of prostate basal cells," *The American Journal of Surgical Pathology*, vol. 27, no. 3, pp. 365–371, 2003.

[8] R. B. Shah, L. P. Kunju, R. Shen, M. LeBlanc, M. Zhou, and M. A. Rubin, "Usefulness of basal cell cocktail (34βE12 + p63) in the diagnosis of atypical prostate glandular proliferations," *American Journal of Clinical Pathology*, vol. 122, no. 4, pp. 517–523, 2004.

[9] P. Thorson, R. T. Vollmer, C. Arcangeli, D. W. Keetch, and P. A. Humphrey, "Minimal carcinoma in prostate needle biopsy specimens: diagnostic features and radical prostatectomy follow-up," *Modern Pathology*, vol. 11, no. 6, pp. 543–551, 1998.

[10] J. I. Epstein, "Diagnostic criteria of limited adenocarcinoma of the prostate on needle biopsy," *Human Pathology*, vol. 26, no. 2, pp. 223–229, 1995.

[11] L. Egevad, W. C. Allsbrook Jr., and J. I. Epstein, "Current practice of diagnosis and reporting of prostatic intraepithelial neoplasia and glandular atypia among genitourinary pathologists," *Modern Pathology*, vol. 19, no. 2, pp. 180–185, 2006.

[12] F. Algaba, J. I. Epstein, H. C. Aldape et al., "Workgroup 5: assessment of prostate carcinoma in core needle biopsy—definition of minimal criteria for the diagnosis of cancer in biopsy material," *Cancer*, vol. 78, no. 2, pp. 376–381, 1996.

[13] K. Watson, C. Wang, A. Yilmaz, T. A. Bismar, and K. Trpkov, "Use of immunohistochemistry in routine workup of prostate needle biopsies: a tertiary academic institution experience," *Archives of Pathology and Laboratory Medicine*, vol. 137, no. 4, pp. 541–545, 2013.

[14] O. Hameed and P. A. Humphrey, "Immunohistochemistry in diagnostic surgical pathology of the prostate," *Seminars in Diagnostic Pathology*, vol. 22, no. 1, pp. 88–104, 2005.

[15] M. Herawi, A. V. Parwani, J. Irie, and J. I. Epstein, "Small glandular proliferations on needle biopsies: most common benign mimickers of prostatic adenocarcinoma sent in for expert second opinion," *American Journal of Surgical Pathology*, vol. 29, no. 7, pp. 874–880, 2005.

[16] H. Kahane, J. W. Sharp, G. B. Shuman, G. Dasilva, and J. I. Epstein, "Utilization of high molecular weight cytokeratin on prostate needle biopsies in an independent laboratory," *Urology*, vol. 45, no. 6, pp. 981–986, 1995.

[17] M. B. Amin, D. S. Schultz, and R. J. Zarbo, "Analysis of cribriform morphology in prostatic neoplasia using antibody to high-molecular-weight cytokeratins," *Archives of Pathology and Laboratory Medicine*, vol. 118, no. 3, pp. 260–264, 1994.

[18] C. Schlesinger, D. G. Bostwick, and K. A. Iczkowski, "High-grade prostatic intraepithelial neoplasia and atypical small acinar proliferation: predictive value for cancer in current practice," *The American Journal of Surgical Pathology*, vol. 29, no. 9, pp. 1201–1207, 2005.

[19] D. Tacha, R. Bremer, T. Haas, and W. Qi, "An immunohistochemical analysis of a newly developed, mouse monoclonal p40 (BC28) antibody in lung, bladder, skin, breast, prostate, and head and neck cancers," *Archives of Pathology & Laboratory Medicine*, vol. 138, no. 10, pp. 1358–1364, 2014.

[20] K. J. Butnor and J. L. Burchette, "P40 (ΔNp63) and keratin 34βE12 provide greater diagnostic accuracy than p63 in the evaluation of small cell lung carcinoma in small biopsy samples," *Human Pathology*, vol. 44, no. 8, pp. 1479–1486, 2013.

[21] R. Sarda and J. Taylor, "P40 (ΔNp63), a lung squamous cell marker, can also be used to label breast myoepithelial cells," *Archives of Pathology and Laboratory Medicine*, vol. 138, no. 5, article 584, 2014.

24

Molecular Events in Primary and Metastatic Colorectal Carcinoma

Rani Kanthan,[1,2] Jenna-Lynn Senger,[1] and Selliah Chandra Kanthan[3]

[1] Department of Pathology and Laboratory Medicine, University of Saskatchewan, Saskatoon, SK, Canada S7N 0W8
[2] Royal University Hospital, Room 2868 G-Wing, 103 Hospital Drive, Saskatoon, SK, Canada S7N 0W8
[3] Department of Surgery, University of Saskatchewan, Saskatoon, SK, Canada S7N 0W8

Correspondence should be addressed to Rani Kanthan, rani.kanthan@saskatoonhealthregion.ca

Academic Editor: Marco Volante

Colorectal cancer (CRC) is a heterogeneous disease, developing through a multipathway sequence of events guided by clonal selections. Pathways included in the development of CRC may be broadly categorized into (a) genomic instability, including chromosomal instability (CIN), microsatellite instability (MSI), and CpG island methylator phenotype (CIMP), (b) genomic mutations including suppression of tumour suppressor genes and activation of tumour oncogenes, (c) microRNA, and (d) epigenetic changes. As cancer becomes more advanced, invasion and metastases are facilitated through the epithelial-mesenchymal transition (EMT), with additional genetic alterations. Despite ongoing identification of genetic and epigenetic markers and the understanding of alternative pathways involved in the development and progression of this disease, CRC remains the second highest cause of malignancy-related mortality in Canada. The molecular events that underlie the tumorigenesis of primary and metastatic colorectal carcinoma are detailed in this manuscript.

1. Introduction

Despite increased general awareness, colorectal cancer (CRC) remains the second leading cause of cancer-related death in Canadian men and women combined [1], with a third of CRC patients dying from this disease [2]. These are grim statistics given that this cancer is a well-studied malignancy with defined risk factors, a slow progression, and preneoplastic lesions that can be detected and treated by colonoscopic polypectomy [3]. Though 5-year survival rates for early stage cancers (Dukes A and B) is up to 95% and 60–80% respectively, survival rates drop dramatically to 35% with lymph node involvement (Dukes C), indicating early detection and treatment is imperative for best patient management [4].

Recognition that histologically identical tumours may have drastically different prognosis and/or response to treatment prompted the theory that, rather than a single malignancy, CRC is a heterogenous, multifactorial disease [5, 6]. It is theorized, perhaps, that individual tumours are initiated and progress in a unique manner that is not necessarily identical amongst all tumours [7]. As a result, the focus of CRC research is shifting from a clinical perspective towards developing an understanding of the molecular basis of this malignancy, including individual susceptibility, development, progression, response, and resistance to antitumour treatment and metastatic spread [8]. Cancer develops through multiple and sequential genetic alterations [3, 9], and some patients may have synchronous alterations in two or three different pathways [10]. Through clonal selections, the cancer cell "chooses" the genetic alterations most conducive to growth through proliferation of cells that possess the desired qualities with apoptosis of those that do not [2]. A more thorough understanding of these molecular pathways may contribute to improved strategies for prevention, screening, diagnosis, and therapy. The following is an overview of the molecular events in primary and metastatic CRC.

2. Materials and Methods

A detailed review was conducted in the published English literature limited to the past five years (since 2006). The search was performed using PubMed and Google Scholar with the text phrases "molecular pathway" and "colorectal." Articles were read, analyzed, and screened with a focus on colorectal cancer/carcinoma. Primary reference lists from these manuscripts as well as PubMed's "Related Articles" feature were used to identify additional relevant articles.

The aim of this review is to discuss molecular changes occurring in

(a) primary CRC, including genomic instability, genomic modifications, microRNA, epigenetic changes,

(b) metastatic CRC (mCRC) including growth factors and epithelial-mesenchymal transitions (EMTs).

3. Genomic Instability

The first model of colorectal tumorigenesis put forward by Fearon and Vogelstein outlined a four-step sequential pathway for the development of cancer, in which

Step 1: *APC* inactivation causes adenoma development,

Step 2: *KRAS* mutations promote adenomatous growth,

Step 3: genetic alterations of chromosome 18q allowed progression with biallelic loss,

Step 4: p53 inactivation triggers the final transition to carcinoma [11, 12].

Recent insights suggest this pathway, now over twenty years old, requires refinement to include new findings [13]. Further, this sequence is thought to occur in only 60% of cases [14]. In the process of elucidating the true pathogenesis of CRC, controversy has emerged between those postulating that genomic instability is necessary to elucidate the multiple mutations present in CRC and those disagreeing, hypothesizing instead that cells continuously produce genetic changes with those that confer a survival advantage being selected through clonal expansion [12].

Only 5% of adenomas will progress to cancer development, indicating that carcinogenesis requires additional molecular modifications, with greater emphasis on increased proliferation [15, 16]. It is suggested CRC is initiated by "cancer-initiating stem cells" with the ability to self-renew, perpetuate, and generate a variety of differentiated cells. These cells are proposed to harbour the initial mutation of *APC* in one of the 10^7 crypts of the gastrointestinal tract which then colonize the crypt with mutated cells [13].

Carcinogenesis is now viewed as an imbalance between mutation development and cell-cycle control mechanisms. When the cell-cycle is no longer capable of controlling the mutation rate, it is referred to as "genomic instability." Three separate pathways have been identified that contribute to this imbalance:

(1) chromosomal instability (CIN),

(2) microsatellite instability (MSI),

(3) CpG island methylator phenotype (CIMP).

These groupings are created in order to facilitate prediction of (a) patient prognosis, (b) response/resistance to therapies, and (c) possible etiological factors to optimize prevention [7].

3.1. Chromosomal Instability. The chromosomal instability (CIN) pathway, also known as the suppressor pathway, is the most common type of genomic instability [8], encompassing 50–85% of CRCs [5, 17]. This pathway is characterized by karyotypic variability resulting from gains and/or losses of whole/portions of chromosomes [13]. Various mechanisms that contribute to CIN have been identified and categorized to include (a) sequence changes, (b) chromosome number alterations, (c) chromosome rearrangements, and (d) gene amplification [18]. Additional changes identified include chromosomal segregation defects/microtubule dysfunction, abnormal centrosome number, telomere dysfunction/telomerase overexpression, DNA damage, and loss of heterozygosity (LOH) [13, 18, 19]. Chromosomes that attach improperly to the mitotic spindle confer a higher risk of mis-segregation. This may be due to *APC* mutations, which normally interact with microtubule-binding-protein EB-1 to assure proper chromosomal attachment [20]. Telomerase dysfunction occurs when cells with shortened telomeres do not undergo apoptosis, leading to breakage-fusion-bridge cycles that can lead to genomic reorganization [13].

A common finding in chromosomally instable neoplasms is loss of 18q, a finding identified in up to 70% of primary CRCs [13]. Genes on this chromosome include *deleted in colorectal carcinoma (DCC)*, *SMAD2*, and *SMAD4*. The product of *DCC* is a cell-surface receptor for neuronal protein netrin-1 and is important in cell adhesion and apoptosis [5]. Mutations to this gene are rare (6% CRCs) [13]. *SMAD2* and *SMAD4* function in the TGF-β-signalling pathway (Section 4.1.3) [3]. 18q loss of heterozygosity (LOH) has been correlated with poor prognosis; however, the extent of the prognostic value requires further validation [5]. The "two-hit hypothesis" for LOH states that both alleles of a tumour suppressor gene must be inactivated in order to contribute to tumourigenesis. Often, this is accomplished by loss of one allele with inactivation by a point mutation of the other [21].

CIN can be detected early in a dysplastic crypt foci [3] and is more commonly found in the distal colon; however, whether or not it precedes *APC* inactivation remains unclear. Detection of these genomic changes often includes cytometry, karyotyping, LOH analysis, fluorescent *in situ* hybridization (FISH), and comparative genomic hybridization (CGH) [13]. This pathway results in a change in both the chromosomal copy number and structure [8] and are characterized by aneuploidy, transformations, and LOH that contribute to the inactivation of tumour suppressor genes such as *APC*, *DCC*, *SMAD4*, and *TP53* [4, 17, 22]. CIN has additionally been associated with loss of chromosome 5q, 17p, and 18q [3]. Though aneuploidy is recognized as occurring in tumours with CIN, the mechanisms responsible for this remain unknown. Therefore, some authors propose that cancer development through genomic instability may arise without mutations, simply through self-propagation. Cancers with aneuploidy often show mitotic abnormalities including centrosome numbers, multipolar spindles, and lagging chromosomes suggesting mitotic spindle checkpoint dysregulation [18].

There remains no clear evidence to discern whether CIN is a cause or a consequence of malignancy [13, 20]. It is clear, however, that CRC with CIN confers a poor survival regardless of ethnicity, tumour location, and treatment with 5-FU [23]. The majority of CIN tumours are predominantly of the distal colon/left sided tumours present clinically with routine lower gastrointestinal symptoms that include bleeding per rectum and presence of a mass with or without obstruction. Histomorphologically, these lesions are either polypoid exophytic or indurated/ulcerated growths with the characteristic histology of moderately well-differentiated adenocarcinoma with a typical "dirty" necrosis of CRC.

3.2. Microsatellite Instability. Microsatellite instability (MSI) is detected in 15% of CRCs and arises when microsatellites become abnormally long or short due to gain/loss of repeated units [24]. This pathway of genomic instability was first reported in 1993 at the detection of thousands of somatic alterations in a length of DNA from a CRC [25]. A microsatellite is a stretch of DNA containing a pattern of 1–5 nucleotides in length with tandem repeats [22, 24]. Microsatellites are found abundantly throughout the genome and are unique in uniform and length within a tissue of one individual [12]. A minimum of 500,000 microsatellites are estimated within the genome, occurring in the intron, untranslated terminal regions, and the coding exon itself [26]. Microsatellites may be classified as monomorphic (the same number of repeats in all individuals) or polymorphic (varied number of repeats among individuals) [26]. Elongation or shortening of the microsatellite is primarily due to inactivation of DNA mismatch repair (MMR) genes, which are responsible for correcting base-base DNA replication errors. At regions of short repeats within the genome, such as satellites, DNA polymerase is particularly susceptible to making mistakes; therefore, when MMR is inactivated and cannot correct these mistakes, MSI is the result [3]. This inactivation may be genetic or acquired. These tumours usually are not associated with mutations in *KRAS* or *TP53*; however, genes such as TGFβRII, EGFR, and BAX, which contain simple repeats, are often mutated in these tumours [5]. Additional genes affected by MSI include regulators of proliferation (GRB1, TCF-4, WISP3, activin receptor-2 insulin-like growth factor-2 receptor, axin-2, CDX), the cell cycle or apoptosis (caspase-5, RIZ, BCL-10, PTEN, hG4-1, FAS) and DNA repair (MBD-4, BLM, CHK1, MLH3, RAD50, MSH3, MSH6) [12].

MMR inactivation may be due to either an inherited germline mutation to one allele with somatic inactivation of the other or somatic inactivation of both alleles [26]. The most common mechanism of MMR inactivation is through an acquired methylation of the h*MLH1* gene promoter [17]. The MMR system comprises seven proteins (MLH1, MLH3, MSH2, MSH3, MSH6, PMS1, PMS2) which associate and form functional heterodimers [3]. These mutations allow repeats within the microsatellite to accumulate or to be lost through clonal propagation [27]. Standard sequencing for the detection of MSI can miss large deletions/rearrangements that arise in up to 1/3 of MMR mutations [24]. The most common detection mechanism is by length measurement of a PCR amplicon containing the microsatellite. Methylation-specific PCR to test for methylation is another simple test, where loss of h*MLH1* staining by immunohistochemistry correlates with MSI [26]. Though MSI is primarily due to MMR inactivation, some CRCs with intact MMR can develop MSI through frameshift mutations at microsatellites. A standardized panel for MSI testing includes two mononucleotides (BAT25 and BAT26) and three dinucleotide microsatellites (D5S346, D2S123, D17S250) [3]. The MSI expanded panel includes BAT40, myb, TGFβRII, IGF2R, and BAX for a 10-marker panel [27]. Based on these markers, the degree of MSI can be categorized as high MSI (MSI-H) when two or more panel markers are involved, low MSI (MSI-L) if only one marker is involved, and MSS if none. The value of a MSI-L category remains questionable, as it is argued if enough microsatellites in CRC are tested, eventually some instability will be detected [26]. The clinical presentation of MSI-L tumours has yet to be fully determined and this will likely result in acceptance or rejection of this category.

Clinicopathological features defining MSI-positive tumours are not reported consistently in the literature [28]. Most of these tumours usually arise from adenomas, are located proximal to the splenic flexure, and confer a better prognosis for their stage than microsatellite-stable (MSS) tumours [10, 17, 29–31]. Additionally, MSI is more common in females and arise in both younger and older population, though this has not been consistent in all studies. Patients can also present with synchronous and metachronous malignancies [28]. On microscopic examination, these tumours are often poorly differentiated with a mucinous phenotype and are associated with prominent intratumoral and peritumoral lymphocytic infiltration [4]. They often have a lower overall stage of disease but demonstrate deeper invasion [28]. Unlike CIN, these tumours do not have chromosomal abnormalities or allelic loss [4]. Many MSI-H tumours have a Crohn's-like inflammatory response near the tumour edge; however, no universal prognostic pathologic feature has been identified in all MSI-positive CRCs. Distant metastases are less common in MSI-positive CRC [28]. It remains uncertain if the favourable prognosis associated with MSI tumours is intrinsic or rather due to a greater sensitivity to chemotherapy. Adjuvant chemotherapy with 5-FU is not beneficial to MSI-H tumours as they demonstrate an altered response to both chemotherapy and radiotherapy. The use of MSI as a prognostic factor remains uncertain although it is suggested that it may be useful in the selection of individual therapeutic regimes [5].

Hereditary nonpolypsis colorectal cancer, now referred to as Lynch syndrome because of its extraintestinal manifestations, is due to a mutant germline MMR gene causing loss of MMR function with somatic inactivation of the wild-type allele [8]. These patients usually develop multiple tumours between 20–30 years of age in the colon and may have extracolonic manifestations in the rectum, endometrium, renal pelvis, ureter, stomach, ovary, skin, brain, and/or small intestine [12, 32]. It is estimated that 80% of Lynch syndrome carriers remain undetected in the population [25]. This syndrome makes up only 3% of CRCs [24] but is the most common inherited cause of CRC [26]. Germline mutations of *MLH1, MSH2, MSH6*, and *PMS2* have been associated with the development of this hereditary syndrome [32]. The majority of cases are due to autosomal-dominant inheritance of a mutation in either *MLH1* or *MSH2*. Approximately 1/3 of these patients will have no pathogenic mutation in their mismatch repair genes [33]. In these cases, Lynch syndrome arises from germline epimutations inactivating genes through promoter methylation and is usually identified in families that show no MMR gene sequence mutation [12]. This most commonly occurs through hypermethylation at *EPCAM* that inactivates the downstream gene *MSH2* [24]. To confirm the diagnosis, testing for BRAF is indicated, as it is virtually never mutated in Lynch syndrome [26] though it is mutated in 40–50% of sporadic MSI tumours [24].

3.3. CpG Island Methylation Phenotype. The newest of the three genomic instability pathways, the CpG island methylator phenotype (CIMP) was originally grouped together with MSI. CpG islands are regions within the genome rich in CpG (Cytosine-phosphate-guanine) dinucleotides where cytosine DNA methylation does not covalently modify [2]. These islands are especially common in promoter sequences, found in over half of them [2]. In normal tissue cytosine methylation is common outside of the exons [8]. Methylation naturally increases with age, injury, and in patients with chronic inflammation [12].

The epigenetic modification of methylation is well recognized as a crucial event in altering gene expression associated with carcinogenesis and is more frequent in cancer than genetic changes [5]. Methylation of promoter CpG islands occurs in all tissue types in carcinogenesis [34]. Methylation leads to transcriptional silencing of genes involved in tumour suppression, cell cycle control, DNA repair, apoptosis, and invasion [35]. CIMP positivity is found in 35–40% of CRCs and has additionally been identified in adenomas [17]. It is postulated DNA methylation may be altered in normal colorectal mucosa, predisposing the affected tissue to further dysplastic changes. It is the second most common cause of sporadic CRC [3]. Through hypermethylation of histone CpG islands, the chromatin closes into a compact structure such that the gene promoter is inaccessible to transcription factors, thereby inactivating gene transcription. Widespread hypermethylation resulting in greater gene inactivation is characteristics of a CIMP-positive tumour [5]. Tumour suppressors that are frequently inactivated in this epigenetic process include p16, p14, MGMT, and hMLH1 [17].

Clinically, CIMP+ tumours share some characteristics with MSI-H tumours including a proximal location and a poor degree of differentiation. Unlike MSI, however, these tumours may have a particularly poor prognosis [17]. These tumours often have KRAS and/or BRAF mutations [5]. CIMP and CIN positivity are mutually exclusive [17]. Traditionally, CIMP was detected by FISH and LOH analysis studying only selected regions; however, with advances in microarray technologies, a genome-wide, high-resolution scan can be achieved with CGH and SNP arrays [21, 36].

Similar to MSI, the prognostic significance of CIMP remains ill defined, with some studies finding an adverse effect on prognosis and others no effect [5]. As such CIMP+ tumours confer a worse prognosis than MSI tumours, though concurrent MSI with CIMP positivity may improve prognosis compared with an MSI−/CIMP+ tumour. It has been suggested the adverse effect associated with CIMP positivity may not be innate, but rather due to *KRAS* or *BRAF* mutations [5].

3.4. Alternative Serrated Neoplastic Pathway. In recent years, it has been recognized that besides the traditional adenoma-carcinoma sequence of CRC, approximately 35% of carcinomas arise from the serrated pathway, developing from precursor lesions often referred to as the "serrated polyp" [31]. Serrated polyps are lesions composed of epithelial infoldings creating a serrated appearance. Though there is currently no universally accepted nomenclature, these lesions include typical hyperplastic polyps (HPs), sessile serrated adenomas (SSAs), and dysplastic serrated polyps (SSADs). There is ongoing nomenclature wars between groups that hold sessile serrated adenoma as a misnomer as they lack cytological dysplasia but harbour architectural crypt disorder and demonstrate disordered proliferation in contrast to traditional "hyperplastic polyps" versus "sessile serrated polyp" versus "sessile serrated lesion" [29]. Two types of hyperplastic polyps are recognized both by image enhanced endoscopy and histology: (a) goblet cell serrated polyps (GCSPs) and (b) microvesicular serrated polyps (MVSPs). These are also genetically dissimilar as GCSPs are associated with KRAS mutations while MVSPs are linked with BRAF mutations with increased susceptibility to aberrant methylation at the CpG rich island (CIMP) [29]. Dysplastic serrated polyps include (a) sessile serrated adenomas with dysplasia (SSAD), (b) traditional serrated adenomas (TSAs), and (c) conventional adenomas with serrated architecture. It is currently believed that SSADs have a greater risk to progress to MSI-H colorectal cancers. This serrated neoplastic pathway of colorectal carcinogenesis is usually found in females with an average age of 61 years and arise predominantly from precursor MVSPs which differ from traditional hyperplastic polyps as they have crypt architectural alterations that reflect disordered growth with dysmaturation. On endoscopy, serrated polyps may be overlooked as they are often flat or sessile. These lesions are suspected to arise more often in the proximal colon, are more common in females, and generally arise a decade later than the average CRC age [14]. Approximately 20% of CRCs originate from the serrated pathway of neoplasia. In this context, two separate molecular pathways have been proposed.

(a) BRAF-mut with CIMP-H is seen in the majority of syndromic, nonsyndromic cancers, and MSI cancers. 12–15% of MSI cancers occur by epigenetic silencing of the promoter methylation of DNA mismatch repair gene hMLH-1 as the key step leading to MSI with rapid progression from low to high grade dysplasia to invasive cancer.

(b) KRAS-mut are CIMP-low, no hMLH-1 activation, and are MSS with many of them harbouring p53 mutations like conventional CRCs. CIMP-high cancers are seen in the proximal colon, in females, have prominent glandular serrations with mucinous differentiation or poorly differentiated glands (medullary/undifferentiated) with intratumoral lymphocytes and Crohn's-like nodular peritumoral infiltrates.

Currently, no management guidelines for serrated polyps have been formalized [29–31]. The risk of metachronous and synchronous neoplasia in patients with serrated polyps is also not clearly defined; however, most evidence points to large serrated polyps being considered as a marker for synchronous advanced colorectal neoplasia and certain proximal or dysplastic serrated polyps increase the risk of metachronous serrated and/or conventional adenomas. Further, in the context of "interval cancers," these are 2.5x more likely to demonstrate CIMP+, 2.7x more likely to demonstrate MSI and nearly 2x more likely to occur in the proximal colon; thus, MSI, and CIMP were independently associated with interval cancers [37]. It is currently believed that many of these interval cancers originate from the serrated neoplastic pathway outlined above.

Various combinations of these pathways exist. Four molecular subtypes of CRCs and their precursor lesions are identified on the basis of both CIN and MSI statuses: (i/ii) conventional adenomas can give rise to CIMP−/MSI− (75–80% CRCs) or CIMP−/MSI+ (5% CRCs) tumours, (iii) sessile serrated adenomas can give rise to CIMP+/MSI+ (10% CRCs) tumours, and (iv) serrated adenomas (sessile or traditional) can give rise to CIMP+/MSI− (5–10% CRCs). Of these combinations, CIMP+/MSI− tumours confer the worst outcome with metastases being most common in these tumours, in 43%, followed by 18% in CIMP−/MSI−, 6% in CIMP−/MSI+, and none in CIMP+/MSI+ in Kang's study. The clinical outcome for MSI-negative tumours worsens when correlated with methylation. In tumours positive for MSI, those also positive for CIMP conferred a worse prognosis [38]. Chromosomal instability and microsatellite instability are mutually exclusive [17]. Recognition of genomic instability and the subtype is important to guide systemic therapy and affects outcome [23].

4. Genomic Modifications

4.1. Mutational Inactivation of Tumour-Suppressor Genes. Tumour suppressor genes code proteins that act to limit growth and proliferation, the cell cycle, motility, and invasion in normal human tissues [8]. In carcinogenic transformation, tumour growth is often facilitated by inactivation of these genes through deletions, mutations, promoter methylation, or mutation of one allele with loss of the other [12, 39]. Several key players in the carcinogenetic process have been identified and are well elucidated in the literature. These genes include *APC, TP53,* and *TGF-β*.

4.1.1. APC. The *APC* gene codes for the APC protein, a large structure that is involved in the regulation of differentiation, adhesion, polarity, migration, development, apoptosis, and chromosomal segregation [13]. The main action of the APC protein is within the Wnt signalling pathway. The canonical Wnt signalling cascade is a well-studied pathway suspected to play an integral role in the development of cancer. When Wnt proteins bind to and activate the cell-surface receptors, these Frizzled proteins activate Dishevelled family proteins, which inhibits the "destruction complex" that includes Axin, glycogen-synthase kinase-3β, and APC. As such, the β-catenin within the cytoplasm will translocate to the nucleus where it acts as a cofactor for T-cell factor/lymphoid enhancing factor (TCF/LEF) transcription factors and regulates a wide variety of specific cells. Normally, Wnt ligand binding is absent, inhibiting the destruction complex, thus allowing it to carry out its action: the phosphorylation of β-catenin for ubiquitination and proteolytic degradation [2, 40].

Mutations of the *APC* gene result in a protein unable to induce β-catenin phosphorylation. Cytoplasmic β-catenin levels increase and migrate to the nucleus [40]. *APC* mutations, therefore, indirectly induce genes targeted by the TCF/LEF transcription factors including the proto-oncogene c-myc and cyclin D1 and genes encoding membrane factors (MMP-7, CD44), growth factors, and Wnt pathway feedback regulators [2, 22]. Such mutations have been detected in 5% of dysplastic aberrant crypt foci, 30–70% of sporadic adenomas, and up to 72% of sporadic tumours [13]. The altered APC protein is most commonly due to premature truncation during protein synthesis, in 95% due to frameshift or nonsense mutations [2]. Alternatively, β-catenin gain-of-function mutations with a fully intact *APC* gene have been detected in up to 50% of colonic tumours with the same result of increased proto-oncogene expression [13]. A mutation to either the *APC* gene or β-catenin that activates this signalling pathway has been detected in the majority of CRCs [40] and is suspected to be an initiating event of carcinogenesis [8]. This is substantiated by the finding that *APC* mutation is sufficient to cause growth of small benign tumours [41]. It has been suggested *APC* mutations may be a rate-limiting event in the development of most adenomas, and both alleles are often inactivated by this point [2].

The distribution of β-catenin within the cell once the *APC* gene has been mutated appears to be heterogeneous. Moderately well-differentiated adenocarcinomas tend to accumulate nuclear β-catenin at their invasive front as well as scattered in the nearby stroma; however, in the central differentiated areas, the β-catenin is detected on the cellular membrane without translocation. It is postulated the tumour microenvironment may be an important factor in CRC growth and dissemination. Growth factors, chemokines, inflammatory factors, and the extracellular matrix are suspected to interact with the Wnt-signalling pathway resulting in this heterogenous intracellular β-catenin distribution [40]. Recent studies indicate that some sessile serrated adenomas (SSAs) have aberrant β-catenin labelling implicating the Wnt pathway in the molecular progression of SSA to colorectal cancer. In the study by Yachida et al., abnormal β-catenin nuclear labelling is seen as a common features in serrated polyps with neoplastic potential and this correlates with early neoplastic progression following BRAF activation [42].

The *APC* gene has been implicated in the development of familial adenomatous polyposis (FAP), an inherited condition characterized by hundreds to thousands of adenomas lining the large intestine by the second to third decade of life with a high propensity for malignant transformation early in life, between the ages of 40 and 50 [33]. This genetic disease accounts for less than 1% of CRC cases [9]. Patients with FAP carry a germline mutation of *APC* [8] which is autosomally dominant and is associated with almost 100% penetrance [43]. Extraintestinal symptoms include osteoma, dental abnormalities, congenital hypertrophy of retinal pigment epithelium, and extracolonic tumours [9]. Gardner's syndrome is also caused by *APC* mutations, and Turcot syndrome is suspected to be due to *APC* gene mutation or mismatch repair gene mutations [33].

4.1.2. TP53. The tumour suppressor protein p53 and its gene *TP53* is a well-studied element of the carcinogenic pathway, with alterations to its function found in most human cancers. The *TP53* gene is found on the short arm of chromosome 17 and is induced by oncogenic proteins such as c-myc, RAS, and adenovirus E1A [13]. Normally, the p53 protein is negatively regulated by MDM2, E3-ubiquitin ligase, and MDM4 that targets p53 for ubiquination. In the presence of cellular stress, MDM2 and MDM4 have disrupted interactions with activation and transcription of p53 [13]. P53 protein then regulates cell cycle by activating DNA repair when necessary, arresting cells in the G1/S and the G2/M boundary when genetic damage is detected, and initiating apoptosis if the damage cannot be repaired [2]. Thus, p53, often designated as the guardian of the genome, has a key role in maintaining genomic stability.

Inactivation of *TP53* is a key step in the development of CRC [8]. Mutations and LOH of p53 are important with the transition from adenoma to carcinoma [2]. Usually both alleles are inactivated by a missense mutation inactivating transcription and a 17p chromosomal deletion of the second *TP53* allele [8]. This loss of function is found in 4–26% of adenomas, 50% of adenomas with invasive foci, and 50–75% of CRCs [13]. The developing neoplasm places a variety of stresses on the cell, including DNA strand breakage, telomere erosion, hypoxia, reduced nutrient exposure, antiangiogenesis, and cell-cycle arrest. Ineffective p53 function prevents the protein from responding appropriately to these stimuli, thereby facilitating growth and invasion [2].

4.1.3. TGF-β. SMAD is the pathway through which the transforming growth factor beta (TGF-β) protein signals activity. The pathway is initiated by a TGF-β dimer binding to a TGF-β Receptor II that recruits and phosphorylates a type I receptor. This receptor then phosphorylates receptor-regulated SMAD (R-SMAD). The family of R-SMADs includes SMAD1, SMAD2, SMAD3, SMAD5, and SMAD8. This R-SMAD will then bind to SMAD4 to form a complex that enters the nucleus and affects transcription [2]. There, it causes apoptosis and cell cycle regulation.

Approximately one third of CRCs demonstrate somatic mutations inactivating the *TGFBR2* gene. Inactivating mutations of the TGF-β pathway is involved in the adenoma transition to high-grade dysplasia or invasive carcinoma [8].

SMAD2 and *SMAD4* encode the proteins SMAD2 and SMAD4 and are mutated in 5% and 10–15% of CRCs respectively [2]. *SMAD4* germline mutations are implicated in juvenile polyposis syndrome, an autosomal dominant condition in which multiple hamartomas develop throughout the gastrointestinal tract [44].

4.2. Activation of Oncogene Pathways. Oncogenes are genes with the potential to cause cancer. They encode growth factors, growth factor receptors, signalling molecules, regulators of the cell cycle, and additional factors implicated in cellular proliferation and survival. When these genes are mutated, results may include overactive gene products, amplifications altering copy number, alterations that affect promoter function or modified interactions that cause transcription/epigenetic modifications.

4.2.1. RAS and BRAF. The RAS-RAF-MAPK pathway begins with a mitogen (such as EGF) binding to the membrane receptor (such as EGFR), which allows the GTPase Ras to exchange its GDP for a GTP, activating MAP3K (Raf) which activates MAP2K which activates MAPK. MAPK then activates transcription factors that express proteins with a role in cellular proliferation, differentiation, and survival [45].

A key, and well-studied, component of this cascade is the Ras family, comprised of three members: KRAS, HRAS, and NRAS. These isoforms are located on the inner surface of the plasma membrane [45]. A common target of somatic mutations, especially at codons 12 (82–87%), 13 (13–18%), and 61, KRAS has been implicated in many human cancers [46]. KRAS mutations have been reported in 40% of CRCs and contribute to the development of colorectal adenomas and hyperplastic polyps [2]. These mutations are usually single nucleotide point mutations that lock the enzyme bound to ATP, by inhibiting its GTPase activities thus upregulating the Ras function [13, 22]. It, therefore, affects downstream signalling cascades including MAPK and PI3K.

Early KRAS mutations have been identified in left-sided hyperplastic polyps [10]. This mutation is more common in polypoid lesions than nonpolypoid [6]. KRAS mutations are associated with a worse prognosis, in part due to the overexpression of KRAS contributing to metastases through increasing the production of protease to degrade the extracellular matrix. However, the prognostic role of KRAS mutations remains largely ill understood and further studies are required. Attempts have been made at targeting KRAS for cancer treatment including inhibition of protein expression through antisense oligonucleotides and with blockage of posttranslational modifications to inhibit downstream effectors [5].

KRAS mutations have recently gained interest as a negative predictive factor for anti-EGFR therapy response. Blocking EGFR will have no effect if KRAS is mutated as it functions downstream of EGF receptors. Thus, a KRAS mutation allows continual activation of the downstream pathway, thus negating the effects of the drug [41]. As such, anti-EGFR drugs (Section 7.1.2) are not recommended in KRAS-mutated tumours. In this context, it has been suggested that all patients with CRC under consideration for anti-EGFRs should be tested for KRAS mutation status prior to treatment initiation [16, 41].

The Raf family includes three members: ARAF, RAF1, and BRAF. When activated, these serine/threonine kinases activate MEK1 and MEK2 which phosphorylate ERK1 and ERK2. The ERKs continue the cascade by phosphorylating cytosolic and nuclear substrates such as JUN and ELK1 that regulate a wide spectrum of enzymes such as cyclin D1 [13]. Similar to KRAS, BRAF mutations render it continually active, in over 80% of CRCs by substitution of thymine to adenine at nucleotide 1799 that results in a substitution of valine to glutamic acid [5]. These point mutations make BRAF an attractive marker for analysis, as they are present in at least 80% of mutants [22]. Such mutations are more frequent in MSI tumours and are reported in 5–15% of CRCs [5]. Mutations in BRAF and KRAS are mutually exclusive as they are intimately connected in the RAS-RAF-MAPK pathway [45]. In the rare instance of concomitant mutations, they confer a synergistic effect and increase tumour progression [5].

BRAF mutations confer a worse clinical outcome and thus the need for adjuvant therapy [5]. Mutations are associated with a shorter progression free and overall survival [45]. Though controversial, some studies have found that these adverse clinical effects of BRAF are negated in CIMP+ tumours, suggesting the poor prognosis is not attributable to the BRAF mutation itself, but is probably attributable to the genetic pathway in which it occurs [5]. Similar to KRAS, BRAF mutations have also been implicated in anti-EGFR resistance. Approximately 60% of KRAS wild-type metastatic CRC (mCRC) are unresponsive to these drugs, and it is hypothesized that BRAF mutations may confer some of this resistance [41]. As such, BRAF mutation status may also be assessed to determine patients resistant to anti-EGFR therapy.

4.2.2. Phosphatidylinositol 3-Kinase (PI3K). The PI3K-Akt begins with activation of PI3K, which can occur in three ways: (1) a growth factor binds to IGF-1 receptor in the cell membrane, causing dimerization and autophosphorylation of the receptor, IRS-1 then binds to the receptor and acts as a binding site and activator of PI3K; (2) a growth factor binds to a receptor tyrosine kinase embedded in the membrane, again causing dimerization and autophosphorylation, the PI3K then binds directly to the receptor and is activated; (3) the GTPase Ras (as seen above) may bind PI3K and activates it. Once PI3K is activated, it detaches and phosphorylates PIP2 that is a component of the membrane, transforming it to PIP3. PIP3 then activates Akt, a proto-oncogene with functions including growth promotion, proliferation, and apoptosis inhibition [5, 22]. The system is restored by PTEN, which dephosphorylates PIP3 and inhibits Akt signalling.

PI3Ks are a family of enzymes divided into three classes. Of interest in CRC is the class 1A PI3Ks, which are composed of one catalytic subunit (either p110α, p110β, or p110δ) and one regulatory subunit (p85α, p85β or p86γ) [22]. The catalytic subunit p110α, which is encoded by the protein *PIK3CA*, has been of particular attention as it is believed to play a significant role in cancer progression. Its mutation has been detected in approximately a third of CRCs [8]. These gain-of-function mutations cause increased Akt signalling even without the presence of growth factors [45]. Clinically, the prognostic role of *PI3KCA* is under investigation, and it is suspected to confer a poor outcome [5]. It has also been suggested to play a role in resistance to anti-EGFR treatment [45].

Due to its inhibitory effect on Akt, the phosphatase and tensin homolog (PTEN) acts as a tumour suppressor gene in this pathway. In CRC, the *PTEN* gene may be inactivated by somatic mutations, allelic loss or hypermethylation of the enhancer region [45]. Mutation of *PTEN* is a later event in carcinogenesis that is correlated with advanced and metastatic tumours. Though it is clear that *PTEN* mutations in stage II CRC is a poor prognostic marker, its role in other stages of CRC remains uncertain [5]. There remains a discrepancy as to the exact role of *PTEN* in anti-EGFR resistance [45].

5. MicroRNA

MicroRNA (miRNA) is short RNA 8–25 nucleotides in length that binds to mRNA to control translation of complementary genes [47]. Over 1,000 miRNA sequences have been identified, each controlling hundreds of genes for a total of over 5,300 genes, 30% of the human genome [48]. These short RNAs play a regulatory role in development, cellular differentiation, proliferation, and apoptosis. In this context, miRNA dysregulation is suggested to play a role in carcinogenesis when their mRNA targets are tumour suppressor genes or oncogenes through silencing and overexpression respectively [47]. Half miRNAs are located at the breakpoints of chromosomes and, therefore, at a higher risk of dysregulation [48]. Whether or not the microenvironment directly affects miRNA dysregulation remains unclear [49]. Mature miRNA conducive to tumour growth may be upregulated through transcriptional activation and/or amplification of the miRNA encoding gene and those unfavourable to growth are silenced by deletion or epigenetic modifications [47]. Overexpression of miR-31, -183, -17-5, -18a, -20a, and -92 and underexpression of miR-143 and -145 are common in CRC [50]. It remains unclear, however, which miRNA changes are causative and which are a result of carcinogenesis [2]. Many of the pathways explained in this manuscript can be affected by miRNA including [47]

(i) APC: miR-135a, miR-135b cause decreased translation,

(ii) PI3K: miR-126 stabilizes PI3K signal, is lost in CRC,

(iii) PTEN: miR-21 is repressed,

(iv) KRAS: miR-143 causes decreases expression,

(v) p53: miR-34a induces apoptosis, is decreased in 36% of primary CRCs, miR-192, miR-194-2, and miR-215 are involved in cell cycle arrest and are also downregulated in CRC [48],

(vi) EMT: miR-200c overexpression causes inhibition of ZEB1 and induces MET in cells that previously underwent EMT [48].

miRNA has the same potential for identification as mRNA/proteins for the screening, diagnosis, and prognostic prediction of CRC. They appear in both the serum and plasma. Each type of human cancer has a distinct miRNA expression pattern [2]. It has been further proposed that the miRNA pattern could be indicative of prognosis and act as a molecular target for treatment [49].

6. Epigenetic Changes

Epigenetic changes are those that alter genetic expression without modifying the actual DNA. These changes are detected in approximately 40% of CRCs [19]. These factors are conveyed during cellular division. Epigenetic changes, as they relate to CRC, can be subclassified into two broad categories: (1) histone modification and (2) DNA methylation.

6.1. Histone Modification. Histones are proteins that package cellular DNA into nucleosomes and play a role in gene regulation. Covalent modifications, including acetylation, methylation, phosphorylation, and ubiquitinylation of these proteins can cause dense inactive heterochromatin to open to euchromatin and vice versa. Such modifications are reversible, usually occurring at the N- and C-terminal regions [51]. Hypoacetylation and hypermethylation are characteristic of transcriptionally repressed chromatin regions. Mutations in histones are most common at lysine and arginine residues [33]. The mutually exclusive modifications that have been identified in CRC include deacetylation and methylation of lysine 9 in histone H3. If acetylation occurs at this position, the gene is expressed whereas if it is methylated, the gene is silenced. It is suggested that a universal marker for malignant transformation is the loss of monoacetylation from Lys 16 and trimethylation at Lys 20 on histone H4 [51].

6.2. DNA Methylation. The process of hypermethylation of CpG islands is discussed above (Section 3.3); therefore, this section will discuss the process of global DNA hypomethylation, a process not as well understood. Over 40% of human DNA contains short interspersed transposable elements (SINEs) and long interspersed transposable elements (LINEs) that are normally methylated but become hypomethylated in CRC development [35]. Hypomethylation most commonly occurs at repetitive sequences such as satellites or pericentromeric regions [51]. This epigenetic change increases chromosomal susceptibility to breakage, thus creating genomic instability, reactivating retrotransposons that disrupt gene structure and function, or activating oncogenes such as the S100A4 metastasis-associated gene in CRC [51]. These changes are believed to occur early in carcinogenesis, as hypomethylation is detected in benign polyps but is not changed once they become malignant [35].

7. Metastatic Colorectal Cancer

The final stage of CRC involves detachment from the primary cancer, migration, access to the blood/lymph, and development of a secondary tumour [40]. Each step in metastatic spread requires definitive genetic and epigenetic changes; however, the exact mechanisms underlying these changes remain largely unknown. The complex pathway that drives progression cannot be assessed with a single marker that can accurately predict growth progression and prognosis. This indicates that a greater understanding of the multiple pathways and the molecular markers involved is necessary [16]. Growth factors such as prostaglandin E2, EGF, and VEGF as well as molecular mediators of the epithelial-mesenchymal transition have been identified as potentiators of metastatic spread. Biological agents specifically targeting these markers have increased the median survival time of mCRC to 23.5 months. However, this is associated with toxicities, a complex management plan, and a hefty financial burden [46]. Approximately 50% of patients with CRC will die due to complications of metastases; therefore, early recognition of these molecular changes involved in this process with development of therapeutic strategies to combat these events is a high priority in mCRC treatment [48].

7.1. Growth Factor Pathways

7.1.1. Prostaglandin and Cyclooxygenase-2. Prostaglandin E2 is mainly produced and secreted by fibroblasts in the stroma and epithelial cells. Its signal is transduced through interactions of endoprostanoid receptors. Activation of these endoprostanoids initiates a cascade that activates EGFR and PI3K/Akt signalling pathways resulting in β-catenin translocation to the nucleus [52]. Signalling of this prostanoid thus plays an important role in the development of adenoma and is strongly associated with CRC through the regulation of proliferation, survival, migration, and invasion [13]. These high levels may be induced by inflammation or mitogen-associated upregulation of cyclooxygenase-2 (COX-2), the mediator of prostaglandin E2, or due to a loss of 15-prostaglandin dehydrogenase (PDGH), the rate-limiting enzyme catalyzing prostaglandin E2 breakdown. Loss of PDGH is high and is reported in up to 80% of colorectal adenomas and carcinomas [8]. COX-2 upregulation can be induced by growth factors, cytokines, inflammatory mediators, tumour promoters, and is overexpressed in ~43% of adenomas and 86% carcinomas [13]. COX-2 has been implicated in angiogenesis, as overexpression of this enzyme induces the production of proangiogenic factors including VEGF and fibroblast growth factor [13]. The tumorigenic effects of COX-2 overexpression may be inhibited by anti-EGFR therapy [53].

7.1.2. Epidermal Growth Factor (EGF). Epidermal growth factor receptor (EGFR), a member of the HER-erbB family of receptor tyrosine kinases, is a cell-surface receptor that binds epidermal growth factor, transforming growth factor α (TGF-α), amphiregulin, betacellulin, and epiregulin [54, 55]. When bound, EGFR changes its conformation to activate its tyrosine activity and mediates signalling through activation of the RAS-RAF-MAPK and PI3K signalling cascades [55]. It may also activate phospholipase-C, STAT (signal transducer and activators of transcription protein), and SRC/FAK [45]. Dysregulation of EGFR signalling can result at multiple points in this pathway including (a) at the receptor (EGFR mutation, copy number change, overexpression), (b) at the transduction regulators (constitutive activation of RAS, RAF, PI3K), and (c) by methylation/mutations in genes coding these proteins [55]. Downstream targets of EGFR form an interconnected network of phosphorylation reactions that activate transcription factors to elucidate effects including tumour proliferation, angiogenesis, and cell survival [45]. Pathways activated by this receptor have been linked to molecules such as VEGF and hypoxia inducible factor α, both with a well-described role in promoting angiogenesis. Additionally, EGFR activation promotes invasiveness and spread by activating serine protease, which aids in the degradation of the extracellular matrix [53]. Finally, it is an initiating event in the RAS-RAF-MAPK pathway and the PI3K-Akt pathway as described above with prominent roles in carcinogenesis. Overexpression of EGFR occurs in 65–70% of CRCs, and as would be suggested by its effects, it is more commonly seen in advanced stage tumours [5]. In this context, EGFR has been identified as an important therapeutic target in metastatic CRC (mCRC).

Overexpression is associated with an advanced stage, a worse histological grade, and lymphovascular invasion. Especially in the setting of mCRC, EGFR expression is suggested to be a potential prognostic factor; however, its impact on survival remains controversial. Nevertheless, pharmacological inhibitors of EGFR have significantly benefited the CRC patient population through both monoclonal antibodies to interfere with receptor signalling and tyrosine kinase inhibitors to interfere with the catalytic activity of the cytoplasmic domain [5]. Two monoclonal antibody (cetuximab and panitumumab) and two tyrosine-kinase inhibitor (Geftinib and Erlotinic) drugs have been created. The higher the patient's EGFR overexpression, the better the response to anti-EGFR treatment.

Cetuximab is a human-murine immunoglobuin (IgG)G1 mAb that inhibits EGFR by binding to its extracellular domain in both normal and tumour cells. This binding results in receptor internalization, inhibiting it from binding a ligand. The most common toxicity of monotherapy cetuximab is an acneiform rash in 88% of patients followed by a hypersensitivity reaction in 10% [54]. The drug can be taken alone or in combination with other chemotherapies to improve survival of chemorefractory CRC [4]. A longer progression-free survival has been demonstrated in patients with mCRC taking cetuximab combined with FOLFIRI (leuvocovorin, 5-FU, irinotecan) [56].

Panitumumab is a κ IgG2 mAb that binds with high specificity and affinity to the extracellular domain of the EGFR in both normal and tumour cells, whereby it prevents the binding of ligands, dimerization, autophosphorylation, and signalling [54]. When used in combination with chemotherapy or radiotherapy for the treatment of recurrent or first-line mCRC or in an adjuvant setting, both panitumumab and cetuximab drugs act synergistically.

Gefitinib is an orally administered anilinoquinazoline that acts through reversible inhibition of EGFR tyrosine kinase autophosphorylation, thereby inhibiting the downstream signalling [54]. The most common toxicity was diarrhoea in two thirds of patients and neutropenia in 60% [54]. It does not mix well with irinotecan-based chemotherapies, and studies have shown no objective response to this drug [54].

Erlotinib is a quinazolinamine that also reversibly inhibits its EGFR tyrosine kinase to prevent receptor autophosphorylation. It has shown no meaningful activity as a single agent treatment for mCRC; however, its effects seem more promising when combined with oxaliplatin and fluoropyrimidine [54].

A common risk of these targeted therapies is resistance in patients who initially responded to monoclonal antibodies or tyrosine kinase treatments. The mechanism behind this resistance remains poorly understood [41]. As noted in Section 4.2.1, the presence of KRAS or BRAF mutations has been found to limit the activity of these anti-EGFR drugs. As such, screening of CRC patients for treatment suitability is suggested in order to avoid unnecessary exposure to the drugs and to reduce treatment costs.

7.1.3. Vascular Endothelial Growth Factor. Angiogenesis, the development of new blood vessels from preexisting ones, is normally a vital process during development and wound healing; however, in carcinogenesis, angiogenesis is necessary to transport oxygen and nutrients into a growing neoplasm. These two processes differ in the balance between pro- and antiangiogenic signals. Proangiogenic factors include vascular endothelial growth factor (VEGF), fibroblast-growth factor (FGF), platelet-derived growth factors (PDGFs), insulin-like growth factor (IlGF), and transforming growth factor (TGF), and antiangiogenic factors include thrombospondin-1, angiostatin, and endostatin [54]. In carcinogenesis, the balance between these factors is lost, with proangiogenic factors predominating. In CRC, neovascularization is driven by hypoxia stimulating the production of angiogenic factors such as VEGF [48].

Vascular endothelial growth factor (VEGF) is a key component of this process in both normal and pathologic tissues, activating endothelial cell growth, migration, differentiation, and vascular permeability [56]. This family of angiogenic and lymphangiogenic factors includes five VEGF glycoproteins (A-E) and placental growth factors (PGFs) 1 and 2 [54]. These ligands bind to the VEGF receptor (VEGFR 1–3), a tyrosine kinase transmembrane protein, to activate pathways such as RAF/MEK, ERK, AKT, mTOR, and PI3K [56]. Specific glycoproteins bind to specific receptors with varying affinity. VEGFR1 is a receptor for VEGF-B and PGF with a role in hematopoiesis, endothelial progenitor recruitment, and growth factor induction. VEGFR2 is a receptor for VEGF-A and -F that increases microvascular permeability, proliferation of endothelial cells, migration, and invasion. Finally, VEGFR3 binds to VEGF-C and -D to mediate embryonic cardiovascular development [54]. High serum levels of VEGF are associated with a poor prognosis [56], and *VEGFR1* gene expression may be predictive of tumour recurrence [16].

Based on the important role that angiogenesis and VEGF play in advanced CRCs, a monoclonal antibody therapy was created to inhibit this process. Bevacizumab works against all isoforms of VEGF-A that inhibit binding to its receptor, causing regression of microvessels and inhibiting the formation of new vessels [54]. The only toxicity reported associated with its use is hypertension that is manageable with pharmaceuticals [56]. Additionally, it is suggested that Bevacizumab impacts vascular flow, facilitating the increased delivery of chemotherapy to the tumour [57]. Bevacizumab may be combined with the FOLFOX (leucovorin, 5-FU, oxaliplatin) or FOLFIRI (leuvocovorin, 5-FU, irinotecan) treatment regimens [56]. This drug combined with chemotherapy increases survival of patients with mCRC when compared with chemotherapy or bevacizumab alone [4]. Three VEGF tyrosine kinase inhibitors have additionally been created: Vatalanib, Afibercept, and Sunitinib [54, 56]. To this point, no other anti-VEGFs have shown efficacy in the treatment of mCRC.

7.2. Epithelial-Mesenchymal Transition. Epithelial-mesenchymal transition (EMT) is a proposed mechanism that facilitates invasion and metastases in which epithelial cells are changed into dedifferentiated mesenchymal cells characterized by decreased E-cadherin, loss of cell adhesion, and increased cell motility [58]. This transition is induced by transcriptional repressor zinc-finger E-box binding homeobox (ZEB1) [47]. ZEB1 causes repression of E-cadherin transcription and is triggered by TGF-β [48]. These cells lose their intercellular connections that are normally mediated by E-cadherin, facilitating association with the extracellular matrix (ECM) for an anchor, and thus propel forward [58]. In this context, ECM remodelling by proteinases such as the urokinase plasminogen activator cascade and matrix metalloproteinases is central to tumour growth, survival, invasiveness, and metastases [47]. EMT signalling additionally causes β-catenin to stabilize and translocate to the nucleus. The EMT is completed when the basement membrane is degraded and the mesenchymal cell is formed as evidenced by loss of β-catenin and E-cadherin membranous expression [59]. These mesenchymal cells are then free to metastasize to distant sites and through mesenchymal-epithelial transition establish colonies histopathologically similar to the primary tumour [59].

This series of events relies on signals from the stroma including hepatocyte growth factor, EGF, placental-derived growth factor, and TGF-β. These signals cause activation of transcription factors to induce EMT, including Snail, Slug, ZEB1, Twist, Goosecoid, and FoxC2 [59]. Hepatocyte growth factor (HGF) promotes the transcriptional activity of β-catenin in a self-amplifying positive feedback loop to promote growth and invasion. EGF, TGF-β, and placental-derived growth factor promote phosphorylation of p68 which binds to β-catenin and inhibits its stabilization by GSK3β [40]. Downstream targets of β-catenin are prometastatic and include galectin-3 and Fascin, both of which are expressed at the invasive margin and confer a poor outcome [40].

In CRC, tumour budding is considered analogous to EMT. Tumour budding is considered the histological mark of EMT and is defined as the presence of dedifferentiated single cells/small clusters at the invasive front of colorectal cancer [60]. This process occurs in 20–40% of CRCs [59]. Tumour budding occurs at the invasive front by a small aggregate of cells detaching and migrating through the stroma and is considered the initiation of invasion and metastases [58, 59]. This process is more common in MSS CRC, which may partially explain the poorer prognosis of MSS when compared with MSI [58]. The Wnt/β-catenin pathway as previously described, as well as the polypeptide subunit of laminin 5 (LAMC2) in the ECM, has been implicated in tumour budding initiation. Budding is independently associated with poor survival [58]. The presence of buds is predictive of metastases to the lymph nodes through the tumour vessels and lymphatics as well as distant metastases, and local recurrence [59]. A study by Zlobec et al. showed that in patients with a KRAS mutation, high-grade tumour budding is predictive of a nonresponse to anti-EGFR therapies with up to 80% accuracy [60].

8. Detection of Molecular Events

Though colonoscopy remains the gold standard for CRC screening, fewer than 60% of those eligible over the age of 50 have undergone this test. Reasons for this may include procedural factors such as test discomfort, invasiveness, embarrassment, and lack of availability of trained personnel/facilities/equipment [61]. Further, despite the uncertainty, the malignant potential serrated lesions is beyond doubt as they represent the precursors to an important proportion of the overall CRC burden. Therefore, such lesions are also regarded as important targets for the development of CRC prevention strategies. As many of these lesions are sessile, and not easily identified on routine colonoscopy, there is a further increased interest in the development of other alternative modalities for the screening of CRC [31]. Blood and feces are the two media in which targets for earlier molecular detection of CRC have been developed.

8.1. Fecal. Fecal occult blood testing (FOBT) is a noninvasive method of testing for blood in the stool that is commonly conducted as a first-line screening for CRC. This screening tool has reduced CRC mortality by 15–33% [62, 63]. Guaiac-based FOBT detects hemoglobin's peroxidase activity. As it will react to the presence of blood from any site, it is not specific for colorectal bleeding and, therefore, false positives may result from upper gastrointestinal bleeding as well as nonhemoglobin sources of peroxidase such as drugs, vegetables, and red meat. As such, patients are asked to withdraw ASA and NSAIDs a week prior to the test, and fresh vegetables/meat 3 days prior. Compliance is, therefore, a problem, and small adenomas that normally do not bleed are often undetected. More recently, with the development of immunological FOBT that uses antibodies against human globin such dietary and medication restrictions are not

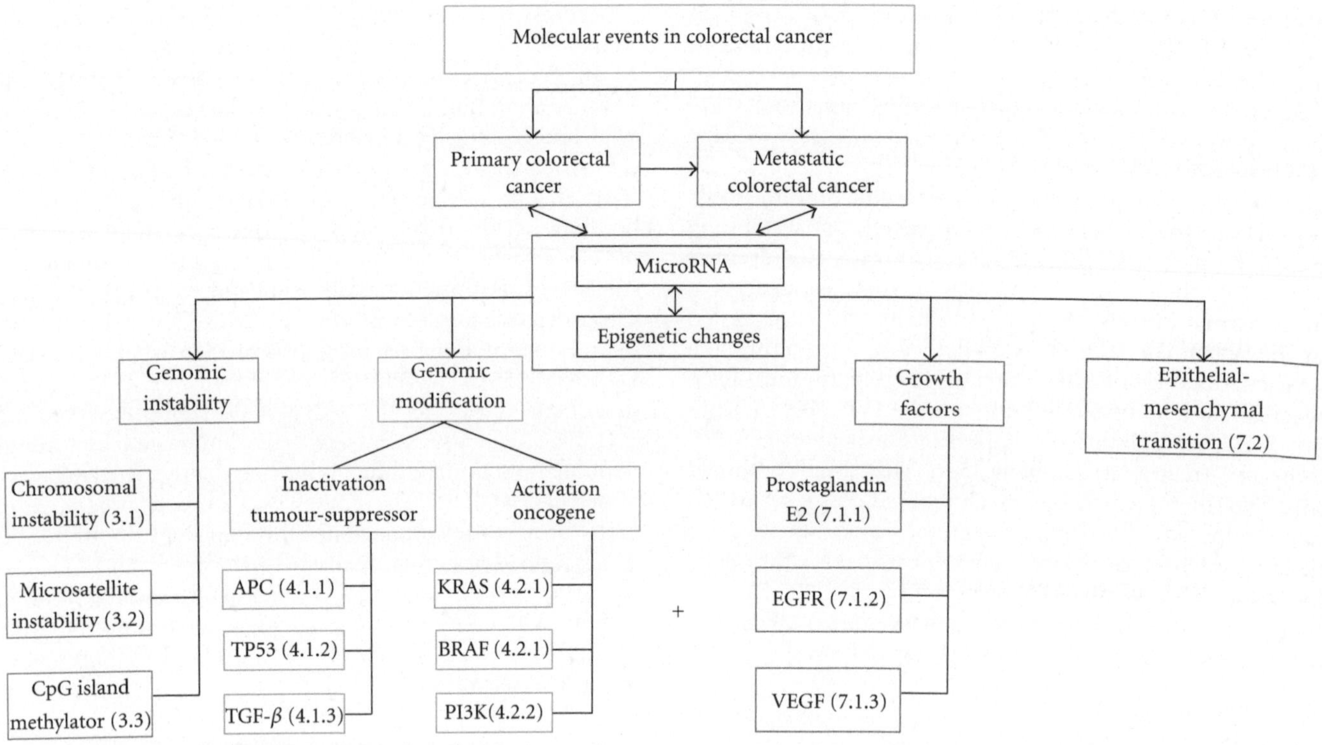

FIGURE 1: Molecular events in colorectal cancer. This is a pictorial representation of the molecular events in primary (blue) and metastatic (red) colorectal carcinoma. The + sign indicates additional molecular events that are recognized in the metastatic progression of this disease. The designated events are referenced to their numerical section within the manuscript.

required. Additionally, as the antibodies in this test are aimed at globin chains that would be degraded if the bleed initiated in the upper gastrointestinal tract, the sensitivity is improved [22].

There has been a recent interest in the detection of molecular markers in fecal specimens as a screening tool for CRC. This detection is based on the natural process of coprocytobiology (colonocytes shedding from the colonic mucosa and being excreted in the stool at a rate of 10^{10} cells/day) [64, 65]. Cells derived from neoplastic lesions are more resistant to destruction and can survive longer in the stool, preserving their genetic aberrations. For the detection of these molecular changes, the fecal samples are stored fresh in a DNA-stabilizing buffer that delays degradation for several days [66, 67]. Once in the laboratory, human genetic materials have to be separated from bacterial, as only 0.01% of the genetic material in feces is human [66]. Genetic material is then amplified with PCR after which genetic molecular markers can be detected through many different methodologies. A wide variety of genetic, epigenetic, and multimarker panels have been suggested as markers to indicate neoplastic growth including *KRAS*, *TP53*, *APC*, and *COX-2*. The role of fecal molecular markers in CRC screening has been recently reviewed from our laboratory and is, therefore, not further discussed in the current manuscript [68].

Stool testing confers a wide spectrum of advantages over flexible sigmoidoscopy/colonoscopy. As colonocytes are shed from the entire length of the colon, fecal genetic material detected is representative of the same; therefore, this screening tool is able to identify lesions undetectable by a flexible sigmoidoscopy that reaches only the distal third [69]. Additionally, patients are more likely to comply with this stool testing, as it is noninvasive, requires no dietary or medicinal restrictions [70], and does not necessitate an office visit [71]. One study found that 91% of patients indicated they would be willing to take the test again in the future [72]. The greatest challenge lies in the identification and selection of a cost-effective single or a select panel of molecular markers with high sensitivity and specificity for CRC.

8.2. Blood. Tumour cells circulating in the peripheral blood may be reflective of tumour genetic characteristics and, therefore, useful in predicting metastatic and recurrence potential [73]. Blood tests are relatively non-invasive and more convenient for the patient than fecal screening. Additionally, blood generally does not contain microflora, reducing interference with genetic material thus facilitating laboratory analysis [73].

More than forty serum proteins have been identified as potential CRC biomarkers, as annotated in Creeden et al.'s recent review [73]. Many of these proteins are for early detection of cancer development. One of the oldest and well-researched markers is carcinoembryonic antigen (CEA) that is positive once a CRC is established; however, it does not readily detect early disease [22]. CEA also has a poor sensitivity and specificity and is clinically used to monitor progression and treatment response in CRC [74]. Studies analyzing methylated DNA detection in the serum/plasma are limited; however, promising results suggest a potential role in the future [74]. The primary challenge remains in the identification of a serum marker specific for colorectal adenoma and carcinoma, as many biomarkers being found are positive in other cancers or in nonneoplastic inflammatory diseases [73].

9. Conclusion

In conclusion, it is, therefore, apparent that, despite many strides in understanding the development and progression of CRC, a lot remains largely unknown due to the multifactorial process of this disease as summarized in Figure 1. Despite the abundance of molecular pathways and markers continually being reported, CRC mortality rates remain high, indicating poor translation from the laboratory to the clinical setting [16]. The goal for the future lies in the development of research tools that can target early detection of many of the ongoing well-recognized subcellular molecular events to improve the burden of mortality and morbidity related to colorectal carcinoma.

References

[1] Colorectal Cancer Statistics at a Glance, http://www.cancer.ca/canada-wide/about%20cancer/cancer%20statistics/stats%20at%20a%20glance/colorectal%20cancer.aspx, 2011.

[2] E. R. Fearon, "Molecular genetics of colorectal cancer," *Annual Review of Pathology*, vol. 6, pp. 479–507, 2011.

[3] D. L. Worthley and B. A. Leggett, "Colorectal cancer: molecular features and clinical opportunities," *The Clinical Biochemist Reviews*, vol. 31, no. 2, pp. 31–39, 2010.

[4] N. Sengupta, K. A. Gill, T. S. MacFie et al., "Management of colorectal cancer: a role for genetics in prevention and treatment?" *Pathology Research and Practice*, vol. 204, no. 7, pp. 469–477, 2008.

[5] V. Deschoolmeester, M. Baay, P. Specenier, F. Lardon, and J. B. Vermorken, "A review of the most promising biomarkers in colorectal cancer: one step closer to targeted therapy," *Oncologist*, vol. 15, no. 7, pp. 699–731, 2010.

[6] L. S. Kahng, "Genetic aspects of non-polypoid colorectal neoplasms," *Gastrointestinal Endoscopy Clinics of North America*, vol. 20, no. 3, pp. 573–578, 2010.

[7] S. Ogino, A. T. Chan, C. S. Fuchs, and E. Giovannucci, "Molecular pathological epidemiology of colorectal neoplasia: an emerging transdisciplinary and interdisciplinary field," *Gut*, 2010.

[8] S. D. Markowitz and M. M. Bertagnolli, "Molecular basis of colorectal cancer," *New England Journal of Medicine*, vol. 361, no. 25, pp. 2404–2460, 2009.

[9] L. Migliore, F. Migheli, R. Spisni, and F. Copped, "Genetics, cytogenetics, and epigenetics of colorectal cancer," *Journal of Biomedicine and Biotechnology*, vol. 2011, Article ID 792362, 19 pages, 2011.

[10] M. Costedio and J. Church, "Pathways of carcinogenesis are reflected in patterns of polyp pathology in patients screened for colorectal cancer," *Diseases of the Colon & Rectum*, vol. 54, no. 10, pp. 1224–1228, 2011.

[11] E. R. Fearon and B. Vogelstein, "A genetic model for colorectal tumorigenesis," *Cell*, vol. 61, no. 5, pp. 759–767, 1990.

[12] C. R. Boland and A. Goel, "Microsatellite instability in colorectal cancer," *Gastroenterology*, vol. 138, no. 6, pp. 2073–e3, 2010.

[13] M. S. Pino and D. C. Chung, "The chromosomal instability pathway in colon cancer," *Gastroenterology*, vol. 138, no. 6, pp. 2059–2072, 2010.

[14] J. Perea, M. Lomas, and M. Hidalgo, "Molecular basis of colorectal cancer: towards an individualized management," *Revista Espanola de Enfermedades Digestivas*, vol. 103, no. 1, pp. 29–35, 2011.

[15] A. H. Sillars-Hardebol, B. Carvalho, M. De Wit et al., "Identification of key genes for carcinogenic pathways associated with colorectal adenoma-to-carcinoma progression," *Tumor Biology*, vol. 31, no. 2, pp. 89–96, 2010.

[16] T. Winder and H. J. Lenz, "Molecular predictive and prognostic markers in colon cancer," *Cancer Treatment Reviews*, vol. 36, no. 7, pp. 550–556, 2010.

[17] A. Goel, T. Nagasaka, C. N. Arnold et al., "The CpG island methylator phenotype and chromosomal instability are inversely correlated in sporadic colorectal cancer," *Gastroenterology*, vol. 132, no. 1, pp. 127–138, 2007.

[18] W. M. Grady and J. M. Carethers, "Genomic and epigenetic instability in colorectal cancer pathogenesis," *Gastroenterology*, vol. 135, no. 4, pp. 1079–1099, 2008.

[19] H. Ashktorab, A. A. Schäffer, M. Daremipouran, D. T. Smoot, E. Lee, and H. Brim, "Distinct genetic alterations in colorectal cancer," *PLoS ONE*, vol. 5, no. 1, Article ID e8879, 2010.

[20] W. B. Dalton and V. W. Yang, "Mitotic origins of chromosomal instability in colorectal cancer," *Current Colorectal Cancer Reports*, vol. 3, no. 2, pp. 59–64, 2007.

[21] B. M. Brenner and D. Rosenberg, "High-throughput SNP/CGH approaches for the analysis of genomic instability in colorectal cancer," *Mutation Research*, vol. 693, no. 1-2, pp. 46–52, 2010.

[22] R. A. Booth, "Minimally invasive biomarkers for detection and staging of colorectal cancer," *Cancer Letters*, vol. 249, no. 1, pp. 87–96, 2007.

[23] A. Walther, R. Houlston, and I. Tomlinson, "Association between chromosomal instability and prognosis in colorectal cancer: a meta-analysis," *Gut*, vol. 57, no. 7, pp. 941–950, 2008.

[24] K. B. Geiersbach and W. S. Samowitz, "Microsatellite instability and colorectal cancer," *Archives of Pathology & Laboratory Medicine*, vol. 125, pp. 1269–1277, 2011.

[25] B. Iacopetta, F. Grieu, and B. Amanuel, "Microsatellite instability in colorectal cancer," *Asia-Pacific Journal of Clinical Oncology*, vol. 6, no. 4, pp. 260–269, 2010.

[26] A. de la Chapelle and H. Hampel, "Clinical relevance of microsatellite instability in colorectal cancer," *Journal of Clinical Oncology*, vol. 28, no. 20, pp. 3380–3387, 2010.

[27] K. L. Yim, "Microsatellite instability in metastatic colorectal cancer: a review of pathology, response to chemotherapy and clinical outcome," *Medical Oncology*. In press.

[28] C. P. Raut, T. M. Pawlik, and M. A. Rodriguez-Bigas, "Clinicopathologic features in colorectal cancer patients with microsatellite instability," *Mutation Research*, vol. 568, no. 2, pp. 275–282, 2004.

[29] C. S. Huang, F. A. Farraye, S. Yang, and M. J. O'Brien, "The Clinical Significance of Serrated Polyps," *American Journal of Gastroenterology*, 2010.

[30] J. R. Jass, "Classification of colorectal cancer based on correlation of clinical, morphological and molecular features," *Histopathology*, vol. 50, no. 1, pp. 113–130, 2007.

[31] D. C. Snover, "Update on the serrated pathway to colorectal carcinoma," *Human Pathology*, vol. 42, no. 1, pp. 1–10, 2011.

[32] A. M. Bellizzi and W. L. Frankel, "Colorectal cancer due to deficiency in DNA mismatch repair function: a review," *Advances in Anatomic Pathology*, vol. 16, no. 6, pp. 405–417, 2009.

[33] R. Venkatachalam, M. J. Ligtenberg, N. Hoogerbrugge, D. R. de Bruijn, R. P. Kuiper, and A. Geurts van Kessel, "The epigenetics of (hereditary) colorectal cancer," *Cancer Genetics and Cytogenetics*, vol. 203, no. 1, pp. 1–6, 2010.

[34] J. H. Kim, S. H. Shin, H. J. Kwon, N. Y. Cho, and G. H. Kang, "Prognostic implications of CpG island hypermethylator phenotype in colorectal cancers," *Virchows Archiv*, vol. 455, no. 6, pp. 485–494, 2009.

[35] Y. S. Kim and G. Deng, "Epigenetic changes (aberrant DNA methylation) in colorectal neoplasia," *Gut and Liver*, vol. 1, no. 1, pp. 1–11, 2007.

[36] Y. W. Cheng, H. Pincas, M. D. Bacolod et al., "CpG island methylator phenotype associates with low-degree chromosomal abnormalities in colorectal cancer," *Clinical Cancer Research*, vol. 14, no. 19, pp. 6005–6013, 2008.

[37] ARAIN.

[38] G. H. Kang, "Four molecular subtypes of colorectal cancer and their precursor lesions," *Archives of Pathology and Laboratory Medicine*, vol. 135, no. 6, pp. 698–703, 2011.

[39] R. Melcher, E. Hartmann, W. Zopf et al., "LOH and copy neutral LOH (cnLOH) act as alternative mechanism in sporadic colorectal cancers with chromosomal and microsatellite instability," *Carcinogenesis*, vol. 32, no. 4, pp. 636–642, 2011.

[40] D. Huang and X. Du, "Crosstalk between tumor cells and microenvironment via Wnt pathway in colorectal cancer dissemination," *World Journal of Gastroenterology*, vol. 14, no. 12, pp. 1823–1827, 2008.

[41] W. de Roock, B. Biesmans, J. De Schutter, and S. Tejpar, "Clinical biomarkers in oncology: focus on colorectal cancer," *Molecular Diagnosis and Therapy*, vol. 13, no. 2, pp. 103–114, 2009.

[42] S. Yachida, S. Mudali, S. A. Martin, E. A. Montgomery, and C. A. Iacobuzio-Donahue, "Beta-catenin nuclear labeling is a common feature of sessile serrated adenomas and correlates with early neoplastic progression after BRAF activation," *American Journal of Surgical Pathology*, vol. 33, no. 12, pp. 1823–1832, 2009.

[43] N. S. Fearnhead, M. P. Britton, and W. F. Bodmer, "The ABC of APC," *Human Molecular Genetics*, vol. 10, no. 7, pp. 721–733, 2001.

[44] G. R. van den Brink, "Linking pathways in colorectal cancer," *Nature Genetics*, vol. 36, no. 10, pp. 1038–1039, 2004.

[45] A. Lièvre, H. Blons, and P. Laurent-Puig, "Oncogenic mutations as predictive factors in colorectal cancer," *Oncogene*, vol. 29, no. 21, pp. 3033–3043, 2010.

[46] U. Asghar, E. Hawkes, and D. Cunningham, "Predictive and prognostic biomarkers for targeted therapy in metastatic colorectal cancer," *Clinical Colorectal Cancer*, vol. 9, no. 5, pp. 274–281, 2010.

[47] O. Slaby, M. Svoboda, J. Michalek, and R. Vyzula, "MicroRNAs in colorectal cancer: translation of molecular biology into clinical application," *Molecular Cancer*, vol. 8, p. 102, 2009.

[48] I. de Krijger, L. J. M. Mekenkamp, C. J. A. Punt, and I. D. Nagtegaal, "MicroRNAs in colorectal cancer metastasis," *Journal of Pathology*, vol. 224, no. 4, pp. 438–447, 2011.

[49] L. Yang, N. Belaguli, and D. H. Berger, "MicroRNA and colorectal cancer," *World Journal of Surgery*, vol. 33, no. 4, pp. 638–646, 2009.

[50] A. Goel and C. R. Boland, "Recent insights into the pathogenesis of colorectal cancer," *Current Opinion in Gastroenterology*, vol. 26, no. 1, pp. 47–52, 2010.

[51] J. J. L. Wong, N. J. Hawkins, and R. L. Ward, "Colorectal cancer: a model for epigenetic tumorigenesis," *Gut*, vol. 56, no. 1, pp. 140–148, 2007.

[52] D. S. Early, L. Fontana, and N. O. Davidson, "Translational approaches to addressing complex genetic pathways in colorectal cancer," *Translational Research*, vol. 151, no. 1, pp. 10–16, 2008.

[53] R. Kumar, "Commentary: targeting colorectal cancer through molecular biology," *Seminars in Oncology*, vol. 32, no. 9, pp. S37–S39, 2005.

[54] T. Winder and H. J. Lenz, "Vascular endothelial growth factor and epidermal growth factor signaling pathways as therapeutic targets for colorectal cancer," *Gastroenterology*, vol. 138, no. 6, pp. 2163–2176, 2010.

[55] S. Barton, N. Starling, and C. Swanton, "Predictive molecular markers of response to epidermal growth factor receptor (EGFR) family-targeted therapies," *Current Cancer Drug Targets*, vol. 10, no. 8, pp. 799–812, 2010.

[56] A. Pohl, W. Zhang, Y. Ning, P. C. Manegold, G. Lurje, and H. J. Lenz, "Targeting metastatic colorectal cancer in 2008: a long way from 5-FU," *Oncology*, vol. 22, no. 4, pp. 456–462, 2008.

[57] A. Cercek and L. Saltz, "Evolving treatment of advanced colorectal cancer," *Current Oncology Reports*, vol. 12, no. 3, pp. 153–159, 2010.

[58] D. Kevans, L. M. Wang, K. Sheahan et al., "Epithelial-mesenchymal transition(EMT) protein expression in a cohort of stage II colorectal cancer patients with characterized tumor budding and mismatch repair protein status," *International Journal of Surgical Pathology*, vol. 20, no. 10, pp. 1–10, 2011.

[59] I. Zlobec and A. Lugli, "Epithelial mesenchymal transition and tumor budding in aggressive colorectal cancer: tumor budding as oncotarget," *Oncotarget*, vol. 1, no. 7, pp. 651–661, 2010.

[60] I. Zlobec, F. Molinari, V. Martin et al., "Tumor budding predicts response to anti-EGFR therapies in metastatic colorectal cancer patients," *World Journal of Gastroenterology*, vol. 16, no. 38, pp. 4823–4831, 2010.

[61] S. Itzkowitz, R. Brand, L. Jandorf et al., "A simplified, noninvasive Stool DNA test for colorectal cancer detection," *American Journal of Gastroenterology*, vol. 103, no. 11, pp. 2862–2870, 2008.

[62] D. E. Brenner and G. Rennert, "Fecal DNA biomarkers for the detection of colorectal neoplasia: attractive, but is it feasible?" *Journal of the National Cancer Institute*, vol. 97, no. 15, pp. 1107–1109, 2005.

[63] K. Lenhard, G. T. Bommer, S. Asutay et al., "Analysis of promoter methylation in stool: a novel method for the detection of colorectal cancer," *Clinical Gastroenterology and Hepatology*, vol. 3, no. 2, pp. 142–149, 2005.

[64] F. E. Ahmed, P. Vos, S. IJames et al., "Transcriptomic molecular markers for screening human colon cancer in stool and tissue," *Cancer Genomics and Proteomics*, vol. 4, no. 1, pp. 1–20, 2007.

[65] P. Nair, S. Lagerholm, S. Dutta et al., "Coprocytobiology: on the nature of cellular elements from stools in the pathophysiology of colonic disease," *Journal of Clinical Gastroenterology*, vol. 36, no. 5, pp. S84–S93, 2003.

[66] D. A. Ahlquist, "Molecular detection of colorectal neoplasia," *Gastroenterology*, vol. 138, no. 6, pp. 2127–2139, 2010.

[67] S. H. Itzkowitz, L. Jandorf, R. Brand et al., "Improved fecal DNA test for colorectal cancer screening," *Clinical Gastroenterology and Hepatology*, vol. 5, no. 1, pp. 111–117, 2007.

[68] R. Kanthan, J. L. Senger, and S. C. Kanthan, "Fecal molecular markers for colorectal cancer screening," *Gastroenterology Research & Practice*, vol. 2012, Article ID 184343, 15 pages, 2012.

[69] B. Greenwald, "The stool DNA test: an emerging technology in colorectal cancer screening," *Gastroenterology Nursing*, vol. 28, no. 1, pp. 28–32, 2005.

[70] A. Loganayagam, "Faecal screening of colorectal cancer," *International Journal of Clinical Practice*, vol. 62, no. 3, pp. 454–459, 2008.

[71] D. A. Ahlquist, "Molecular stool screening for colorectal cancer. Using DNA markers may be beneficial, but large scale evaluation is needed," *British Medical Journal*, vol. 321, no. 7256, pp. 254–255, 2000.

[72] B. M. Berger, P. C. Schroy, J. L. Rosenberg et al., "Colorectal cancer screening using stool DNA analysis in clinical practice: early clinical experience with respect to patient acceptance and colonoscopic follow-up of abnormal tests," *Clinical Colorectal Cancer*, vol. 5, no. 5, pp. 338–343, 2006.

[73] J. Creeden, F. Junker, S. Vogel-Ziebolz, and D. Rex, "Serum tests for colorectal cancer screening," *Molecular Diagnosis and Therapy*, vol. 15, no. 3, pp. 129–141, 2011.

[74] M. S. Kim, J. Lee, and D. Sidransky, "DNA methylation markers in colorectal cancer," *Cancer and Metastasis Reviews*, vol. 29, no. 1, pp. 181–206, 2010.

25

Noninvasive Follicular Thyroid Neoplasm with Papillary-Like Nuclear Features: An Evidence-Based Nomenclature Change

Rachel Jug and Xiaoyin Jiang

Duke Health, DUMC 3712, Durham, NC 27710, USA

Correspondence should be addressed to Xiaoyin Jiang; jiang009@mc.duke.edu

Academic Editor: Marco Volante

A consensus panel recently used clinical evidence and pathologic parameters to rename noninvasive encapsulated follicular variant of papillary thyroid carcinoma to noninvasive follicular thyroid neoplasm with papillary-like nuclear features (NIFTP) to better reflect the indolent course of this tumor. NIFTP has stringent histopathologic diagnostic criteria established by the panel, including papillary-like nuclear features, and submission of the entire tumor capsule to exclude invasion. From a molecular standpoint, NIFTP is often characterized by RAS-type mutations, similar to other follicular-patterned lesions. While there has been prior evidence in the literature for the low malignant potential of these tumors, projects moving forward will help to independently reinforce the reliability of these criteria and nomenclature. With planned inclusion of NIFTP into the latest World Health Organization endocrine tumor classification scheme, this nomenclature shift provides a model for pathology efforts to refine diagnostic classifications to better guide treatment. In this review we discuss this nomenclature change and review the current literature.

1. Introduction

A group of experts in endocrine neoplasia were led by Dr. Nikiforov to formally assess the tumor previously known as "noninvasive encapsulated follicular variant of papillary thyroid carcinoma (FVPTC)" to develop diagnostic criteria and study prognosis. Based on the group's consensus findings, the new term "noninvasive follicular thyroid neoplasm with papillary-like nuclear features (NIFTP)" was announced at the meeting of the Endocrine Pathology Society in March 2015 [1], and the study was published in April 14, 2016, in an online publication of JAMA Oncology [2]. This name change made headlines in the medical community and mainstream media alike [3]. The terminology is planned for inclusion in the new World Health Organization classification system for endocrine tumors. The reclassification of NIFTP was undertaken to further characterize the clinical behavior of this lesion in an effort to prognosticate and manage patients appropriately to prevent potential overtreatment and reduce the burden to patients of a "cancer" diagnosis [4]. Pathological classification criteria accompanying the new name were developed [2, 5]. Beyond changing the classification of a small but significant proportion of thyroid cancers, this movement has provided a model for the reclassification of other low grade malignancies.

2. Clinical Presentation

Clinically, NIFTP presents similarly to most thyroid neoplasms by detection of a nodule on routine or focused physical examination or incidentally during unrelated diagnostic imaging. If NIFTP grows large enough, it can also potentially present by mass effect on surrounding structures, leading to dysphonia, globus sensation, or airway compromise [6].

3. Histopathological Findings

Grossly, NIFTP appears as a solid well-circumscribed or encapsulated nodule. The capsule may be thin and difficult to discern; however, a clear demarcation between the lesion and surrounding thyroid tissue will be readily appreciated. The cut surface is often paler than normal surrounding thyroid tissue and necrosis and hemorrhage are unlikely to be seen. In the NIFTP series studied by Nikiforov et al., the 109 tumors ranged in size from 1.1 to 9 cm [2].

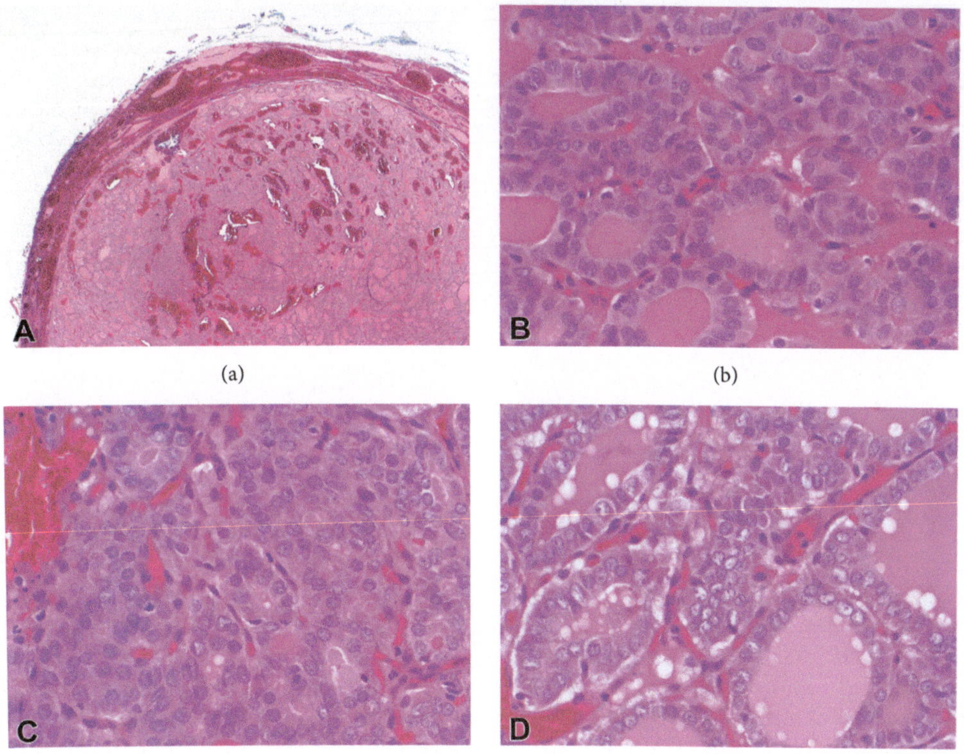

(a) (b) (c) (d)

FIGURE 1: H&E images of NIFTP: (a) low-power (2x) view demonstrating a well-circumscribed lesion with follicular architecture. No vascular or capsular invasion is present. (b, c, d) High-power (40x) images demonstrating nuclear enlargement, crowding, optical clearing, and grooves.

The histological diagnosis of NIFTP is made using strict inclusion and exclusion criteria following submission of the entire tumor capsule for histology and careful examination of nuclear features, as well as overall architecture. The name NIFTP aptly conveys this lesion's prognosis and histologic features. Beginning with "noninvasive," the capsule or tumor/normal interface must be entirely examined microscopically to rule out invasion as capsular or vascular invasion would exclude the tumor from a NIFTP classification (Figure 1(a)). Next, a follicular growth pattern defined as less than 1% papillae, <30% of the lesion composed of a solid, trabecular, or insular growth pattern, and a lack of psammoma bodies helps to classify this lesion as "follicular." Acceptable follicular growth patterns include microfollicular, macrofollicular, and normofollicular with colloid. "Papillary-like nuclear features" must be present, with an overall qualifying score of 2-3 based upon a consensus grading system. Include 1 point each for the presence of either (1) nuclear enlargement/overlapping/crowding or elongation, (2) nuclear membrane irregularities, grooves, or pseudoinclusions, or (3) glassy nuclei/cleared chromatin with margination (Figures 1(b), 1(c), and 1(d)). Finally, there must be no tumor necrosis and mitoses must number less than 3 per 10 high-power fields (400x). These histological features are similar to those used formerly to diagnose the noninvasive encapsulated FVPTC, with the study authors proposing a nuclear scoring system with a 94.3% classification accuracy [2]. In addition, the current requirement of complete microscopic examination of the tumor-normal interface to make the diagnosis of NIFTP imposes standards for grossing of these specimens as well. Immunohistochemical stains apart from hematoxylin and eosin are not required for the diagnosis of NIFTP; however, HBME-1, galectin-3, and CK19 are positive in follicular-patterned tumors which could support a differential diagnosis including NIFTP and EFVPTC [7].

4. Impact on Cytopathology

The introduction of the NIFTP nomenclature has posed a potential problem for cytopathologists. Often, the first specimens obtained from thyroid nodules for review by a pathologist are fine needle aspirates (FNA), on which evaluation of capsular invasion is not possible, and differentiating nuclear features of NIFTP and papillary thyroid carcinoma can be challenging. Many worry that making the diagnosis of PTC on cytopathology now carries the risk of a false-positive result in NIFTP. The Bethesda System for Reporting Thyroid Cytopathology (BSRTC) assigns a risk of malignancy to each of the possible diagnostic categories into which biopsies are placed by the pathologist. The creation of NIFTP has introduced a shift to the currently described risk of malignancy for each of these categories. Early studies seem to indicate that the risk of false-positive for a Bethesda VI diagnosis is low, with most NIFTPs being classified on preoperative FNA into

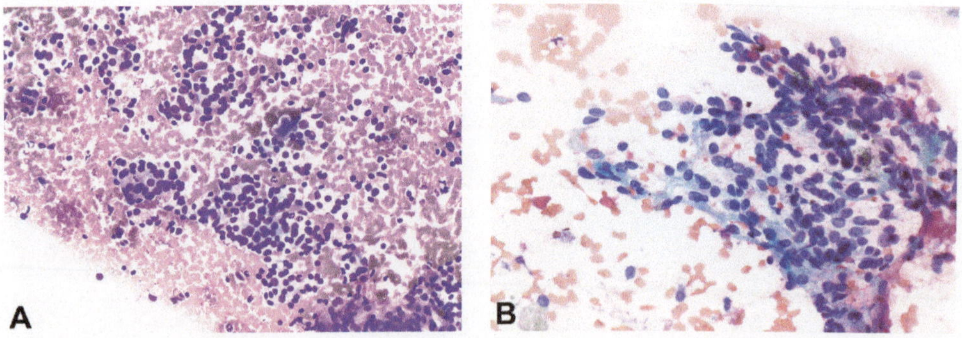

(a) (b)

Figure 2: Cytology images of NIFTP: (a) high-power (20x, Diff-Quik) view demonstrating a cellular lesion with microfollicles. (b) High-power (40x, Papanicolaou stain) view showing nuclear elongation and grooves.

indeterminate categories. Strickland et al. performed a single institution study correlating FNA biopsies to surgical specimens (655-patient cohort) and found NIFTP was most often classified into the indeterminate categories of the BSRTC (including atypia of undetermined significance/follicular lesion of undetermined significance, follicular neoplasm, and suspicious for malignancy) and thus correspondingly significantly lowered the risk of malignancy associated with each of these indeterminate categories. Most significantly, the risk of malignancy in the suspicious for malignancy category decreased by 41.5% [8]. Faquin et al. performed a multi-institutional group study with a cohort of 6943 thyroid lesions biopsied by FNA with 1827 surgical specimens available for diagnostic correlation and similarly found NIFTP lesions were assigned the three indeterminate diagnostic categories of the BSRTC and likewise lowered the associated risk of malignancy in each category. Most significantly, the suspicious for malignancy category had a decreased rate of malignancy by 17.6–23.4% with the addition of NIFTP lesions [9]. Similarly, Maletta et al. reviewed the cytology of 96 histologically proven NIFTP samples and they were proportionately assigned to the following Bethesda categories: 56% Bethesda IV, 27% Bethesda V, 15% Bethesda III, and 2% Bethesda VI [10]. These findings elucidate the need to revisit guidelines for surgical management since they are currently based on the risk of malignancy associated with BSRTC diagnostic categories that do not take NIFTP into account. On FNA specimens with nuclear features of PTC and/or follicular architecture, NIFTP is now on the differential diagnosis, just as was EFVPTC [11] (Figures 2(a) and 2(b)). Overall, the evaluation of NIFTP lesions and EFVPTC by FNA has proven difficult with a 29% false-positive rate and 9–58% true predictive value on preoperative assessment of follicular variant tumors [7].

5. Molecular Findings in NIFTP

Driving clonal alterations have been found in NIFTP tumors, though to date data is limited on the specific entity of NIFTP as such [2]. The genetic alterations responsible for NIFTP include RAS oncogene alterations, similar to those driving follicular adenoma and follicular carcinoma tumors, in contrast to the BRAF oncogenes mutated in the classic papillary thyroid cancer pathway [2]. In the literature on encapsulated follicular variant of PTC, Rivera et al. demonstrated genotypic abnormalities in 11 of 28 encapsulated FVPTC tumors of which 26% of the invasive tumors and 0% of noninvasive tumors harbored a BRAF mutation. In comparison, 36% of encapsulated FVPTC harbored RAS mutations in contrast to 10% of invasive FVPTC tumors [12]. Howitt et al. observed a similar rate (46%) of RAS mutations in a series of partially encapsulated or well-circumscribed FVPTC tumors [13]. Eszlinger et al. demonstrated BRAF mutations in 50% of [invasive] FVPTC [14]. These findings support the theory that NIFTP may be genetically distinct from classical PTC or the more aggressive [infiltrative] FVPTC.

Given the recent description of the entity, the diagnostic criteria for NIFTP do not include a characteristic mutation, much like other thyroid tumors. Molecular studies are much more likely to play a critical role in guiding management at the time of FNA of these lesions. The presence of RAS mutations may contribute supportive evidence favoring a diagnosis of NIFTP, follicular adenoma, or follicular carcinoma, in contrast to BRAF mutations which are more commonly observed in association with classical papillary thyroid carcinoma [12–14]. The presence of a BRAF V600E mutation would not be compatible with NIFTP.

The utility, predictive value, and reporting schemes of currently available molecular tests will need to be reassessed in the era of NIFTP. Early work confirms that the shift in nomenclature will alter test specificity and overall rate of malignancy [8, 15–17]. Wong et al. reviewed a cohort of 63 cases that had been tested with the Afirma Gene Expression Classifier (GEC) in which FNA biopsies yielded diagnoses of atypia/follicular lesion of undetermined significance or suspicious for a follicular neoplasm and corresponding surgical resection specimens were reviewed. They found that NIFTP accounted for 64% of the carcinomas ("suspicious" test results) detected by the Afirma GEC [17]. Valderrabano et al. assessed the performance of the ThryoSeq v2 at their institution by retrospectively reviewing results on Bethesda category III and IV specimens and extrapolated their results to predict the impact on the overall rate of malignancy presuming NIFTPs as a benign diagnosis. They estimated that the overall rate of malignancy would drop from 24% to 15%, the negative predictive value would increase from 88% to 94%, and the positive predictive value would decrease from 50% to 34% overall in both indeterminate categories [18]. At our institution, we have reviewed results of molecular testing from thyroid nodules subsequently diagnosed as NIFTP on surgical resection and showed that all of the surgically confirmed NIFTPs showed molecular alterations on both the ThyroSeq and GEC. Expectedly, all of the NIFTP cases were called Bethesda category III or IV on cytology and all harbored RAS mutations [19]. More independent work is clearly needed in this area to better characterize molecular test performance under the new nomenclature.

6. Differential Diagnosis

The main differential diagnosis for NIFTP is invasive encapsulated FVPTC as this lesion shares the well-circumscribed, often encapsulated structure, follicular architecture and papillary-like nuclear features with NIFTP and differs only with as much as a single focus of capsular or vascular invasion. Invasive encapsulated FVPTC harbors similar RAS-type mutations as NIFTP, follicular adenoma, and follicular carcinoma. In order to differentiate these diagnoses, the tumor capsule must be entirely submitted for microscopic examination to exclude invasion in the case of NIFTP [12].

Follicular adenoma is another entity that shares a similar morphological appearance and molecular genotype to NIFTP [4]. Follicular adenomas are well-circumscribed, partially, or completely encapsulated and composed of follicles that can be arranged in various growth patterns (microfollicular, macrofollicular, trabecular, etc.) and lack nuclear features of papillary thyroid carcinoma [20]. The establishment of a clear scheme for nuclear diagnostic criteria for NIFTP was helpful to attempt to address the considerable interobserver variability when pathologists were tasked with diagnosing FVPTC [21]. With a 94.3% classification accuracy reported for NIFTP using the nuclear scoring system, differentiating between NIFTP and follicular adenomas based on nuclear features may become more reproducible [2].

7. Prognosis and Treatment

While there is little in the literature assessing clinical outcome in NIFTP by the NIFTP name, there has been much in the literature describing the indolent clinical characteristics of EFVPTC without invasion [8, 9]. Ghossein conducted a clinicopathological study of 78 patients with follicular variant of papillary thyroid carcinoma at Memorial Sloan Kettering and found no recurrences or metastases after 11 years in all 42 patients with noninvasive encapsulated FVPTC. In contrast, 6% of participants with invasive FVPTC experienced adverse outcomes [22]. The seemingly benign behavior of the lesion was observed, but the evidence and nomenclature were not in place to appropriately label and simultaneously prognosticate it as various names were proposed, including tumor of uncertain malignant potential or multifocal papillary thyroid carcinoma [22]. Nikiforov et al. clarified the confusion surrounding classification of this lesion by demonstrating the excellent prognosis associated with the diagnosis of NIFTP. After 10–26 years of follow-up, all 109 patients in the NIFTP group were alive without evidence of disease recurrence. In contrast, 12% of 101 patients in the encapsulated FVPTC with invasion experienced an adverse event within 1–18 years of follow-up [2]. In a series of 94 patients with encapsulated follicular variant of papillary thyroid carcinoma, Thompson found no evidence of recurrence or lymph node metastasis (42 patients underwent lymph node sampling) after a median follow-up time of 11.8 years [4].

Early reports suggest that nodal metastasis is a rare event in NIFTP, with one series presented at the 2016 American Thyroid Association meeting demonstrating no NIFTPs with nodal metastases [23] and another demonstrating a low rate (2.2%) of metastasis of NIFTPs at presentation [24]. Hahn et al. identified central nodal metastasis in 1 of 34 cases of NIFTP in their series [25]. It is unclear whether these cases of NIFTP with potential metastasis all underwent complete histopathologic evaluation of the entire tumor capsule, which is currently required to make a definite determination of NIFTP. Another limitation is the potential for occult microcarcinoma metastasis from another area of the thyroid giving rise to metastases then attributed to the NIFTP. We have reported in our series a case of potential lymph node metastasis from an entirely submitted NIFTP to a central lymph node [19], in which the remainder of the thyroid was submitted entirely, excluding the possibility of an occult microcarcinoma. This case suggests that caution and further study are required to better characterize the behavior of NIFTPs.

Prior to the reclassification of NIFTP, there was a lack of evidence to support conservative management (lobectomy alone) of noninvasive encapsulated FVPTC, and if the lesion measured greater than 1.5 cm, many physicians recommended completion thyroidectomy with subsequent radioactive iodine therapy and extensive follow-up, similar to conventional papillary thyroid carcinoma [22]. In addition to demonstrating the indolent clinical course of the pathologically defined NIFTP, Nikiforov et al. found that none of the 101 patients classified in the NIFTP group received radioactive iodine and 67 of them were treated solely by lobectomy [2]. Subsequently, Thompson of the Southern California Permanente Medical Group studied a series of 101 cases of encapsulated FVPTC, including 24 invasive and 77 noninvasive tumors, and of the 69 patients managed with surgery alone, there was an 11.8-year event-free median survival [4].

The American Thyroid Association strongly recommends follow-up of differentiated thyroid cancer by means of serial serum thyroglobulin measurement, serum thyroid stimulating hormone (in patients on thyroid hormone therapy), cervical/neck ultrasonography, and other tests depending on the clinical scenario [26]. Under the name of noninvasive encapsulated FVPTC, NIFTP was traditionally managed this way postoperatively due to a lack of evidence to support a more conservative approach. According to Thompson, NIFTP would fit into the lowest point on the "Risk Continuum" which corresponds to the treatment recommendation of surgical lobectomy without radiotherapy, a prophylactic central neck lymph node staging, or staging since NIFTP is not considered malignant [7]. This nomenclature shift has the potential to begin to reduce the burdens, with more studies adding to the evidence for these tumors' good prognosis. The diagnosis of cancer, treatment, and follow-up places financial strain on healthcare systems and patients and causes both financial and emotional consequences for patients.

8. Conclusions

The rigorous evidence-based efforts made by the expert panel convened to reclassify noninvasive encapsulated FVPTC to NIFTP have paved the way for reframing our approach to diagnosis and treatment of indolent thyroid lesions. They provided clear criteria for diagnosis and supporting evidence with long-term follow-up demonstrating benign behavior in the population they studied [2]. NIFTP, at least in initial reports, shares molecular alterations with follicular lesions of the thyroid (RAS oncogenes) as opposed to those found in PTC (BRAF oncogenes) [2, 12–14]. The establishment of NIFTP has prognostic implications that will modify clinical decision-making and the risk of malignancy associated with BSRTC diagnostic categories on thyroid FNA specimens. Early data suggest the majority of NIFTP fall into the indeterminate categories, thus while the concern of NIFTP leading to false-positive Bethesda VI diagnoses is a valid one, it does not appear to be a frequent occurrence [8, 9]. With widespread acceptance by inclusion of NIFTP in the latest World Health Organization endocrine tumor classification scheme, more research moving forward will be useful to better characterize the molecular findings of this lesion and build the literature on the long-term follow-up of these tumors. Large-scale population based studies are needed to further characterize the behavior of these tumors since small retrospective studies have demonstrated a possible low risk of nodal and distant metastatic disease in tumors classified as NIFTP [24].

Competing Interests

The authors declare that there is no conflict of interests regarding the publication of this paper.

References

[1] G. Tallini, V. Nose, S. Fish, P. Vielh, Y. E. Nikiforov, and R. Ghossein, "Encapsulated follicular cell-derived tumors of the thyroid gland, a practical update," in *Proceedings of the Endocrine Pathology Society Meeting*, Boston, Mass, USA, March 2015.

[2] Y. E. Nikiforov, R. R. Seethala, G. Tallini et al., "Nomenclature revision for encapsulated follicular variant of papillary thyroid carcinoma," *JAMA Oncology*, vol. 2, no. 8, pp. 1023–1029, 2016.

[3] G. Kolata, "It's not cancer: doctors reclassify a thyroid tumor," The New York Times, April 2016.

[4] L. D. Thompson, "Ninety-four cases of encapsulated follicular variant of papillary thyroid carcinoma: a name change to Noninvasive Follicular Thyroid Neoplasm with Papillary-like Nuclear Features would help prevent overtreatment," *Modern Pathology*, vol. 29, no. 7, pp. 698–707, 2016.

[5] K. Titus, "For certain thyroid lesions, the shift is on," *CAP Today*, vol. 30, no. 7, pp. 1–30, 2016.

[6] R. M. Tuttle, "Overview of papillary thyroid cancer," UpToDate, 2016, http://www.uptodate.com/contents/overview-of-papillary-thyroid-cancer.

[7] L. D. R. Thompson, "Update on follicular variant of papillary thyroid carcinoma with an emphasis on new terminology: Noninvasive follicular thyroid neoplasm with papillary-like nuclear features," *Diagnostic Histopathology*, vol. 22, no. 5, pp. 171–178, 2016.

[8] K. C. Strickland, B. E. Howitt, E. Marqusee et al., "The impact of noninvasive follicular variant of papillary thyroid carcinoma on rates of malignancy for fine-needle aspiration diagnostic categories," *Thyroid*, vol. 25, no. 9, pp. 987–992, 2015.

[9] W. C. Faquin, L. Q. Wong, A. H. Afrogheh et al., "Impact of reclassifying noninvasive follicular variant of papillary thyroid carcinoma on the risk of malignancy in the Bethesda System for Reporting Thyroid Cytopathology," *Cancer Cytopathology*, vol. 124, no. 3, pp. 181–187, 2016.

[10] F. Maletta, F. Massa, L. Torregrossa et al., "Cytological features of 'noninvasive follicular thyroid neoplasm with papillary-like nuclear features' and their correlation with tumor histology," *Human Pathology*, vol. 54, pp. 134–142, 2016.

[11] S. Logani, P. K. Gupta, V. A. LiVolsi, S. Mandel, and Z. W. Baloch, "Thyroid nodules with FNA cytology suspicious for follicular variant of papillary thyroid carcinoma: follow-up and management," *Diagnostic Cytopathology*, vol. 23, no. 6, pp. 380–385, 2000.

[12] M. Rivera, J. Ricarte-Filho, J. Knauf et al., "Molecular genotyping of papillary thyroid carcinoma follicular variant according to its histological subtypes (encapsulated vs infiltrative) reveals distinct BRAF and RAS mutation patterns," *Modern Pathology*, vol. 23, no. 9, pp. 1191–1200, 2010.

[13] B. E. Howitt, Y. Jia, L. M. Sholl, and J. A. Barletta, "Molecular alterations in partially-encapsulated or well-circumscribed follicular variant of papillary thyroid carcinoma," *Thyroid*, vol. 23, no. 10, pp. 1256–1262, 2013.

[14] M. Eszlinger, S. Piana, A. Moll et al., "Molecular testing of thyroid fine-needle aspirations improves presurgical diagnosis and supports the histologic identification of minimally invasive follicular thyroid carcinomas," *Thyroid*, vol. 25, no. 4, pp. 401–409, 2015.

[15] D. N. Johnson, N. A. Cipriani, and T. Antic, "The role of molecular testing in thyroid FNA practice," *Journal of the American Society of Cytopathology*, vol. 5, no. 2, 2016.

[16] R. R. Lastra, M. R. Pramick, C. J. Crammer, V. A. LiVolsi, and Z. W. Baloch, "Implications of a suspicious afirma test result in thyroid fine-needle aspiration cytology: an institutional experience," *Cancer Cytopathology*, vol. 122, no. 10, pp. 737–744, 2014.

[17] K. S. Wong, T. E. Angell, K. C. Strickland et al., "Noninvasive Follicular variant of papillary thyroid carcinoma and the afirma gene-expression classifier," *Thyroid*, vol. 26, no. 7, pp. 911–915, 2016.

[18] P. Valderrabano, L. Khazai, M. E. Leon et al., "Single center independent validation of ThyroSeq v2 performance: impact of reclassifying the encapsulated non-invasive follicular variant papillary thryoid carcinoma as non-invasive follicular thyroid neoplasms with papillary-like nuclear features (NIFTP)," *Thyroid*, vol. 26, supplement 1, Article ID P-1-A-129, 2016.

[19] X. Jiang, G. P. Harrison, and M. B. Datto, "Young investigator challenge: molecular testing in noninvasive follicular thyroid neoplasm with papillary-like nuclear features," *Cancer Cytopathology*, vol. 124, no. 12, pp. 893–900, 2016.

[20] Z. W. Baloch and V. A. LiVolsi, "Our approach to follicular-patterned lesions of the thyroid," *Journal of Clinical Pathology*, vol. 60, no. 3, pp. 244–250, 2007.

[21] K. N. Patel, "Noninvasive Encapsulated Follicular Variant of Papillary Thyroid 'Cancer' (or Not): time for a name change," *JAMA Oncology*, vol. 2, no. 8, pp. 1005–1006, 2016.

[22] R. Ghossein, "Problems and controversies in the histopathology of thyroid carcinomas of follicular cell origin," *Archives of Pathology and Laboratory Medicine*, vol. 133, no. 5, pp. 683–691, 2009.

[23] M. Kossaï, M. Kordahi, A. Berdelou et al., "Histological analysis of 183 cases of thyroid cancer with distant metastasis looking for NIFTP," *Thyroid*, vol. 26, Supplement 1, Article ID P-1-A-129, 2016.

[24] P. Valderrabano, L. Khazai, M. E. Leon et al., "Non-invasive follicular thyroid neoplasms with papillary-like nuclear features (NIFTP) have very low but real malignant potential," *Thyroid*, vol. 26, supplement 1, Article ID P-1-A-129, 2016.

[25] S. Y. Hahn, J. H. Shin, H. K. Lim et al., "Preoperative differentiation between noninvasive follicular thyroid neoplasm with papillary-like nuclear features (NIFTP) and non-NIFTP," *Clinical Endocrinology*, 2016.

[26] B. R. Haugen, E. K. Alexander, K. C. Bible et al., "2015 American thyroid association management guidelines for adult patients with thyroid nodules and differentiated thyroid cancer: the American thyroid association guidelines task force on thyroid nodules and differentiated thyroid cancer," *Thyroid*, vol. 26, no. 1, pp. 1–133, 2016.

Leishmaniasis in Central Morocco: Seasonal Fluctuations of Phlebotomine Sand Fly in Aichoun Locality, from Sefrou Province

Fatima Zahra Talbi,[1,2] Abdelhakim El Ouali Lalami,[3] Abdellatif Janati Idrissi,[1] Faiza Sebti,[4] and Chafika Faraj[2]

[1] *Analysis and Modelisation of Continental Ecosystems Laboratory, Faculty of Sciences Dhar El Mehraz, Sidi Mohamed Ben Abdellah University, 30000 Fes, Morocco*
[2] *Laboratory of Medical Entomology, National Institute of Hygiene, 27 Avenue Ibn Battuta, Agdal, 11400 Rabat, Morocco*
[3] *Regional Diagnostic Laboratory Epidemiological and Environmental Health, Regional Health Directorate, EL Ghassani Hospital, 30000 Fes, Morocco*
[4] *National Reference Laboratory of Leishmaniasis, National Institute of Hygiene, 27 Avenue Ibn Battuta, Agdal, 11400 Rabat, Morocco*

Correspondence should be addressed to Abdelhakim El Ouali Lalami; eloualilalami@yahoo.fr

Academic Editor: Shahid Pervez

Cutaneous leishmaniases (CL) are endemic in Morocco. They are common in the human population in different localities such as Aichoun in Sefrou province, Morocco. This study was carried out in Aichoun locality from April to October 2012 in order to study the spatiotemporal trends of the main *Leishmania* phlebotomine vectors in this focus. Overall, 1171 sand flies, belonging to four species, were collected by sticky traps. *Phlebotomus sergenti* was the predominant species (78.4%) followed by *Ph. perniciosus* (10.5%), *Ph. papatasi* (7.94%), and *Ph. longicuspis* (3.16%). Sandflies were active during 6 months (May–October). *Ph. sergenti, Ph. perniciosus*, and *Ph. papatasi* displayed a bimodal distribution with a first peak in July and a second peak in September, while *Ph. longicuspis* showed a monophasic trend with a peak in August. The high abundance and the lengthy period of activity of *Ph. sergenti* and *Ph. perniciosus*, vectors of *L. tropica* and *L. infantum*, respectively, are a cause for concern as they indicate the high potential risk of *Leishmania* transmission in the studied areas.

1. Introduction

Cutaneous Leishmaniasis (CL) is an increasingly public health problem in Morocco. Three forms are present: anthroponotic leishmaniasis caused by *Leishmania tropica* and zoonotic leishmaniasis caused by *L. major* and less frequently by *Leishmania infantum* [1]. The parasites are transmitted by phlebotomine sand flies, namely, *Phlebotomus sergenti* for ACL and *Ph. papatasi* and phlebotomines from *Larrousius* subgenus for *L. major* and *L. infantum*, respectively, for ZCL [2]. The main reservoir host for *L. major* is considered to be the rodent *Meriones shawi* [1].

CL caused by *L. tropica* is the most widespread in semiarid areas in central and south-western Morocco. This disease was reported for the first time in Azilal province in 1989 [3], then in other focus in central and southern areas of the country such as Guelmim, Agadir, Essaouira [4], and Taza [5]. CL due to *L. infantum* was reported in Taounate province in 1996, within an active focus of visceral leishmaniasis [6]. *L. infantum* is also responsible for widespread visceral leishmaniasis in the north-eastern slope of the Rif Mountains when dog is the main domestic reservoir of the parasite [7].

Each year, we witness the emergence of new foci, extending the disease distribution and increasing its total impact. In 2011 and 2012, the Ministry of Health recorded, respectively, 4426 and 2990 cases with 4.92% and 7.19% in the region of Fes-Boulmane [8, 9]. The region of Fes-Boulmane recorded the first outbreak of CL in 2001 with 1600 cases in the province

TABLE 1: Sandflies collected in Aichoun locality, 2012.

Subgenus (R. Ab. %)	Species	Mal	Female	Total	R. Ab. (%)
Larroussius (13.74)	*Phlebotomus longicuspis*	13	24	**37**	3.16
	Phlebotomus perniciosus	113	10	**123**	10.50
Paraphlebotomus (78.28)	*Phlebotomus sergenti*	845	73	**918**	**78.4**
Phlebotomus (7.98)	*Phlebotomus papatasi*	63	30	**93**	7.94

R. Ab.: Relative Abundance.

of Moulay Yacoub alone [10, 11]. The outbreak was rapidly stopped by insecticides use, but the disease has persisted since that under endemic and epidemic forms in other provinces of the region with more than 100 cases each year despite a strong monitoring plan.

The control of the disease is mainly based on case detection and treatment of human cases and on vector control. This is based essentially on environmental management including promotion of improved solid waste disposal practices. The use of bed nets and local residual indoor spraying with synthetic pyrethroids are often applied in newly emerged epidemic foci. Nevertheless, few data are available on the vector *Ph. sergenti*, especially seasonal fluctuations of its abundance. This information is essential for the success of vector control. In this context, we have conducted this study for the first time in a village belonging to the region of Sefrou province in center of Morocco.

This study also allows a better understanding of the dynamics of the transmission of leishmaniasis in the area of Aichoun and, therefore, contributes to the future design of surveillance strategies.

2. Materials and Methods

2.1. Study Area and Environment. The entomological study was conducted in the locality of Aichoun (33°39′N, 04°38′W) situated in the northwest of the Moroccan Middle Atlas, a part of the province of Sefrou that belongs to the territory pastoral village of Tazouta with a cold semiarid climate. The mean altitude is 750 m. The average annual rainfall is 400 mm, the main minimum of the coldest month is 2°C, and maximum of the hottest month is 40°C.

The locality of Aichoun is characterized by the presence of cowsheds, caves, and accumulation of animal waste that creates an environment favorable to the biological cycle of sand flies. The vegetation is characterized by a covering more or less degraded because of overgrazing and overexploitation for domestic uses (*Tetraclinis articulata, Pistacia lentiscus, Olea oleaster, Olea europaea,* and *Juniperus phoenicea*).

2.2. Sand Fly Collection and Identification. Sand flies were collected bimonthly during their optimum development period in Morocco, between May and October. Five collecting sites were chosen in Aichoun locality. Collections were performed by using sticky papers (21 × 27,3 cm) coated with castor oil. We used 40 traps in each trapping campaign. The traps were installed in different habitats during the day and were removed the next day. Collected sand flies were transferred in glass tubes containing a solution of ethanol at 70°. After sex determination, all sand flies collected were identified by examining the morphology of the pharyngeal armature and spermathecae of female flies and the external genitalia of males using the morphological key [12, 13]. Morphological differentiation of the two sympatric species *Ph. longicuspis* and *Ph. perniciosus* was made according to description of Berchi et al. [14].

3. Results

3.1. Taxonomic Inventory of Sand Flies. This study has established a faunal inventory of Aichoun revealing the presence of four species belonging to the genus *Phlebotomus*. The sex ratio indicated that more males were collected; the male/female ratio was 7.54.

The collections accounted for 1171 sand fly specimens. *Ph. sergenti* was the predominant and the most frequently collected species with 918 individuals (78.4%). In second place comes *Ph. perniciosus* Newstead with 123 (10.50%) followed by *Ph. papatasi* Scopoli with 93 individuals (7.94%). *Ph. longicuspis* Nitzulescu was represented by 3.16% (Table 1).

3.2. Seasonal Fluctuations of Sand Flies Species. Seasonal activity of sand flies extended from May to the end of October, with variation in the monthly evolution according to species. *Ph. sergenti, Ph. Perniciosus,* and *Ph. papatasi* displayed a bimodal distribution with a first peak in July, where *Ph. sergenti* dominates (29.46%), and a second peak in September with 13.83%, while *Ph. longicuspis* showed a monophasic trend with a slight peak in August (1.11%) (Figure 1).

4. Discussion

Over the last years, incidence of *L. tropica* CL has continuously increased in the province of Sefrou [15]. Between 1997 and 2011, 1242 cases were declared [16]. The majority of cases were reported mainly in El Menzel, Sefrou, Aghbalou, Tazouta, Sidi Lahcen, and Ain Chegag communes [17].

Ph. sergenti is confirmed as vector of *L. tropica* in northern Africa, Middle East, and Central Asia [18, 19], the same in Morocco [4]. It dominates in arid and semiarid areas [20]. In this study area, *Ph. sergenti* was largely widespread; it was present throughout the whole period of our surveys, showing a biphasic course evolution with two peaks in July and September, respectively. Its activity period was investigated in Taza, a semiarid area in northern Morocco, where it was collected from June to November showing two density

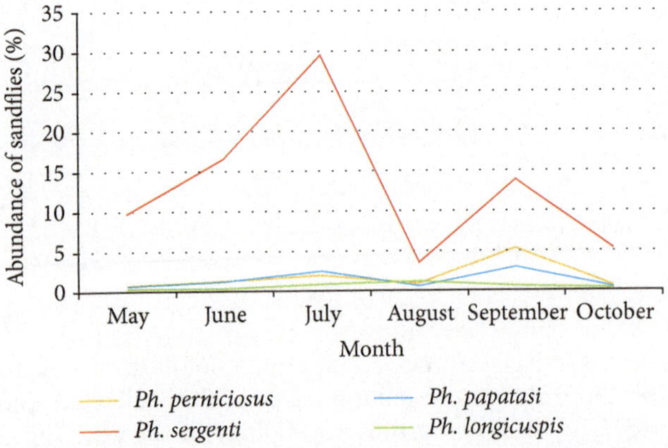

Figure 1: Seasonal variation of sand flies collected in Aichoun by sticky paper traps.

peaks [21]. *Ph. sergenti* was the dominant species compared to other species, which confirms the results obtained in 2011 [22] and with a maximum activity in July confirming the results obtained in Marrakech province [23].

Ph. perniciosus, one of the most competent *L. infantum* vectors in the Mediterranean foci [24], was present during all the period of our study. This species showed a biphasic activity and dominating in September (5.29%). This is in line with the results obtained by Guernaoui et al. [25] in the province of Chichaoua, southwest of Morocco.

Ph. papatasi was also present in our study even if it is considered to be adapted to arid climate [26]; *Ph. papatasi* populations were present from May to October with two peaks. These results are in accordance with the data obtained in Marrakech area in southwestern Morocco [27].

Ph. longicuspis was collected in Aichoun locality. The highest density of this species was observed in August. This result is in accordance with Guernaoui et al. [28] in Chichaoua province where this species showed a monophasic cycle, with one density peak in August-September.

In the region of Fez Boulmane one similar study of the species inventory sand flies in a focus of cutaneous leishmaniasis nominated Ouled aid and belonging to a neighboring province than that Sefrou was realized in 2011 during a year between April 2011 and March 2012 [29, 30]. If we compare our results with those found in this study, we can infer that the same species were encountered but not in the same abundance. Indeed, the most abundant species found were, respectively, *Phlebotomus papatasi* (50.52%), *Phlebotomus sergenti* (24.7%), *Phlebotomus perniciosus* (9.69%), and *Phlebotomus longicuspis* (5.54%) [29].

According Lahouiti et al. [30], the destruction of vectors' habitats, the improvement of human habitats, the treatment of scraps, animal drop-pings, dung, and the separation between animal and human dwellings could be an efficient way to get rid of sand flies and consequently diminish the risks of contamination.

In addition to means mentioned above, we must remember that the companions of information-education-communication and the process of integrated management of vector control piloted together by the health services are very efficient tools to prevent cases of leishmaniasis.

Also, these means will be very efficient not only to fight the mosquito sand fly vector of such diseases but also to combat the parasite tanks such as rats and stray dogs who are increasingly responsible for many emerging zoonoses [31, 32].

5. Conclusion

This study, conducted in Aichoun locality during the months of April to October 2012, was aimed at studying the spatial and temporal trends of the main vectors of *Leishmania* in sand flies in this focus. 1171 sand flies, belonging to the four species, were collected by sticky traps. *Phlebotomus sergenti* was the predominant species (78.4%) followed by *Ph. perniciosus* (10.5%), *Ph. papatasi* (7.94%), and *Ph. longicuspis* (3.16%). Sand flies were active during 6 months (May–October).

The large distribution and the long activity period of *Ph. sergenti* and species of the subgenus *Larroussius* in Aichoun locality indicate the high potential risk of *L. tropica* and *L. infantum* transmission in this area.

Conflict of Interests

The authors declare that they have no conflict of interests.

Acknowledgments

The authors thank Mr. El Kohli Mohamed, M. Adlaoui El Bachir, Lakraa Lhoussine, El Rhazi Mohamed, and Ouahabi Souad Laboratory Medical Entomology, for the constant support made during this study. Likewise, the authors thank the regional direction of the Fes-Boulemane Health, provincial delegate of Ministry of Health, Sefrou province, and staff of Aichoun locality for their cooperation, assistance, information, and help.

References

[1] J. A. Rioux, F. Petter, O. Akalay et al., "*Meriones shawi* (Duvernoy, 1842) (Rodentia, Gerbillidae), reservoir of *Leishmania major*, Yakimoff and Schokhor, 1914 in South Morocco," *Rendered Accounts of Meetings of the Academy of Sciences, Series III: Life Sciences*, vol. 294, pp. 515–517, 1982.

[2] E. Guilvard, J. A. Rioux, M. Gallego et al., "*Leishmania tropica* in Morocco. III—the vector of *Phlebotomus sergenti*. Apropos of 89 isolates," *Annales de Parasitologie Humaine et Comparee*, vol. 66, no. 3, pp. 96–99, 1991.

[3] P. Marty, Y. Le Fichoux, F. Pratlong, J. A. Rioux, G. Rostain, and J. P. Lacour, "Cutaneous leishmaniasis due to *Leishmania tropica* in a young Moroccan child observed in Nice, France," *Transactions of the Royal Society of Tropical Medicine & Hygiene*, vol. 83, no. 4, p. 510, 1989.

[4] F. Pratlong, J. A. Rioux, J. Dereure et al., "*Leishmania tropica* in Morocco. IV—Intrafocal enzyme diversity," *Annales de Parasitologie Humaine et Comparee*, vol. 66, no. 3, pp. 100–104, 1991.

[5] N. Guessous-Idrissi, A. Hamdani, A. Rhalem et al., "Epidemiology of human visceral leishmaniasis in Taounate, a northern province of Morocco," *Parasite*, vol. 4, no. 2, pp. 181–185, 1997.

[6] J. A. Rioux, J. Mahjoub, M. Gallego et al., "Leishmaniose cutanée humaine à *Leishmania infantum* Mon-24 au Maroc," *Bulletin de la Societe Francaise de Parasitologie*, vol. 14, pp. 179–183, 1996.

[7] R. Nejjar, M. Lemrani, A. Malki, S. Ibrahimy, H. Amarouch, and A. Benslimane, "Canine leishmaniasis due to *Leishmania infantum* MON-1 in northern Morocco," *Parasite*, vol. 5, no. 4, pp. 325–330, 1998.

[8] DELM 2011, Department of Planning and Financial Resources, Directorate of Planning and Research Services Research and Health Information, Health Digit Edit, 2012.

[9] DELM 2012, Department of Planning and Financial Resources, Directorate of Planning and Research Services Research and Health Information, Health Digit Edit, 2013.

[10] H. Fellah, M. Rhajaoui, S. Ouahabi, D. Belghiti, and M. Lyagoubi, "Occurrence of human cutaneous leishmaniasis in Zouagha My Yacoub province (Morocco)," *International Journal of Agriculture and Biology*, vol. 9, no. 1, pp. 197–198, 2007.

[11] M. Rhajaoui, "Human leishmaniases in Morocco: a nosogeographical diversity," *Pathologie Biologie*, vol. 59, no. 4, pp. 226–229, 2011.

[12] D. J. Lewis, "The phlebotomine sandflies (Diptera: Psychodidae) of the Oriental Region," *Bulletin of the British Museum (Natural History) (Entomology)*, vol. 37, pp. 217–343, 1978.

[13] Ministry of Health (MS), *Fight against Leishmaniasis, Activity Guide*, Ministry of Health (MS), Rabat, Morocco, 2010.

[14] S. Berchi, A. Bounamous, K. Louadi, and B. Pesson, "Morphological distinction between two sympatric species: *Phlebotomus pernlciosus* and *Phlebotomus longicuspis* (Diptera: Psychodidae)," *Annales de la Societe Entomologique de France*, vol. 43, no. 2, pp. 201–203, 2007.

[15] DELM and Directorate of Epidemiology and Disease Control, "Eco epidemiology of leishmaniasis in Morocco," *Epidemiological Bulletin*, no. 65–68, pp. 1–15, 2006.

[16] Moroccan Ministry of Health, *Etat d'Avancement des Programmes de Lutte Contre les Maladies Parasitaires*, Direction de l'Épidémiologie et de Lutte Contre les Maladies, Rabat, Morocco, 2011.

[17] H. Asmae, A. Fatima, F. Hajiba et al., "Coexistence of *Leishmania tropica* and *Leishmania infantum* in Sefrou province, Morocco," *Acta Tropica*, vol. 130, no. 1, pp. 94–99, 2014.

[18] M. A. Al-Zahrani, W. Peters, D. A. Evans, C. Chin, V. Smith, and R. P. Lane, "*Phlebotomus sergenti*, a vector of *Leishmania tropica* in Saudi Arabia," *Transactions of the Royal Society of Tropical Medicine and Hygiene*, vol. 82, no. 3, article 416, 1988.

[19] A. Tabbabi, N. Bousslimi, A. Rhim, K. Aoun, and A. Bouratbine, "First report on natural infection of *Phlebotomus sergenti* with *Leishmania* promastigotes in the cutaneous leishmaniasis focus in southeastern Tunisia," *The American Journal of Tropical Medicine and Hygiene*, vol. 85, no. 4, pp. 646–647, 2011.

[20] J. A. Rioux, "Eco-epidemiology of leishmaniasis in Morocco: review of 30 years of cooperation. D.E.L.M," *Epidemiological Bulletin*, vol. 37, pp. 2–10, 1999.

[21] N. Guessous-Idrissi, S. Chiheb, A. Hamdani et al., "Cutaneous leishmaniasis: an emerging epidemic focus of *Leishmania tropica* in north Morocco," *Transactions of the Royal Society of Tropical Medicine and Hygiene*, vol. 91, no. 6, pp. 660–663, 1997.

[22] C. Faraj, A. El Bachir, S. Ouahabi et al., "Distribution and bionomic of sand flies in five ecologically different cutaneous Leishmaniasis foci in Morocco," *ISRN Epidemiology*, vol. 2012, Article ID 145031, 8 pages, 2012.

[23] S. Boussaa, S. Guernaoui, and A. Boumezzough, "Periodicity pf phlebotomine sand flies (h) in an urban area of Marrakech, Morocco," in *Proceedings of the European Multicolloquium of Parasitology*, pp. 18–23, 2004.

[24] R. Benikhlef, Z. Harrat, M. Toudjine, A. Djerbouh, S. Bendali-Braham, and M. Belkaid, "Detection of Leishmania infantum MON-24 in the dog," *Medecine Tropicale: Revue du Corps de Santé Colonial*, vol. 64, no. 4, pp. 381–383, 2004.

[25] S. Guernaoui, A. Boumezzough, and A. Laamrani, "Altitudinal structuring of sand flies (Diptera: Psychodidae) in the High-Atlas mountains (Morocco) and its relation to the risk of leishmaniasis transmission," *Acta Tropica*, vol. 97, no. 3, pp. 346–351, 2006.

[26] J. A. Rioux, O. Akalay, J. Périères et al., "The ecoepidemiological evolution of risk leishmanien Moroccan Atlantic Sahara. Heuristic interest bioclimates sandflies relationship," *Mediterranean School*, vol. 23, pp. 73–92, 1997.

[27] S. Boussaa, S. Guernaoui, B. Pesson, and A. Boumezzough, "Seasonal fluctuations of phlebotomine sand fly populations (Diptera: Psychodidae) in the urban area of Marrakech, Morocco," *Acta Tropica*, vol. 95, no. 2, pp. 86–91, 2005.

[28] S. Guernaoui, A. Boumezzough, B. Pesson, and G. Pichon, "Entomological investigations in Chichaoua: an emerging epidemic focus of cutaneous leishmaniasis in Morocco," *Journal of Medical Entomology*, vol. 42, no. 4, pp. 697–701, 2005.

[29] K. Lahouiti, A. El Ouali Lalami, H. Hmamouch, and K. Bakht, "Phototropism of sand flies species (Diptera: Psychodidae) collected in a rural locality in Central Morocco," *Journal of Parasitology and Vector Biology*, vol. 6, no. 5, pp. 66–74, 2014.

[30] K. Lahouiti, A. El Ouali Lalami, S. Maniar, and K. Bekhti, "Seasonal fluctuations of phlebotomines sand fly populations (Diptera: Psychodidae) in the Moulay Yacoub province, centre Morocco: effect of ecological factors," *African Journal of Environmental Science and Technology*, vol. 7, no. 11, pp. 1028–1036, 2013.

[31] K. T. Wong and K. C. Ong, "Pathology of acute henipavirus infection in humans and animals," *Pathology Research International*, vol. 2011, Article ID 567248, 12 pages, 2011.

[32] H. I. Al-Sadi and S. S. Al-Mahmood, "Pathology of experimental *Encephalitozoon cuniculi* infection in immunocompetent and immunosuppressed mice in Iraq," *Pathology Research International*, vol. 2014, Article ID 857036, 6 pages, 2014.

27

The Regulation of Inflammatory Pathways and Infectious Disease of the Cervix by Seminal Fluid

Anthonio Adefuye, Arieh Anthony Katz, and Kurt Jason Sales

MRC/UCT Receptor Biology Research Unit, Institute of Infectious Disease and Molecular Medicine and Division of Medical Biochemistry, Faculty of Health Sciences, University of Cape Town, Room No. 2.02 Wernher and Beit North, Observatory 7925, South Africa

Correspondence should be addressed to Kurt Jason Sales; kurtjsales@gmail.com

Academic Editor: Runjan Chetty

The connection between human papillomavirus (HPV) infection and the consequent sequelae which establishes cervical neoplastic transformation and invasive cervical cancer has redefined many aspects of cervical cancer research. However there is still much that we do not know. In particular, the impact of external factors, like seminal fluid in sexually active women, on pathways that regulate cervical inflammation and tumorigenesis, have yet to be fully understood. HPV infection is regarded as the initiating noninflammatory cause of the disease; however emerging evidence points to resident HPV infections as drivers of inflammatory pathways that play important roles in tumorigenesis as well as in the susceptibility to other infections such as human immunodeficiency virus (HIV) infection. Moreover there is emerging evidence to support a role for seminal fluid, in particular, the inflammatory bioactive lipids, and prostaglandins which are present in vast quantities in seminal fluid in regulating pathways that can exacerbate inflammation of the cervix, speed up tumorigenesis, and enhance susceptibility to HIV infection. This review will highlight some of our current knowledge of the role of seminal fluid as a potent driver of inflammatory and tumorigenic pathways in the cervix and will provide some evidence to propose a role for seminal plasma prostaglandins in HIV infection and AIDS-related cancer.

1. Introduction

Cervical cancer is a malignant neoplasm arising from the cervical squamous or columnar and glandular epithelial cells that line the cervix-uteri in women. Neoplastic transformation of these cells is initiated by infection of the cervical epithelium with high risk oncogenic types of human papillomavirus (HPV) and is largely regarded as an infectious disease [1, 2]. Around 180 different types of HPV have been described to date [3]. Of these, around 40 types are known to infect the anogenital tract, giving rise to genital warts, condylomata or cancers, and their precursor lesions [4]. The primary route for genital infection is via exposure of the mucosa (vaginal, oral, or anal) to HPV present in bodily fluids (mainly seminal fluid, but can also be passed on by saliva) or via skin to skin contact and transmission during sexual intercourse [4].

HPV infects the basal keratinocyte [4]. After infection the cell divides and the life cycle of the virus closely follows that of the keratinocyte as it differentiates and matures. Early viral genes, such as the E6 and E7 oncogene, are expressed in the undifferentiated basal and parabasal layers, whilst expression of the late genes and viral DNA replication occurs in the upper more differentiated granular or cornified layers of the epithelium [4, 5]. The virus is a molecular "hitchhiker" completely lacking any ability to facilitate its own replication and hence is solely reliant on the cellular machinery of its host for propagation. As the cell differentiates, the viral capsid forms and the resultant virion can be released at the cell surface to infect other host cells [4–6] or to be passed on during sexual intercourse to infect another individual. During the initial phase of infection, the HPV E6 and E7 oncogenes are transcribed and translated and it is the E6 and E7 oncoproteins that do most of the cancer-transformation of the infected cell. Recent studies have now shown that HPV mediated transformation occurs by chromosomal alterations, due in part to the actions of the HPV E6 and E7 oncogene, which induce epigenetic changes and changes in miRNA expression to facilitate cellular immortality and neoplastic transformation [7–11].

HPV infections are nonlytic and as such, the host does not mount an inflammatory response at the onset of infection. However, it is emerging that resident HPV oncogenes can regulate cellular effectors, including miRNAs and genes involved in tissue remodeling events in neoplastic cervical epithelial cells, which are critical regulators of the inflammatory processes in cancerous tissue [12, 13].

Emerging evidence points to a role for resident HPV oncogenes in driving tumor-associated inflammation in immortalized cells by inducing the inflammatory cyclooxygenase- (COX-) prostaglandin (PG) axis and elevating cytokine networks [14–16]. Two isoforms of cyclooxygenase enzymes have been described in humans, namely, COX-1 and COX-2, which catalyze the rate limiting conversion of arachidonic acid, derived by de-esterification of plasma membrane phospholipids or dietary polyunsaturated fatty acids, to eicosanoids (prostaglandins, thromboxanes, and prostacyclins) [17]. Many chronic inflammatory diseases and cancers are all associated with upregulation in COX enzyme expression and aberrant biosynthesis of proinflammatory eicosanoids [18, 19]. Elevated signaling of prostaglandins has been observed in uterine-cervical cancers and is considered a key modulator of tumor progression [19–22].

Prostaglandins mediate their effects via coupling to specific prostanoid G protein-coupled receptors (GPCRs) [23]. In the past two decades, many studies have highlighted that prostaglandins, produced as a consequence of elevated COX enzyme expression, can act via these prostanoid GPCRs to promote extensive tissue remodeling within tumours by evoking all the classical hallmarks of cancer, namely, cellular proliferation, angiogenesis, inhibition of apoptosis, and alteration in vascular permeability, to allow immune cell extravasation from the vasculature and inflammation [19, 24]. These hallmarks of cancer in cervical cancer cells have now all been shown to be driven by HPV oncogenes via the induction of potent proinflammatory pathways—in particular, by inducing expression of the immediate early oncogene COX-2 and expression of the E-series prostaglandin receptors (PTGER) such as PTGER2 and PTGER4 [14–16]. In addition to the regulation of tumorigenic pathways by endogenous prostaglandins, produced in cervical cells after HPV infection and neoplastic transformation, the cervix (and vagina) can also be regulated by seminal fluid and in particular seminal plasma prostaglandins, like PGE_2 [25–27].

2. The Role of Seminal Fluid in Regulating Cervical Inflammation and Tumorigenesis

The male ejaculate is a complex organic fluid comprising of secretions of multiple bioactive molecules derived from the Cowper's and Littre's glands (5%), prostate (15–30%), and the seminal vesicles (65–70%) [28]. Secretions from each of these reproductive organs are biochemically distinct and on mixing, as occurs at ejaculation, give rise to the complex biochemical nature of the seminal plasma (SP; also called seminal fluid), the main constituent of the ejaculate. The spermatozoa during ejaculation are bathed in this fluid, which has conventionally been viewed as a nutritive, protective, and transport medium for the mammalian spermatozoa [29]. Semen deposition into the female reproductive tract results in modulated immunity and introduction of an inflammatory response in the mucosa, which promotes conditions for favorable conception and pregnancy [29, 30]. In rodents and humans, studies have shown that SP contains signaling molecules which can bind to cognate epithelial receptors in the female reproductive tract to trigger inflammatory gene expression, modifications in cellular structure, and tissue remodeling events in a sequence that closely resembles an inflammatory response [29].

In mammals, the most striking physiological effects of this inflammatory response can be observed after insemination, where a prompt and dramatic influx of inflammatory cells can be observed to infiltrate the site of semen deposition [29]. These cellular changes have been studied in detail in rodents, where a surge in inflammatory cytokines and chemokines can be seen in cervical and uterine epithelial cells after administration of seminal plasma [31–33]. These proinflammatory mediators stimulate the extravasation and infiltration of cervical subepithelial stroma by immune cells. Similarly, in humans coitus elicits immune cell (neutrophils, macrophages, dendritic cells, and lymphocytes) recruitment into the superficial epithelial and deep stroma tissues of the female reproductive tract [34].

In sexually active women, the degree at which SP normally activates the secretion of these proinflammatory components in any compartment of the female reproductive tract is poorly understood. However, exposure of the cervix to seminal plasma during coitus has been shown to elicit substantial changes in the leukocyte populations within the cervix, initiating a reaction reminiscent of the inflammatory response with effects that penetrate through the stratified epithelial layer and deep into the stroma of the ectocervix [35]. The role of seminal plasma in these studies in mediating leukocyte influx in the cervix was confirmed in control subjects where an absence of inflammatory response was seen with condom-protected coitus or in women abstaining from coitus [35].

Seminal plasma is thought to control the influx of immune cells and expand inducible regulatory T cell population to produce immune tolerance for conception [35–37] via the activation of proinflammatory cytokine/chemokine networks [38]. Under pathological conditions or in women with neoplastic cervical lesions—post-HPV infection—the inflammatory response initiated by SP could be exaggerated and could drive pathways which regulate tumorigenesis. Indeed, *in vitro* studies have shown that SP induces the expression of inflammatory COX-1 and COX-2, interleukin (IL)-6, IL-11, and chemokines CXCL1 and CXCL8 in cervical adenocarcinoma cells [26, 39] *in vitro* and in animal models *in vivo* to regulate blood vessel recruitment and angiogenesis

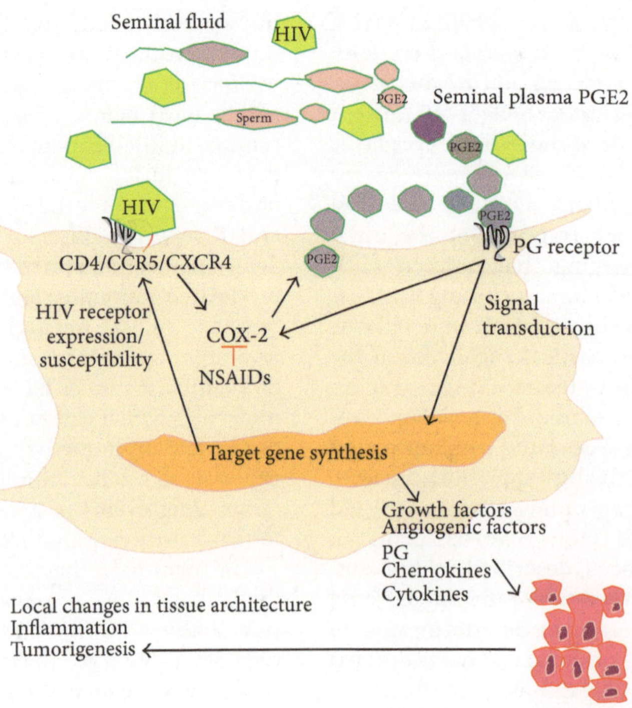

FIGURE 1: A cartoon highlighting the role of seminal plasma and seminal plasma prostaglandins (PG) such as PGE_2 in regulating inflammatory and tumorigenic pathways in cervical cancer cells. Seminal plasma PGE_2, or PGE_2 endogenously produced by COX enzymes in response to inflammation or HIV infection via the induction of COX-2, binds to PG receptors on the surface of the cell to activate intracellular signal transduction pathways and target gene transcription and biosynthesis. Target genes which are known to be regulated in this manner include HIV chemokine receptors like CXCR4 as well as growth factors, angiogenic factors, chemokines, and cytokines. These latter factors all act in an autocrine/paracrine manner in the tumour microenvironment to facilitate local changes in tissue architecture, inflammation and enhance tumorigenesis. Elevated expression of HIV receptors could enhance virus entry into cells and enhance susceptibility to infection. HIV is also known to enhance inflammation by inducing COX-2 expression. The activity of COX-2 and subsequent inflammation can be inhibited by nonsteroidal anti-inflammatory drugs (NSAIDs). The activity of specific PG receptors can also be inhibited with selective receptor antagonists to inhibit subsequent activation of signal transduction pathways.

(Figure 1) [26, 39]. The induced expression of these effector molecules in neoplastic cervical epithelial cells by direct stimulation with seminal plasma suggests that repeated exposure of the cervix to seminal fluid in the absence of barrier contraception could exacerbate tumour-associated inflammation and could enhance disease progression (Figure 1).

In addition to direct exposure of the epithelial layer surrounding the anterior and posterior vaginal fornix, ecto- and endocervix to seminal fluid during intercourse, direct absorption of components of seminal plasma can enter into the endometrial or peritoneal bed. The intravaginal absorption of male hormones has been described [40], and vaginal absorption of molecules is widely regarded as a potential means of drug delivery in women. Absorption may occur as a result of hematogenous dissemination or direct tissue perfusion through the anterior or posterior vaginal fornix [41]. Although it is likely that the concentrations of inflammatory mediators in SP in the recipient woman after intercourse would be orders of magnitude lower than that found in semen, concentrations of inflammatory mediators would nevertheless be greater in sexually active women and could impact *in situ* on inflammation and tumour growth. Indeed, prostaglandins, especially PGE_2, are present in seminal plasma in orders of magnitude greater than at the site of infection or endogenously regulated inflammation [42]. PGE_2 has recently been described as the main constituent of seminal fluid responsible for regulating inflammatory gene expression in vaginal epithelial cells [27]. Since expression of the PGE_2 receptors is elevated in cervical cancers [21, 22], it is likely that seminal plasma (and in particular the PGE_2 present in seminal plasma) can regulate inflammatory and tumorigenic pathways directly via paracrine interactions with their cognate GPCRs in the cervix to regulate many of the hallmarks of tumorigenesis, including angiogenesis (Figure 1) [43, 44], cellular proliferation, and immune cell regulation.

3. The Role of Seminal Plasma in Regulating HIV Infection and Its Potential Contribution to AIDS-Related Cervical Cancer

The origins of human immunodeficiency virus (HIV) are thought to predate the first half of the 20th century, where zoonotic transmission of simian immunodeficiency virus (SIV), found in chimpanzees, occurred, giving rise to HIV, as we know it today [45]. To date, HIV has infected more than 60 million people and caused more than 25 million deaths [46].

Current data estimate that approximately 35 million people currently live with HIV worldwide [46]. In 2012 alone there were around 2.3 million new infections and 1.6 million deaths due to HIV/AIDS worldwide [46]. These figures highlight that 30 years on, after the first reported cases of HIV/AIDS, HIV still remains a major global health pandemic and one of the leading causes of death and disease in women of reproductive age [47]. Morbidity is driven by depletion of the immune system. HIV attacks the immune system by targeting $CD4^+$ cells and increases the risk of acquiring opportunistic infections. In 1993, cervical cancer was classified as an AIDS-defining disease in women infected with HIV [48], highlighting HIV as an important risk factor/cofactor in the development of invasive cervical cancer.

It has been well documented that unprotected sexual intercourse is the major route of HIV infection with infected seminal plasma being the major transmission vector [49–51]. After deposition of semen into the female genital tract, dramatic tissue remodeling events occur [29, 52, 53]. Although these events are thought to promote fertilization and pregnancy, the alterations to the local cellular environment could also enhance HIV susceptibility. Some of the alterations in the local environment which could impact on HIV susceptibility include immune cell recruitment and activation; alterations in epithelial integrity; alterations in the mucous barrier in the genital tract; alterations in the levels of naturally occurring flora and antimicrobials in the genital tract; and alterations in the balance of inflammatory/anti-inflammatory mediators in the genital mucosa [54].

Once HIV has been deposited within the genital tract, infectious virus must cross the mucosal epithelium to interact with macrophages, $CD4^+$ T lymphocytes, and dendritic cells (DCs). Transmission occurs via transcytosis of virions through the genital epithelium [50, 55] or through exposed genital lesions in the mucosa [56–58] or microabrasions in the vagina [59].

HIV infects cells via receptors on the host cell surface. Initially, the virus attaches to the surface of the host cells. This can occur via heparin sulphate proteoglycans [60]. The initial step in membrane fusion begins with binding of the viral envelope protein (Env, consisting of a trimer of gp120-gp41 heterodimers) to the CD4 cell surface protein and a chemokine coreceptor present on the host cell [61]. Most HIV-1 variants use CCR5 and CXCR4 as the main coreceptor *in vivo*; however up to 12 other chemokine coreceptors for HIV infection have been identified *in vitro* [62, 63].

The cervicovaginal epithelium displays heterogeneous tissue architecture, comprising a multilayered stratified squamous epithelium at the vaginal-ectocervical interface, whilst the endocervix is lined with a single layered columnar epithelium. The epithelial surface expresses all the receptors necessary for HIV infection including CD4, CCR5, CXCR4 [64, 65], and various other G protein-coupled coreceptors (GPCRs) known to mediate entry of HIV into cells (including CCR2b, CXCR6, and GPR1) [63, 66], indicating a vast area of the female genital tract that can potentially be infected. Furthermore the transformation zone (the interface between the squamous ectocervix and columnar endocervical canal) is thought to be particularly susceptible to HIV infection as it has an enhanced population of $CD4^+$ T cells [55, 67]. Recent studies have highlighted that cervical epithelium can become productively infected and behave as viral reservoirs, which sequester virus and facilitate introduction of virus to leukocytes present in the submucosa [68, 69].

4. The Role of Semen in Modulating HIV Infectivity

Beyond its role as a carrier for delivery of HIV during receptive vaginal or anal intercourse, semen has been suggested to play a more major role in HIV transmission. In addition to local changes in tissue architecture, inflammatory cell recruitment, and secretion of inflammatory mediators in the female genital tract, semen may facilitate or inhibit mucosal HIV infection via multiple mechanisms to impact on susceptibility.

One mechanism by which semen could enhance sexual transmission of HIV was demonstrated by Munch and colleagues in 2007 [70]. To identify natural agents that might play a role in sexual transmission of HIV, Munch and colleagues developed a complex peptide/protein library derived from human seminal plasma which was screened for novel inhibitors and enhancers of HIV infection. They found that naturally occurring fragments of the prostatic acidic phosphatase (PAP) dramatically enhance HIV infection [70]. Functional and structural analyses showed that PAP forms amyloid fibrils, termed semen-derived enhancer of virus infection (SEVI), which markedly increased HIV infection [70]. SEVI capture HIV and promote the attachment and fusion of the virus to the cell surface to increase infection of both R5 and X4 tropic HIV-1 to peripheral blood mononuclear cells (PBMCs), DCs, and macrophages *in vitro*. In an *in vivo* experiment to demonstrate the enhancing effect mediated by SEVI, using hCD4/hCCR5-transgenic rats challenged with HIV-1 or SEVI-treated HIV-1 by tail vein injection, it was discovered that pretreatment of HIV with SEVI resulted in a 5-fold increase in the number of HIV cDNA copies found in the splenocyte extracts from infected rats [70]. The increase in HIV infectivity when treated with SEVI *in vitro* suggests that it might favor sexual transmission of HIV. This, however, has been shown to be highly dependent on the individual semen donor and correlates with the level of SEVI [71].

Another study highlighting a role for semen in enhancing HIV-1 infections has been reported by Bouhlal and colleagues (2002) [72]. These authors showed that opsonization of HIV-1 by semen complement fragments enhances infection in human epithelial cells. In this study, it was demonstrated that both R5- and X4-tropic viruses could infect epithelial cells and that infection of cells was enhanced 2-fold when virus was added to semen prior to incubation with the epithelial cells and that this effect was complement dependent [72]. There is also evidence that semen can raise the pH of the vaginal fluid from a normally acidic pH to a neutral pH 7. This natural buffering capacity of semen might further enhance HIV stability and create an environment conducive to infection [73, 74]. Other proposed mechanisms of semen-mediated HIV transmission include the role of spermatozoa in efficient transmission of HIV to dendritic cells [75], semen-mediated inflammation [76], semen-mediated immunomodulation, and suppression of both innate and adaptive immune response against HIV [77], and more recently semen lactoferrin has been shown to promote expression of CCL20 in epithelial cells to potentially enhance HIV transmission [78].

Although semen has been shown to be permissive to infection of certain cell types there is also evidence that certain constituents of seminal plasma can impede HIV infectivity. For example, mucin-6 can prevent the capture of HIV-1 by dendritic cells (DC) such as DC-SIGN (DC-specific-intracellular-adhesion-molecule-3-grabbing-nonintegrin) [79, 80]. Productive infection of certain DC *in vivo* is still a matter of debate; however, they are important for early HIV pathogenesis and transfer of virus to $CD4^+$ T cells [81, 82]. In addition cationic polypeptides [83] contained in seminal plasma and reactive oxygen species produced by leukocytes and spermatozoa are known to provide antiviral activity against HIV [84]. More research is needed to elucidate the collective effects of all these effectors in semen in modulating the cervico-vaginal environment after intercourse and the impact on HIV susceptibility in women.

5. The Role of Semen in Regulation of Cell Surface Receptors and Signaling

Constituents of seminal plasma, including TGFβ, EGF, prostaglandins, and soluble complement components could directly regulate HIV susceptibility via the interaction with or modulation of expression of cell surface receptors present on mucosal epithelial and immune cells [19, 25, 29, 52, 85]. For example, Bouhlal and colleagues showed that complement activation in seminal fluid generates C3 cleavage and augments HIV-1 infection in epithelial cells via a complement receptor type 3- (CR3-) mediated mechanism [72]. CR3 is expressed on the apical surface of epithelial cells including cells of the ecto- and endocervix, endometrium, and fallopian tube [86]. This suggests that opsonization of HIV with complement is important in the early events surrounding mucosal transmission of HIV [87]. Furthermore as highlighted earlier, the epithelial surface expresses all the receptors necessary for HIV infection including CD4, CCR5, CXCR4 [64, 65], and various other G protein-coupled coreceptors (GPCRs) known to mediate entry of HIV into cells (including CCR2b, CXCR6, and GPR1) [63, 66]. Some of these receptors display cyclical variations during the menstrual cycle indicating that susceptibility of cells could be different in women, depending on the phase of the menstrual cycle [65]. In women with genital tract pathologies, and cervical cancers in particular, expression of chemokine receptors such as CXCR4 and CCR5 is elevated [88, 89]. Chemokine receptors like CXCR4 are known to play a role in lymph node metastasis during advanced-stage disease [89]; however their elevated expression in cervical cancers could potentially be hijacked by HIV for entry. Furthermore, CXCR4 expression can be regulated by HPV oncogenes [90] and prostaglandins (PGE_2) [91] in the female genital tract (Figure 1) and could potentially be enhanced following sexual exposure to semen and seminal plasma PGE_2. Indeed, seminal plasma has been shown to increase CCR5 expression in target lymphocytes [92], and seminal plasma and PGE_2 have been shown to increase CCR5 expression in cervical epithelial cells via induction of the PGE_2 receptor signalling pathway [88], indicating the potential for enhancing the preferential transmission of R5 tropic HIV. These observations suggest that HPV infection, inflammatory mediators, and semen can drive expression of HIV coreceptors on cervical epithelial cells. Elevated HIV receptors, which can themselves be regulated by seminal plasma prostaglandins [88], could then enhance the susceptibility of these women to HIV infection.

As highlighted earlier, cervical cancer is an AIDS-related disease. Recently Fitzgerald and colleagues have demonstrated that HIV infection in women with HPV positive cervical cancers increases COX-2 expression and systemic PGE_2 levels [93]. In cervical cancers, expression of the PGE_2 receptors is elevated in cervical epithelial cells [21]. In the case of women with dual HPV and HIV infection, where PGE_2 receptor expression is elevated together with elevated circulating PGE_2 concentrations, the enhanced ligand-receptor signalling mediated by PGE_2 could potentially exacerbate inflammation and drive tumour progression and morbidity. These data provide some compelling evidence into a possible mechanism whereby HIV infection can increase AIDS-related cervical cancer progression in women with cervical cancer.

6. Conclusions

There is significant evidence that the cervicovaginal microenvironment is modified during sexual intercourse by semen to enhance conception and pregnancy via the remodeling of multiple tissue compartments. Opportunistic infections and HIV present during intercourse can hijack the pathways mediating this response to seminal fluid and can be enhanced by factors present in seminal fluid. As demonstrated schematically in Figure 1, there is further evidence for a role for seminal plasma and seminal plasma prostaglandins, like PGE_2, in regulating inflammation and pathways which regulate tumor progression in cervical cancers. Furthermore, there is evidence that seminal plasma and PGE_2 can increase susceptibility to HIV infection by modulating the local inflammatory response in the cervix and elevating expression of HIV receptors in cervical epithelial cells and lymphocytes. Once infected, HIV can potentially enhance tumorigenesis by increasing systemic PGE_2, which has been shown to promote tumour progression. Nonsteroidal anti-inflammatory drugs (NSAIDs) that inhibit the synthesis of PGE_2, or drugs that inhibit the actions of PGE_2, like specific PGE_2 receptor antagonists, have demonstrated dramatic anti-inflammatory and antineoplastic activity for a variety of cancers [94, 95] by inhibition of the COX-prostaglandin pathway. These compounds may prove useful in reducing inflammation and the progression of AIDS-related cervical cancer in women and may also prevent the semen-induced upregulation in cellular machinery that could enhance HIV infection. More research is needed to determine the potential effectiveness of such interventions in women's health.

Conflict of Interests

The authors declare that there are no conflicts of interests regarding the publication of this paper.

Acknowledgments

Arieh A. Katz and Kurt J. Sales were supported by grant funding to the MRC/UCT Receptor Biology Research Unit by the Medical Research Council of South Africa (MRC). Kurt J. Sales was supported by the following grants: Poliomyelitis Research Foundation of South Africa (PRF), Cancer Association of South Africa (CANSA), National Research Foundation of South Africa (NRF), and University of Cape Town Research Committee (URC). The funders played no role in the design or interpretation of the paper or the decision to publish.

References

[1] H. Zur Hausen, "Immortalization of human cells and their malignant conversion by high risk human papillomavirus genotypes," *Seminars in Cancer Biology*, vol. 9, no. 6, pp. 405–411, 1999.

[2] H. zur Hausen, "Papillomaviruses in the causation of human cancers—a brief historical account," *Virology*, vol. 384, no. 2, pp. 260–265, 2009.

[3] H. Bernard, R. D. Burk, Z. Chen, K. van Doorslaer, H. Z. Hausen, and E. de Villiers, "Classification of papillomaviruses (PVs) based on 189 PV types and proposal of taxonomic amendments," *Virology*, vol. 401, no. 1, pp. 70–79, 2010.

[4] M. A. Stanley, "Human papillomavirus and cervical carcinogenesis," *Best Practice and Research: Clinical Obstetrics and Gynaecology*, vol. 15, no. 5, pp. 663–676, 2001.

[5] M. A. Stanley, "Epithelial cell responses to infection with human papillomavirus," *Clinical Microbiology Reviews*, vol. 25, no. 2, pp. 215–222, 2012.

[6] M. A. Stanley, "Genital human papillomavirus infections: current and prospective therapies," *Journal of General Virology*, vol. 93, no. 4, pp. 681–691, 2012.

[7] R. D. M. Steenbergen, J. De Wilde, S. M. Wilting, A. A. T. P. Brink, P. J. F. Snijders, and C. J. L. M. Meijer, "HPV-mediated transformation of the anogenital tract," *Journal of Clinical Virology*, vol. 32, supplement 1, pp. S25–S33, 2005.

[8] A. Botezatu, C. D. Goia-Rusanu, I. V. Iancu et al., "Quantitative analysis of the relationship between microRNA-124a, -34b and -203 gene methylation and cervical oncogenesis," *Molecular Medicine Reports*, vol. 4, no. 1, pp. 121–128, 2011.

[9] S. M. Wilting, P. J. F. Snijders, W. Verlaat et al., "Altered microRNA expression associated with chromosomal changes contributes to cervical carcinogenesis," *Oncogene*, vol. 32, no. 1, pp. 106–116, 2013.

[10] M. Bierkens, S. M. Wilting, W. N. van Wieringen et al., "Chromosomal profiles of high-grade cervical intraepithelial neoplasia relate to duration of preceding high-risk human papillomavirus infection," *International Journal of Cancer*, vol. 131, no. 4, pp. E579–E585, 2012.

[11] S. M. Wilting, R. A. A. van Boerdonk, F. E. Henken et al., "Methylation-mediated silencing and tumour suppressive function of hsa-miR-124 in cervical cancer," *Molecular Cancer*, vol. 9, article 167, 2010.

[12] B. Kaczkowski, M. Morevati, M. Rossing, F. Cilius, and B. Norrild, "A decade of global mRNA and miRNA profiling of HPV-positive Cell lines and clinical specimens," *The Open Virology Journal*, vol. 6, pp. 216–231, 2012.

[13] B. Kaczkowski, M. Rossing, D. K. Andersen et al., "Integrative analyses reveal novel strategies in HPV11,-16 and -45 early infection," *Scientific Reports*, vol. 2, article 515, 2012.

[14] K. Subbaramaiah and A. J. Dannenberg, "Cyclooxygenase-2 transcription is regulated by human papillomavirus 16 E6 and E7 oncoproteins: evidence of a corepressor/coactivator exchange," *Cancer Research*, vol. 67, no. 8, pp. 3976–3985, 2007.

[15] J. Oh, S. Kim, E. Cho, Y. Song, W. Kim, and Y. Juhnn, "Human papillomavirus type 16 E5 protein inhibits hydrogen peroxide-induced apoptosis by stimulating ubiquitin-proteasome-mediated degradation of Bax in human cervical cancer cells," *Carcinogenesis*, vol. 31, no. 3, pp. 402–410, 2010.

[16] J. Oh, S. Kim, Y. Lee et al., "Human papillomavirus E5 protein induces expression of the EP4 subtype of prostaglandin E2 receptor in cyclic AMP response element-dependent pathways in cervical cancer cells," *Carcinogenesis*, vol. 30, no. 1, pp. 141–149, 2009.

[17] M. T. Rizzo, "Cyclooxygenase-2 in oncogenesis," *Clinica Chimica Acta*, vol. 412, no. 9-10, pp. 671–687, 2011.

[18] M. P. Wymann and R. Schneiter, "Lipid signalling in disease," *Nature Reviews Molecular Cell Biology*, vol. 9, no. 2, pp. 162–176, 2008.

[19] H. N. Jabbour, K. J. Sales, R. D. Catalano, and J. E. Norman, "Inflammatory pathways in female reproductive health and disease," *Reproduction*, vol. 138, no. 6, pp. 903–919, 2009.

[20] H. S. Ryu, K. H. Chang, H. W. Yang, M. S. Kim, H. C. Kwon, and K. Oh, "High cyclooxygenase-2 expression in stage IB cervical cancer with lymph node metastasis or parametrial invasion," *Gynecologic Oncology*, vol. 76, no. 3, pp. 320–325, 2000.

[21] K. J. Sales, A. A. Katz, M. Davis et al., "Cyclooxygenase-2 expression and prostaglandin E2 synthesis are up-regulated in carcinomas of the cervix: a possible autocrine/paracrine regulation of neoplastic cell function via EP2/EP4 receptors," *Journal of Clinical Endocrinology and Metabolism*, vol. 86, no. 5, pp. 2243–2249, 2001.

[22] K. J. Sales, A. A. Katz, B. Howard, R. P. Soeters, R. P. Millar, and H. N. Jabbour, "Cyclooxygenase-1 is up-regulated in cervical carcinomas: autocrine/paracrine regulation of cyclooxygenase-2, prostaglandin E receptors, and angiogenic factors by cyclooxygenase-1," *Cancer Research*, vol. 62, no. 2, pp. 424–432, 2002.

[23] S. Narumiya, Y. Sugimoto, and F. Ushikubi, "Prostanoid receptors: structures, properties, and functions," *Physiological Reviews*, vol. 79, no. 4, pp. 1193–1226, 1999.

[24] H. N. Jabbour and K. J. Sales, "Prostaglandin receptor signalling and function in human endometrial pathology," *Trends in Endocrinology and Metabolism*, vol. 15, no. 8, pp. 398–404, 2004.

[25] K. J. Sales, A. A. Katz, R. P. Millar, and H. N. Jabbour, "Seminal plasma activates cyclooxygenase-2 and prostaglandin E2 receptor expression and signalling in cervical adenocarcinoma cells," *Molecular Human Reproduction*, vol. 8, no. 12, pp. 1065–1070, 2002.

[26] K. J. Sales, J. R. Sutherland, H. N. Jabbour, and A. A. Katz, "Seminal plasma induces angiogenic chemokine expression in cervical cancer cells and regulates vascular function," *Biochimica et Biophysica Acta—Molecular Cell Research*, vol. 1823, no. 10, pp. 1789–1795, 2012.

[27] T. Joseph, I. A. Zalenskaya, L. C. Sawyer, N. Chandra, and G. F. Doncel, "Seminal plasma induces prostaglandin-endoperoxide synthase (PTGS) 2 expression in immortalized human vaginal cells: involvement of semen prostaglandin E2 in PTGS2 upregulation," *Biology of Reproduction*, vol. 88, no. 1, article 13, 2013.

[28] D. H. Owen and D. F. Katz, "A review of the physical and chemical properties of human semen and the formulation of a semen simulant," *Journal of Andrology*, vol. 26, no. 4, pp. 459–469, 2005.

[29] S. A. Robertson, "Seminal plasma and male factor signalling in the female reproductive tract," *Cell and Tissue Research*, vol. 322, no. 1, pp. 43–52, 2005.

[30] H. J. Schuberth, U. Taylor, H. Zerbe, D. Waberski, R. Hunter, and D. Rath, "Immunological responses to semen in the female genital tract," *Theriogenology*, vol. 70, no. 8, pp. 1174–1181, 2008.

[31] M. De, R. Choudhuri, and G. W. Wood, "Determination of the number and distribution of macrophages, lymphocytes, and granulocytes in the mouse uterus from mating through implantation," *Journal of Leukocyte Biology*, vol. 50, no. 3, pp. 252–262, 1991.

[32] M. T. McMaster, R. C. Newton, S. K. Dey, and G. K. Andrews, "Activation and distribution of inflammatory cells in the mouse uterus during the preimplantation period," *Journal of Immunology*, vol. 148, no. 6, pp. 1699–1705, 1992.

[33] S. A. Robertson, V. J. Mau, K. P. Tremellen, and R. F. Seamark, "Role of high molecular weight seminal vesicle proteins in eliciting the uterine inflammatory response to semen in mice," *Journal of Reproduction and Fertility*, vol. 107, no. 2, pp. 265–277, 1996.

[34] I. J. Pandya and J. Cohen, "The leukocytic reaction of the human uterine cervix to spermatozoa," *Fertility and Sterility*, vol. 43, no. 3, pp. 417–421, 1985.

[35] D. J. Sharkey, K. P. Tremellen, M. J. Jasper, K. Gemzell-Danielsson, and S. A. Robertson, "Seminal fluid induces leukocyte recruitment and cytokine and chemokine mRNA expression in the human cervix after coitus," *Journal of Immunology*, vol. 188, no. 5, pp. 2445–2454, 2012.

[36] S. A. Robertson, L. R. Guerin, J. J. Bromfield, K. M. Branson, A. C. Ahlström, and A. S. Care, "Seminal fluid drives expansion of the CD4+CD25+ T regulatory cell pool and induces tolerance to paternal alloantigens in mice," *Biology of Reproduction*, vol. 80, no. 5, pp. 1036–1045, 2009.

[37] L. M. Moldenhauer, K. R. Diener, D. M. Thring, M. P. Brown, J. D. Hayball, and S. A. Robertson, "Cross-presentation of male seminal fluid antigens elicits T cell activation to initiate the female immune response to pregnancy," *Journal of Immunology*, vol. 182, no. 12, pp. 8080–8093, 2009.

[38] D. J. Sharkey, A. M. Macpherson, K. P. Tremellen, D. G. Mottershead, R. B. Gilchrist, and S. A. Robertson, "TGF-β mediates proinflammatory seminal fluid signaling in human cervical epithelial cells," *Journal of Immunology*, vol. 189, no. 2, pp. 1024–1035, 2012.

[39] J. R. Sutherland, K. J. Sales, H. N. Jabbour, and A. A. Katz, "Seminal plasma enhances cervical adenocarcinoma cell proliferation and tumour growth in vivo," *PLoS ONE*, vol. 7, no. 3, Article ID e33848, 2012.

[40] P. G. Ney, "The intravaginal absorption of male generated hormones and their possible effect on female behaviour," *Medical Hypotheses*, vol. 20, no. 2, pp. 221–231, 1986.

[41] L. Klemmt and A. R. Scialli, "The transport of chemicals in semen," *Birth Defects Research B—Developmental and Reproductive Toxicology*, vol. 74, no. 2, pp. 119–131, 2005.

[42] R. W. Kelly, "Immunosuppressive mechanisms in semen: implications for contraception," *Human Reproduction*, vol. 10, no. 7, pp. 1686–1693, 1995.

[43] S. Battersby, K. J. Sales, A. R. Williams, R. A. Anderson, S. Gardner, and H. N. Jabbour, "Seminal plasma and prostaglandin E2 up-regulate fibroblast growth factor 2 expression in endometrial adenocarcinoma cells via E-series prostanoid-2 receptor-mediated transactivation of the epidermal growth factor receptor and extracellular signal-regulated kinase pathway," *Human Reproduction*, vol. 22, no. 1, pp. 36–44, 2007.

[44] M. Muller, K. J. Sales, A. A. Katz, and H. N. Jabbour, "Seminal plasma promotes the expression of tumorigenic and angiogenic genes in cervical adenocarcinoma cells via the E-series prostanoid 4 receptor," *Endocrinology*, vol. 147, no. 7, pp. 3356–3365, 2006.

[45] B. Korber, M. Muldoon, J. Theiler et al., "Timing the ancestor of the HIV-1 pandemic strains," *Science*, vol. 288, no. 5472, pp. 1789–1796, 2000.

[46] UNAIDS, UNAIDS Report on Global AIDS epidemic. Geneva, UNAIDS, 2013, http://www.unaids.org/en/Dataanalysis/Epidemiology/.

[47] *WHO Women's Health Fact Sheet No. 334*, WHO, Geneva, Switzerland, 2013.

[48] A. M. Levine, "AIDS-related malignancies: the emerging epidemic," *Journal of the National Cancer Institute*, vol. 85, no. 17, pp. 1382–1397, 1993.

[49] C. J. Miller and R. J. Shattock, "Target cells in vaginal HIV transmission," *Microbes and Infection*, vol. 5, no. 1, pp. 59–67, 2003.

[50] K. Gupta and P. J. Klasse, "How do viral and host factors modulate the sexual transmission of HIV? Can transmission be blocked?" *PLoS Medicine*, vol. 3, no. 2, article 79, 2006.

[51] A. T. Haase, "Targeting early infection to prevent HIV-1 mucosal transmission," *Nature*, vol. 464, no. 7286, pp. 217–223, 2010.

[52] S. A. Robertson, "Seminal fluid signaling in the female reproductive tract: lessons from rodents and pigs.," *Journal of Animal Science*, vol. 85, no. 13, pp. E36–E44, 2007.

[53] D. J. Sharkey, A. M. Macpherson, K. P. Tremellen, and S. A. Robertson, "Seminal plasma differentially regulates inflammatory cytokine gene expression in human cervical and vaginal epithelial cells," *Molecular Human Reproduction*, vol. 13, no. 7, pp. 491–501, 2007.

[54] C. L. Rametse, A. J. Olivier, L. Masson, S. Barnabas, and L. R. McKinnon, "Role of semen in altering the balance between inflammation and tolerance in the female genital tract: does it contribute to HIV risk?" *Viral Immunology*, vol. 27, pp. 200–206, 2014.

[55] F. Hladik and M. J. McElrath, "Setting the stage: host invasion by HIV," *Nature Reviews Immunology*, vol. 8, no. 6, pp. 447–457, 2008.

[56] S. R. Galvin and M. S. Cohen, "The role of sexually transmitted diseases in HIV transmission," *Nature Reviews Microbiology*, vol. 2, no. 1, pp. 33–42, 2004.

[57] P. Piot and M. Laga, "Genital ulcers, other sexually transmitted diseases, and the sexual transmission of HIV. The first two may

be important risk factors for the third," *British Medical Journal*, vol. 298, no. 6674, pp. 623–624, 1989.

[58] D. Serwadda, R. H. Gray, N. K. Sewankambo et al., "Human immunodeficiency virus acquisition associated with genital ulcer disease and herpes simplex virus type 2 infection: a nested case-control study in Rakai, Uganda," *Journal of Infectious Diseases*, vol. 188, no. 10, pp. 1492–1497, 2003.

[59] M. K. Norvell, G. I. Benrubi, and R. J. Thompson, "Investigation of microtrauma after sexual intercourse," *Journal of Reproductive Medicine for the Obstetrician and Gynecologist*, vol. 29, no. 4, pp. 269–271, 1984.

[60] I. Mondor, S. Ugolini, and Q. J. Sattentau, "Human immunodeficiency virus type 1 attachment to HeLa CD4 cells is CD4 independent and gp120 dependent and requires cell surface heparans," *Journal of Virology*, vol. 72, no. 5, pp. 3623–3634, 1998.

[61] C. B. Wilen, J. C. Tilton, and R. W. Doms, "Molecular mechanisms of HIV entry," *Advances in Experimental Medicine and Biology*, vol. 726, pp. 223–242, 2012.

[62] B. J. Doranz, Z. H. Lu, J. Rucker et al., "Two distinct CCR5 domains can mediate coreceptor usage by human immunodeficiency virus type 1," *Journal of Virology*, vol. 71, no. 9, pp. 6305–6314, 1997.

[63] N. Shimizu, A. Tanaka, A. Oue et al., "Broad usage spectrum of G protein-coupled receptors as coreceptors by primary isolates of HIV," *AIDS*, vol. 23, no. 7, pp. 761–769, 2009.

[64] G. R. Yeaman, S. Asin, S. Weldon et al., "Chemokine receptor expression in the human ectocervix: Implications for infection by the human immunodeficiency virus-type I," *Immunology*, vol. 113, no. 4, pp. 524–533, 2004.

[65] G. R. Yeaman, A. L. Howell, S. Weldon et al., "Human immunodeficiency virus receptor and coreceptor expression on human uterine epithelial cells: regulation of expression during the menstrual cycle and implications for human immunodeficiency virus infection," *Immunology*, vol. 109, no. 1, pp. 137–146, 2003.

[66] H. Blaak, P. H. M. Boers, R. A. Gruters, H. Schuitemaker, M. E. van der Ende, and A. D. M. E. Osterhaus, "CCR5, GPR15, and CXCR6 are major coreceptors of human immunodeficiency virus type 2 variants isolated from individuals with and without plasma viremia," *Journal of Virology*, vol. 79, no. 3, pp. 1686–1700, 2005.

[67] J. Pudney, A. J. Quayle, and D. J. Anderson, "Immunological microenvironments in the human vagina and cervix: mediators of cellular immunity are concentrated in the cervical transformation zone," *Biology of Reproduction*, vol. 73, no. 6, pp. 1253–1263, 2005.

[68] C. S. Dezzutti, P. C. Guenthner, J. E. Cummins Jr. et al., "Cervical and prostate primary epithelial cells are not productively infected but sequester human immunodeficiency virus type 1," *Journal of Infectious Diseases*, vol. 183, no. 8, pp. 1204–1213, 2001.

[69] D. Maher, X. Wu, T. Schacker, J. Horbul, and P. Southern, "HIV binding, penetration, and primary infection in human cervicovaginal tissue," *Proceedings of the National Academy of Sciences of the United States of America*, vol. 102, no. 32, pp. 11504–11509, 2005.

[70] J. Münch, E. Rücker, L. Ständker et al., "Semen-derived amyloid fibrils drastically enhance HIV infection," *Cell*, vol. 131, no. 6, pp. 1059–1071, 2007.

[71] K. Kim, M. Yolamanova, O. Zirafi et al., "Semen-mediated enhancement of HIV infection is donor-dependent and correlates with the levels of SEVI," *Retrovirology*, vol. 7, article 55, 2010.

[72] H. Bouhlal, N. Chomont, N. Haeffner-Cavaillon, M. D. Kazatchkine, L. Belec, and H. Hocini, "Opsonization of HIV-1 by semen complement enhances infection of human epithelial cells," *Journal of Immunology*, vol. 169, no. 6, pp. 3301–3306, 2002.

[73] C. Tevi-Benissan, L. Belec, M. Levy et al., "In vivo semen-associated pH neutralization of cervicovaginal secretions," *Clinical and Diagnostic Laboratory Immunology*, vol. 4, pp. 367–374, 1997.

[74] J. Ongradi, L. Ceccherini-Nelli, M. Pistello, S. Specter, and M. Bendinelli, "Acid sensitivity of cell-free and cell-associated HIV-1: clinical implications," *AIDS Research and Human Retroviruses*, vol. 6, no. 12, pp. 1433–1436, 1990.

[75] A. Ceballos, F. R. Lenicov, J. Sabatté et al., "Spermatozoa capture HIV-1 through heparan sulfate and efficiently transmit the virus to dendritic cells," *The Journal of Experimental Medicine*, vol. 206, no. 12, pp. 2717–2733, 2009.

[76] S. A. Robertson, S. O'Leary, and D. T. Armstrong, "Influence of semen on inflammatory modulators of embryo implantation," *Society of Reproduction and Fertility supplement*, vol. 62, pp. 231–245, 2006.

[77] R. W. Kelly and H. O. Critchley, "Immunomodulation by human seminal plasma: a benefit for spermatozoon and pathogen?" *Human Reproduction*, vol. 12, no. 10, pp. 2200–2207, 1997.

[78] A. G. Lourenco, M. C. Komesu, A. A. Machado, S. M. Quintana, and T. Bourlet, "Semen lactoferrin promotes CCL20 production by epithelial cells: involvement in HIV transmission," *World Journal of Virology*, vol. 3, pp. 11–17, 2014.

[79] J. Sabatté, A. Ceballos, S. Raiden et al., "Human seminal plasma abrogates the capture and transmission of human immunodeficiency virus type 1 to CD4+ T cells mediated by DC-SIGN," *Journal of Virology*, vol. 81, no. 24, pp. 13723–13734, 2007.

[80] M. J. Stax, T. van Montfort, R. R. Sprenger et al., "Mucin 6 in seminal plasma binds DC-SIGN and potently blocks dendritic cell mediated transfer of HIV-1 to $CD4^+$ T-lymphocytes," *Virology*, vol. 391, no. 2, pp. 203–211, 2009.

[81] R. M. Steinman, A. Granelli-Piperno, M. Pope et al., "The interaction of immunodeficiency viruses with dendritic cells," *Current Topics in Microbiology and Immunology*, vol. 276, pp. 1–30, 2003.

[82] C. Trumpfheller, C. G. Park, J. Finke, R. M. Steinman, and A. Granelli-Piperno, "Cell type-dependent retention and transmission of HIV-1 by DC-SIGN," *International Immunology*, vol. 15, no. 2, pp. 289–298, 2003.

[83] J. A. Martellini, A. L. Cole, N. Venkataraman et al., "Cationic polypeptides contribute to the anti-HIV-1 activity of human seminal plasma," *The FASEB Journal*, vol. 23, no. 10, pp. 3609–3618, 2009.

[84] A. Agarwal and S. A. Prabakaran, "Mechanism, measurement, and prevention of oxidative stress in male reproductive physiology," *Indian Journal of Experimental Biology*, vol. 43, no. 11, pp. 963–974, 2005.

[85] O. A. Vanderpuye, C. A. Labarrere, and J. A. McIntyre, "The complement system in human reproduction," *The American Journal of Reproductive Immunology*, vol. 27, no. 3-4, pp. 145–155, 1992.

[86] J. L. Edwards, E. J. Brown, K. A. Ault, and M. A. Apicella, "The role of complement receptor 3 (CR3) in Neisseria gonorrhoeae infection of human cervical epithelia," *Cellular Microbiology*, vol. 3, no. 9, pp. 611–622, 2001.

[87] H. Stoiber, I. Frank, M. Spruth et al., "Inhibition of HIV-1 infection in vitro by monoclonal antibodies to the complement

receptor type 3 (CR3): an accessory role for CR3 during virus entry?" *Molecular Immunology*, vol. 34, no. 12-13, pp. 855–863, 1997.

[88] K. J. Sales, A. Adefuye, L. Nicholson, and A. A. Kat, "CCR5 expression is elevated in cervical cancer cells and is upregulated by seminal plasma," *Molecular Human Reproduction*, 2014.

[89] J. Kodama, T. Kusumoto, N. Seki et al., "Association of CXCR4 and CCR7 chemokine receptor expression and lymph node metastasis in human cervical cancer," *Annals of Oncology*, vol. 18, no. 1, pp. 70–76, 2007.

[90] A. Amine, S. Rivera, P. Opolon et al., "Novel anti-metastatic action of cidofovir mediated by inhibition of E6/E7, CXCR4 and Rho/ROCK signaling in HPV+ tumor cells," *PLoS ONE*, vol. 4, no. 3, Article ID e5018, 2009.

[91] K. J. Sales, V. Grant, R. D. Catalano, and H. N. Jabbour, "Chorionic gonadotrophin regulates CXCR4 expression in human endometrium via E-series prostanoid receptor 2 signalling to PI3K-ERK1/2: implications for fetal-maternal crosstalk for embryo implantation," *Molecular Human Reproduction*, vol. 17, no. 1, Article ID gaq069, pp. 22–32, 2011.

[92] E. Balandya, S. Sheth, K. Sanders, W. Wieland-Alter, and T. Lahey, "Semen protects CD4+ target cells from HIV infection but promotes the preferential transmission of R5 tropic HIV," *The Journal of Immunology*, vol. 185, no. 12, pp. 7596–7604, 2010.

[93] D. W. Fitzgerald, K. Bezak, O. Ocheretina et al., "The effect of HIV and HPV coinfection on cervical COX-2 expression and systemic prostaglandin E2 levels," *Cancer Prevention Research*, vol. 5, no. 1, pp. 34–40, 2012.

[94] T. Hida, J. Leyton, A. N. Makheja et al., "Non-small cell lung cancer cycloxygenase activity and proliferation are inhibited by non-steroidal antiinflammatory drugs," *Anticancer Research*, vol. 18, no. 2A, pp. 775–782, 1998.

[95] J. Burn, A. Gerdes, F. Macrae et al., "Long-term effect of aspirin on cancer risk in carriers of hereditary colorectal cancer: an analysis from the CAPP2 randomised controlled trial," *The Lancet*, vol. 378, no. 9809, pp. 2081–2087, 2011.

28

The Possible Role of Mast Cells in the Odontogenic Cyst's Pathogenesis: A Comparative Study between Dentigerous Cyst and Keratocystic Odontogenic Tumor

Sareh Farhadi,[1] Fatemeh Shahsavari,[1] and MirMahdi Davardan[2]

[1] *Oral & Maxillofacial Pathology Department, Islamic Azad University, Dental Branch of Tehran, Tehran 16686 49911, Iran*
[2] *Islamic Azad University, Dental Branch of Tehran, Tehran 16686 49911, Iran*

Correspondence should be addressed to Fatemeh Shahsavari; shaahsavari@gmail.com

Academic Editor: Marco Volante

Background. Recently, mast cells were recognized in the pathogenesis of more aggressive pathologic lesions. This study was aimed to evaluate and compare the density of mast cells in Dentigerous cyst (DC) and Keratocystic odontogenic tumor (KCOT) regarding their different clinical behavior. *Method.* This study was conducted on 23 and 26 cases of DC and KCOT, respectively. Four-micron sections were prepared for Toluidine blue staining and mast cell densities in two desired cysts were studied. Final data was analyzed via t-test and Mann-Whitney U test method regarding the significant level lower than 0.05. *Results.* Mast cell densities were significantly higher in KCOTs for deep and superficial layers and both layers ($P < 0.05$). The density of degranulated mast cells in the deeper layers and both layers was significantly higher in KCOTs ($P < 0.05$). However, the density of degranulated mast cells in the superficial layer had no significant difference ($P > 0.05$). *Conclusion.* It seems that mast cells may be involved in the pathogenesis of KCOT, but, regarding wide range of mast cell's biologic activities, further investigations are recommended to confirm the issue and prepare the details.

1. Introduction

Dentigerous cyst is the most common developmental odontogenic cyst with excellent prognosis and low recurrence [1]. Keratocystic odontogenic tumor was described first time by Philipsen in 1956 [2] as an odontogenic cyst. Recently, due to aggressive behavior and tendency to high recurrence of these lesions, the new classification of WHO placed it in the category of the benign odontogenic tumor [3–5] which can invade into cranial, zygomatic, and orbital bone or conflict sinus [6].

Several types of cells are associated with the development of cysts and tumors. Many efforts have been made to understand the pathogenesis of odontogenic cysts, but many of them have been unsuccessful [7]. Several mechanisms have been proposed for the growth and expansion of odontogenic cysts; however, the exact mechanism of enlargement is not known [8]. Recently, among inflammatory cells, mast cells have been considered. First, these cells were described by Paul Ehrlich in 1877 with Mastzellan [9]. These cells are elliptical to circular with a diameter of about 20 to 30 micrometers and are containing basophilic secretory granules of 0.5 to 0.2 micrometers. These secretory cells diffuse around blood vessels, nerves, and lymph throughout the body, but especially in the skin; digestive mucosa and respiratory systems can be seen in abundance [10–12]. Mast cells can have an inhibitory role on the development of pathological lesions. However, stimulatory role of mast cells in the growth of pathological lesions is more prevalent and obvious than their inhibitory effect [13]. It seems that the stimulatory role depends on many factors and conditions.

The mast cell granules contain numerous active components as histamine, tryptase, and kinase with stimulatory or inhibitory effects. Also, some of them, such as heparin, would be able to present both stimulatory and inhibitory agents for microenvironment signalling pathway [14]. On the other hand, the other mediators produced by stromal cells adjacent to mast cells as fibroblasts and endothelial cells may

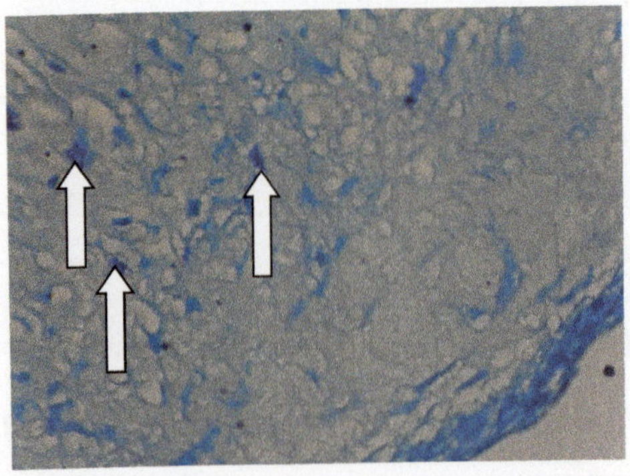

Figure 1: Mast cells (arrow tip) in a deep area of Dentigerous cyst wall stained with Toluidine blue by 400x magnification.

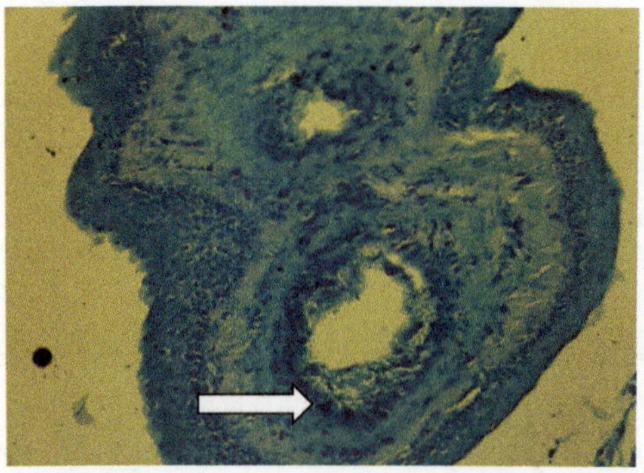

Figure 2: Many mast cells in the wall of Keratocystic odontogenic tumor stained with Toluidine blue by 200x magnification; one of them marks with arrow tip.

potentially influence the pathogenesis of the lesions through a variety of mechanisms such as cyclooxygenase metabolites and heparinizes [14].

Mast cells may be associated with the pathogenesis of cysts too. Previous studies have identified mast cells in odontogenic cysts [8], but there were limited studies about the role of mast cells in the pathogenesis of odontogenic cysts. So, this study was aimed to evaluate and compare the density of mast cells in Dentigerous cysts (DC) and Keratocystic odontogenic tumor (KCOT).

2. Material and Methods

This experimental study evaluates the pathologic records of patients with final diagnosis of Dentigerous cyst and Keratocystic odontogenic tumor from the year 2006 to the year 2014 selected from the archive of Oral Pathology Department, Dental Branch of Tehran, Islamic Azad University, Tehran, Iran. 49 cases include 23 cases of Dentigerous cyst, and 26 cases of Keratocystic odontogenic tumor were chosen after the evaluation of paraffin blocks and related slides. The samples with no sufficient tissue for microscopic evaluation, bleeding, and/or necrosis were excluded from the study.

Four-micron sections from the selected blocks were prepared for Toluidine blue staining to assess and count mast cell. Each slide was examined by two observers by Olympus optical microscope with a magnification of 400 times. For each sample, the granulated mast cells were counted in five view of the deep layer and five view of the superficial layer and also the degranulated mast cells were counted again in five view of the deep layer and five view of the superficial layer. Then, the number of granulated and degranulated mast cells in the total of two layers and also the total number of mast cells in both layers were calculated and the average amounts of the counted cells were recorded (Figures 1–4). The extracting data was analyzed using statistical software SPSS Version 22 via t-test otherwise Mann-Whitney U test and significant level of 0.05 was set.

3. Results

As Table 1 showed, the densities of mast cells in the deep layer of Dentigerous cyst and Keratocystic odontogenic tumor were 8 ± 5 and 23 ± 10, respectively. On the other hand, the densities of degranulated mast cells in the deep layer of the Dentigerous cyst and Keratocystic odontogenic tumor were 1 ± 2 and 2 ± 2, respectively.

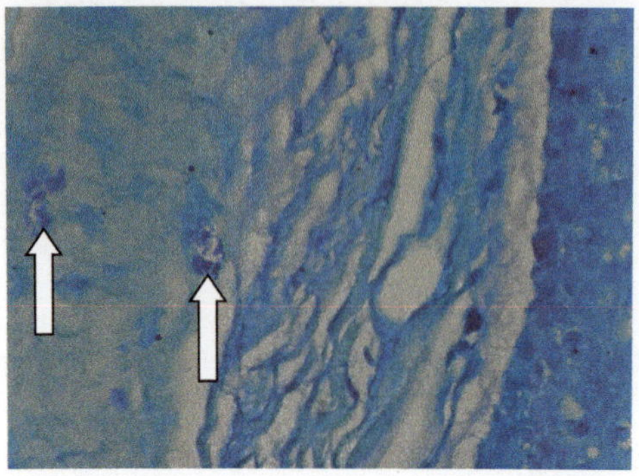

Figure 3: Degranulated mast cells (arrow tip) in the superficial area of the Keratocystic odontogenic tumor wall, stained with Toluidine blue by 400x magnification.

Also, the densities of mast cells in the superficial layer of Dentigerous cyst and Keratocystic odontogenic tumor were 8 ± 5 and 16 ± 8, respectively. Furthermore, the densities of degranulated mast cells in the superficial layer of Dentigerous cyst and Keratocystic odontogenic tumor were 0 ± 1 and 1 ± 1, respectively. Finally, the densities of degranulated mast cells in both layers of Dentigerous cyst and Keratocystic odontogenic tumors were 2 ± 2 and 2 ± 3, respectively.

According to Table 2, the density of mast cells in deep and superficial layer and both layers of Dentigerous cyst and Keratocystic odontogenic tumor had significant differences, presenting that the density of mast cells was higher in all cases of Keratocystic odontogenic tumor (P value < 0.05).

Regarding Table 3, the densities of degranulated mast cells in deep layer and both layers in Dentigerous cyst and Keratocystic odontogenic tumor have significant differences, presenting that the density of mast cells was higher in all cases of Keratocystic odontogenic tumor (P value < 0.05). But the density of degranulated mast cells in the superficial layer of Dentigerous cyst and Keratocystic odontogenic tumor had not significant differences (P value > 0.05).

TABLE 1: Mast cell densities in all layers of cyst wall of Keratocystic odontogenic tumors and Dentigerous cysts.

Mast cell density (mean ± SD)	Cyst type	
	Dentigerous cyst	Keratocystic odontogenic tumor
Density of mast cells in deep layer	8 ± 5	23 ± 10
Density of degranulated mast cells in deep layer	1 ± 2	2 ± 2
Density of mast cells in superficial layer	8 ± 5	16 ± 8
Density of degranulated mast cells in superficial layer	0 ± 1	1 ± 1
Density of degranulated mast cells in both of the two layers	2 ± 3	2 ± 2

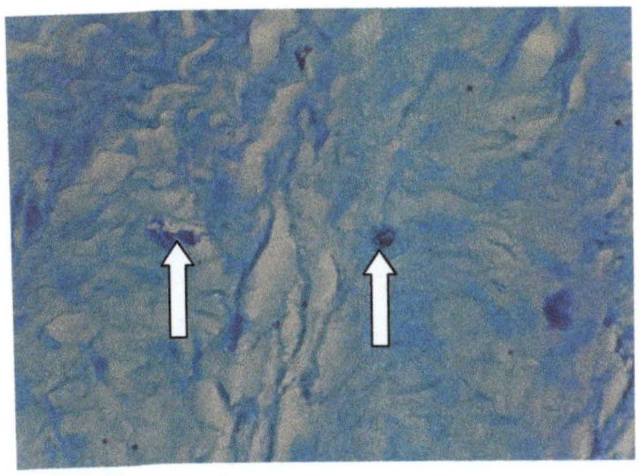

FIGURE 4: Degranulated mast cells (arrow tip) in a deep area of Dentigerous cyst wall stained with Toluidine blue by 400x magnification.

TABLE 2: Comparative results of mast cells densities in Dentigerous cyst and Keratocystic odontogenic tumor.

Statistical points	Mast cell densities					
	Deep layer		Superficial layer		Both layers	
P value	0.000	0.000	0.000	0.000	0.000	0.000
Mean difference	14.30		8.32		22.47	

TABLE 3: Comparative results of Mann Whitney *U* test for degranulated mast cells in the superficial and deep layers and both layers.

Statistical points	Degranulated mast cell densities		
	Deep layer	Superficial layer	Both layers
P value	0.025	0.628	0.031

4. Discussion

The present study showed that the average density of mast cells in deep and superficial layer and both layers was significantly higher in odontogenic keratocyst versus Dentigerous cyst (P value < 0.05). Also, the average density of degranulated mast cells in the deep layer and both layers was significantly higher in Keratocystic odontogenic tumors versus Dentigerous cyst (P value < 0.05). But the average density of degranulated mast cells in superficial layer of Dentigerous cyst and Keratocystic odontogenic tumors had no significant difference (P value > 0.05).

In the study of de Noronha Santos Netto et al., in 2012, inflammatory Dentigerous cysts and Keratocystic odontogenic tumors have more average of mast cells as compared to noninflammatory lesions in all sectors. Along with this present study, deep sections of all cysts showed greater average of degranulated mast cells [8]. On the other hand, in the study of Teronen et al., in 1996, compared with the results of the present study, the majority of mast cells had been detected in inflammatory areas and just below the epithelium of cyst, but the majority of mast cells in periphery of the lesion have been degranulated [15]. Also, Rajabi-Moghaddam et al. could not find any significant difference between DC, RC, and KCOTs. Their little sample volume might be the notable explanation for this result [16].

Smith et al., in 1989, showed that the density of mast cells had significant difference in keratinized and nonkeratinized odontogenic cysts. They concluded that mast cells participated in inflammatory procedures in nonkeratinized cysts, with inverse action in keratinized cysts [17]. Patidar et al., in 2012, reported the highest number of mast cells in radicular cyst and the lowest number for KCOT, in contrast to the present results presenting subepithelial areas of all cysts with more mast cells compared to deeper areas [7].

Prior to this, the presence of mast cells in odontogenic cysts and tumors, especially in the periapical and Dentigerous cysts and Keratocystic odontogenic tumors, was reported [17]. Also, it was suggested previously that degranulation productions of mast cells can correlate with the increase of extracellular matrix destruction in cystic wall by stimulating cytokine production and thus can facilitate the expansion of the lesion [18]. Regarding the results of the studies of Teronen et al. [15] and de Noronha Santos Netto et al. [8], the presence of mast cells specifically in the wall of connective tissue and also in close proximity with the inflammatory cells resulted in the participation of these cells in the expansion of cyst by the secretion of heparin and other hydrolytic enzymes. This procedure was accompanied by dissolution facilitates of glycosaminoglycan and proteoglycan in the cystic fluid conduit with the increase of osmotic and hydrostatic pressure [19, 20]. Also degranulated mast cells release tryptases and prostaglandins, two substances that can participate in bone loss in the joint line between the cyst and bone, which results in the growing cyst [18].

Regarding the present results, higher density of mast cells was observed in the deepest area of the cyst wall in both lesions. This result may show more activities of these cells in the outer layer of the cystic wall with close vicinity of perilesional bone. It is suggested that these cells may relate to bone loss phenomenon similar to osteoporosis and mastocytosis [21]. Mast cells have been known to participate in bone resorption in the pathogenesis of osteoporosis. Also, it has been shown that these cells can adjust osteoclast activity through releasing their granule related to stem cells factor [20]. Furthermore, it has been shown that these cells can increase bone loss with the production of heparin and TNF-A and can stimulate osteoclast activity [22].

This information accompanied by evidences from the results of the present study suggests that mast cells can affect the pathogenesis of Odontogenic cysts, contributing to bone destruction and cystic growth [15]. So, it seems that the presence and degranulation of mast cells may explain the growth potential of Keratocystic odontogenic tumors. However, the accomplishment of further studies is recommended to illustrate the details.

5. Conclusion

The results of this study suggest that mast cells may be involved in the pathogenesis of Keratocystic odontogenic tumors, but, regarding wide range of mast cell's biologic activities, further investigations are recommended to confirm the issue and prepare the details.

Conflict of Interests

The authors declare that there is no conflict of interests regarding the publication of this paper.

Acknowledgment

The authors appreciate Dr. Aghdas Forouzandeh for her close cooperation and scientific support in this study.

References

[1] M. C. Z. Deboni, M. A. Brozoski, A. A. Traina, R. R. Acay, and M. da Graça Naclério-Homem, "Surgical management of dentigerous cyst and keratocystic odontogenic tumor in children: a conservative approach and 7-year follow-up," *Journal of Applied Oral Science*, vol. 20, no. 2, pp. 282–285, 2012.

[2] H. P. Philipsen, "On keratocysts in the jaws," *Tandleagebladet*, vol. 60, pp. 963–980, 1956.

[3] B. Neville, D. Damm, C. Allen, and J. Bouquot, *Oral & Maxillofacial Pathology*, chapters 3, 15, WB Saunders, Philadelphia, Pa, USA, 2th edition, 2009.

[4] K. Forssell, "The primordial cyst. A clinical and radiographic study," *Proceedings of the Finnish Dental Society*, vol. 76, no. 3, pp. 129–174, 1980.

[5] J. Madras and H. Lapointe, "Keratocystic odontogenic tumour: reclassification of the odontogenic keratocyst from cyst to tumour," *The Journal of the Canadian Dental Association*, vol. 74, no. 2, pp. 165–165h, 2008.

[6] T. P. Williams and F. A. Connor Jr., "Surgical management of the odontogenic keratocyst: aggressive approach," *Journal of Oral and Maxillofacial Surgery*, vol. 52, no. 9, pp. 964–966, 1994.

[7] K. A. Patidar, R. N. Parwani, S. P. Wanjari, and A. P. Patidar, "Mast cells in human odontogenic cysts," *Biotechnic and Histochemistry*, vol. 87, no. 6, pp. 397–402, 2012.

[8] J. de Noronha Santos Netto, F. R. Pires, E. C. da Fonseca, L. E. Silva, and S. de Queiroz Chaves Lourenço, "Evaluation of mast cells in periapical cysts, dentigerous cysts, and keratocystic odontogenic tumors," *Journal of Oral Pathology and Medicine*, vol. 41, no. 8, pp. 630–636, 2012.

[9] D. A. Kessler, R. S. Langer, N. A. Pless, and J. Folkman, "Mast cells and tumor angiogenesis," *International Journal of Cancer*, vol. 18, no. 5, pp. 703–709, 1976.

[10] J. Glowacki and J. B. Mulliken, "Mast cells in hemangiomas and vascular malformations," *Pediatrics*, vol. 70, no. 1, pp. 48–51, 1982.

[11] T. J. Poole and B. R. Zetter, "Stimulation of rat peritoneal mast cell migration by tumor-derived peptides," *Cancer Research*, vol. 43, no. 12, pp. 5857–5861, 1983.

[12] W. R. Roche, "The nature and significance of tumour-associated mast cells," *Journal of Pathology*, vol. 148, no. 2, pp. 175–182, 1986.

[13] L. M. Coussens, W. W. Raymond, G. Bergers et al., "Inflammatory mast cells up-regulate angiogenesis during squamous epithelial carcinogenesis," *Genes and Development*, vol. 13, no. 11, pp. 1382–1397, 1999.

[14] M. Samoszuk, E. Kanakubo, and J. K. Chan, "Degranulating mast cells in fibrotic regions of human tumors and evidence that mast cell heparin interferes with the growth of tumor cells through a mechanism involving fibroblasts," *BMC Cancer*, vol. 5, article 121, 2005.

[15] O. Teronen, J. Hietanen, C. Lindqvist et al., "Mast cell-derived tryptase in odontogenic cysts," *Journal of Oral Pathology & Medicine*, vol. 25, no. 7, pp. 376–381, 1996.

[16] M. Rajabi-Moghaddam, H. Abbaszadeh-Bidokhty, and A. Bijani, "Comparison of mast cells count in odontogenic cysts using histochemical staining," *Iranian Journal of Pathology*, vol. 10, no. 2, pp. 105–110, 2015.

[17] G. Smith, A. J. Smith, and M. K. Basu, "Mast cells in human odontogenic cysts," *Journal of Oral Pathology and Medicine*, vol. 18, no. 5, pp. 274–278, 1989.

[18] S. Chatterjee, S. Mahajan, K. Boaz, and T. George, "Quantitative role of mast cells in odontogenic cystic enlargement," *Brazilian Journal of Oral Sciences*, vol. 7, no. 27, pp. 1662–1665, 2008.

[19] G. Smith, A. J. Smith, and R. M. Browne, "Glycosaminoglycans in fluid aspirates from odontogenic cysts," *Journal of Oral Pathology*, vol. 13, no. 6, pp. 614–621, 1984.

[20] G. Smith, A. J. Smith, and R. M. Browne, "Histochemical studies on glycosaminoglycans of odontogenic cysts," *Journal of Oral Pathology*, vol. 17, no. 2, pp. 55–59, 1988.

[21] N. Chiappetta and B. Gruber, "The role of mast cells inosteoporosis," *Seminars in Arthritis and Rheumatism*, vol. 36, no. 1, pp. 32–36, 2006.

[22] R. Dražić, J. Sopta, and A. J. Minić, "Mast cells in periapical lesions: potential role in their pathogenesis," *Journal of Oral Pathology and Medicine*, vol. 39, no. 3, pp. 257–262, 2010.

Genetic and Epigenetic Events Generate Multiple Pathways in Colorectal Cancer Progression

Massimo Pancione,[1] Andrea Remo,[2] and Vittorio Colantuoni[1]

[1] *Department of Biological, Geological and Environmental Sciences, University of Sannio, Via Port'Arsa 11, 82100 Benevento, Italy*
[2] *Department of Pathology, "Mater Salutis" Hospital, ULSS21 Legnago, Verona, Italy*

Correspondence should be addressed to Massimo Pancione, massimo.pancione@unisannio.it and Vittorio Colantuoni, colantuoni@unisannio.it

Academic Editor: Ka F. To

Colorectal cancer (CRC) is one of the most common causes of death, despite decades of research. Initially considered as a disease due to genetic mutations, it is now viewed as a complex malignancy because of the involvement of epigenetic abnormalities. A functional equivalence between genetic and epigenetic mechanisms has been suggested in CRC initiation and progression. A hallmark of CRC is its pathogenetic heterogeneity attained through at least three distinct pathways: a traditional (adenoma-carcinoma sequence), an alternative, and more recently the so-called serrated pathway. While the alternative pathway is more heterogeneous and less characterized, the traditional and serrated pathways appear to be more homogeneous and clearly distinct. One unsolved question in colon cancer biology concerns the cells of origin and from which crypt compartment the different pathways originate. Based on molecular and pathological evidences, we propose that the traditional and serrated pathways originate from different crypt compartments explaining their genetic/epigenetic and clinicopathological differences. In this paper, we will discuss the current knowledge of CRC pathogenesis and, specifically, summarize the role of genetic/epigenetic changes in the origin and progression of the multiple CRC pathways. Elucidation of the link between the molecular and clinico-pathological aspects of CRC would improve our understanding of its etiology and impact both prevention and treatment.

1. Background: The Molecular Basis of Colon Carcinogenesis

Colorectal cancers (CRCs) arise through a multistep process in which genetic and epigenetic alterations accumulate in a sequential order. Three different pathogenetic pathways have been implicated in the development of these tumors: (1) chromosomal instability (CIN); (2) microsatellite instability (MSI); (3) CpG island methylator phenotype (CIMP).

The CIN pathway is associated with the sequential deregulation of tumor suppressor genes (TSGs) and oncogenes such as, *APC*, *KRAS*, *DCC/SMAD4*, and *TP53*. It generally occurs within inherited tumors, such as familial adenomatous polyposis (FAP), but it has also been associated with the majority of sporadic CRCs. Microsatellite instability is responsible for the Lynch syndrome and sporadic tumors and is mainly caused by inactivation of the DNA mismatch repair genes (*hMLH1*, *hMSH2*, *hMSH6*, and *hPMS2*). CRCs displaying MSI tend to be rightsided, generally have high histological grades, a mucinous phenotype, and diagnosed at lower pathological stages than CIN cancers. The CpG island methylator phenotype (CIMP) refers to the widespread hypermethylation of CpG islands at several loci. Typically, one type of molecular signature predominates suggesting that the three pathways rarely overlap; a complex interplay occurs in some tumors whereby one pathway is a result of one other (i.e., CIMP and MSI due to *hMLH1* promoter hypermethylation).

2. Introduction

More than one million of individuals develop CRC every year worldwide [1, 2]. Despite the remarkable accomplishments in new therapeutic options, CRC remains one of the most

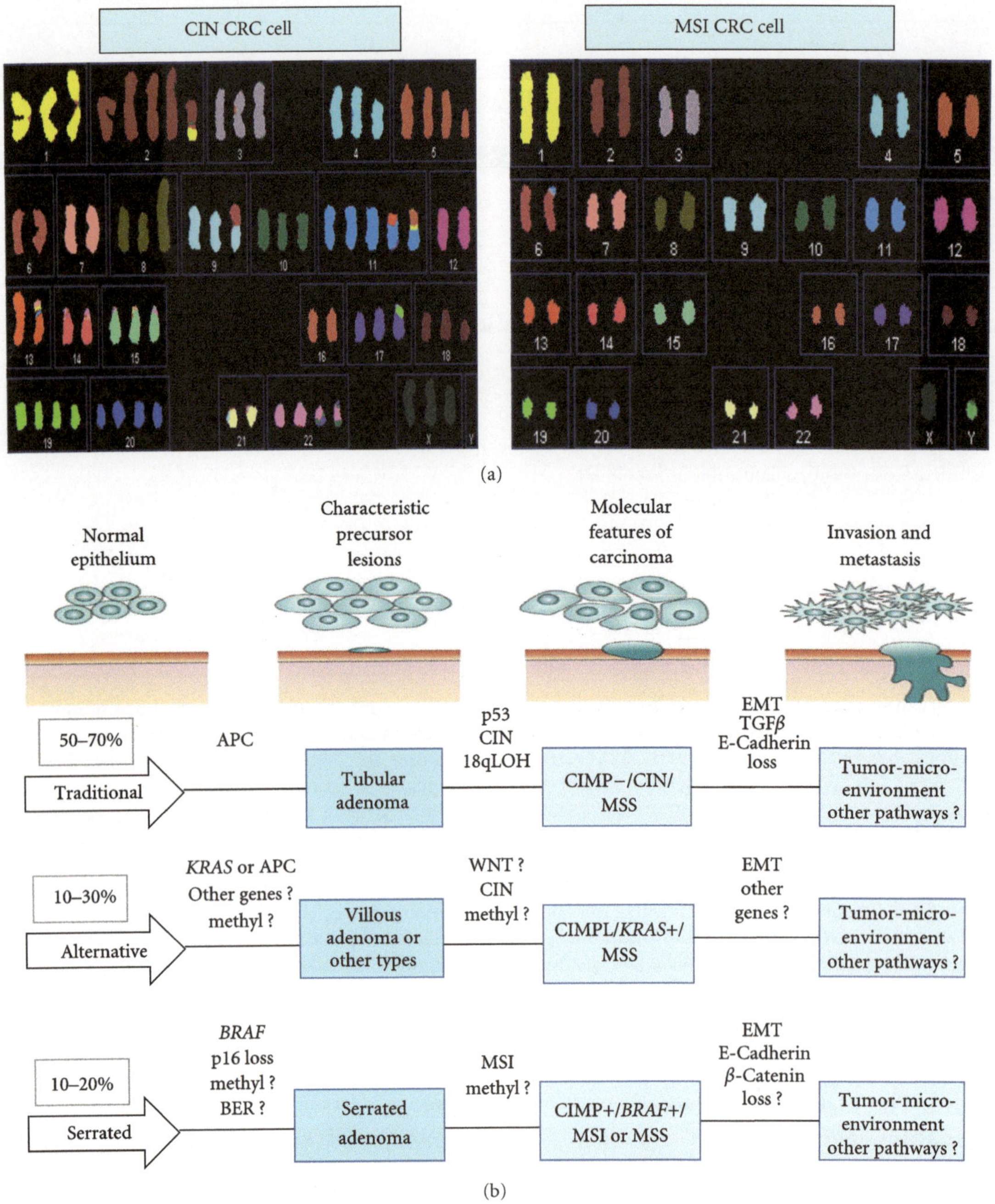

FIGURE 1: Genomic instability and multiple pathways in colorectal cancer pathogenesis. (a) Comparison of the numerical chromosomal abnormalities between two representative colon cancer cell lines characterized by CIN (highly rearranged aneuploid karyotype) and MSI (diploid karyotype), respectively. The images are publicly available on the web at: http://www.path.cam.ac.uk. (b) Three distinct parallel pathways with the approximate indicated prevalence are implicated in colon cancer pathogenesis: traditional, alternative, and serrated. The sequential of genetic and epigenetic changes occurring in each pathway are simplified, along with the characteristic precursor lesions (adenomas) and distinctive molecular features of the corresponding carcinomas. The traditional and serrated pathways are more homogeneous and clearly distinguishable; the alternative is more heterogeneous. The best known genetic/epigenetic alterations are indicated in bold, the poorly understood or hypothetical pathways are indicated in italics. APC, adenomatous polyposis coli; MSI, microsatellite instability; CIMP, CpG island methylator phenotype; CIMPL, CIMP-low; CIN, chromosomal instability; MSS, microsatellite stable; BER, base excision repair pathway; Methyl, DNA methylation silencing in yet unknown genes; WNT, wingless pathway; EMT, epithelial mesenchymal transition; TGFβ, transforming growth factor-beta; LOH, loss-of-heterozigosity. Note: tumor microenvironment indicates the crosstalk between cancer cells and cells of the neoplastic stroma.

common malignancies [3, 4]. Intriguingly, during the last decade, CRC incidence in the Asian population increased from two- to four-times, whereas it progressively diminished in western countries, implying yet undefined gene-environment interactions [4, 5]. CRC occurs sporadically in the majority of cases and only in 5–10% is due to inherited mutations in well-known cancer-related genes [6]; about 25% of patients, however, reveal a family history of the disease, suggesting a specific contribution by yet unidentified genes [6]. In 1990, Fearon and Vogelstein proposed a model whereby CRC proceeds through a series of morphological steps due to specific genetic alterations [7]. The model emphasizes the central role of the adenomatous polyp as the precursor lesion and provides evidence that in the majority of CRCs the primary event is the aberrant activation of the APC/β-catenin pathway, followed by *RAS/RAF* mutations and loss of p53 function at later stages [7]. Ten years later, only 7% of CRCs have been shown to bear mutations in all three genes, implying that multiple pathways may be involved in the tumorigenic process [8]. Recently, the development of CRC has been considered from a different point of view [9–12]. Genetic alterations are, in fact, only a piece of a more complex puzzle [13]; epigenetic variations in cancer-related genes and noncoding RNAs play also a role contributing to the malignant status [14, 15]. The timing and combinations of genetic and epigenetic events rather than the mere accumulation of genetic disorders appear to confer cancer cells a selective advantage resulting in the activation of distinct pathways [11, 14, 16]. Genomic instability is emerging as a fundamental process in colorectal tumorigenesis [17], as highlighted by a number of inherited CRCs such as FAP, MYH associated polyposis (MAP), and hereditary nonpolyposis colon cancer (HNPCC). They are caused, in fact, by germline mutations in cancer-related genes involved in DNA duplication or repair, respectively [2, 6]. CIN, a hallmark of these events, is a process that generates gene deletions, duplications, and chromosomal rearrangements [18]. CRC development has also been associated with frequent mutations at simple sequence repeats or microsatellites, generating MSI [19]. Recently, it has been hypothesized that point mutation instability (PIN), a process that increases spontaneous mutations in random nucleotide sequences, could contribute to both CIN and MSI [20, 21]. In the last decade, a novel type of instability has been suggested to influence CRC pathogenesis. It is merely epigenetic and referred as CIMP [22–24]. Current evidences indicate that only one type of genomic instability predominates, providing the main "genetic or epigenetic signature" to the development of a specific CRC [23]. Although the molecular bases of genomic instability remain elusive, the global genomic/epigenomic aberrations differentially mark three distinct developmental pathways: traditional, alternative, and serrated [10, 12]. This suggests that not a single but multiple pathogenetic mechanisms account for colorectal tumorigenesis. One attractive question is to establish the relative contribution of each of these pathways to tumor development and the effects they exert on the phenotype and clinical behaviour. In this paper we will examine the achievements in our understanding of CRC pathogenesis with a special focus on the molecular basis of its heterogeneity.

3. Genomic and Epigenomic Instability Associate with Different CRC Pathogenetic Pathways

Genomic stability is strictly controlled in order to maintain cell homeostasis [17]. Hence, any defect in the mechanisms governing this event will promote mutational processes, selection, and clonal expansion of the mutated cells, contributing to cancer progression. CIN is the most common type of genomic instability occurring in 60% of CRCs, mainly in tumors proficient in DNA mismatch repair [18]. CIN positive tumors are characterized by frequent loss-of-heterozygosity (LOH) at tumor suppressor gene loci, chromosomal rearrangements, and numerical abnormalities "manifested as aneuploidy" (Figure 1(a)). MSI accounts, instead, for approximately 15–20% of sporadic CRCs with a well-defined phenotype resulting from loss of DNA mismatch repair functions [19]. The characteristic signature of MSI is the deletion of one element in a repetitive region of DNA that generates a frameshift in the coding sequence and hence gene inactivation, generally at tumor suppressor genes loci [19]. Interestingly, most MSI-CRCs are apparently diploid or near-diploid (Figure 1(a)). In association with mutations in cancer-related genes, CIN has been proposed for long time as the driving force to achieve the malignant status [7]. During the last decade, also epigenetic events, that is heritable changes in gene expression not accompanied by changes in the DNA sequence, have been recognized to play a crucial role in CRC development [25]. The term encompasses histone modification, nucleosome location, noncoding RNAs, and DNA methylation [13, 14]. DNA hypermethylation at specific regulatory sites, enriched in CpG motifs (CpG islands) in the promoter regions of tumor suppressor genes, has been linked to transcription repression in human tumors [14]. In 1999, Toyota et al. proposed the term CIMP to describe a subset of CRCs that consistently show widespread CpG island hypermethylation at seven different loci defined methylated in tumors (MINT) [22]. Subsequently, methylation at least three MINT loci has strongly been correlated with *CDKN2A* (p16) and *hMLH1* methylation constituting the so-called "classic panel" and providing a simplified approach to CIMP definition [22–25]. Using these markers, CIMP positive tumors are more frequently associated with MSI-CRCs than the MSS counterpart and localized to the right colon (up to 40%) than left colon and rectum (3–12%). The CIMP phenotype is, however, uncommon in HNPCC that exhibits MSI, suggesting distinct underlying molecular processes [24–26]. The existence of such a phenotype has largely been debated and a consensus on which markers should be used for its definition has not been reached yet. To overcome this difficulty and support the CIMP phenotype as a distinct CRC molecular trait,Curtin et al. proposed alternative markers (*CACNA1G, IGF2, NEUROG1, RUNX3* and *SOCS1)* to the classic list of genes [26]. Based on this new panel, CIMP positive tumors do not have any relationship with *KRAS* mutations but strongly correlate with the *BRAF* V600E mutation [25, 26]. According to the number of methylated CIMP markers, CRCs can be divided in three epigenotypes: CIMP-high, -low and -negative [9]. CIMP positive tumors are also referred as CIMP-high CRCs [26]. The CIMP phenotype has recently been validated as an independent pathway using a whole-methylome sequencing approach [27–29]. CIMP tumors show differentially methylated CpG sites as compared to CIMP negative tumors and normal matched controls. Many of these CpG sites appear to be more prone to methylation and uniquely methylated in CIMP tumors with respect to non-CIMP tumors [27–29]. Moreover, DNA methylation spreading appears to be preferentially unidirectional and likely due to the binding of specific transcription factors [27]. According to Berman et al., the hypermethylated areas of CIMP tumors are focal (the so-called partially methylated domains (PMDs)) and associated with long-range hypomethylated regions [29]. Consequently, the CRC genome can be divided into four clusters: (1) methylation-prone, that is, regions "methylated in tumor," but not in normal tissues; (2) methylation resistant, that is, regions "no methylated in either cell type;" (3) methylation-loss, that is regions "methylated in normal, but not in tumor tissue;" (4) constitutively methylated loci, that is, regions "methylated either in normal and in tumor tissue." Interestingly, the methylation prone elements are highly enriched for marks with polycomb repressive complex 1 and 2 activity, resembling human embryonic stem cells (hES) [27, 29]. These studies support the notion that widespread DNA methylation changes in colon cancer are linked to specific silencing programs, suggesting the CIMP phenotype as part of a specific pathway of intense DNA hypermethylation, defined "epigenomic instability" [25–29].

Based on these new concepts, Issa revised the model of CRC development: instead of a linear progression of single events, he proposes three distinct multiple pathways, each of which based on different molecular mechanisms and variable prognosis [30]. These pathways are illustrated in (Figure 1(b)) that takes into consideration the current understanding and the novel hypotheses. Out of the three pathways proposed, the alternative one is the most heterogeneous as it originates mainly from villous but also from serrated adenomas (Figure 1(b)). It is characterized by a CIMP-low phenotype, predominant *KRAS* but occasional *BRAF* mutations, and no CIN and is associated with a worse prognosis [9, 10, 30]. In contrast, the traditional and serrated pathways appear to be clearly distinct (Figure 2(a)). Based on their molecular and pathological characteristics, the major distinction between the serrated and traditional pathways resides in their epigenomic instability (CIMP positive versus negative) and subsequently in gene alterations (*BRAF* versus *APC*, MSI versus CIN) (Figure 2(a)). We propose that the specific identity of these two pathways is established at an early evolutionary stage and fully enforced within precancerous lesions. Tumor development through the traditional pathway is, in fact, relatively slow (5–20 years), probably due to the fact that the initial events occur in the fully differentiated cells of the colonic crypt (Figure 2(b)). APC mutations, generally, are detected in the cells of the upper crypt compartment according to the top-down morphogenetic model [31]. The causal events underlying the serrated pathway, instead, may take place in the cells of the lower crypt compartment, whose functions are finely regulated by epigenetic mechanisms carried out by the components of the PcG polycomb repressive complexes (PRCs) [13, 32–34]. An "epigenetic memory" might operate at this compartment predisposing to the epigenetic characteristics of the adult cancer cells [32–35]. Albeit speculative, the present model integrates both morphological and molecular evidences and would explain why the precursor lesions of the traditional pathway originate in the upper part of the crypt tend to grow upward while those of the serrated pathway grow downward or laterally, are rapidly progressive and prone to CIMP (Figure 2(b)) [12, 30, 36]. Among the genetic alterations associated with these events, *BRAF* mutations have been proposed as the earliest genetic event, followed by inactivation of p16/INK4a [36, 37]. Whether this is the seminal genetic lesion and which are the subsequent ones occurring in serrated adenomas remain to be established (Figure 1(b)). Also the nature and characteristics of the tumor-initiating cells (TICs) from which the different pathogenetic pathways originate are not known yet, although they are the focus of intense research [34, 38]. TICs are able to form a malignant stem-cell compartment with a hierarchical organization and a specialized microenvironment "niche," resembling the normal stem-cell system at the bottom of the crypt (Figure 2(b)). TICs are constituted by at least three different subtypes and only one of them has recently been demonstrated to be truly tumorigenic [38]. Cells of this subfraction are defined long-term TICs (LT-TICs), because they can initiate tumor formation, maintain self-renewal, and promote distant metastasis [38]. Genetic heterogeneity does not significantly contribute to the functional differences between distinct types of TICs. As mentioned above, the methylation profile of hypermethylated regions in CIMP tumors appears to be very similar to normal stem cells, as it is enriched in repressive marks of the PRC family and in specific transcription factors. The relative extent of CpG island hyper- and hypomethylation in tumors may reflect different features of the TICs subclone of origin (i.e., long-term stem cells versus transient amplifying precursors or differentiated cells). We hypothesize that the early appearance of CIMP and higher CpG island hypermethylation present in the serrated pathway could be related to the specific chromatin organization program of the cell of origin (Figure 2(b)). The "hierarchy model" hypothesizes that cancer stem cells initiate the malignant process and provide a continuous source of transformed cells expanding the tumor mass and tumor heterogeneity. Moreover, they display an increased ability to survive genotoxic stress and injury, suggesting that they are responsible for chemo- and radioresistance, for metastasis and, ultimately, patient demise [38]. The discovery of different types of TICs suggests a distinct contribution of the stem-cell-like population to tumor formation and progression; however, the molecular link between the "cell of origin" and the specific pathogenetic pathway remains to be demonstrated [13, 30, 34, 38]. Cancers related to chronic

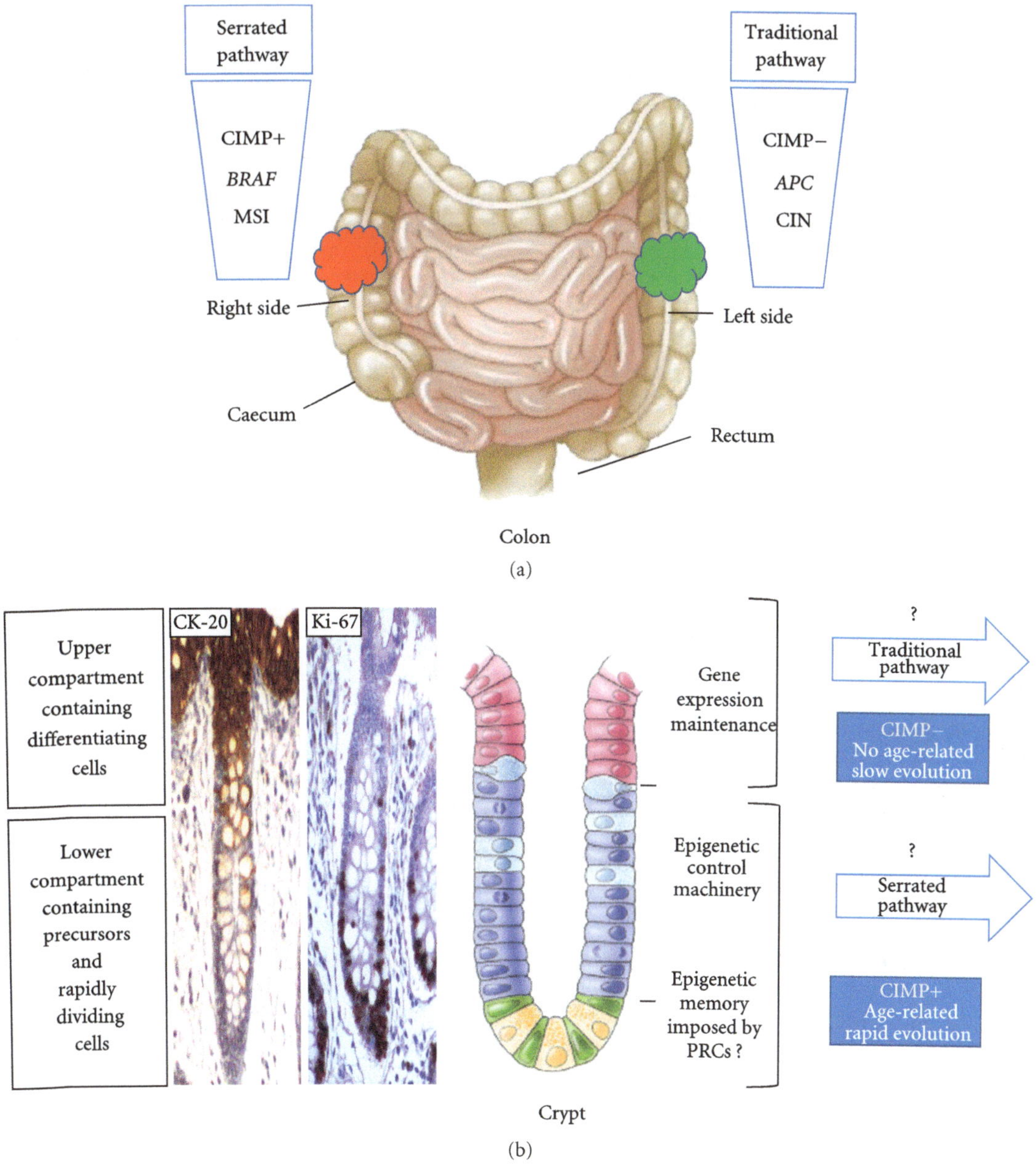

Figure 2: Epigenetic alterations may differentiate the traditional and serrated pathway at early stage of tumor development. (a) The serrated and traditional pathways show clinical differences, especially when referred to the site of origin of the tumor. The serrated pathway tends to be localized to the proximal (right) colon; the traditional to the distal (left) colon. The main molecular alterations that clearly distinguish the two pathways are the presence (+)/absence (−) of the CIMP phenotype and different genetic characteristics (*BRAF*/MSI versus *APC*/CIN). (b) The colonic epithelium consists of spatially separated, nonproliferative/differentiated cells at the tip of the villi, marked by cytokeratin 20 and proliferative/undifferentiated cell populations marked by Ki67. The molecular mechanisms underlying CIMP and CIN are still unknown; however, these alterations may evolve in a nonrandom fashion. According to the top-down model [31], the traditional pathway may arise from genetic lesions (*APC* mutations) confined to the upper crypt compartment. In contrast, the serrated pathway may originate in the lower crypt compartment by yet uncharacterized genetic and/or epigenetic lesions. Current evidences support the idea that the specific functions played in the lower compartment are maintained by an epigenetic program finely regulated by PRCs [13, 32–35]. Initial lesions in cells of this compartment may predispose to the epigenetic characteristics of the adult cancer through an "epigenetic memory." This may explain why these specific precursor lesions proliferate downward or laterally, are age-related, rapidly progressive, and prone to CIMP. APC, adenomatous polyposis coli; MSI, microsatellite instability; CIMP, CpG island methylator phenotype; CIN, chromosomal instability; polycomb repressive complexes (PRCs).

inflammation processes, such as colitis-associated cancers (CAC), follow an alternative pathway, generally initiated by mutations in *PT53* or by COX2 overexpression and followed by *APC* inactivation in later stages [39].

Although these pathways represent a simplification of our current knowledge on colon tumorigenesis, they provide evidence to support a revision of the classical adenoma-carcinoma sequence. The complete elucidation of the

Table 1: Components of the SWI/SNF complex and their biological roles in colorectal cancer.

SWI/SNF components in mammals			
Members	Gene	Biological relevance	References
BRM	*SMARCA2*	(i) Mutated or lost in CRC cell lines (ii) TSG	[45, 46, 49, 54]
BRG1	*SMARCA4*	(i) Mutated or lost in CRC cell lines (ii) EMT in CRC (iii) TSG	[48–50, 52, 53]
BAF170	*SMARCC2*	(i) CRC? (ii) ESC self-renewal pluripotency	[46, 47]
BAF155	*SMARCC1*	(i) CRC? (ii) ESC self-renewal pluripotency	[46, 47]
HLTF	*SMARCA3*	(i) TSG in CRC	[61]
BAF47	*SMARCB1*	(i) CRC? (ii) TSG	[46, 55–58]

SWI: mating-type switching; SNF: sucrose nonfermenting; BRM: brahma; BRG1: brahma-related gene-1; BAFs: BRG- and BRM- associated factors; TSG: tumor suppressor gene; CRC: colorectal cancer; HLTF: helicase-like transcription factor; EMT: epithelial mesenchymal transition; ESC: embryonic stem cells. CRC? indicates a yet unknown role in colorectal cancer.
Note: representative SWI/SNF components are shown; at least 15 subunits have been described in mammals so far.

molecular modifications underlying these multiple pathogenetic pathways, in association with lifestyle and genetic polymorphisms, will likely change our understanding of the molecular basis of colorectal tumorigenesis.

4. Chromatin Remodeling and Epigenetic Abnormalities in Colon Carcinogenesis

Epigenetic events play a role in tumorigenesis as they activate oncogenes and inactivate tumor suppressor genes according to the multistep origin of the process [13, 14]. They do not involve changes in DNA sequences but rather are self-propagating and potentially reversible molecular signatures [13, 14]. The notion of epigenetic variations of DNA along with the identification of the CIMP phenotype and, more recently, the discovery of various classes of noncoding (ncRNA) and micro-RNAs (miRNA) have significantly modified our knowledge on carcinogenesis [27, 40, 41]. Gene silencing occurring after DNA hypermethylation is a complex process mediated either by direct inhibition of transcription factors binding or by methyl-DNA binding proteins (MBD) [42]. These latter proteins, in turn, recruit other transcriptional repressors such as histone deacetylases (HDACs) and histone methyl transferases (HMT), generating a transcriptionally inactive chromatin [42, 43]. Nucleosome positioning is also relevant in determining accessibility of transcription factors to their target DNA sequences [44]. A series of protein complexes, known as chromatin remodelers, mediate this event as they can slide, destabilize, or relocate nucleosomes in an ATP-dependent manner [44, 45]. The SWI/SNF mating-type switching (SWI) and sucrose nonfermenting (SNF) subfamily has particularly been investigated in cancer research [46]. The complex contains two subunits with ATPase activity, Brahma-(Brm), Brahma-related gene-1 (*BRG1*) and several Brahma associated factors (BAFs) (Table 1) [44–46]. Loss-of-function of SWI/SNF components impairs normal chromatin remodeling in human cancers [46, 47]. *BRG1* is mutated in several cancer cell lines including those derived from colon [48], and loss of *BRG1* is observed in a wide variety of solid tumors [49]. Mice heterozygous for mutations at *Brg1* are cancer-prone; the precise role of *Brg1* in CRC is, however, still controversial [48–53]. Loss of *Brm* expression is observed in several tumors and appears to occur at the posttranscriptional level [46, 49]; recent evidences show that *Brm* promotes the differentiation of gastric cancer cells [54]. SNF5 (also called SMARCB1, INI1, BAF47), localized to the 22q11.2 chromosome region, is the most extensively studied subunit of the SWI/SNF complex for its critical role in tumorigenesis (Table 1) [46, 55]. In fact, *SNF5* is inactivated either at germline or at somatic level in malignant rhabdoid tumors (MRTs), a pediatric and highly lethal neoplasm of the kidney and brain [55–58]. Despite their extremely aggressive behaviour, most of these tumors display a normal karyotype and the so-called rhabdoid cells [58]. They are characterized by an eccentrically located and large nucleus, prominent nucleoli, eosinophilic cytoplasm with a spheroid perinuclear inclusion body, and aggregates of intermediate filaments, including both vimentin and cytokeratins. MRTs have also been described in extrarenal organs including the large intestine [58], giving rise to rhabdoid colorectal Tumor (RCT) a rare, highly aggressive neoplasm frequently observed at the right colon of elderly patients [59, 60]. hSNF5/INI1 inactivation does not appear to be determinant in RCT development implying the involvement of other yet unknown loci. Its role in sporadic CRCs remains to be determined (Table 1). We have recently suggested that RCTs commonly present a combination of *BRAF* mutations, CIMP-high, and MSI-high phenotype [59, 60]. Further studies are needed to understand the complex interplay between chromatin remodelers CIMP tumors and CRC progression.

5. Epigenetic Changes and Epithelial Mesenchymal Transition in Colorectal Cancer Metastasis

Metastatic dissemination represents one of the key determinants of poor patients' prognosis in colon carcinogenesis. MSI-CRCs have been shown to be associated with a better prognosis than MSS-CRCs or CIN tumors [62], likely due to the lower metastatic potential, although the molecular bases have not been clearly established yet [62]. Among the processes involved in tumor invasion and metastasis, epithelial mesenchymal transition (EMT) has been proposed as a critical step in the acquisition of a more aggressive phenotype [62, 63]. EMT is a highly conserved process required for embryonic development, tissue remodeling, and wound repair. Activation of the EMT program in adult epithelia represses cell adhesion molecules (E-cadherin, cytokeratin, zona occludens 1 (ZO-1)) and induces mesenchymal markers (vimentin, N-cadherin, fibronectin) [64, 65]. Consequently, cells acquire a fibroblast-like appearance [64]. These biochemical and morphological changes enhance the migratory potential of cancer cells, promoting invasiveness, resistance to apoptosis, and synthesis of extracellular matrix components (ECM) [64–66]. Hepatocyte growth factor (HGF), epidermal growth factor (EGF), placental-derived growth factor (PDGF), or transforming growth factor-β (TGF-β) appears to be responsible for the induction or functional activation of a series of EMT-inducing transcription factors such as Snail, Slug, ZEB1, Twist, Goosecoid, and FoxC2 [64–69]. Their effects onto the EMT program depend upon the activation of a series of intracellular signaling networks involving ERK, MAPK, PI3K, AKT, SMADs, and integrins [70]. The WNT/β-catenin signaling pathway and E-cadherin loss are considered the major effectors of EMT and implicated in CRC metastatic progression [71–74]. The serrated pathway is associated with a lower frequency of nuclear β-catenin localization than the traditional one, suggesting that noncanonical Wnt/β-catenin pathways may influence metastasis formation especially in right-sided tumors (Figure 1(b)) [74, 75]. TGF-β1 has recently been demonstrated to induce EMT only in colon cancer cell lines bearing a wild type TGFBR2 receptor type II *(TGFBR2)* [76]. This gene contains an (A)10 repeat which is mutated in 80% of MSI-positive tumors, compared with just 0.6% of CIN tumors. Thus, it has been postulated that CIN-CRCs show an increased incidence of EMT and consequently shorter survival rates than MSI-tumors [76]. Recently, it has been suggested that the CIMP positive phenotype, in combination with MSI-CRCs, is usually associated with specific histological features and a poorer patients' prognosis, suggesting that the interplays of genomic instability with epigenetic variations are crucial events in metastatic dissemination [77, 78].

CRCs could then be classified according to their epithelial or mesenchymal subtype; by doing so, it would be possible to predict disease progression and recurrence even at early stages of tumorigenesis [79–81]. Consistent with this, cells that have undergone EMT histologically constitute cell buds that is single cells or small clusters of dedifferen- tiated cells at the invasive tumor front [82–85]. Tumor budding has been recognized as an independent prognostic factor to predict lymph node and distant metastasis or local recurrence and poor patient survival [82–85]. The EMT program has been identified as a possible unifying molecular signature in CRC clinical behavior and thus as a dominant pathway in metastatic progression (Figure 1(b)) [81]. According to this notion, our own data suggest that some CRC tumors presenting MSI, CIMP, and $BRAF^{(V600E)}$ mutation are extremely aggressive, characterized by a diffuse and intense EMT and resemble those originated via the serrated pathway (our unpublished data) [59, 60, 86]. These results support the existence of crosstalks between EMT and epigenetic modifications in the MSI-CRC group. That multiple pathways operate within apparently homogenous CRC subtypes cannot be excluded.

6. Molecular and Phenotypic Heterogeneity of CRC

Accumulating evidences indicate that human cancer cells harbor global epigenetic abnormalities and in CRC the number of genes inactivated by CpG island promoter hypermethylation is greater than the mutated genes [87, 88]. The three distinct pathways involving genomic instability (MSI, CIN, and CIMP) appear, in fact, to enhance the diversity of gene expression and phenotypic changes in CRC [87, 88]. They are generally present in a mutually exclusive fashion, rarely overlap, and provide a distinctive molecular signature of CRC development; for instance, MSI versus CIN or alternatively CIN versus CIMP (Figure 2(a)) [87, 88]. Sporadic cases with MSI can frequently be attributed to CIMP-related silencing of the mismatch repair gene MLH1 [89]. Some CRCs, however, present both MSI and CIN or no MSI or CIN at all: so it remains to be established whether they represent other subgroups [88, 90].

Based on the stringent link between molecular, pathological, and clinical features, Jass classifies CRCs into 5 types [10], the approximate frequencies of each subgroup are reported in (Figure 3(a)). This classification is based on the correct identification of CIN, a survey that poses many problems because the currently used criteria are not uniform. It has been, then, proposed to classify CRCs into only 4 molecular subtypes taking into account MSI and CIMP only, as they are relatively more defined than CIN Figure 3(b) [77, 78]. Interestingly, the frequency of the CIMP+/MSI+ subtype versus CIMP−/MSI+ subtype differs substantially between Western and Asian populations [77]. People of Anglo-Celtic origin have a higher risk of cancers with CIMP and *BRAF* mutations than people of southern European origin [91, 92]. In line with this, in our CRC series of about 200 patients of southern European origin, *BRAF* mutations occur at a frequency even lower ($\leq$5%) than that reported in the literature. Accumulating evidences suggest that CIMP+/MSI+ CRCs (10% of total) arise through the serrated pathway and are characterized by a high frequency of *BRAF* mutations (Figure 1(b)). We propose that, within the MSI-CRC group, the combination CIMP+/BRAF+ may constitute a new subtype associated

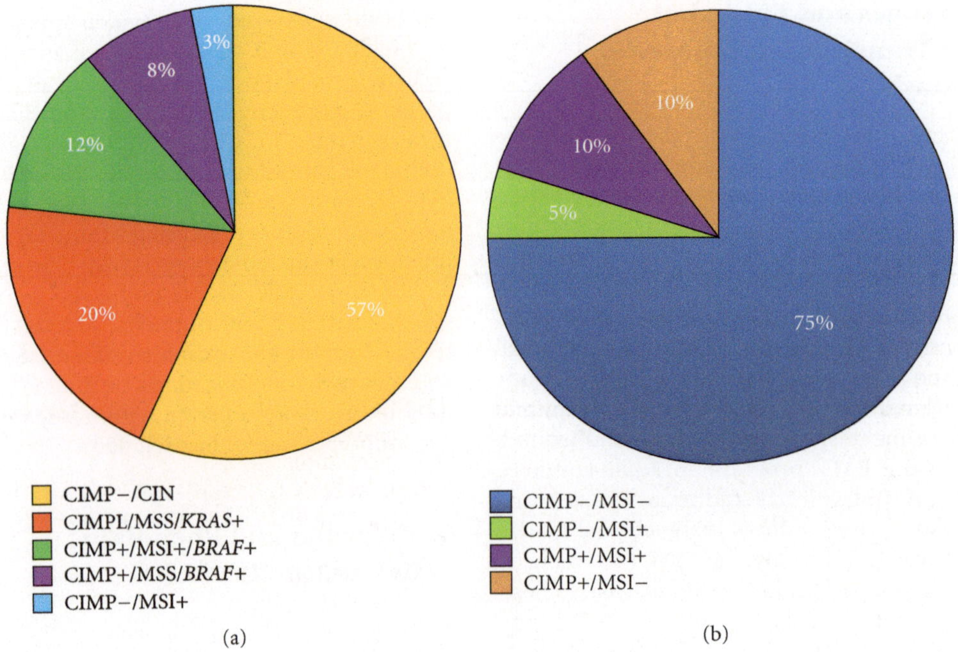

Figure 3: CRC classification in molecular subgroups. (a) Five molecular colorectal cancer subgroups have been proposed, stratified on the basis of genomic instability, presence/absence of CIMP [10]. The approximate frequencies of each CRC subtype in the Western population are illustrated. (b) Because the currently used criteria for CIN analysis are not uniform, as compared to MSI and CIMP, a classification into only 4 molecular subtypes has been proposed [77, 78]. The approximate frequencies in the Western population are illustrated. The distribution of the CIMP subgroup appears to correlate with ethnic differences (see text), suggesting that predisposition to the CIMP pathway may be tied to the contribution of yet unknown gene-environment interactions. MSI, microsatellite instability; CIMP, CpG Island methylator phenotype; CIN, chromosomal instability; CIMPL, CIMP Low.

with the worst clinical outcome [59, 60, 93]. Interestingly, the MSI+/CIMP+/BRAF+ subgroup is associated with synchronous colorectal cancers and exhibits a sarcomatoid dedifferentiation profile, due to the intense expression of mesenchymal markers [59, 60]. These data suggest that the variable predisposition observed among different populations to develop tumors through the serrated pathway may be tied to the specific contribution of yet unidentified gene-environment interactions. Further genetic and epigenetic studies of this pathway are needed to understand the reasons of these differences.

7. Final Remarks and Future Challenges

The multistep model of colorectal tumorigenesis has been seminal and paradigmatic in cancer biology. One of the most intriguing but still unanswered questions is to understand the precise molecular events and their temporal occurrences that lead to tumor initiation, abnormal cellular expansion, and phenotypic changes. Likewise, the cell of origin and initial hit in a specific colon crypt compartment that determine the different CRC pathogenetic pathways remain obscure. Cancer stem cells have been proposed as the cellular drivers of subclonal expansion and probably vary in frequency and phenotypic features among different CRC pathways.

In this paper we have summarized the role of genetic/epigenetic changes in the origin of the multiple CRC pathways. Growing evidence suggests that the rate of epigenetic changes is estimated to be higher than that of genetic changes and could be a major determinant in the origin of tumor, clonal evolution, and tumor heterogeneity. These studies have, in fact, expanded our understanding of the pathogenetic mechanisms involved in tumor progression. The recognition and attempts to define the multiple pathogenetic pathways in CRC as reported here account for all these new accomplishments.

The identification and characterization of the CIMP positive phenotype, along with that of the full array of genes modified in CRC, have further deepened our knowledge and made even more complex the resulting picture. Whole epigenome sequencing supports the existence of a CIMP phenotype and epigenomic instability as a distinct molecular pathway prone to aberrant methylation in cancer.

We hypothesize that the pathogenetic pathway of a specific CRC appears to be imposed at an early stage of the neoplastic evolution, through an "epigenetic memory" of the cell of origin. This condition may predispose the adult cancer cell to distinct degrees of epigenetic abnormalities, explaining the differences between the serrated and traditional pathway. So the acquisition of genomic and epigenomic instability (CIN, MSI, CIMP) are crucial features in tumor development. A better definition of the molecular mechanisms that initiate each of these alterations will be critical for the understanding of CRC pathogenesis and feasibility of targeting cancer cells specifically. In hereditary cancers, genomic instability can be attributed to mutations in DNA repair genes; however, the relationship between DNA repair systems, chromatin-remodelling complexes, and molecular basis of genomic instability in sporadic cancers remains unclear. Elucidation of these pathways will be relevant to improve the clinical management of patients. Age-dependent DNA methylation may drive gene expression changes associated with carcinogenesis. Elucidation of the link between age, environmental risk, and carcinogenesis will help to define the impact of epigenomic/genomic instability on multiple CRC pathways. These findings may have broad implications for cancer prevention, risk prediction, and prognosis. Moreover, they could provide new therapeutic targets or reliable biomarkers of chemo- or radiotherapy and ultimately could be a promising basis towards personalized therapeutic treatments.

Acknowledgments

The authors would like to thank Associazione Italiana per la lotta ai linfomi e leucemie (AIL) for financial support to V. Colantuoni.

References

[1] D. Cunningham, W. Atkin, H. J. Lenz et al., "Colorectal cancer," *The Lancet*, vol. 375, no. 9719, pp. 1030–1047, 2010.

[2] A. Tenesa and M. G. Dunlop, "New insights into the aetiology of colorectal cancer from genome-wide association studies," *Nature Reviews Genetics*, vol. 10, no. 6, pp. 353–358, 2009.

[3] A. Jemal, M. M. Center, E. Ward, and M. J. Thun, "Cancer occurrence," *Methods in Molecular Biology*, vol. 471, pp. 3–29, 2009.

[4] A. Jemal, R. Siegel, E. Ward et al., "Cancer statistics, 2008," *CA Cancer Journal for Clinicians*, vol. 58, no. 2, pp. 71–96, 2008.

[5] J. J. Y. Sung, J. Y. W. Lau, K. L. Goh et al., "Increasing incidence of colorectal cancer in Asia: implications for screening," *The Lancet Oncology*, vol. 6, no. 11, pp. 871–876, 2005.

[6] A. K. Rustgi, "The genetics of hereditary colon cancer," *Genes and Development*, vol. 21, no. 20, pp. 2525–2538, 2007.

[7] E. R. Fearon and B. Vogelstein, "A genetic model for colorectal tumorigenesis," *Cell*, vol. 61, no. 5, pp. 759–767, 1990.

[8] G. Smith, F. A. Carey, J. Beattie et al., "Mutations in APC, Kirsten-ras, and p53—alternative genetic pathways to colorectal cancer," *Proceedings of the National Academy of Sciences of the United States of America*, vol. 99, no. 14, pp. 9433–9438, 2002.

[9] S. Ogino and A. Goel, "Molecular classification and correlates in colorectal cancer," *Journal of Molecular Diagnostics*, vol. 10, no. 1, pp. 13–27, 2008.

[10] J. R. Jass, "Classification of colorectal cancer based on correlation of clinical, morphological and molecular features," *Histopathology*, vol. 50, no. 1, pp. 113–130, 2007.

[11] S. D. Markowitz and M. M. Bertagnolli, "Molecular basis of colorectal cancer," *The New England Journal of Medicine*, vol. 361, no. 25, pp. 2404–2460, 2009.

[12] J. Young, M. Jenkins, S. Parry et al., "Serrated pathway colorectal cancer in the population: genetic consideration," *Gut*, vol. 56, no. 10, pp. 1453–1459, 2007.

[13] S. Sharma, T. K. Kelly, and P. A. Jones, "Epigenetics in cancer," *Carcinogenesis*, vol. 31, no. 1, pp. 27–36, 2009.

[14] M. Esteller, "Molecular origins of cancer: epigenetics in cancer," *The New England Journal of Medicine*, vol. 358, no. 11, pp. 1148–1096, 2008.

[15] R. Bonasio, S. Tu, and D. Reinberg, "Molecular signals of epigenetic states," *Science*, vol. 330, no. 6004, pp. 612–616, 2010.

[16] D. Hanahan and R. A. Weinberg, "Hallmarks of cancer: the next generation," *Cell*, vol. 144, no. 5, pp. 646–674, 2011.

[17] R. A. Beckman and L. A. Loeb, "Genetic instability in cancer: theory and experiment," *Seminars in Cancer Biology*, vol. 15, no. 6, pp. 423–435, 2005.

[18] M. S. Pino and D. C. Chung, "The chromosomal instability pathway in colon cancer," *Gastroenterology*, vol. 138, no. 6, pp. 2059–2072, 2010.

[19] C. R. Boland and A. Goel, "Microsatellite instability in colorectal cancer," *Gastroenterology*, vol. 138, no. 6, pp. 2073–2087, 2010.

[20] L. A. Loeb, C. F. Springgate, and N. Battula, "Errors in DNA replication as a basis of malignant changes," *Cancer Research*, vol. 34, no. 9, pp. 2311–2321, 1974.

[21] C. A. Klein, "Random mutations, selected mutations: a PIN opens the door to new genetic landscapes," *Proceedings of the National Academy of Sciences of the United States of America*, vol. 103, no. 48, pp. 18033–18034, 2006.

[22] M. Toyota, N. Ahuja, M. Ohe-Toyota, J. G. Herman, S. B. Baylin, and J. P. J. Issa, "CpG island methylator phenotype in colorectal cancer," *Proceedings of the National Academy of Sciences of the United States of America*, vol. 96, no. 15, pp. 8681–8686, 1999.

[23] C. R. Boland, N. L. Komarova, and A. Goel, "Chromosomal instability and cancer: not just one CINgle mechanism," *Gut*, vol. 58, no. 2, pp. 163–164, 2009.

[24] W. S. Samowitz, H. Albertsen, J. Herrick et al., "Evaluation of a large, population-based sample supports a CpG island methylator phenotype in colon cancer," *Gastroenterology*, vol. 129, no. 3, pp. 837–845, 2005.

[25] J. P. J. Issa, L. Shen, and M. Toyota, "CIMP, at last," *Gastroenterology*, vol. 129, no. 3, pp. 1121–1124, 2005.

[26] K. Curtin, M. L. Slattery, and W. S. Samowitz, "CpG island methylation in colorectal cancer: past, present and future," *Pathology Research International*, vol. 2011, Article ID 902674, 8 pages, 2011.

[27] Y. Xu, B. Hu, A. J. Choi et al., "Unique DNA methylome profiles in CpG island methylator phenotype colon cancers," *Genome Research*, vol. 22, no. 2, pp. 283–291, 2012.

[28] T. Hinoue, D. J. Weisenberger, C. P. Lange et al., "Genome-scale analysis of aberrant DNA methylation in colorectal cancer," *Genome Research*, vol. 22, no. 2, pp. 271–282, 2012.

[29] B. P. Berman, D. J. Weisenberger, J. F. Aman et al., "Regions of focal DNA hypermethylation and long-range hypomethylation in colorectal cancer coincide with nuclear lamina-associated domains," *Nature Genetics*, vol. 44, no. 1, pp. 40–46, 2012.

[30] J. P. Issa, "Colon cancer: it's CIN or CIMP," *Clinical Cancer Research*, vol. 14, no. 19, pp. 5939–5940, 2008.

[31] I. M. Shih, T. L. Wang, G. Traverso et al., "Top-down morphogenesis of colorectal tumors," *Proceedings of the National Academy of Sciences of the United States of America*, vol. 98, no. 5, pp. 2640–2645, 2001.

[32] A. P. Feinberg, R. Ohlsson, and S. Henikoff, "The epigenetic progenitor origin of human cancer," *Nature Reviews Genetics*, vol. 7, no. 1, pp. 21–33, 2006.

[33] R. A. Irizarry, C. Ladd-Acosta, B. Wen et al., "The human colon cancer methylome shows similar hypo- and

hypermethylation at conserved tissue-specific CpG island shores," *Nature Genetics*, vol. 41, no. 2, pp. 178–186, 2009.

[34] J. E. Ohm, K. M. McGarvey, X. Yu et al., "A stem cell-like chromatin pattern may predispose tumor suppressor genes to DNA hypermethylation and heritable silencing," *Nature Genetics*, vol. 39, no. 2, pp. 237–242, 2007.

[35] H. P. Mohammad, Y. Cai, K. M. McGarvey et al., "Polycomb CBX7 promotes initiation of heritable repression of genes frequently silenced with cancer-specific DNA hypermethylation," *Cancer Research*, vol. 69, no. 15, pp. 6322–6330, 2009.

[36] D. C. Snover, "Update on the serrated pathway to colorectal carcinoma," *Human Pathology*, vol. 42, no. 1, pp. 1–10, 2011.

[37] B. Leggett and V. Whitehall, "Role of the serrated pathway in colorectal cancer pathogenesis," *Gastroenterology*, vol. 138, no. 6, pp. 2088–2100, 2010.

[38] S. M. Dieter, C. R. Ball, C. M. Hoffmann et al., "Distinct types of tumor-initiating cells form human colon cancer tumors and metastases," *Cell Stem Cell*, vol. 9, no. 4, pp. 375–365, 2011.

[39] J. Terzic, S. Grivennicov, E. Karin, and M. Karin, "Inflammation and colon cancer," *Gastroenterology*, vol. 138, no. 6, pp. 2101–2114, 2010.

[40] A. P. Feinberg and B. Vogelstein, "Hypomethylation distinguishes genes of some human cancers from their normal counterparts," *Nature*, vol. 301, no. 5895, pp. 89–92, 1983.

[41] R. J. Taft, K. C. Pang, T. R. Mercer, M. Dinger, and J. S. Mattick, "Non-coding RNAs: regulators of disease," *Journal of Pathology*, vol. 220, no. 2, pp. 126–139, 2010.

[42] A. Portela and M. Esteller, "Epigenetic modifications and human disease," *Nature Biotechnology*, vol. 28, no. 10, pp. 1057–1068, 2010.

[43] M. Pancione, L. Sabatino, A. Fucci et al., "Epigenetic silencing of peroxisome proliferator- activated receptor γ is a biomarker for colorectal cancer progression and adverse patients' outcome," *PLoS ONE*, vol. 5, no. 12, article e14229, 2010.

[44] R. K. Chodavarapu, S. Feng, Y. V. Bernatavichute et al., "Relationship between nucleosome positioning and DNA methylation," *Nature*, vol. 466, no. 7304, pp. 388–392, 2010.

[45] K. N. Harikrishnan, M. Z. Chow, E. K. Baker et al., "Brahma links the SWI/SNF chromatin-remodeling complex with MeCP2-dependent transcriptional silencing," *Nature Genetics*, vol. 37, no. 3, pp. 254–264, 2005.

[46] D. Reisman, S. Glaros, and E. A. Thompson, "The SWI/SNF complex and cancer," *Oncogene*, vol. 28, no. 14, pp. 1653–1668, 2009.

[47] L. Ho, J. L. Ronan, J. Wu et al., "An embryonic stem cell chromatin remodeling complex, esBAF, is essential for embryonic stem cell self-renewal and pluripotency," *Proceedings of the National Academy of Sciences of the United States of America*, vol. 106, no. 13, pp. 5181–5186, 2009.

[48] P. P. Medina and M. Sanchez Cespedes, "Involvement of the chromatin-remodeling factor BRG1/SMARCA4 in human cancer," *Epigenetics*, vol. 3, no. 2, pp. 64–68, 2008.

[49] D. N. Reisman, M. W. Strobeck, B. L. Betz et al., "Concomitant down-regulation of BRM and BRG1 in human tumor cell lines: differential effects on RB-mediated growth arrest vs CD44 expression," *Oncogene*, vol. 21, no. 8, pp. 1196–1207, 2002.

[50] A. K. C. Wong, F. Shanahan, Y. Chen et al., "BRG1, a component of the SWI-SNF complex, is mutated in multiple human tumor cell lines," *Cancer Research*, vol. 60, no. 21, pp. 6171–6177, 2000.

[51] S. Bultman, T. Gebuhr, D. Yee et al., "A Brg1 null mutation in the mouse reveals functional differences among mammalian SWI/SNF complexes," *Molecular Cell*, vol. 6, no. 6, pp. 1287–1295, 2000.

[52] T. Watanabe, S. Semba, and H. Yokozaki, "Regulation of PTEN expression by the SWI/SNF chromatin-remodelling protein BRG1 in human colorectal carcinoma cells," *British Journal of Cancer*, vol. 104, no. 1, pp. 146–154, 2011.

[53] E. Sánchez-Tilló, A. Lázaro, R. Torrent et al., "ZEB1 represses E-cadherin and induces an EMT by recruiting the SWI/SNF chromatin-remodeling protein BRG1," *Oncogene*, vol. 29, no. 24, pp. 3490–3500, 2010.

[54] N. Yamamichi, K. I. Inada, M. Ichinose et al., "Frequent loss of Brm expression in gastric cancer correlates with histologic features and differentiation state," *Cancer Research*, vol. 67, no. 22, pp. 10727–10735, 2007.

[55] C. G. Sansam and C. W. M. Roberts, "Epigenetics and cancer: altered chromatin remodeling via Snf5 loss leads to aberrant cell cycle regulation," *Cell Cycle*, vol. 5, no. 6, pp. 621–624, 2006.

[56] N. Sévenet, A. Lellouch-Tubiana, D. Schofield et al., "Spectrum of hSNF5/INI1 somatic mutations in human cancer and genotype-phenotype correlations," *Human Molecular Genetics*, vol. 8, no. 13, pp. 2359–2368, 1999.

[57] J. A. Biegel, J. Y. Zhou, L. B. Rorke, C. Stenstrom, L. M. Wainwright, and B. Fogelgren, "Germ-line and acquired mutations of INI1 in atypical teratoid and rhabdoid tumors," *Cancer Research*, vol. 59, no. 1, pp. 74–79, 1999.

[58] C. W. M. Roberts and J. A. Biegel, "The role of SMARCB1/INI1 in development of rhabdoid tumor," *Cancer Biology and Therapy*, vol. 8, no. 5, pp. 412–416, 2009.

[59] A. Remo, C. Zanella, E. Molinari et al., "Rhabdoid carcinoma of the colon, a distinct entity with a very aggressive behaviour. A case report, associated with a polyposis coli and review of the Literature," *International Journal of Surgical Pathology*, vol. 2, no. 20, pp. 185–190, 2012.

[60] M. Pancione, A. Di Blasi, L. Sabatino et al., "A novel case of rhabdoid colon carcinoma associated with a positive CpG island methylator phenotype and BRAF mutation," *Human Pathology*, vol. 42, no. 7, pp. 1047–1052, 2011.

[61] H. R. Moinova, W. D. Chen, L. Shen et al., "HLTF gene silencing in human colon cancer," *Proceedings of the National Academy of Sciences of the United States of America*, vol. 99, no. 7, pp. 4562–4567, 2002.

[62] S. Popat, R. Hubner, and R. S. Houlston, "Systematic review of microsatellite instability and colorectal cancer prognosis," *Journal of Clinical Oncology*, vol. 23, no. 3, pp. 609–618, 2005.

[63] A. Lugli, I. Zlobec, P. Minoo et al., "Prognostic significance of the wnt signalling pathway molecules APC, β-catenin and E-cadherin in colorectal cancer—a tissue microarray-based analysis," *Histopathology*, vol. 50, no. 4, pp. 453–464, 2007.

[64] R. Kalluri and R. A. Weinberg, "The basics of epithelial-mesenchymal transition," *Journal of Clinical Investigation*, vol. 119, no. 6, pp. 1420–1428, 2009.

[65] J. G. Clohessy and P. P. Pandolfi, "β-tting on p63 as a Metastatic Suppressor," *Cell*, vol. 137, no. 1, pp. 28–30, 2009.

[66] G. Moreno-Bueno, H. Peinado, P. Molina et al., "The morphological and molecular features of the epithelial-to-mesenchymal transition," *Nature Protocols*, vol. 4, no. 11, pp. 1591–1613, 2009.

[67] M. Guarino, B. Rubino, and G. Ballabio, "The role of epithelial-mesenchymal transition in cancer pathology," *Pathology*, vol. 39, no. 3, pp. 305–318, 2007.

[68] M. J. Larriba, J. Casado-Vela, N. Pendás-Franco et al., "Novel snail1 target proteins in human colon cancer identified by

proteomic analysis," *PLoS ONE*, vol. 5, no. 4, article e10221, 2010.

[69] G. Moreno-Bueno, E. Cubillo, D. Sarrió et al., "Genetic profiling of epithelial cells expressing E-cadherin repressors reveals a distinct role for snail, Slug, and E47 Factors in epithelial- mesenchymal transition," *Cancer Research*, vol. 66, no. 19, pp. 9543–9556, 2006.

[70] M. Amano, M. Nakayama, and K. Kaibuchi, "Rho-kinase/ROCK: a key regulator of the cytoskeleton and cell polarity," *Cytoskeleton*, vol. 67, no. 9, pp. 545–554, 2010.

[71] P. Ortega, A. Morán, C. De Juan et al., "Differential Wnt pathway gene expression and E-cadherin truncation in sporadic colorectal cancers with and without microsatellite instability," *Clinical Cancer Research*, vol. 14, no. 4, pp. 995–1001, 2008.

[72] H. Suzuki, N. Masuda, T. Shimura et al., "Nuclear β-catenin expression at the invasive front and in the vessels predicts liver metastasis in colorectal carcinoma," *Anticancer Research*, vol. 28, no. 3, pp. 1821–1830, 2008.

[73] D. Horst, S. Reu, L. Kriegl, J. Engel, T. Kirchner, and A. Jung, "The intratumoral distribution of nuclear β-catenin is a prognostic marker in colon cancer," *Cancer*, vol. 115, no. 10, pp. 2063–2070, 2009.

[74] M. Pancione, N. Forte, A. Fucci et al., "Prognostic role of β-catenin and p53 expression in the metastatic progression of sporadic colorectal cancer," *Human Pathology*, vol. 41, no. 6, pp. 867–876, 2010.

[75] J. García-Solano, P. Conesa-Zamora, J. Trujillo-Santos et al., "Immunohistochemical expression profile of β-catenin, E-cadherin, P-cadherin, laminin-5γ2 chain, and SMAD4 in colorectal serrated adenocarcinoma," *Human Pathology*, vol. 43, no. 7, pp. 1094–1102, 2012.

[76] M. S. Pino, H. Kikuchi, M. Zeng et al., "Epithelial to mesenchymal transition is impaired in colon cancer cells with microsatellite instability," *Gastroenterology*, vol. 138, no. 4, pp. 1406–1417, 2010.

[77] G. H. Kang, "Four molecular subtypes of colorectal cancer and their precursor lesions," *Archives of Pathology and Laboratory Medicine*, vol. 135, no. 6, pp. 698–703, 2011.

[78] J. M. Bae, M. J. Kim, J. H. Kim et al., "Differential clinicopathological features in microsatellite instability-positive colorectal cancers depending on CIMP status," *Virchows Archiv*, vol. 459, no. 1, pp. 55–63, 2011.

[79] R. N. Jorissen, P. Gibbs, M. Christie et al., "Metastasis-associated gene expression changes predict poor outcomes in patients with Dukes stage B and C colorectal cancer," *Clinical Cancer Research*, vol. 15, no. 24, pp. 7642–7651, 2009.

[80] J. J. Smith, N. G. Deane, F. Wu et al., "Experimentally derived metastasis gene expression profile predicts recurrence and death in patients with colon cancer," *Gastroenterology*, vol. 138, no. 3, pp. 958–968, 2010.

[81] A. Loboda, M. V. Nebozhyn, J. W. Watters et al., "EMT is the dominant program in human colon cancer," *BMC Medical Genomics*, vol. 4, article 9, 2011.

[82] F. Prall, "Tumour budding in colorectal carcinoma," *Histopathology*, vol. 50, no. 1, pp. 151–162, 2007.

[83] E. Karamitopoulou, A. Lugli, I. Panayiotides et al., "Systematic assessment of protein phenotypes characterizing high-grade tumour budding in mismatch repair-proficient colorectal cancer," *Histopathology*, vol. 57, no. 2, pp. 233–243, 2010.

[84] I. Zlobec, F. Molinari, V. Martin et al., "Tumor budding predicts response to anti-EGFR therapies in metastatic colorectal cancer patients," *World Journal of Gastroenterology*, vol. 16, no. 38, pp. 4823–4831, 2010.

[85] I. Zlobec and A. Lugli, "Epithelial mesenchymal transition and tumor budding in aggressive colorectal cancer: tumor budding as oncotarget," *Oncotarget*, vol. 1, no. 7, pp. 651–661, 2010.

[86] W. S. Samowitz, C. Sweeney, J. Herrick et al., "Poor survival associated with the BRAF V600E mutation in microsatellite-stable colon cancers," *Cancer Research*, vol. 65, no. 14, pp. 6063–6070, 2005.

[87] M. S. Kim, J. Lee, and D. Sidransky, "DNA methylation markers in colorectal cancer," *Cancer and Metastasis Reviews*, vol. 29, no. 1, pp. 181–206, 2010.

[88] W. M. Grady and J. M. Carethers, "Genomic and epigenetic instability in colorectal cancer pathogenesis," *Gastroenterology*, vol. 135, no. 4, pp. 1079–1099, 2008.

[89] J. J. L. Wong, N. J. Hawkins, R. L. Ward, and M. P. Hitchins, "Methylation of the 3p22 region encompassing MLH1 is representative of the CpG island methylator phenotype in colorectal cancer," *Modern Pathology*, vol. 24, no. 3, pp. 396–411, 2011.

[90] I. B. Georgiades, L. J. Curtis, R. M. Morris, C. C. Bird, and A. H. Wyllie, "Heterogeneity studies identify a subset of sporadic colorectal cancers without evidence for chromosomal or microsatellite instability," *Oncogene*, vol. 18, no. 56, pp. 7933–7940, 1999.

[91] D. R. English, J. P. Young, J. A. Simpson et al., "Ethnicity and risk for colorectal cancers showing somatic BRAF V600E mutation or CpG island methylator phenotype," *Cancer Epidemiology Biomarkers and Prevention*, vol. 17, no. 7, pp. 1774–1780, 2008.

[92] L. S. Rozek, C. M. Herron, J. K. Greenson et al., "Smoking, gender, and ethnicity predict somatic BRAF mutations in colorectal cancer," *Cancer Epidemiology Biomarkers and Prevention*, vol. 19, no. 3, pp. 838–843, 2010.

[93] S. Ogino, K. Nosho, G. J. Kirkner et al., "CpG island methylator phenotype, microsatellite instability, BRAF mutation and clinical outcome in colon cancer," *Gut*, vol. 58, no. 1, pp. 90–96, 2009.

Permissions

All chapters in this book were first published in PRI, by Hindawi Publishing Corporation; hereby published with permission under the Creative Commons Attribution License or equivalent. Every chapter published in this book has been scrutinized by our experts. Their significance has been extensively debated. The topics covered herein carry significant findings which will fuel the growth of the discipline. They may even be implemented as practical applications or may be referred to as a beginning point for another development.

The contributors of this book come from diverse backgrounds, making this book a truly international effort. This book will bring forth new frontiers with its revolutionizing research information and detailed analysis of the nascent developments around the world.

We would like to thank all the contributing authors for lending their expertise to make the book truly unique. They have played a crucial role in the development of this book. Without their invaluable contributions this book wouldn't have been possible. They have made vital efforts to compile up to date information on the varied aspects of this subject to make this book a valuable addition to the collection of many professionals and students.

This book was conceptualized with the vision of imparting up-to-date information and advanced data in this field. To ensure the same, a matchless editorial board was set up. Every individual on the board went through rigorous rounds of assessment to prove their worth. After which they invested a large part of their time researching and compiling the most relevant data for our readers.

The editorial board has been involved in producing this book since its inception. They have spent rigorous hours researching and exploring the diverse topics which have resulted in the successful publishing of this book. They have passed on their knowledge of decades through this book. To expedite this challenging task, the publisher supported the team at every step. A small team of assistant editors was also appointed to further simplify the editing procedure and attain best results for the readers.

Apart from the editorial board, the designing team has also invested a significant amount of their time in understanding the subject and creating the most relevant covers. They scrutinized every image to scout for the most suitable representation of the subject and create an appropriate cover for the book.

The publishing team has been an ardent support to the editorial, designing and production team. Their endless efforts to recruit the best for this project, has resulted in the accomplishment of this book. They are a veteran in the field of academics and their pool of knowledge is as vast as their experience in printing. Their expertise and guidance has proved useful at every step. Their uncompromising quality standards have made this book an exceptional effort. Their encouragement from time to time has been an inspiration for everyone.

The publisher and the editorial board hope that this book will prove to be a valuable piece of knowledge for researchers, students, practitioners and scholars across the globe.

List of Contributors

Qiu-ping Liu
ThirdWard of VIP, 323 Hospital of PLA, Xi'an 710054, China

Dang-xia Zhou and Shui-ping Han
Pathology Department, Medical School, Xi'an Jiaotong University, Xi'an 710061, China

Li Sun
Ward of VIP, Shaanxi People's Hospital, Xi'an 710068, China

Luo Ling
Department of Endocrinology, The First Hospital of PLA, Lanzhou 730000, China

Chang-gui Wu
Department of Respiratory Medicine, Xijing Hospital, Fourth Military Medical University, Xi'an 710038, China

Pu Lin
Electric Power Science Research Institute of Shaanxi Province, Xi'an 710054, China

Shahzad Iqbal, David Friedel and Stavros N. Stavropoulos
Division of Gastroenterology, Department of Medicine, Winthrop-University Hospital, Mineola, NY 1150, USA

Lorna Ogden and Mala Gupta
Department of Pathology, Winthrop-University Hospital, Mineola, NY 1150, USA

Kanupriya Gupta and Rashmi Metgud
Department of Oral and Maxillofacial Pathology, Pacific Dental College and Hospital, Udaipur, Rajasthan 313001, India

Marisa D. Santos, Cristina Silva, Anabela Rocha and Carlos Nogueira
Department of Surgery, Digestive Surgery Service, Hospital de Santo António, Centro Hospitalar do Porto, Largo Abel Salazar, 4099-003 Porto, Portugal

Eduarda Matos
Department of Community Health, Instituto de Ciências Biomédicas Abel Salazar, Rua Jorge Viterbo Ferreira, No. 228, 4050-313 Porto, Portugal

Carlos Lopes
Department of Pathology, Pathological Anatomy Service, Hospital de Santo António, Centro Hospitalar do Porto, Largo Professor Abel Salazar, 4099-003 Porto, Portugal
Department of Pathology and Molecular Immunology, Instituto de Ciências Biomédicas Abel Salazar, Rua Jorge Viterbo Ferreira, No. 228, 4050-313 Porto, Portugal

Nikolaos Koletsas and Spyros Choidas
Urology Department, Interbalkan Medical Center, Thessaloniki, Greece

Triantafyllia Koletsa, Thomas Zaramboukas and Georgia Raptou
Pathology Department, Medical School, Aristotle University of Thessaloniki, Thessaloniki, Greece

Konstantinos Anagnostopoulos
Laboratory of Biochemistry, School of Medicine, Democritus University of Thrace, Alexandroupolis, Greece

Stavros Touloupidis
Urology Department, School of Medicine, Democritus University ofThrace, Alexandroupolis, Greece

Nikolaos Papadopoulos and Maria Lambropoulou
Laboratory of Histology-Embryology, School of Medicine, Democritus University ofThrace, Alexandroupolis, Greece

Marilin Rosa
Department of Pathology and Laboratory Medicine, College of Medicine, University of Florida, Jacksonville, FL 32209, USA
Anatomic Pathology and Women's Oncology, Moffitt Cancer Center and Research Institute, 12902 Magnolia Drive, Tampa, FL 33612, USA

Amir Mohammadi
Department of Pathology and Laboratory Medicine, College of Medicine, University of Florida, Jacksonville, FL 32209, USA

Sas Leen
Translational Cancer Research Unit, GZA Hospitals Sint-Augustinus, Oosterveldlaan 24, 2610 Antwerp, Belgium

Department of Medical Oncology, University of Antwerp, Universiteitsplein 1, 2610 Antwerp, Belgium

Van Laere Steven
Translational Cancer Research Unit, GZA Hospitals Sint-Augustinus, Oosterveldlaan 24, 2610 Antwerp, Belgium
Department of Oncology, KU Leuven, Herestraat 49, 3000 Leuven, Belgium

Dierick Anne Marie and Duwel Valérie
Department of Pathology, AZ Klina Hospital, Augustijnslei 100, 2930 Brasschaat, Belgium

De Pauw Annemie
Department of Pathology, AZ Nikolaas Hospital, Moerlandstraat 1, 9100 Sint-Niklaas, Belgium

Van Den Eynden Gert, Dirix Luc and Vermeulen Peter
Translational Cancer Research Unit, GZA Hospitals Sint-Augustinus, Oosterveldlaan 24, 2610 Antwerp, Belgium

Van Dam Peter and Lardon Filip
Department of Medical Oncology, University of Antwerp, Universiteitsplein 1, 2610 Antwerp, Belgium

O. H. Radhika Krishna, Geetha Kayla, Mohammed Abdul Aleem and Ramani Malleboyina
Department of Pathology, Niloufer Hospital forWomen and Children, Red Hills, Hyderabad, Telangana 500004, India

Ramesh Reddy Kota
Department of Pediatric Surgery, Niloufer Hospital forWomen and Children, Red Hills, Hyderabad, Telangana 500004, India

Prashant Goyal, Shelly Sehgal, Soumyesh Ghosh, Deepti Mittal, Awanindra Kumar and Sompal Singh
Department of Pathology, Swami Dayanand Hospital, Dilshad Garden, Delhi 110095, India

Vasu Reddy Challa, Basavanna Goud Yale Guru, Poornima Rangappa, Vijayalakshmi Deshmane
Department of Surgical Oncology, Kidwai Memorial Institute of Oncology, Bangalore, Karnataka 560029, India

Devi. M. Gayathri
Department of Pathology, Kidwai Memorial Institute of Oncology, Bangalore, Karnataka 560029, India

Rancés Blanco, Mercedes Cedeño and Enrique Rengifo
Laboratory of Recognition and Biological Activity Assays, Center of Molecular Immunology, 216 Street and 15th Avenue, Atabey, Playa, P.O. Box 16040, 11600 Havana, Cuba

Elizabeth Domínguez
Laboratory of Biochemistry, Department of Quality Control, Center of Molecular Immunology, 216 Street and 15th Avenue, Atabey, Playa, P.O. Box 16040, 11600 Havana, Cuba

Orlando Morales
Process Development Direction, Center of Molecular Immunology, 216 Street and 15th Avenue, Atabey, Playa, P.O. Box 16040, 11600 Havana, Cuba

Damián Blanco
Department of Cell Biology and Tissues Banking, National Institute of Oncology and Radiobiology, 29 and F Street, Vedado, Plaza de la Revolución, 10400 Havana, Cuba

DarelMartínez
Tumor Immunology Direction, Center of Molecular Immunology, 216 Street and 15th Avenue, Atabey, Playa, P.O. Box 16040, 11600 Havana, Cuba

Charles E. Rengifo
Department of Pathology, Manuel Fajardo General Hospital, Zapata and D Street, Vedado, Plaza de la Revolución, 10400 Havana, Cuba

Carmen Viada
Clinical Trials Direction, Center of Molecular Immunology, 216 Street and 15th Avenue, Atabey, Playa, P.O. Box 16040, 11600 Havana, Cuba

Adriana Carr
Research and Development Direction, Center of Molecular Immunology, 216 Street and 15th Avenue, Atabey, Playa, P.O. Box 16040, 11600 Havana, Cuba

Nabeel Al-Brahim
Department of Pathology, Farwaniya Hospital, P.O. Box 3313, 22034 Salmiya, Kuwait

Ibrahim Al-Kandari and Musaad Munahai
Department of Surgery, Farwaniya Hospital, 81004 Sabah Al-Naser, Kuwait

Prem Sharma
Faculty of Medicine, Kuwait University, P.O. Box 24923, 13110 Safat, Kuwait

Taylor Chomiak, Nathanael Turner and Bin Hu
Department of Clinical Neurosciences, Hotchkiss Brain Institute, Faculty of Medicine, University of Calgary 3280 Hospital Drive NW, Calgary, AB, Canada T2N 4N1

Romano Oguić
Department of Urology, Clinical Hospital Centre Rijeka, Krešimirova 42, 51000 Rijeka, Croatia

Vladimir Mozetič
Medico Polyclinic, Agaticéva 8, 51000 Rijeka, Croatia

Eleonora Cini Tešar
Department of Oncology, Clinical Hospital Centre Rijeka, Krešimirova 42, 51000 Rijeka, Croatia

Dora Fulkar HupiT, Elvira MustaT and Gordana YorZeviT
Department of Pathology, School of Medicine, University of Rijeka, Braće Branchetta 20, 51000 Rijeka, Croatia

Mamta Gupta
Department of Pathology, Subharti Medical College, Swami Vivekananda Subharti University, Meerut, Uttar Pradesh 250002, India

Flora D. Lobo and Deepa Sowkur Anandarama Adiga
Department of Pathology, Kasturba Medical College, Mangalore, Manipal University, Karnataka 575001, India

Abhishek Gupta
Department of Medicine, Subharti Medical College, Swami Vivekananda Subharti University, Meerut, Uttar Pradesh 250002, India

Saeeda Almarzooqi
Nationwide Children's Hospital, 700 Children's Drive, Columbus, OH 43205, USA

Ronald H. Houston
Anatomic Pathology ChildLab, Nationwide Children's Hospital, 700 Children's Drive, Columbus, OH 43205, USA

Vinay Prasad
Nationwide Children's Hospital, Clinical Ohio State University, 700 Children's Drive, Columbus, OH 43205, USA

Azadeh Andisheh Tadbir
Department of Oral and Maxillofacial Pathology, School of Dentistry, Shiraz University of Medical Sciences, Ghom Abad, Ghasrodasht Avenue, Shiraz 71956-15878, Iran

Bijan Khademi
Department of Otolaryngology, Khalili Hospital, Shiraz Institute for Cancer Research, Shiraz University of Medical Sciences, Shiraz 71348-45794, Iran

Mahyar Malekzadeh
Shiraz Institute for Cancer Research, Shiraz University of Medical Sciences, Shiraz 71348-45794, Iran

Maryam Mardani
Department of Oral Medicine, School of Dentistry, Shiraz University of Medical Sciences, GhomAbad, Ghasrodasht Avenue, Shiraz 71956-15878, Iran

Bahar Khademi
School of Dentistry, Shiraz University of Medical Sciences (International Branch), Azadi Square, Jahad Sazandegi Street, Shiraz 71447-16699, Iran

Hafidh I. Al-Sadi
Department of Oral and Maxillofacial Surgery, College of Dentistry, University of Mosul, Mosul, Iraq

Saevan S. Al-Mahmood
Department of Pathology and Poultry Diseases, College of Veterinary Medicine, University of Mosul, Mosul, Iraq

Brijesh Thakur
Department of Pathology, SGRRIM & HS, Patel Nagar Industrial Area, Niranjanpur, Dehradun, Uttarakhand 248001, India

Ravi Mehrotra
Institute of Cytology and Preventive Oncology (ICPO), I-7 Sector 39, Noida, Uttar Pradesh 201303, India

Jitendra Singh Nigam
Department of Pathology, Deen Dayal Upadhyay Hospital, Harinagar, New Delhi 110066, India

Shefali Chopra and Mark Li-cheng Wu
Department of Pathology and Laboratory Medicine, University of California Irvine School of Medicine, Irvine, CA 92868, USA

Amita Negi
Department of Oral Pathology & Microbiology, Himachal Dental College, Sunder Nagar, District Mandi, Himachal Pradesh 175002, India

Abhiney Puri, Rakhi Gupta, Rajat Nangia, Alisha Sachdeva and Megha Mittal
Department of Oral Pathology & Microbiology, Himachal Institute of Dental Sciences, Paonta Sahib, District Sirmour, Himachal Pradesh 173025, India

Atul Bhardwaj and Thomas J.McGarrity
Division of Gastroenterology and Hepatology, Penn State Milton S. Hershey Medical Center, 500 University Drive, P.O. Box 850, HU33, Hershey, PA 17033, USA

Douglas B. Stairs and HareshMani
Department of Pathology, Penn State Milton S. Hershey Medical Center, 500 University Drive, P.O. Box 850, HO83, Hershey, PA 17033, USA

Hermann Brustmann
Department of Pathology, Landesklinikum Baden-Moedling,Wimmergasse 19, 2500 Baden, Austria

Rani Kanthan
Department of Pathology and Laboratory Medicine, University of Saskatchewan, Saskatoon, SK, Canada S7N 0W8
Royal University Hospital, Room 2868 G-Wing, 103 Hospital Drive, Saskatoon, SK, Canada S7N 0W8

Jenna-Lynn Senger
Department of Pathology and Laboratory Medicine, University of Saskatchewan, Saskatoon, SK, Canada S7N 0W8

Selliah Chandra Kanthan
Department of Surgery, University of Saskatchewan, Saskatoon, SK, Canada S7N 0W8

Rachel Jug and Xiaoyin Jiang
Duke Health, DUMC 3712, Durham, NC 27710, USA

Fatima Zahra Talbi
Analysis and Modelisation of Continental Ecosystems Laboratory, Faculty of Sciences Dhar El Mehraz, Sidi Mohamed Ben Abdellah University, 30000 Fes, Morocco
Laboratory of Medical Entomology, National Institute of Hygiene, 27 Avenue Ibn Battuta, Agdal, 11400 Rabat, Morocco

Abdelhakim El Ouali Lalami
Regional Diagnostic Laboratory Epidemiological and Environmental Health, Regional Health Directorate, EL Ghassani Hospital, 30000 Fes, Morocco

Abdellatif Janati Idrissi
Analysis and Modelisation of Continental Ecosystems Laboratory, Faculty of Sciences Dhar El Mehraz, Sidi Mohamed Ben Abdellah University, 30000 Fes, Morocco

Faiza Sebti
National Reference Laboratory of Leishmaniasis, National Institute of Hygiene, 27 Avenue Ibn Battuta, Agdal, 11400 Rabat, Morocco

Chafika Faraj
Laboratory of Medical Entomology, National Institute of Hygiene, 27 Avenue Ibn Battuta, Agdal, 11400 Rabat, Morocco

Anthonio Adefuye, Arieh Anthony Katz and Kurt Jason Sales
MRC/UCT Receptor Biology Research Unit, Institute of Infectious Disease and Molecular Medicine and Division of Medical Biochemistry, Faculty of Health Sciences, University of Cape Town, Room No. 2.02Wernher and Beit North, Observatory 7925, South Africa

Sareh Farhadi and Fatemeh Shahsavari
Oral & Maxillofacial Pathology Department, Islamic Azad University, Dental Branch of Tehran, Tehran 16686 49911, Iran

MirMahdi Davardan
Islamic Azad University, Dental Branch of Tehran, Tehran 16686 49911, Iran

Massimo Pancione and Vittorio Colantuoni
Department of Biological, Geological and Environmental Sciences, University of Sannio, Via Port'Arsa 11, 82100 Benevento, Italy

Andrea Remo
Department of Pathology, "Mater Salutis" Hospital, ULSS21 Legnago, Verona, Italy

Index